# Handbook of
# APPLIED BIOCHEMISTRY
# NUTRITION AND DIETETICS

# Handbook of APPLIED BIOCHEMISTRY NUTRITION AND DIETETICS

(for Nursing and Allied Health Students)
As per Revised INC BSc Syllabus 2021

**Fifth Edition**

### Shivananda Nayak B
MSc PhD FAGE NRCC-CC (USA) FACB (USA) FABM PGDCHC

Professor of Biochemistry
Department of Preclinical Sciences
Faculty of Medical Sciences
The University of the West Indies
Trinidad and Tobago, West Indies

Visiting Professor
Department of Biochemistry
Sri Ramachandra University
Chennai, Tamilnadu, India
and
Subbaiah Institute of Medical Sciences
Shivamogga, Karnataka, India

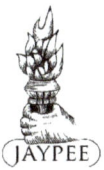

**JAYPEE BROTHERS MEDICAL PUBLISHERS**
*The Health Sciences Publisher*
New Delhi | London

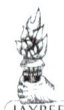 **Jaypee Brothers Medical Publishers (P) Ltd**

**Headquarters**

Jaypee Brothers Medical Publishers (P) Ltd
EMCA House, 23/23-B
Ansari Road, Daryaganj
New Delhi 110 002, India
Landline: +91-11-23272143, +91-11-23272703
+91-11-23282021, +91-11-23245672
Email: jaypee@jaypeebrothers.com

**Corporate Office**

Jaypee Brothers Medical Publishers (P) Ltd
4838/24, Ansari Road, Daryaganj
New Delhi 110 002, India
Phone: +91-11-43574357
Fax: +91-11-43574314
Email: jaypee@jaypeebrothers.com

**Overseas Office**

J.P. Medical Ltd
83 Victoria Street, London
SW1H 0HW (UK)
Phone: +44 20 3170 8910
Fax: +44 (0)20 3008 6180
Email: info@jpmedpub.com

Website: www.jaypeebrothers.com
Website: www.jaypeedigital.com

© 2022, Jaypee Brothers Medical Publishers

The views and opinions expressed in this book are solely those of the original contributor(s)/author(s) and do not necessarily represent those of editor(s) of the book.

All rights reserved. No part of this publication may be reproduced, stored or transmitted in any form or by any means, electronic, mechanical, photocopying, recording or otherwise, without the prior permission in writing of the publishers.

All brand names and product names used in this book are trade names, service marks, trademarks or registered trademarks of their respective owners. The publisher is not associated with any product or vendor mentioned in this book.

Medical knowledge and practice change constantly. This book is designed to provide accurate, authoritative information about the subject matter in question. However, readers are advised to check the most current information available on procedures included and check information from the manufacturer of each product to be administered, to verify the recommended dose, formula, method and duration of administration, adverse effects and contraindications. It is the responsibility of the practitioner to take all appropriate safety precautions. Neither the publisher nor the author(s)/editor(s) assume any liability for any injury and/or damage to persons or property arising from or related to use of material in this book.

This book is sold on the understanding that the publisher is not engaged in providing professional medical services. If such advice or services are required, the services of a competent medical professional should be sought.

Every effort has been made where necessary to contact holders of copyright to obtain permission to reproduce copyright material. If any have been inadvertently overlooked, the publisher will be pleased to make the necessary arrangements at the first opportunity.

**Inquiries for bulk sales may be solicited at:** jaypee@jaypeebrothers.com

*Handbook of Applied Biochemistry, Nutrition and Dietetics*

*First Edition :* 2007

*Second Edition :* 2010

*Third Edition :* 2015

*Fourth Edition*: 2021

*Fifth Edition*: 2022

ISBN: 978-93-5465-654-5

**Dedicated to**

*My parents and family*

# Message

The publication of this handbook is particularly welcome since it provides coverage of all aspects of the undergraduate course of study in biochemistry. Given its scope and given that the study of the chemical substances and vital processes in living organisms is an integral part of the syllabus for medical, allied health and nursing students, it is the most useful teaching and learning tool.

It is a source of pride that this book has been produced by a member of the teaching staff of the faculty of medical sciences of the University of the West Indies. It is the hallmark of the best academic institutions that their members disseminate their knowledge and the results of research to the wider public. Moreover, that process benefits considerably from the lessons gained from the pedagogical process and the interaction between lecturer and students and thus ensures that the information that is transmitted is relevant and up-to-date.

Good academic texts are critical to teaching and learning. This is particularly important in the field of medical, allied health and nursing since those who are trained in those disciplines play a critical role in providing health care for the population and in undertaking research that addresses many of the medical problems prevalent in the wider society. Topics discussed in the book are highly relevant to the allied and nursing professions. These conform to the curricular requirements of the allied and nursing councils and allied nursing institutions in India and abroad. Chapters are concise, well-written, and the contents are easy to understand. Information provided is also examination oriented; hence, students of allied and nursing would find the book very useful to prepare for examinations. Although this book is targeted primarily at the undergraduate allied and nursing students, medical students and others would also find the contents useful for quick revision.

I compliment Professor Shivananda Nayak B for taking the initiative in producing a student-friendly textbook that facilitates training and education in this most important field and fulfils a genuine need in biochemistry for this particular target group.

**Bhoendradatt Tewarie**
Republic of Trinidad and Tobago, West Indies

# Message

This fifth edition of the *Handbook of Applied Biochemistry, Nutrition and Dietetics* indicates the popularity of this handbook with the nursing and allied health students. The author has taken great pains to incorporate in this edition. The comments and suggestions coming from the students and the teachers, so that the handbook is made more comprehensive. More chapters have been included and some of the earlier chapters have been revised to keep pace with the advances made by the biochemistry branch of medicine. Lucid explanations and illustrations have added value to the handbook, which shall certainly benefit the students in understanding of the subject with ease and perfection.

My congratulations to Professor Shivananda Nayak B on bringing out this fourth edition of the handbook which, I am sure, will meet with a favorable reception.

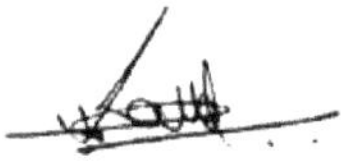

**HS Ballal** MD DMRD
Pro-Vice-Chancellor
Manipal University
Manipal, Karnataka, India

# Preface to the Fifth Edition

I have great pleasure in presenting this Fifth edition of the *Handbook of Applied Biochemistry, Nutrition and Dietetics*. All the previous editions of this title has been popular among the nursing and allied health students and it has been recommended by various nursing and allied health colleges as a reference book. The overwhelming response from the student community and support from the teachers of various institutions has encouraged me to bring out this fifth edition. The simple, concise, diagram-based explanation and self-assessment question format has been maintained in this revised edition. The suggestions and criticisms of teachers and the students to my previous editions have been used as a basis of revision. I tried best to incorporate new contents which are essential for both allied health and nursing students. Attempted to incorporate diagram-based explanation, self-assessment questions and additional multiple choice questions in each chapter.

Content of the handbook is divided into 22 chapters. A number of new illustrations and figures have been included to facilitate understanding the contents easily. The vitamins, minerals and nutrition chapters are completely revised to suit the revised syllabus of Indian Nursing Council (INC).

I am always trying to keep up my promise of bringing revised edition whenever required. I hope my efforts will be appreciated by the teachers and students community at large. Please feel free to send your comments, suggestions and constructive criticisms to my e-mail address as: ***shiv25@gmail.com.*** Your feedback always helps in including new things whenever I am revising this handbook

**Shivananda Nayak B**

# Preface to the First Edition

I am glad to present the book entitled *Handbook of Biochemistry (for Allied and Nursing Students)*. There are ample textbooks, which deal with the theory aspects of biochemistry in a simple way. My experience of more than 15 years in teaching biochemistry to medical, dental, allied health and nursing students in India as well as abroad stimulated me to write this book in a simple way that can be easily understood by the student community. I tried my level best to incorporate diagram-based explanation wherever necessary that may help the readers. Also I presented self-assessment questions at the end of each chapter for self-evaluation. The encouragement and support both from the teacher and the student community inspired me to bring out this book with interesting diagrams.

I take this opportunity to thank all those who warmly received my other book Manipal Manual of Clinical Biochemistry which was published by M/s Jaypee Brothers Medical Publishers (P) Ltd, New Delhi. I am always grateful to Dr Ramdas M Pai (Chancellor, Manipal University), Dr R Phaneendra Rao (Dean, Kasturba Medical College), Dr Sudhakar Nayak (Head, Department of Biochemistry), Dr Shivaraj (Professor, Department of Biochemistry, Manipal), and Dr S Gurumadva Rao (Vice-Chancellor, RAK Medical and Health Sciences, UAE), for their inspirations and support throughout my service in Kasturba Medical College. I am indebted to Dr Bhoendradatt Tewarie (Principal and Pro-Vice-Chancellor, The University of the West Indies) for writing Foreword to this book. Last but not the least; I thank each and everyone who encouraged me to bring out this book in time.

A textbook will be improved only by successive revisions. I will try to revise this book in every two years. The comments, suggestions and constructive criticisms from the faculty, students and other readers are always welcome. Please feel free to communicate at my e-mail address as: shiv25@gmail.com if you have any suggestions. The success of the book was due to the active participation of the M/s Jaypee Brothers Medical Publishers (P) Ltd, New Delhi, India.

This is to record my appreciation for the support extended by Shri Jitendar P Vij (Group Chairman), Mr Ankit Vij (Managing Director), Mr MS Mani (Group President), Mr Venugopal, Branch Manager, Bengaluru branch and their associates of M/s Jaypee Brothers Medical Publishers (P) Ltd., New Delhi, India, for readily conceding my request to publish the book in color and taking all pains to bring out this book to my utmost satisfaction.

**Shivananda Nayak B**

# Acknowledgments

I sincerely thank all those who warmly received the Previous edition. I am always grateful to Dr Ramdas M Pai (President, Manipal University), Professor Sudhakar Nayak (Department of Biochemistry) Manipal for their inspirations and support throughout my service at Kasturba Medical College. I am indebted to Dr Bhoendradatt Tewarie, Ex-Member of Parliament, Republic of Trinidad and Tobago wrote message to this title. I would like to thank Dr HS Ballal, Pro-Vice-Chancellor, Manipal Academy of Higher Education, Manipal for writing message to this title. Last but not the least; I thank each and every one who encouraged me to bring out this book on time.

I am grateful to Dr Geetha Samanth, DVS College Shimoga; for contributing chapter—Cell. My special thanks to Dr Geetha Bhaktha, who helped in editing and providing additional information on nutrition which is mainly required for nursing students.

A textbook will be improved only by successive revisions. As per my promise, I am bringing this fourth edition on right time. The comments, suggestions and constructive criticisms from the faculty, students and other readers are always welcome. The success of the book was due to the active participation of the Publishers. This is to record my appreciation for the support extended by Shri Jitendar P Vij (Group Chairman), Mr Ankit Vij (Managing Director), Mr MS Mani (Group President), Dr Madhu Choudhary (Publishing Head–Education), Ms Pooja Bhandari (Production Head), Ms Sunita Katla (Executive Assistant to Group Chairman and Publishing Manager), Ms Samina Khan (Executive Assistant to Publishing Head–Education), Mr Rajesh Sharma (Production Coordinator), Ms Seema Dogra (Cover Visualizer), Mr Kulwant Singh (Typesetter), Mr Laxmidhar Padhiary (Proofreader), Mr Deepak Goel (Graphic Designer), Mr Venugopal, Branch Manager, Bengaluru Branch and their associates of M/s Jaypee Brothers Medical Publishers (P) Ltd., New Delhi, India, for readily conceding my request to publish the book in color and taking all pains to bring out this book to my utmost satisfaction.

# Contents

**Chapter 1: The Cell** — 1
- Plasma Membrane  *1*
- Prokaryotic and Eukaryotic Cells  *4*
- Transport Across Membrane  *5*
- Cell Fractionation  *8*

**Chapter 2: Enzymes** — 13
- Chemical Nature of Enzymes  *13*
- Energy of Activation of Catalyzed and Uncatalyzed Reactions  *14*
- Mechanism of Enzyme Catalysis  *16*
- Enzyme Inhibition  *20*
- Isoenzymes  *23*

**Chapter 3: Chemistry of Carbohydrates** — 33
- Classification  *33*
- Isomerism in Carbohydrates  *35*

**Chapter 4: Metabolism of Carbohydrates** — 43
- Digestion and Absorption of Carbohydrates  *43*
- Metabolism of Carbohydrates  *46*
- Glycolysis  *47*

**Chapter 5: Chemistry of Amino Acids and Proteins** — 90
- Definition of an $\alpha$-Amino Acid  *90*
- Classification of Amino Acids  *93*
- Chromatography  *104*

**Chapter 6: Metabolism of Amino Acids** — 114
- Digestion and Absorption of Proteins  *114*
- Catabolism of Amino Acids  *115*
- Urea Cycle (Krebs–Henseleit Cycle)  *117*
- Metabolism of Important Amino Acids  *118*

**Chapter 7: Chemistry of Lipids** — 133
- Definition  *133*
- Functions of Lipids  *133*
- Classification of Lipids  *133*

**Chapter 8: Metabolism of Lipids** — 148
- Digestion and Absorption of Lipids  *148*
- Oxidation of Fatty Acids  *151*
- Alcohol Metabolism  *163*
- Risk Factors for Cardiovascular Disease  *171*

## Chapter 9: Integration of Metabolism and Homeostasis — 181
- Pathways of Metabolism  *182*
- Hormonal Regulation of Metabolism During Well-fed State  *184*
- Hormonal Regulation of Metabolism During Fasting/Starvation  *185*

## Chapter 10: Hemoglobin Metabolism — 194
- Structure of Hemoglobin  *194*
- Compare Myoglobin and Hemoglobin  *195*
- Thalassemia  *198*
- Sickle Cell Hemoglobin  *199*
- Detection of Abnormal Hemoglobin  *200*
- Jaundice  *205*

## Chapter 11: Acid–Base Balance — 209
- Buffers  *209*
- Acid–Base Disorders  *213*
- Mixed Acid–Base Disorders  *216*

## Chapter 12: Biological Oxidation — 222
- Principles of Reduction–Oxidation Reactions  *222*
- Structural Organization of Respiratory Chain and Electron Transport Structure of the Mitochondria  *223*
- Organization of the Chain  *223*

## Chapter 13: Hormones — 229
- Pituitary Hormones  *231*
- Thyroid Hormones  *233*
- Hyperthyroid Diseases  *234*
- Parathyroid Hormones  *234*
- Adrenal Gland  *235*
- Glucocorticoids  *235*
- Pancreas  *240*
- Female Sex Hormones  *240*
- Ovary  *241*
- Testes  *242*

## Chapter 14: Immunochemistry — 249
- Humoral and Cellular Immunity  *249*
- Vaccine Development  *250*
- Immunoglobulin  *250*
- Mechanism of Antibody Production  *252*
- Human Leukocyte Antigen  *257*

## Chapter 15: Free Radicals and Antioxidants — 261
- Reactive Oxygen Species  *262*
- Antioxidants  *263*
- Oxidative Stress in Disease  *266*

## Chapter 16: Specialized Proteins — 268
- Collagen  *268*
- Elastin  *269*
- Keratin  *270*
- Actin  *270*
- Myosin  *270*
- Lens Protein  *271*

## Chapter 17: Vitamins — 273
- Fat-soluble Vitamins  *273*
- Water-soluble Vitamins  *279*
- B-complex Vitamins  *280*

## Chapter 18: Minerals — 294
- Calcium ($Ca^{2+}$)  *294*
- Magnesium ($Mg^{2+}$)  *298*
- Sodium ($Na^+$)  *298*
- Osmolality  *299*
- Atrial Natriuretic Peptide  *300*
- Potassium ($K^+$)  *302*
- Chloride ($Cl^-$)  *306*
- Iron (Fe)  *306*
- Copper ($Cu^{2+}$)  *309*
- Zinc (Zn)  *310*
- Manganese ($Mn^{2+}$)  *310*
- Molybdenum (Mo)  *311*
- Cobalt (Co)  *311*
- Selenium (Se)  *311*
- Fluoride (F)  *311*
- Chromium (Cr)  *312*
- Iodine ($I_2$)  *312*

## Chapter 19: Water and Electrolyte Balance — 317
- Water Balance  *317*
- Electrolyte Balance  *321*

## Chapter 20: Nutrition and Dietetics — 329
- Dietary Fiber  *332*
- Measurement of Metabolic Rate or Energy  *334*
- Nutrition-related Diseases  *337*
- Cookery Rules and Preservation of Nutrients  *345*
- Balanced Diet  *348*
- Supplementary/Complementary Foods  *358*
- RDA  *358*
- Types of Infant Feeding  *359*
- Diet for Obesity  *360*
- Diet for Liver Disease  *360*

- Diet for Underweight  *360*
- Diet for Renal Disease  *361*
- Diet for Pre- and Postoperative Period  *361*

**Chapter 21:  Organ Function Tests**  364
- Liver Function Tests  *364*
- Renal Function Tests  *368*
- Thyroid Function Tests  *371*

**Chapter 22:  Laboratory Values**  386
- Blood  *386*
- Urine  *389*

Index  *391*

# APPLIED BIOCHEMISTRY

(Revised INC BSc Nursing Syllabus 2021)

**PLACEMENT:** II SEMESTER

**THEORY:** 2 credits (40 hours) (includes lab hours also)

**DESCRIPTION:** The course is designed to assist the students to acquire knowledge of the normal biochemical composition and functioning of human body, its alterations in disease conditions and to apply this knowledge in the practice of nursing.

**COMPETENCIES:** On completion of the course, the students will be able to
- Describe the metabolism of carbohydrates and its alterations.
- Explain the metabolism of lipids and its alterations.
- Explain the metabolism of proteins and amino acids and its alterations.
- Explain clinical enzymology in various disease conditions.
- Explain acid base balance, imbalance and its clinical significance.
- Describe the metabolism of hemoglobin and its clinical significance.
- Explain different function tests and interpret the findings.
- Illustrate the immunochemistry.

## Course Outline
### T – Theory

| Unit | Time (Hrs) | Learning Outcomes | Content | Teaching/ Learning Activities | Assessment Methods |
|---|---|---|---|---|---|
| I | 8 (T) | Describe the metabolism of carbohydrates and its alterations | **Carbohydrates**<br>• Digestion, absorption and metabolism of carbohydrates and related disorders<br>• Regulation of blood glucose<br>• Diabetes Mellitus – type 1 and type 2, symptoms, complications and management in brief<br>• Investigations of Diabetes Mellitus<br>• OGTT – Indications, Procedure,<br>• Interpretation and types of GTT curve<br>• Mini GTT, extended GTT, GCT, IVGTT<br>• HbA1c (Only definition)<br>• Hypoglycemia – Definition and causes | • Lecture cum Discussion<br>• Explain using charts and slides<br>• Demonstration of laboratory tests | • Essay<br>• Short answer<br>• Very short answer |

| Unit | Time (Hrs) | Learning Outcomes | Content | Teaching/Learning Activities | Assessment Methods |
|---|---|---|---|---|---|
| II | 8 (T) | Explain the metabolism of lipids and its alterations | **Lipids**<br>• Fatty acids – Definition, classification<br>• Definition and Clinical significance of MUFA and PUFA, Essential fatty acids, Trans fatty acids<br>• Digestion, absorption and metabolism of lipids and related disorders<br>• Compounds formed from cholesterol<br>• Ketone bodies (name, types and significance only)<br>• Lipoproteins – types and functions (metabolism not required)<br>• Lipid profile<br>• Atherosclerosis (in brief) | • Lecture cum Discussion<br>• Explain using charts and slides<br>• Demonstration of laboratory tests | • Essay<br>• Short answer<br>• Very short answer |
| III | 9 (T) | • Explain the metabolism of amino acids and proteins<br><br>• Identify alterations in disease conditions | **Proteins**<br>• Classification of amino acids based on nutrition, metabolic rate with examples<br>• Digestion, absorption and metabolism of protein and related disorders<br>• Biologically important compounds synthesized from various amino acids (only names)<br>• In born errors of amino acid metabolism—only aromatic amino acids (in brief)<br>• Plasma protein – types, function and normal values<br>• Causes of proteinuria, hypoproteinemia, hyper-gamma globinemia<br>• Principle of electrophoresis, normal and abnormal electrophoretic patterns (in brief) | • Lecture cum Discussion<br>• Explain using charts, models and slides | • Essay<br>• Short answer<br>• Very short answer |
| IV | 4 (T) | Explain clinical enzymology in various disease conditions | **Clinical Enzymology**<br>• Isoenzymes – Definition and properties<br>• Enzymes of diagnostic importance in<br>• Liver Diseases – ALT, AST, ALP, GGT<br>• Myocardial infarction – CK, cardiac troponins, AST, LDH<br>• Muscle diseases – CK, Aldolase<br>• Bone diseases – ALP<br>• Prostate cancer – PSA, ACP | • Lecture cum Discussion<br>• Explain using charts and slides | • Essay<br>• Short answer<br>• Very short answer |
| V | 3 (T) | Explain acid base balance, imbalance and its clinical significance | **Acid base maintenance**<br>• pH – definition, normal value<br>• Regulation of blood pH – blood buffer, respiratory and renal<br>• ABG – normal values<br>• Acid base disorders – types, definition and causes | • Lecture cum Discussion<br>• Explain using charts and slides | • Short answer<br>• Very short answer |

| Unit | Time (Hrs) | Learning Outcomes | Content | Teaching/ Learning Activities | Assessment Methods |
|---|---|---|---|---|---|
| VI | 2 (T) | Describe the metabolism of hemoglobin and its clinical significance | **Heme catabolism**<br>• Heme degradation pathway<br>• Jaundice – type, causes, urine and blood investigations (van den berg test) | • Lecture cum Discussion<br>• Explain using charts and slides | • Short answer<br>• Very short answer |
| VII | 3 (T) | Explain different function tests and interpret the findings | **Organ function tests (biochemical parameters and normal values only)**<br>• Renal<br>• Liver<br>• Thyroid | • Lecture cum Discussion<br>• Visit to Lab<br>• Explain using charts and slides | • Short answer<br>• Very short answer |
| VIII | 3 (T) | Illustrate the immunochemistry | **Immunochemistry**<br>• Structure and functions of immunoglobulin<br>• Investigations and interpretation – ELISA | • Lecture cum Discussion<br>• Explain using charts and slides<br>• Demonstration of laboratory tests | • Short answer<br>• Very short answer |

*Note:* Few lab hours can be planned for observation and visits (Less than 1 credit, lab hours are not specified separately).

# APPLIED NUTRITION AND DIETICS
(Accd to Revised INC Syllabus 2021)

**PLACEMENT:** II SEMESTER
**THEORY:** 3 credits (60 hours)
**Theory:** 45 hours
**Lab:** 15 hours

**DESCRIPTION:** The course is designed to assist the students to acquire basic knowledge and understanding of the principles of Nutrition and Dietetics and apply this knowledge in the practice of Nursing.

**COMPETENCIES:** On completion of the course, the students will be able to
- Identify the importance of nutrition in health and wellness.
- Apply nutrient and dietary modifications in caring patients.
- Explain the principles and practices of Nutrition and Dietetics.
- Identify nutritional needs of different age groups and plan a balanced diet for them.
- Identify the dietary principles for different diseases.
- Plan therapeutic diet for patients suffering from various disease conditions.
- Prepare meals using different methods and cookery rules

## Course Outline
### T – Theory

| Unit | Time (Hrs) | Learning Outcomes | Content | Teaching/ Learning Activities | Assessment Methods |
|---|---|---|---|---|---|
| I | 2 (T) | Define nutrition and its relationship to Health | **Introduction to Nutrition** *Concepts* <br>• Definition of Nutrition and Health <br>• Malnutrition – Under Nutrition and Over Nutrition <br>• Role of Nutrition in maintaining health <br>• Factors affecting food and nutrition <br>**Nutrients** <br>• Classification <br>• Macro and Micronutrients <br>• Organic and Inorganic <br>• Energy Yielding and Non-Energy Yielding <br>**Food** <br>• Classification – Food groups <br>• Origin | • Lecture cum Discussion <br>• Charts/Slides | • Essay <br>• Short answer <br>• Very short answer |

# Applied Biochemistry, Nutrition and Dietics (Revised INC BSc Nursing Syllabus)

| Unit | Time (Hrs) | Learning Outcomes | Content | Teaching/ Learning Activities | Assessment Methods |
|---|---|---|---|---|---|
| II | 3 (T) | • Describe the classification, functions, sources and recommended daily allowances (RDA) of carbohydrates<br>• Explain BMR and factors affecting BMR | **Carbohydrates**<br>• Composition – Starches, sugar and cellulose<br>• Recommended Daily Allowance (RDA)<br>• Dietary sources<br>• Functions<br>**Energy**<br>• Unit of energy – Kcal<br>• Basal Metabolic Rate (BMR)<br>• Factors affecting BMR | • Lecture cum Discussion<br>• Charts/Slides<br>• Models<br>• Display of food items | • Essay<br>• Short answer<br>• Very short answer |
| III | 3 (T) | • Describe the classification,<br>• Functions, sources and RDA of proteins. | **Proteins**<br>• Composition<br>• Eight essential amino acids<br>• Functions<br>• Dietary sources<br>• Protein requirements – RDA | • Lecture cum Discussion<br>• Charts/Slides<br>• Models<br>• Display of food items | • Essay<br>• Short answer<br>• Very short answer |
| IV | 2 (T) | • Describe the classification,<br>• Functions, sources and RDA of fats | **Fats**<br>• Classification – Saturated and unsaturated<br>• Calorie value<br>• Functions<br>• Dietary sources of fats and fatty acids<br>• Fat requirements – RDA | • Lecture cum Discussion<br>• Charts/Slides<br>• Models<br>• Display of food items | • Essay<br>• Short answer<br>• Very short answer |
| V | 3 (T) | Describe the classification, functions, sources and RDA of vitamins | **Vitamins**<br>Classification – fat soluble and water soluble<br>• Fat soluble – Vitamins A, D, E, and K<br>• Water soluble – Thiamine (vitamin B1), Riboflavin (vitamin B2), Nicotinic acid, Pyridoxine (vitamin B6), Pantothenic acid, Folic acid, Vitamin B12, Ascorbic acid (vitamin C)<br>• Functions, Dietary Sources and Requirements – RDA of every vitamin | • Lecture cum Discussion<br>• Charts/Slides<br>• Models<br>• Display of food items | • Essay<br>• Short answer<br>• Very short answer |
| VI | 3 (T) | Describe the classification, functions, sources and RDA of minerals | **Minerals**<br>• Classification – Major minerals (Calcium, phosphorus, sodium, potassium and magnesium) and Trace elements<br>• Functions<br>• Dietary Sources<br>• Requirements – RDA | • Lecture cum Discussion<br>• Charts/Slides<br>• Models<br>• Display of food items | • Short answer<br>• Very short answer |

| Unit | Time (Hrs) | Learning Outcomes | Content | Teaching/ Learning Activities | Assessment Methods |
|---|---|---|---|---|---|
| VII | 7 (T) 8 (L) | Describe and plan balanced diet for different age groups, pregnancy, and lactation | **Balanced diet**<br>• Definition, principles, steps<br>• Food guides – Basic Four Food Groups<br>• RDA – Definition, limitations, uses<br>• Food Exchange System<br>• Calculation of nutritive value of foods<br>• Dietary fibre<br>• Nutrition across life cycle<br>• Meal planning/Menu planning – Definition, principles, steps<br>• Infant and Young Child Feeding (IYCF) guidelines – breast feeding, infant foods<br>• Diet plan for different age groups – Children, adolescents and elderly<br><br>• Diet in pregnancy – nutritional requirements and balanced diet plan<br>• Anemia in pregnancy – diagnosis, diet for anemic pregnant women, iron and folic acid supplementation and counseling<br>• Nutrition in lactation – nutritional requirements, diet for lactating mothers, complementary feeding/ weaning | • Lecture cum Discussion<br>• Meal planning<br>• Lab session on Preparation of balanced diet for different categories<br>• Low cost nutritious dishes | • Short answer<br>• Very short answer |
| VIII | 6 (T) | Classify and describe the common nutritional deficiency disorders and identify nurses' role in assessment, management and prevention | **Nutritional deficiency disorders**<br>• Protein energy malnutrition – magnitude of the problem, causes, classification, signs and symptoms, Severe acute malnutrition (SAM), management and prevention and nurses' role<br>• Childhood obesity – signs and symptoms, assessment, management and prevention and nurses' role<br>• Vitamin deficiency disorders – vitamin A, B, C and D deficiency disorders –causes, signs and symptoms, management and prevention and nurses' role<br>• Mineral deficiency diseases – iron, iodine and calcium deficiencies –causes, signs and symptoms, management and prevention and nurses' role | • Lecture cum Discussion<br>• Charts/Slides<br>• Models | • Essay<br>• Short answer<br>• Very short answer |
| IX | 4 (T) 7 (L) | Principles of diets in various diseases | **Therapeutic diets**<br>• Definition, Objectives, Principles<br>• Modifications – Consistency, Nutrients,<br>• Feeding techniques.<br>• Diet in Diseases – Obesity, Diabetes Mellitus, CVD, Underweight, Renal diseases, Hepatic disorders Constipation, Diarrhea, Pre and Post-operative period | • Lecture cum Discussion<br>• Meal planning<br>• Lab session on preparation of therapeutic diets | • Essay<br>• Short answer<br>• Very short answer |

## Applied Biochemistry, Nutrition and Dietics (Revised INC BSc Nursing Syllabus)

| Unit | Time (Hrs) | Learning Outcomes | Content | Teaching/Learning Activities | Assessment Methods |
|---|---|---|---|---|---|
| X | 3 (T) | Describe the rules and preservation of nutrients | **Cookery rules and preservation of nutrients**<br>• Cooking – Methods, Advantages and Disadvantages<br>• Preservation of nutrients<br>• Measures to prevent loss of nutrients during preparation<br>• Safe food handling and Storage of foods<br>• Food preservation<br>• Food additives and food adulteration<br>• Prevention of Food Adulteration Act (PFA)<br>• Food standards | • Lecture cum Discussion<br>• Charts/Slides | • Essay<br>• Short answer<br>• Very short answer |
| XI | 4 (T) | Explain the methods of nutritional assessment and nutrition education | **Nutrition assessment and nutrition education**<br>• Objectives of nutritional assessment<br>• Methods of assessment – clinical examination, anthropometry, laboratory and biochemical assessment, assessment of dietary intake including Food frequency questionnaire (FFQ) method<br>• Nutrition education – purposes, principles and methods | • Lecture cum Discussion<br>• Demonstration<br>• Writing nutritional assessment report | • Essay<br>• Short answer<br>• Evaluation of Nutritional assessment report |
| XII | 3 (T) | Describe nutritional problems in India and nutritional programs | **National Nutritional Programs and role of nurse**<br>• Nutritional problems in India<br>• National nutritional policy<br>• *National nutritional programs* – Vitamin A Supplementation, Anemia Mukt Bharat Program, Integrated Child Development Services (ICDS), Mid-day Meal Scheme (MDMS), National Iodine Deficiency Disorders Control Program (NIDDCP), Weekly Iron Folic Acid Supplementation (WIFS) and others as introduced<br>• Role of nurse in every program | • Lecture cum Discussion | • Essay<br>• Short answer<br>• Very short answer |
| XIII | 2 (T) | • Discuss the importance of food hygiene and food safety<br>• Explain the Acts related to food safety | **Food safety**<br>• Definition, Food safety considerations and measures<br>• Food safety regulatory measures in India – Relevant Acts<br>• Five keys to safer food<br>• Food storage, food handling and cooking<br>• General principles of food storage of food items (ex. milk, meat)<br>• Role of food handlers in food borne diseases<br>• Essential steps in safe cooking practices | • Guided reading on related acts | • Quiz<br>• Short answer |

**Food borne diseases and food poisoning are dealt in Community Health Nursing I.**

# The Cell

## Chapter 1

## LEARNING OBJECTIVES

*At the end of this chapter students should be able to:*
- ❖ Know about ultrastructure of the cell
- ❖ State the different organelles of the cell and their individual function
- ❖ Know the marker enzymes to identify the organelles of the cell

## ■ Introduction

Cells are the structural and functional units of all living organisms. Humans are a multicellular organism, which contains at least $10^{14}$ cells. These cells differ considerably in shape, structure, and function as a result of specialization. An aggregation of cells, which are similar in origin, structure, and function forms tissue. Most of the metabolic activities occur at cellular level.

A typical cell, as seen by the light microscope, is illustrated in **Figure 1.1**. It contains two compartments, inner nucleus and outer cytoplasm. Nucleus contains nucleoplasm suspended with genetic material. Nuclear envelope separates nucleus from cytoplasm. Cytoplasm composed of aqueous cytosol is suspended with particles and membrane-bound organelles. Externally cytoplasm is limited by plasma membrane.

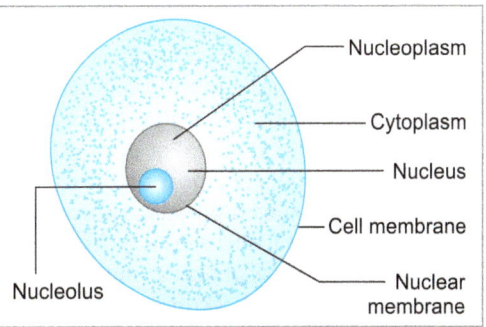

**Fig. 1.1:** Structure of the cell as seen with light microscope.

Normal cell ranges between 10 and 30 μm in diameter. **Figure 1.2** shows the ultrastructure or finer details of typical cell, which has been revealed by the electron microscope.

**Briefly explain the structural and functional aspects of cell organelles.**

## ■ Plasma Membrane

- ❖ The cell membrane, which completely envelops the cell, is a thin (75-100 A°), living, dynamic, and selectively permeable membrane.
- ❖ It has specialized surface structures for attachment and communication. Those are (1) tight junctions—produce seal between adjacent cells and (2) gap junctions—allow ions and electric current between adjacent cells. They may also include certain modifications to carry out physiological functions such as microvilli for absorption and invagination or infoldings to carry out transportation.
- ❖ All biological membranes, including the plasma membrane and internal membranes, which form the subcellular structures such as endoplasmic reticulum (ER), mitochondria, lysosomes nuclear envelope, peroxisomes, and Golgi complex, are similar in structure, lipoprotein in nature, and consist of lipids (60-40%), proteins (40-60%), and carbohydrates (1-10%).

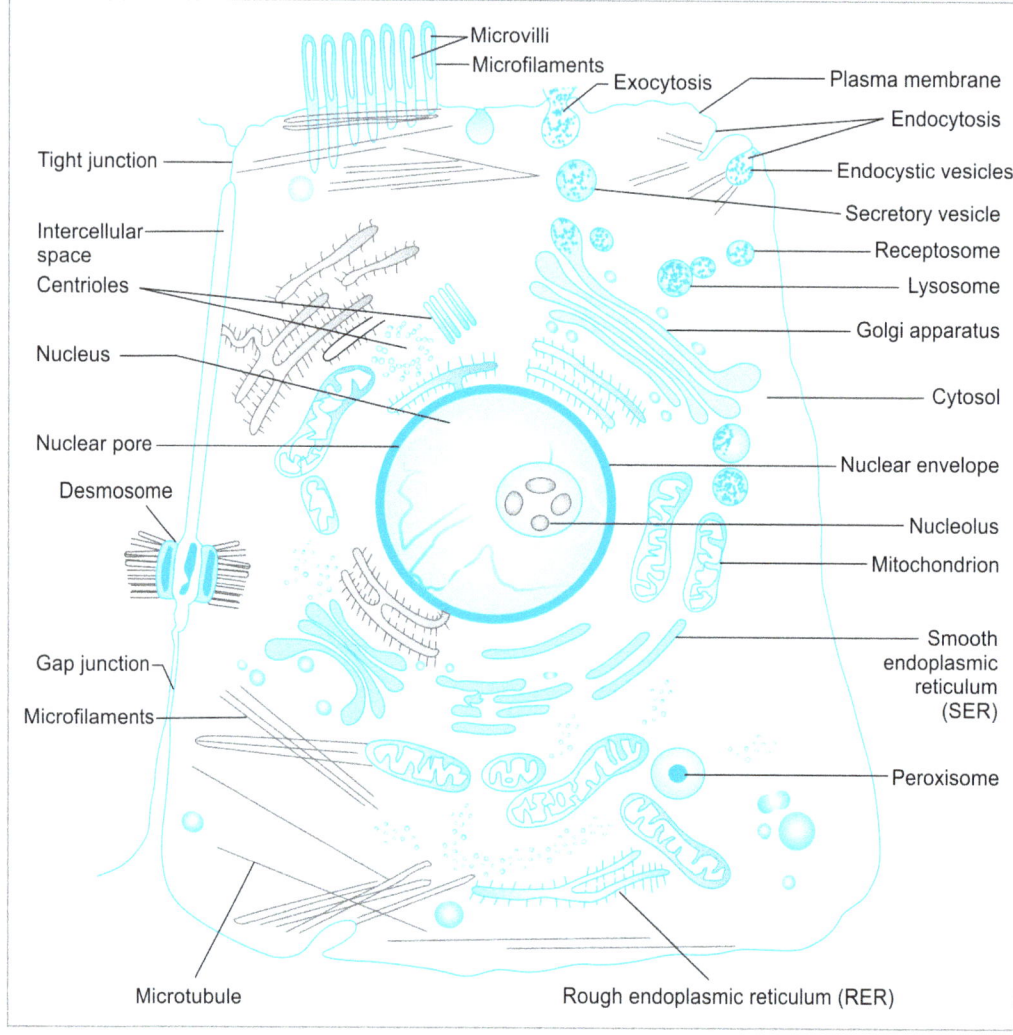

**Fig. 1.2:** Ultrastructure of typical cell showing all cell organelles as seen in the electron microscope.

- The membranes separate the cell from external environment and separates different parts of the cell from one another, so that cellular activities are compartmentalized.

### Endoplasmic Reticulum

- Cytoplasm is traversed by extensive network of interconnecting membrane-bound channels or cisternae (diameter of 40–50 µm), vesicles (diameter 25–500 µm), and tubules (diameter 50–190 µm), which form ER **(Fig. 1.3)**.

- Membranes of ER are continuous with plasma membrane and outer nuclear envelope.
- There are two basic morphological types: (1) rough ER (RER)—it possesses rough surface due the attachment of ribosomes. RER occurs mainly in the form of cisternae and concerned with protein synthesis and (2) smooth ER (SER)—it lacks ribosomes on their surface and occurs mainly in the form of tubules. SER is concerned with lipid synthesis.
- ER provides skeletal framework to cells and gives mechanical support to the colloidal

# CHAPTER 1: The Cell

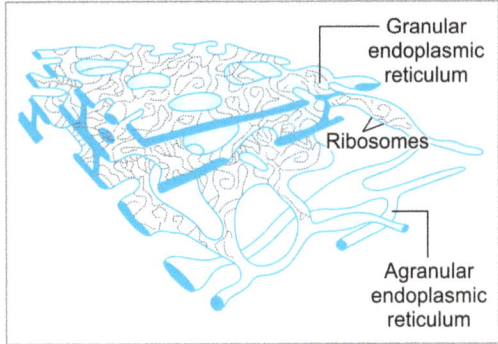

Fig. 1.3: Endoplasmic reticulum.

cytoplasm. It also plays a role in detoxifying the xenobiotic.

## Golgi Complex
- Golgi complex is membrane-bound structure similar to ER, discovered in 1873 by Camillo Golgi.
- It is a stack of flattened-membrane vesicles (cisternae) surrounded by networking of tubules of 300-500 A° diameters.
- Cisternae gently curved, convex part *cis* side faces ER and concave part *trans* side locates near plasma membrane (**Fig. 1.4**).
- Golgi complex functions in association with ER and is a center of reception, finishing, packaging, and transportation of variety of materials.

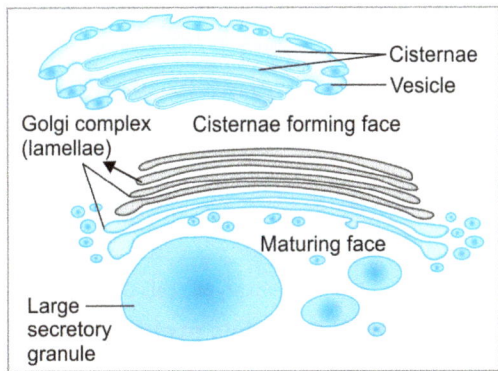

Fig. 1.4: Golgi apparatus.

- Proteins synthesized in ER is added with sulfate, carbohydrates, lipid moieties, etc. and dispatched in the form of secretory vesicles.
- Golgi complex also gives rise to lipoprotein of plasma membrane and lysosomes.

## Lysosomes
- Lysosomes are packets of hydrolases.
- These are spherical in shape and 1 µm in diameter surrounded by tough carbohydrate-rich lipoprotein membrane enclosing about 50 types of hydrolases such as proteases, lipases, nucleases, transferases, and sulfatases.
- Lysosomes provide an intracellular digestive system through which macromolecules, foreign bodies, and worn-out unwanted structures are digested.

## Peroxisomes
- Circular membrane-bound organelle having about 0.25 µm diameters contains enzymes, peroxidases and catalase.
- Peroxisomes detoxify various toxic substances and metabolites through peroxidative reactions catalyzed by peroxidases. Catalase degrades $H_2O_2$, which resulted from the breakdown of fatty acid and amino acids.

## Mitochondria
- They are spherical, oval, or rod-like bodies, about 0.5–1 µm in diameter and up to 7 µm in length. There are DNA molecules, which encode information for certain mitochondrial proteins (**Fig. 1.5**).

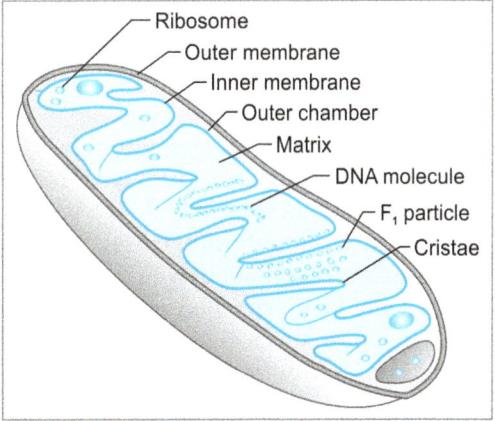

Fig. 1.5: Longitudinal section of mitochondrion.

- Mitochondria are considered to be the powerhouse of the cell, where energy released from oxidation of foodstuffs is trapped as chemical energy in the form of ATP.
- Mitochondria are respiratory center of cell where pyruvate oxidation, citric acid cycle, electron transport chain, and ATP generation take place. In addition, beta-oxidation of fatty acid and ketone body synthesis also take place.

## Centrioles

- Two cylindrical rod-shaped structures of 0.3–0.7 μm length and 0.1–0.25 μm diameters, lying at right angle to one another near nucleus, are called centrioles.
- Centriole is an array of nine-triplet microtubules equally spaced from central axis, made up of structural protein tubulin. Centrioles form mitotic poles during cell division.
- They also give rise to cilia and tail of sperm.

## Nucleus

- Nucleus is the command center of cells, which are spherical structure where genetic material is confined.
- All cells in the human body contain nucleus, except matured red blood cells (RBCs) and upper dead skin cells.
- Generally, nucleus is spherical or oval in shape and of 3–25 μm in diameter. But squamous epithelial cells contain discoidal and multilobed nucleus as in polymorphonuclear leukocytes.
- Nuclear envelope, which encircles the nucleus, consists of outer and inner nuclear membranes, which is a typical lipoprotein membrane. Outer nuclear membrane is continuous with membranes of ER and found attached with ribosomes on its outer surface. Nuclear envelope contains numerous nuclear pores of 100–1,000 A° diameter, which regulates nucleocytoplasmic trafficking of ions, nucleotides, proteins, mRNA, tRNA, and ribosomal subunits.
- Nucleoplasm is the gelatinous substance within the nuclear envelope also called karyoplasm and consists of genetic material (chromosomes) and nucleolus. It regulates the passage of molecules between the nucleoplasm and the cytoplasm.
- Nucleolus is made up of proteins and ribonucleic acids (RNA) and is the site of the formation of ribosomal subunits. The main components are nucleoproteins, proteins, enzymes, minerals, and organic and inorganic substances.

## ■ Prokaryotic and Eukaryotic Cells

Cells are of two types, prokaryotes and eukaryotes. "Karyose" comes from a Greek word, which means "kernel," as in a kernel of grain. In biology, we use this word root to refer to the nucleus of a cell. "Pro" means "before," and "eu" means "true," or "good." So "prokaryotic" means "before a nucleus," and "eukaryotic" means "possessing a true nucleus." Prokaryotic cells have no nuclei, while eukaryotic cells do have true nuclei **(Fig. 1.6)**.

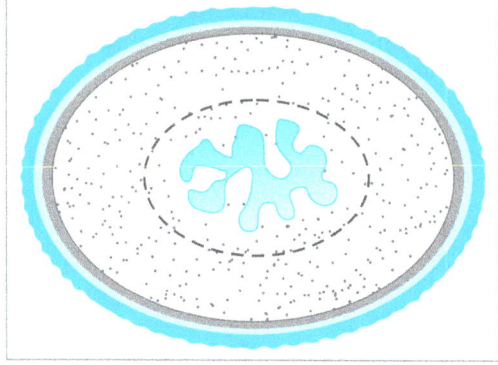

Fig. 1.6: Prokaryotic cell.

**How do you differentiate prokaryotic cells from eukaryotic cells?**

### Differences between Eukaryotic and Prokaryotic Cells

1. Eukaryotic cells have a true nucleus, bound by a double membrane **(Fig. 1.7)**.

## CHAPTER 1: The Cell

are composed of only 3 kinds of rRNA and about 50 kinds of protein.
5. The cytoplasm of eukaryotic cells is filled with a large, complex collection of organelles, many of them enclosed in their own membranes; the prokaryotic cell contains no membrane-bound organelles, which are independent of the plasma membrane.

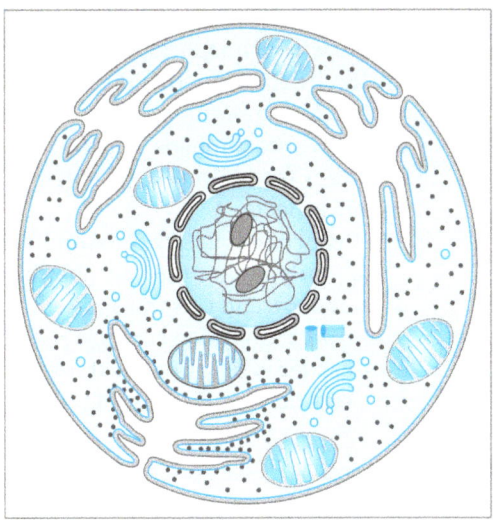

Fig. 1.7: Eukaryotic cell.

Prokaryotic cells have no nucleus. The purpose of the nucleus is to sequester the DNA-related functions of the big eukaryotic cell into a smaller chamber, for the purpose of increased efficiency. This function is unnecessary for the prokaryotic cell, because it is much smaller size and closer appearance of all materials. Prokaryotic cells also have DNA and DNA functions.
2. Eukaryotic DNA is linear; prokaryotic DNA is circular.
3. Eukaryotic DNA is complexed with proteins called "histones" and is organized into chromosomes; prokaryotic DNA is "naked" (no histones), and it is not formed into chromosomes. A eukaryotic cell contains a number of chromosomes; a prokaryotic cell contains only one circular DNA molecule and a varied assortment of much smaller circlets of DNA called "plasmids."
4. Both cell types have many ribosomes, but the ribosomes of the eukaryotic cells are larger and more complex than those of the prokaryotic cell.
A eukaryotic ribosome is composed of 5 kinds of rRNA and about 80 kinds of proteins, while prokaryotic ribosomes

## ▎Transport Across Membrane

Biological membranes are lipoprotein viscous barriers. This exists around all living cell and also form structural and functional component of all cell organelles. The membranes contain mainly lipids, proteins, and very little amount of carbohydrates. The contents of these vary according to the nature of the membrane. Lipids are mainly amphipathic phospholipids, glycolipids, and cholesterol. Proteins are of two types: (1) peripheral or extrinsic proteins and (2) integral or intrinsic proteins.

### What is a fluid mosaic model? Explain briefly?

Organization of biological membranes, the arrangement of lipids and proteins was best explained in fluid mosaic model of Singer and Nicolson (1972) **(Fig. 1.8)**. According to this model, membrane is viscous fluid with phospholipid bilayer, in which globular proteins are inserted in a mosaic pattern. Amphipathic phospholipid consists of polar phosphate head, glycerol neck, and nonpolar two fatty

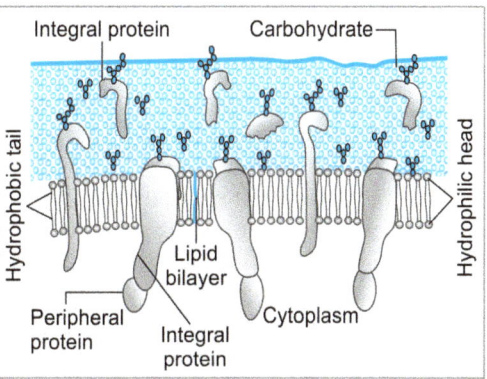

Fig. 1.8: Fluid mosaic model of plasma membrane.

acid tails. The hydrophobic tails or fatty acids form the middle core of lipid bilayer. The hydrophilic heads line both the sides. Both phospholipids and proteins are amphipathic and form permeability barrier. The degree of saturation and unsaturation of fatty acids, presence of cholesterol and carbohydrates regulate the fluidity and movement of molecules. Hydrophilic heads of inner and outer surface keep constant circulation of water. But hydrophobic fatty acid core acts as selective permeable barrier, protecting the cells and cell organelles from osmotic shocks.

**Explain the different transport mechanisms that occur in the membranes.**

Important function of the membrane is to withhold unwanted molecules but permit entry of molecules necessary for cellular metabolism. Transport across the membrane occurs in following ways:
- Passive transport
- Active transport
- Exocytosis
- Endocytosis

## Passive Transport

- Passive transport of molecules across the membrane is along the concentration gradient without using energy.
- Movement of molecules from higher concentration to lower concentration takes place without using energy.
- Solutes and gases enter the cells passively.
- They are driven by the concentration gradient.
- The rate of transport is directly proportional to the concentration gradient of that solute across the membrane.
- Passive transport of molecules across the biomembranes is in two ways:
  1. *Simple diffusion*: Small uncharged molecules such as $H_2O_2$, $O_2$, $CO_2$, $CH_4$, other gases, urea, and move ethanol across lipid bilayer by simple diffusion.
  2. *Facilitated diffusion or carrier-mediated passive transport*: Diffusion of molecules across the membrane along the concentration gradient through carrier proteins or permeases. It differs from simple diffusion in certain aspects.
     - The process is stereospecific, i.e., only one of the two possible isomers, L and D, is transported.
     - It shows saturation kinetics.
     - A carrier is required for transport across the membranes (**Fig. 1.9**).

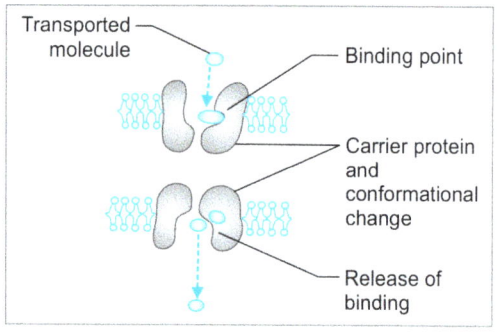

**Fig. 1.9:** Mechanism of facilitated diffusion.

The carrier proteins or permeases are specific integral membrane proteins and are highly specific for molecules, which they transport. Carrier proteins are specific for individual sugars, amino acids, phosphate, etc. As a concentration gradient of a solute across the membrane exists, solute molecules from hypertonic side bind to specific permease of the membrane. This binding triggers some conformational change, producing a pore or tunnel in carrier protein through which ions, glucose, etc., may cross. Following this permease regains its original structure.

## Uniport, Symport, and Antiport

Carrier proteins, which simply transport a single solute from one side of the membrane to the other, are called uniports. Transport of one solute depends on the simultaneous transfer of a second solute, either in the same direction (symport) or in the opposite direction (antiport). Both symport and antiport are collectively called cotransport **(Fig. 1.10)**.

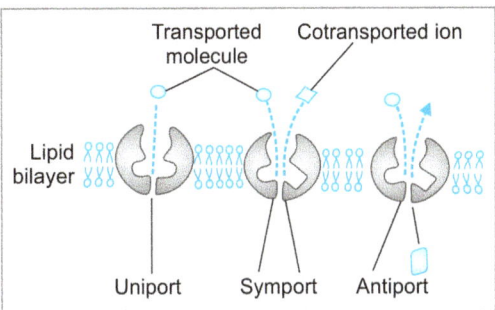

**Fig. 1.10:** Carrier proteins of membrane functioning as uniports, symports, and antiports.

*Symport:* Glucose-Na+ symport protein in intestinal epithelial cell.

*Antiport:* Na$^+$-K$^+$-ATPase pump, Cl$^-$/HCO$_3^-$ anion exchange permease in erythrocytes.

## Active Transport

- The transport of molecules across the membrane against the concentration gradient using energy. Molecules are transported from lower concentration (hypotonic) to higher concentration (hypertonic) with the use of energy **(Fig. 1.11)**.
- In all cells, a significant portion of energy goes in maintaining concentration gradient of ions across plasma membrane and intracellular membranes.

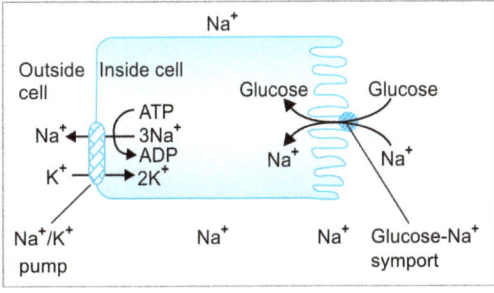

**Fig. 1.11:** Active transport.

- In human RBC, 50% of (cellular metabolism) energy is used for the above purpose.
- Active transport is mainly of two types:
  1. *ATP-driven active transport or primary active transport*: Transmembrane proteins or carrier proteins form channels to bring the transport of molecules and ions across biological membranes using energy from ATP. The most important active transport in cells is Na$^+$/K$^+$-ATPase pump. All cells maintain high internal concentration of K$^+$ and low concentration of Na$^+$. This Na$^+$/K$^+$ gradient across the membrane is maintained using energy from hydrolysis of ATP. ATPase is large carrier protein, hydrolysis of ATP brings the binding of 3Na$^+$ to ATPase, causing some conformational changes in ATPase, resulting in pumping of 3Na$^+$ outside in exchange of 2K$^+$ pumped in opposite direction.
  2. *Ion-driven active transport or secondary active transport*: Secondary active transport takes place in the presence of ionic gradient maintained across the membrane by primary active transport. Example: glucose absorption in intestinal epithelial cells. Concentration gradient maintained by Na$^+$/K$^+$-ATPase pump across the cell brings the symport of Na$^+$ and glucose molecules into the cell.

## Exocytosis

Secretions of cell such as proteins, lipids, and carbohydrates are released out of the cell through exocytosis. These secretions are packed in the form of secretory vesicles. As per necessary stimulation, these vesicles move toward and fuse with plasma membrane. In this way, materials inside the vesicles are externalized. Examples: release of acetylcholine from synaptic vesicles in presynaptic cholinergic nerves; release of trypsinogen by pancreatic cells; release of insulin by β cells of Langerhans, etc.

## Endocytosis

Endocytosis is the mechanism by which cells uptake macromolecules in the form of endocytic vesicles. Plasma membrane invaginates and encloses the materials, which results into vesicles. There are two types **(Fig. 1.12)**:

1. *Phagocytosis:* Ingestion of large particles such as bacteria and cell debris and plasma membrane invaginates in the form of pseudopodia and encloses particles in the form of phagosome. Materials of phagosomes will be digested by lysosomes. Examples: engulfment of bacteria by macrophages and granulocytes.
2. *Pinocytosis:* Uptake of nonspecific or specific extracellular molecules in the form of endocytic vesicles. Later it is termed "receptor-mediated endocytosis." Plasma membranes internalize these receptor-attached molecules in the form of vesicles. Examples: uptake of chylomicrons by liver cells and internalization of LDL through LDL receptors of plasma membrane.

## Cell Fractionation

The study of biochemical properties of individual organelles requires subcellular fractionation. The subcellular fractionation involves breaking of cell by means of mechanical force to purify organelles.

The steps involved are **(Figs. 1.13 and 1.14)**:

- Mince the tissue using a buffer.
- Tissue is carefully broken up in homogenizer using isotonic 0.25 M sucrose solution (the sucrose solution is preferred because it is not metabolized and does not readily pass through the membranes and does not cause interorganelles to swell).
- The gentle homogenization with an isotonic sucrose solution ruptures the cell membrane and keeps most of the organelles intact. But ER is broken into small pieces that form microsomes.

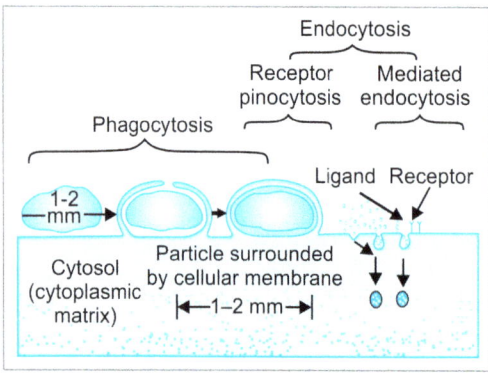

**Fig. 1.12:** The process of phagocytosis and endocytosis.

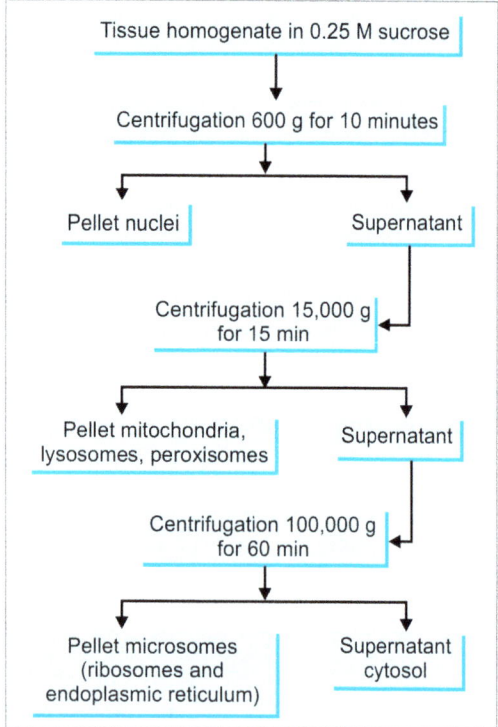

**Fig. 1.13:** Subcellular fractionation of cell by differential centrifugation.

# CHAPTER 1: The Cell

by differential centrifugation. The dense nuclei are sedimented first, followed by the mitochondria and finally by the microsomal fraction. The soluble remnant is the cytosolic portion.

The mitochondria isolated in this way are contaminated with lysosome and peroxisomes. These may be separated by isopycnic centrifugation technique. In this technique, a density gradient is set up in a centrifuge tube (the density of the solution in the tube increases from top to the bottom). Sucrose is used as medium and colloidal materials such as Pecroll, which form density gradients with a low osmotic pressure, are often used. Particles are sedimented to an equilibrium position at which their density equals that of the medium at that point in the tube. Different organelles are separated according to their density.

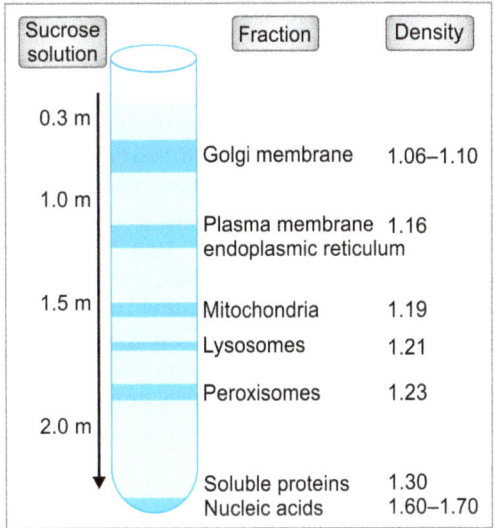

Fig. 1.14: Organelle separation by isopycnic centrifugation.

- Homogenate is drained to remove connective tissue and fragments of blood vessels by stainless steel sieve.
- The homogenate thus obtained is centrifuged at a series of increasing centrifugal force.

The nuclei and mitochondria differ in size and specific gravity and therefore sediment at different rates in a centrifugal field. This can be isolated from the homogenate

The purity of the isolated subcellular fraction is assessed by the analysis of marker enzymes. These marker enzymes are located exclusively in a particular fraction and are specific to that fraction. Analysis of marker enzymes confirms the degree of purity and contamination **(Table 1.1)**.

**List the enzymes that can be used to identify the cell organelles.**

**Table 1.1:** Marker enzymes of subcellular fractions.

| Fraction | Enzyme |
| --- | --- |
| Plasma membrane | $5^1$ nucleotidase and $Na^+$-$K^+$ ATPase |
| Golgi membrane | Galactosyltransferase and mannosidase |
| Endoplasmic reticulum | Glucose-6-phosphatase and cytochrome b reductase |
| Mitochondria | Succinate dehydrogenase and cytochrome C oxidase |
| Cytosol | Lactate dehydrogenase and glucose-6-phosphate dehydrogenase |
| Lysosomes | Acid phosphatase |
| Peroxisomes | Catalase |
| Nucleus | DNA polymerase and RNA polymerase |

## SUMMARY

Humans are a multicellular organism, which contains at least $10^{14}$ cells. Cell contains two compartments, inner nucleus and outer cytoplasm. Nucleus contains nucleoplasm suspended with genetic material. Nuclear envelope separates nucleus from cytoplasm. Cytoplasm is composed of aqueous cytosol, suspended with particles and membrane-bound organelles. Normal cell ranges between 10 and 30 μm in diameter. The various cell organelles are endoplasmic reticulum, Golgi complex, lysosomes, peroxisomes, mitochondria, nucleus, and centrioles. Biological membranes (lipoprotein viscous barriers) exist around all the living cells and also form structural and functional component of all the cell organelles. A membrane contains mainly lipids, proteins, and very little amount of carbohydrates. Important function of the membrane is to withhold unwanted molecules but permit entry of molecules necessary for cellular metabolism. Transport across the membrane occurs through passive transport, active transport, exocytosis, and endocytosis. Subcellular fraction of individual organelles of cell allows to study the biochemical properties in them individually.

## SELF-ASSESSMENT QUESTIONS

1. Briefly discuss the ultrastructure of a typical cell.
2. Add a note on the structural aspects of mitochondria and mention the metabolism that takes place in mitochondria.
3. Explain the fluid mosaic model of plasma membrane.
4. Write the features and importance of active transport mechanism.
5. How do you explain the ATP-driven active transport and ion-driven active transport?
6. Mention significances of endocytosis and exocytosis.
7. What is ion-driven active transport? Explain with an example.
8. Explain uniport and antiport transport mechanism with an example.
9. Why do we call mitochondrion as a powerhouse of the cell?

## MULTIPLE CHOICE QUESTIONS

1. Concerning plasma membrane, one of the following statements is not true:
   (a) Plasma membrane consists of specialized surface structures for attachment and for communication
   (b) Tight junctions produce seal between adjacent cells
   (c) Gap junctions does allow ions and electric current between adjacent cells
   (d) Consists of proteins, lipids, and carbohydrates
2. Cytoplasm is traversed by extensive network of interconnecting membrane-bound channels or cisternae, vesicles, and tubules form:
   (a) Endoplasmic reticulum
   (b) Golgi complex
   (c) Ribosomes
   (d) Microsomes
3. Concerning the Golgi complex, all of the following statements are true, *except*:
   (a) It is a membrane-bound structure
   (b) It is a stack of flattened-membrane vesicles
   (c) It does not gives rise to lipoprotein of plasma membrane
   (d) It helps in packaging and transportation of variety of materials
4. Concerning mitochondria, one of the following statements is incorrect:
   (a) It is considered to be the powerhouse of the cell
   (b) They are respiratory center of cell where pyruvate oxidation takes place
   (c) It accommodates for glycolysis
   (d) It has electron transport chain

5. **Nucleus:**
   (a) Presents in all cells of the body
   (b) Does not have nuclear envelope
   (c) Absents in RBCs
   (d) Exists in different shapes
6. **Concerning passive transport, one of the following statements is incorrect:**
   (a) It requires ATP
   (b) It requires carrier protein
   (c) It occurs along the concentration gradient
   (d) Its process is stereospecific
7. **Concerning active transport, one of the following statements is incorrect:**
   (a) Transport of molecules across the membrane is against the concentration gradient
   (b) It is energy dependent
   (c) Most important active transport in cells is Na$^+$–K$^+$-ATPase pump
   (d) 2Na$^+$ pumped outside and in exchange 3K$^+$ pumped in opposite direction
8. **Glucose absorption in intestinal epithelial cells is:**
   (a) Ion-driven active transport
   (b) Facilitated diffusion
   (c) Passive transport
   (d) Does not depend on concentration gradient
9. **Transport of macromolecules takes place through the following mechanisms, except:**
   (a) Diffusion
   (b) Phagocytosis
   (c) Pinocytosis
   (d) Exocytosis
10. **All of the following are the examples for endocytosis, except:**
    (a) Uptake of chylomicrons by liver cells
    (b) Internalization of LDL through LDL receptors of plasma membrane
    (c) Uptake of glucose by intestinal cells
    (d) Engulfment of bacteria by macrophages
11. **The main function of mitochondria is:**
    (a) DNA synthesis
    (b) Protein processing and packaging
    (c) ATP production
    (d) RNA synthesis
12. **The main function of the Golgi apparatus is:**
    (a) DNA synthesis
    (b) Protein processing and packaging
    (c) ATP synthesis
    (d) RNA synthesis
13. **The following are true of plasma membranes, except:**
    (a) They are made up of a double layer of lipid molecules in which proteins are embedded
    (b) The lipid membranes include phospholipids and cholesterol
    (c) The plasma membrane has RNA-binding sites on the inside surface of the membrane resembling rough endoplasmic reticulum
    (d) The plasma membrane has both integral membrane proteins and peripheral membrane proteins
14. **The function of smooth endoplasmic reticulum is:**
    (a) Protein synthesis
    (b) Regulation of intracellular calcium distribution
    (c) Excretion
    (d) Maintain the skeleton of the cell
15. **All of the following are the functions of lysosomes, except:**
    (a) Phagocytosis
    (b) Pinocytosis
    (c) Exocytosis
    (d) Breakdown of some intracellular materials
16. **Hydrolytic enzymes are found in:**
    (a) Golgi apparatus
    (b) RER
    (c) Lysosomes
    (d) Ribosomes
17. **The site of lysosomes can be seen using a specific histochemical reaction called:**
    (a) Alkaline phosphatase
    (b) Acid phosphatase
    (c) Peroxidase
    (d) Succinic dehydrogenase

18. Organelles most notable for producing and degrading hydrogen peroxide are:
    (a) Lysosomes
    (b) Mitochondria
    (c) Golgi bodies
    (d) Peroxisomes
19. The function of attached ribosomes to RER is to synthesize:
    (a) Lipid
    (b) Carbohydrate
    (c) Protein that will be secreted by the cell
    (d) Glycogen
20. Ribosomal RNA is formed in:
    (a) The euchromatin
    (b) The nucleolus
    (c) The RER
    (d) The heterochromatin
21. Glycogen can be demonstrated using:
    (a) Best's carmine
    (b) H and E
    (c) Sudan black
    (d) Silver
22. Euchromatin is predominant in:
    (a) Nuclei of metabolically active cells
    (b) Nuclei of metabolically inactive cells
    (c) Special type of stain
    (d) Type of cell organoids
23. The nucleolus is formed of:
    (a) Protein and DNA
    (b) Protein only
    (c) Chromatin
    (d) Protein and RNA
24. The nuclear pore:
    (a) Is hexagonal in shape
    (b) Is bridged by a unit membrane
    (c) Is a transient structure
    (d) Allows for communication between the nucleus and the cytoplasm
25. The feature of phospholipids that is essential for their role in biological membranes is:
    (a) To form strong rigid membranes
    (b) Extremely hydrophobic
    (c) To possess hydrophilic and hydrophobic portions
    (d) Extremely hydrophilic

## ANSWERS

| | | | | | | | |
|---|---|---|---|---|---|---|---|
| 1. c | 2. a | 3. c | 4. c | 5. c | 6. a | 7. d | 8. a |
| 9. b | 10. c | 11. c | 12. b | 13. c | 14. b | 15. c | 16. c |
| 17. b | 18. d | 19. c | 20. b | 21. a | 22. a | 23. d | 24. d |
| 25. c | | | | | | | |

# Chapter 2: Enzymes

## LEARNING OBJECTIVES

*At the end of this chapter students should be able to:*
- Understand the classification and function of enzymes
- Know about the active site and mechanism of enzyme action
- Explain the factors affecting enzyme activity
- Describe the different types of inhibition and use of competitive inhibition technique in the drug therapy
- Know about the diagnostic importance of enzymes

## ■ Introduction

- Enzymes are biological catalysts produced by the living cells and they catalyze several reactions in the body.
- They are proteins in nature.
- They are specific in action, i.e., each enzyme can catalyze only one type of reaction.
- They are required in very small quantities.
- The loss of catalytic activity was observed when they are subjected to heat or strong acids or bases or organic solvents.
- The enzymes mainly catalyze the metabolic pathways in the human body.
- The deficiency of the enzyme leads to inborn errors of metabolism.
- Most of the enzymes are produced by the cells of a particular tissue and function within that cell. Such enzymes are called *intracellular enzymes*.
- *Example*: Enzymes of glycolysis, tricarboxylic acid (TCA) cycle, and fatty acid synthesis.
- There are certain enzymes, which are produced by the cells of a particular tissue from where these are liberated for use in the other tissues. Such enzymes are called *extracellular enzymes*.

*Example:* Various proteolytic enzymes of gastrointestinal tract (trypsin and chymotrypsin).

The enzyme binds with its specific substrate and forms an enzyme–substrate complex. At the end of the reaction, the substrate is converted into the product and the enzyme remains unchanged.

$$E + S - ES \rightarrow E + Product$$

## ■ Chemical Nature of Enzymes

The chemical nature of enzymes is as follows:
- Enzymes with two or more subunits (polypeptides) are called oligomeric enzymes.
- Several enzymes occur in the form of multienzyme complex. In this case, several enzymes occur in a single complex form, e.g., pyruvate dehydrogenase and fatty acid synthase complex.
- Some enzymes require the presence of certain additional organic or inorganic substances and are *conjugated proteins*. Such enzymes are called **holoenzymes**. The protein part is called *apoenzymes* and the nonprotein part is *prosthetic group*.
- **Holoenzyme:** Apoenzyme+prosthetic group (coenzyme).
- Several apoenzymes require the presence of metal ions such as $Mg^{2+}$ (for hexokinase) and $Zn^{2+}$ (for the activity of carboxypeptidase). Such inorganic ions are called **cofactors**. If the metal ion is the integral part of the enzyme, such enzymes are called **metalloenzymes**.

## Ribozymes

These are RNA molecules that can act as catalysts.

These ribozymes break RNA phosphodiester bonds at certain specific location in the RNA molecules, serving as ribonucleases and as peptidyl transferase (catalyzes the formation of peptide body).

These ribozymes are being considered as possible therapeutic agents for disorders caused by the inappropriate expression of RNA or the expression of a mutated RNA. However, further research is required for this to consider.

**What are proenzymes?**

## Zymogens or Proenzymes

The protein-digesting enzymes (proteolytic enzymes) of gastrointestinal tract are produced in the form of precursor to prevent unwanted degradation of body self-protein. These inactive precursor forms of enzymes (zymogen) are converted into active form by HCl and trypsin.

*For example:*
- Pepsinogen → pepsin (HCl activates the pepsinogen).
- Trypsinogen → trypsin (trypsin and enteropeptidase activate the enzymes).
- Procarboxypeptidase to carboxypeptidase.
- Chymotrypsinogen to chymotrypsin.

**What are coenzymes? Explain with examples.**

## Coenzymes

Coenzymes are dialyzable, thermostable, low-molecular-weight organic substances (also considered as cosubstrate or second substrate) (**Table 2.1**).

They are small organic molecules that transport chemical groups from one enzyme to another.

They are usually regenerated and their concentrations maintained at a steady level inside the cell, e.g., NADPH is regenerated through the pentose phosphate pathway and S-adenosylmethionine by methionine adenosyltransferase.

## Energy of Activation of Catalyzed and Uncatalyzed Reactions

All chemical reactions have an energy barrier, separating the reactants and the products. This barrier, called the free energy of activation, is the energy difference between the energy of the reactant and high-energy intermediates

**Table 2.1:** Common coenzymes and their functions.

| Vitamin | Coenzyme | Function |
| --- | --- | --- |
| Thiamine ($B_1$) | TPP | Oxidative decarboxylation and transketolase reaction |
| Riboflavin ($B_2$) | FAD | Oxidative and reductive reaction |
| | FMN | |
| Niacin | NAD | Oxidative and reductive reaction |
| | NADP | |
| Pyridoxine ($B_6$) | PLP | Transamination, deamination, and decarboxylation reactions |
| Biotin | Biocytin | Carboxylation reactions |
| Folic acid | THF | Carrier of one carbon |
| Pantothenic acid | Coenzyme A | Acyl carrier |
| Cyanocobalamin ($B_{12}$) | Methylcobalamin and deoxyadenosylcobalamin | Transfer of $CH_3$ group and isomerizations |

(FAD: flavin adenine dinucleotide; FMN: flavin mononucleotide; NAD: nicotinamide adenine dinucleotide; NADP: nicotinamide adenine dinucleotide phosphate; PLP: pyridoxal phosphate; THF: tetrahydrofolate; TPP: thiamine pyrophosphate).

# CHAPTER 2: Enzymes

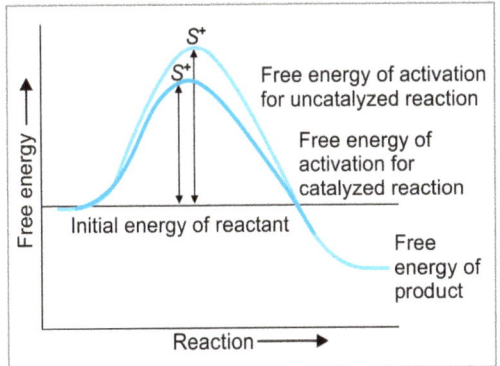

**Fig. 2.1:** Free energy of activation of a catalyzed and uncatalyzed reaction.

that occurs during the formation of a product (Fig. 2.1).

$$S \longleftrightarrow S^* \longleftrightarrow P$$
[Reactant]      [Product]

The peak of free energy activation, represents the transition state, in which the high-energy intermediates ($S^*$) are formed during the conversion of a reactant to a product.

Due to the effect of activation energy, the rates of unanalyzed chemical reactions are slow.

An enzyme lowers the energy required for activation to the transition state.

With an enzyme as a catalyst, the reaction may easily proceed at the normal physiological temperature, otherwise addition of heat energy is required for the reaction to occur.

## Active Site of an Enzyme

* The active site of an enzyme is the region where substrate binds.
* This active site contains the specific amino acid residues (binding and catalytic residues) and possesses three-dimensional structure.
* The amino acid residues at the active site of an enzyme have two functions:
  1. The binding amino acid residues recognize and bind the correct substrate to form enzyme–substrate (ES) complex.
  2. The catalytic residues create a chemical environment that enhances the rate of reaction and ES complex is converted to an enzyme ($E$) and a product ($P$).
* A change in the primary, secondary, tertiary, or quaternary structure may alter the three-dimensional shape of the active site to reduce its binding and catalytic activity.

**List and explain the factors that affect the enzyme activity.**
1. pH
2. Temperature
3. Concentration of substrate
4. Concentration of enzyme.

## Effect of PH

Each enzyme has an optimum pH at which the activity of the enzyme is maximum **(Fig. 2.2)**. Either decreased or increased pH causes a decrease in enzyme activity.

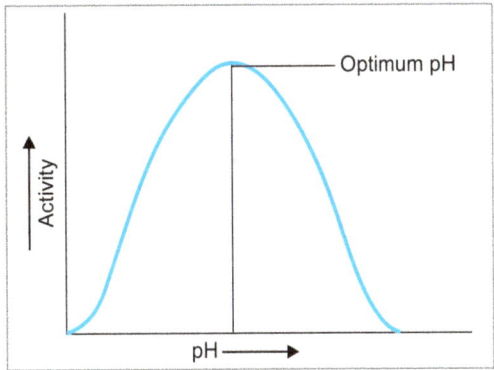

**Fig. 2.2:** Effect of pH on enzyme activity.

For example:
1. Pepsin has an optimum pH at 1.2 (its activity is maximum at this pH).
2. Optimum pH for amylase is 6.8.
3. Optimum pH for alkaline phosphatase (ALP) is 9.0.
4. Optimum pH for acid phosphatases (ACP) is 5.0.

## Effect of Temperature

The temperature at which the enzyme activity is more is called optimum temperature **(Fig. 2.3)**. Any strong change in the optimum temperature results in the loss of enzyme activity.

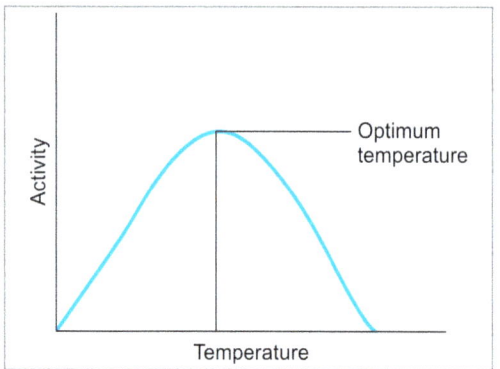

Fig. 2.3: Effect of temperature on enzyme activity.

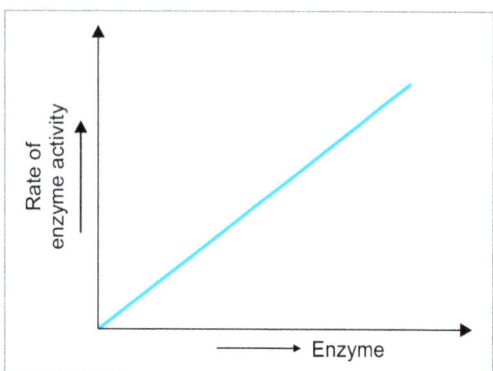

Fig. 2.5: Effect of enzyme concentration.

Optimum temperature of enzymes in the human body is 37°C.

## Effect of Substrate Concentration

At low substrate concentration enzyme, molecules are free initially and the ES complex (ES=enzyme–substrate) formation is proportional to the substrate concentration. This means the rate of velocity is directly proportional to the [S] and follows first-order kinetics. At higher concentration, all the enzyme molecules are saturated with substrate. There will be no change in the activity further (Fig. 2.4) and followed by hyperbolic curve; this is zero-order kinetics.

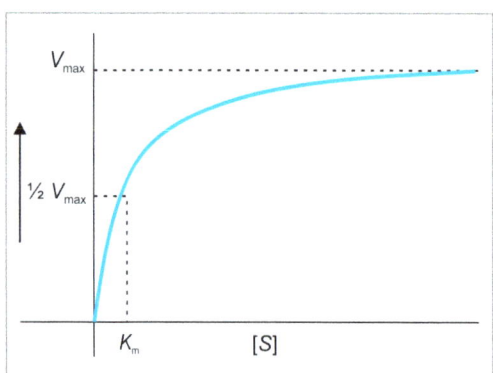

Fig. 2.4: Effect of substrate concentration.

## Effect of Enzyme Concentration

The velocity of the enzyme reaction is directly proportional to the enzyme concentration (Fig. 2.5).

## Classification of Enzymes with Examples

Enzymes are classified into six groups (Table 2.2) according to the International Union of Biochemistry.

## Enzyme Specificity

The most important property of enzyme is its specificity. They exhibit several types of specificity (Table 2.3).

**Briefly explain the mechanism of enzyme actions using different models.**

## Mechanism of Enzyme Catalysis

In the first step in enzyme catalysis, the substrate binds noncovalently at the active site of the enzyme and forms enzyme–substrate (ES) complex. This complex is subsequently converted to product and free enzyme.

Two models have been proposed to explain the binding mechanism of substrate to the active site of the enzyme.
- Lock and key model
- Induced fit model or hand-in glove model of Koshland.

## Lock and Key Model (Proposed by Emil Fischer)

In this model, the enzyme is preshaped and the active site has a rigid structure that is complimentary to substrate.

## Table 2.2: Classification of enzymes.

| Class | Examples |
|---|---|
| *Oxidoreductases:* Enzymes involved in oxidation-reduction reactions | Lactate dehydrogenase and glyceraldehyde-3-phosphate dehydrogenase |
| *Transferases:* Transfer a specific group from one substrate to another | Alanine transaminase and hexokinase |
| *Hydrolases:* Hydrolyze the substrate with the addition of water molecule | Glucose-6-phosphatase amylase and pepsin |
| *Lyases:* Catalyze the removal of a small molecule from a large substrate without the addition of water | Fumarase and enolase |
| *Isomerases:* Isomerize substrates | Racemases and isomerase |
| *Ligases:* Synthesize substance by joining two substrates with the utilization of energy | Glutamine synthetase |

## Table 2.3: Enzyme specificity.

1. *Stereospecificity:* The group of enzyme catalyzes either L- or D-isomer
2. *Reaction specificity:* One enzyme catalyzes only one type of reaction
3. *Substrate specificity:* Pepsin hydrolyzes residues of only aromatic amino acids while trypsin hydrolyzes residues of the basic amino acids only
   a. *Absolute specificity:* Glucokinase acts on glucose only
   b. *Group specificity:* Hexokinase catalyzes hexoses
4. *Bond specificity:* Refers to the action of proteolytic enzymes. Peptidase and glycosidase act on peptide bonds of proteins and glycosidic bonds of carbohydrates, respectively. Lipases act on ester bonds of lipids

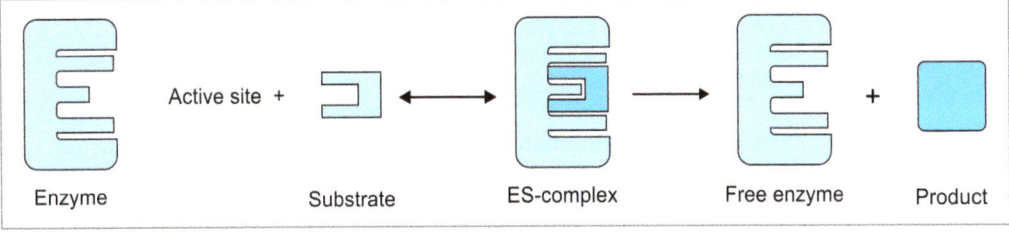

**Fig. 2.6:** Lock and key model.

This model is called lock and key model, because in this model, the substrate fits into the active site in the same way as a key fits into a lock **(Fig. 2.6)**.

This model gives the idea about the specificity of the enzymes, which binds only a specific substrate not another compound with an almost identical structure.

*For example:* The enzymes of glycolysis can bind D-isomer than L-isomer (which differs only in the configuration around a single carbon atom).

### Induced Fit Model

This model explains the specificity of the enzyme as well as the changes taking place during catalysis.

Koshland explained that the enzymes are flexible and shapes of the active site can be modified by the binding of the substrate.

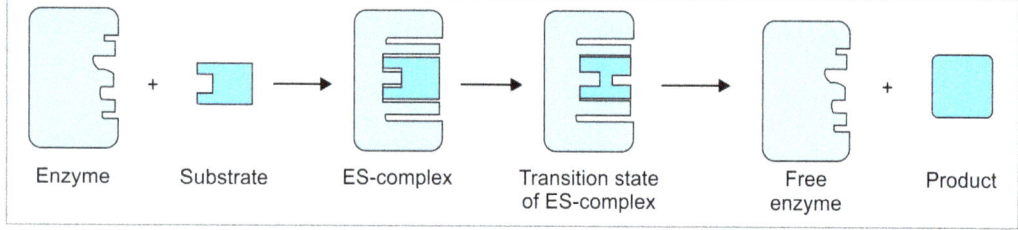

Enzyme  Substrate  ES-complex  Transition state of ES-complex  Free enzyme  Product

**Fig. 2.7:** Induced fit model.

In the induced fit model, the substrate induces a conformational change in the enzyme, in the same way in which placing a hand (substrate) into a glove (enzyme) induces changes in the glove's shape. Therefore, this model is also called a hand-in glove model (Fig. 2.7).

This arranges catalytic residues, which participate in catalysis. The enzyme in turn induces reciprocal changes in its bound substrate that changes their orientation and configuration and strains the structure of the bound substrate. Such changes help to bring the ES complex into its transition state.

The intrinsic binding energy due to the substrate–enzyme interaction is made available for the transformation of the substrate into product.

## Enzyme Kinetics

Study of the impact made on the rate of an enzyme-catalyzed reaction by changes in experimental conditions is known as enzyme kinetics.

Knowledge of kinetics can be a very useful tool in understanding the mechanism by which an enzyme carries out its catalytic activity.

The effect of substrate concentration on the initial rate of an enzyme-catalyzed reaction is the main concept in enzyme kinetics. The substrate concentration is the important factor affecting rate of a reaction catalyzed by enzyme.

The effect on initial velocity ($V_i$) of varying substrate concentration [S], when enzyme

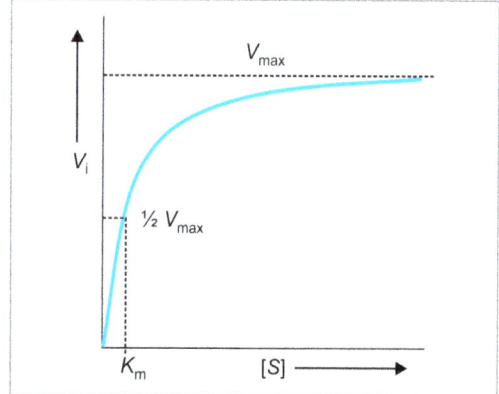

**Fig. 2.8:** Initial reaction velocity versus substrate concentration for Michaelis–Menten equation.

concentration is held constant is shown below (Fig. 2.8).

$V_i$ = initial velocity
[S] = substrate concentration
$V_{max}$ = maximum velocity
$K_m$ = substrate concentration when $V_i$ is one half of $V_{max}$ (Michaelis–Menten constant).

There are several modern ways to explain the way in which the Michaelis–Menten equation is derived, and one is mentioned below.

For most enzymes, if increased the substrate concentration [$S_z$] and hold enzyme concentration [E] constant, the resulting initial velocities, or reaction rates, of the reaction ($V_i$) produce a hyperbolic curve. In other words, $V_i$ increases rapidly at first as we increase substrate concentration [S]. This is first-order kinetics.

At higher substrate concentrations, $V_i$ increases by smaller amounts in response to increase in [S].

Then, the rate of increase in $V_i$ decreases, and $V_i$ approaches a limit of the reaction rate, called $V_{max}$. No further increases in [S] will increase velocity. This condition is known as zero-order kinetics.

We already learned that in an enzyme-catalyzed reaction, the enzyme exists in two forms, that is free [E] and the combined form [ES].

At low substrate concentration, most of enzyme will be in freeform $\dot{E}$. In this condition, the rate is proportional to [S].

The maximum velocity of the catalyzed reaction is observed when the entire enzyme is present as the enzyme-substrate complex and concentration of E is vanishingly low. Therefore, at this condition all the enzymes will be saturated with its substrate, and all the free enzymes will be converted into ES form. So that any increase in the [S] has no effect on the rate and the reaction immediately reaches a steady state, in which [ES] remains approximately constant. The ES complex breaks down to yield the product and the enzyme is free to bind another substrate molecule.

## Michaelis–Menten Equation

With some assumptions, the Michaelis–Menten equation describes the relationship between [S] and reaction rate ($V_i$), which is as follows:

$$V_i = \frac{V_{max}[S]}{K_m+[S]}$$

$K_m$ is Michaelis-Menten constant and is equal to the [S] where $V_i = \frac{V_{max}}{2}$.

$K_m$ is also an indicator of the enzyme's affinity for the substrate. The lower the $K_m$ value, the higher the affinity, so it takes less substrate to reach half of $V_{max}$ and the enzyme is a better catalyst for the reaction.

By considering a simple reaction in which one substrate, S, in the presence of an enzyme, E, converts to one product, P. Michaelis and Menten hypothesized that the enzyme catalyzes the reaction by reacting with the substrate

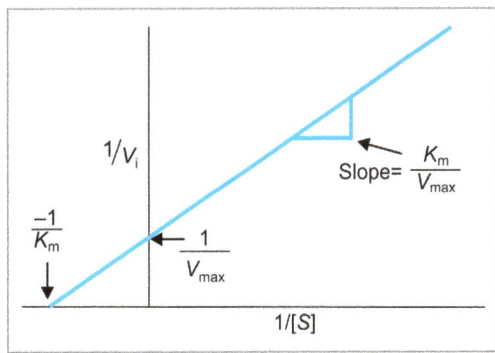

**Fig. 2.9:** Double reciprocal or Lineweaver–Burk plot.

to form an intermediate enzyme-substrate complex, ES. This complex experiences a catalytic reaction to form the enzyme, E, and the product, P. The following diagram represents the situation, where $K_1$, $K_2$, $K_3$, and $K_4$ are rate constants:

$$E+S \xrightarrow[K_2]{K_1} ES \xrightarrow[K_4]{K_3} E+P$$

To derive their model, Michaelis and Menten made the following simplifying assumptions:

Moreover, considering $x = 1/[S]$ to be an independent variable and $y = 1/V_i$ to be a dependent variable, the equation has the form of a line, $y = mx + b$. Thus in the graph **(Fig. 2.9)** of $1/V_i$ versus $1/[S]$, the slope is:

1. The reaction rate is determined before much product is formed. Consequently, the reverse reaction from $E + P$ to ES is negligible.
2. $K_3$ is small in comparison to $K_1$ and $K_2$, i.e., the rate of product formation is slow in comparison to the rate of ES formation and the rate of ES dissociation to $E + S$.
3. [S] is much greater than [E], so that [S] is virtually constant.
4. [E]+[ES] is constant.

Under these assumptions, the Michaelis–Menten equation models reaction (1) as follows:

$$V_i = \frac{K_m[S]}{V_{max}[S]}$$

Although the Michaelis–Menten equation captures the relationship of reaction velocity to substrate concentration, $K_m$ and $V_{max}$ are difficult to ascertain from its graph. Hans Lineweaver and Dean Burk reorganized the equation into a form that is more helpful for determination of these constants. Taking the reciprocal of both sides, they solved for $1/v$ in terms of $1/[S]$, as follows:

$$\frac{1}{V_i} = \frac{K_m[S]}{V_{max}[S]}$$

$$\frac{1}{V_i} = \frac{K_m}{V_{max}[S]} + \frac{[S]}{V_{max}[S]}$$

$$\frac{1}{V_i} = \left(\frac{K_m}{V_{max}}\right) + \frac{1}{[S]} + \frac{1}{V_{max}}$$

$\dfrac{K_m}{V_{max}}$ and $\dfrac{1}{V_{max}}$ are constants

Moreover, considering $x = 1/[S]$ to be an independent variable and $y = 1/V_i$ to be a dependent variable, the equation has the form of a line, $y = mx + b$. Thus in the graph (Fig. 2.9) of $1/V_i$ versus $1/[S]$, the slope is and the vertical intercept is $\dfrac{K_m}{V_{max}}$ and the vertical intercept is $\dfrac{1}{V_{max}}$.

Setting $1/V_i$ equal to zero, we find that the horizontal intercept is $\dfrac{-1}{K_m}$. Such a plot is called double reciprocal or Lineweaver–Burk plot.

**What is enzyme inhibition and what are its types? Explain with specific examples.**

## Enzyme Inhibition

The phenomenon of the decrease in the rate of enzymatic reaction brought about by the addition of a chemical substance is called enzyme inhibition. The substances, which inhibit the enzyme, are called inhibitors.

### Competitive Inhibition

The competitive inhibitor (reversible inhibitor) closely resembles with that of substrate.

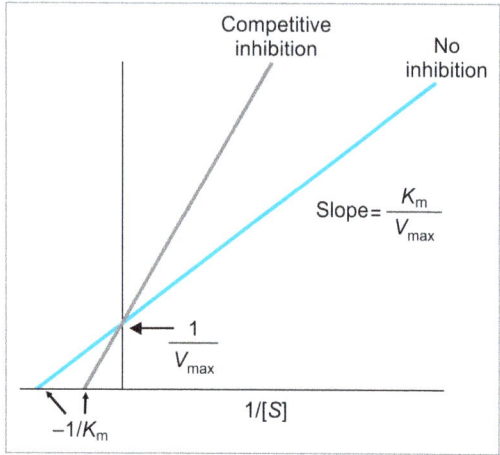

**Fig. 2.10:** Competitive inhibition.

Hence, the inhibitor competes with the substrate for substrate-binding sites of the enzyme. This type of inhibition can be overcome by sufficiently high concentrations of substrate, i.e., by out-competing the inhibitor (Fig. 2.10).

Competitive inhibitors can bind to E, but not to ES. Competitive inhibition increases $K_m$ (i.e., the inhibitor interferes with substrate binding) but does not affect $V_{max}$ (the inhibitor does not hamper catalysis in ES because it cannot bind to ES).

*For example:* Inhibition of succinate dehydrogenase by malonate.

The Michaelis–Menten equation for competitive inhibition is:

$$E + S \xrightarrow{K_m} ES \xrightarrow{K_2} E + P$$
$$I \downarrow K_I$$
$$EI$$

where $K_i$ is the dissociation constant for the EI complex. EI does not react to form $E+P$, and the enzyme is unable to bind both S and I at the same time.

The Michaelis–Menten equation for competitive inhibition is:

$$V = \frac{V_{max}[S]}{[S] + K_m\left(1 + \dfrac{[I]}{K_i}\right)}$$

**Table 2.4:** Commonly used drugs that are competitive inhibitors.

| Drug | Enzyme | Substrate | Therapeutic use |
|---|---|---|---|
| Methotrexate | Dihydrofolate reductase | $FH_2$ | Treatment of cancer |
| Allopurinol | Xanthine oxidase | Hypoxanthine | Treatment of gout |
| Acetazolamide | Carbonic anhydrase | $H_2CO_3$ | To treat hypertension |
| Mevinolin and lovastatin | HMG CoA reductase | HMG CoA | To treat hypercholesterolemia |
| Captopril and enalapril | ACE | Angiotensin | To treat high blood pressure |

(ACE: angiotensin converting enzyme; HMG CoA: β-hydroxy-β-methyl-glutaryl CoA).

The Lineweaver–Burk equation for competitive inhibition is:

$$\frac{1}{V} = \frac{K_m}{V_{max}} \frac{1}{[S]} \left(1 + \frac{[I]}{K_i}\right) + \frac{1}{V_{max}}$$

*For example:* Succinate dehydrogenase is the enzyme catalyzing the conversion of succinate to fumarate.

The malonate has the close structural resemblance to succinate.

That is why the malonate tries to occupy the active site of the enzyme.

Some of the competitive inhibitors made use in the treatment of disorders are as follows:

**List the therapeutic use of competitive inhibition.**

## Competitive Inhibition Technique in Drug Therapy

The competitive inhibitors available are mostly synthetic compounds, which are designed in such a way that it should have similarities with the substances present in the human body. So this similarity helps that compound to inhibit the enzymes that act on the particular substrates and finally block the reaction. Such type of inhibitors or drugs inhibits the important enzyme reactions in a bacteria or virus to control the infection. This type of treatment with chemicals or drugs to control infection is called chemotherapy.

To understand this, we should go through some of the examples **(Table 2.4).**

a. *Treatment with sulfa drugs:* Bacteria can synthesize folic acid from para-aminobenzoic acid (PABA).

- Sulfa drugs such as sulfonamide have a structure similar to PABA.
- When a person is treated with sulfa drugs, it inhibits the synthesis of folic acid in bacteria.
- The folic acid is an important vitamin required for bacterial multiplication.
- When sulfa drugs block the synthesis folic acid, the bacterial multiplication is inhibited and infection is controlled.

b. *Treatment for gout by allopurinol:*
- Allopurinol is the drug of choice for the treatment of gout.
- It has a structure similar to hypoxanthine.
- So allopurinol competitively inhibits xanthine oxidase, the enzyme that converts hypoxanthine to xanthine and then to uric acid.

c. *Control of cancer by amethopterin and aminopterin:*
- Amethopterin and aminopterin are antifolic compounds having structural similarity with folic acid **(Fig. 2.11).**
- Coenzyme (tetrahydrofolic acid) of this folic acid helps in the transfer of one

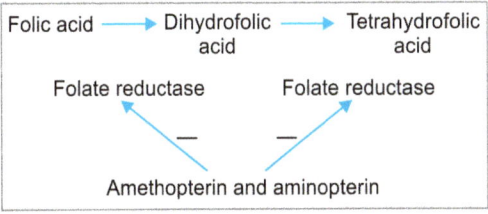

**Fig. 2.11:** Action of amethopterin and aminopterin.

carbon unit (in the reactions like the synthesis of purines and pyrimidines).
- Purines and pyrimidines are required for the synthesis of nucleic acids for growth and cell multiplication.
- Aminopterin or amethopterin competitively inhibits folate reductase and interferes with the synthesis of tetrahydrofolate.
- Thus these compounds are used in the treatment of blood cancer where in there is excessive production of WBC.
- Because of the coenzyme deficiency, the multiplication of WBC is inhibited.

d. *Dicumarol to thromboembolic condition*:
- Vitamin K is involved in the γ-carboxylation (see details in Vitamin K) of glutamic acid residues of the clotting factors such as prothrombin, proconvertin factor, Christmas factor, and Stuart-Prower factor.
- There are various anticoagulants to treat the thromboembolic conditions.
- Important and useful clinically are coumarins and heparins. Dicumarol and warfarin are the coumarins to treat the thromboembolic condition.
- When the patient is treated with dicumarol, it competes with vitamin K and decreases the formation of prothrombin by liver.

e. *Isonicotinic acid hydrazide (INH) treatment for tuberculosis:*
- The INH drug has structural similarity with pyridoxine.
- This drug interferes with the formation of pyridoxal phosphate, a coenzyme of pyridoxine used by TB bacillus. That is the reason why patients treated with INH always supplemented with vitamin $B_6$.

## Noncompetitive Inhibition

In this type, the inhibitor does not resemble the substrate and does not bind to the substrate-binding site of the enzyme. It binds to the enzyme other than the active site **(Fig. 2.12)**, e.g., inhibition of enzymes by heavy metals such as $Hg^{2+}$, iodoacetamide, and diisopropylphosphofluoride (DIPF).

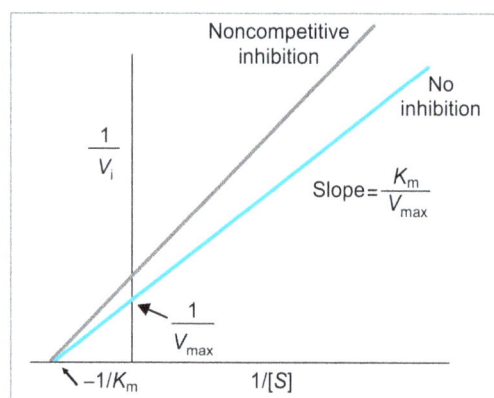

Fig. 2.12: Noncompetitive inhibition.

Iodoacetamide reacts with sulfhydryl groups of cysteine residues or with the imidazole group of histidine residues of the enzyme.

DIPF can inhibit acetylcholine esterase by covalently reacting with the hydroxyl group of a serine residues present at the active site of an enzyme.

A noncompetitive inhibitor lowers the $V_{max}$ with no change in the $K_m$ value.

Noncompetitive inhibitors have identical affinities for $E$ and ES ($K_i = K_i'$). Noncompetitive inhibition does not change $K_m$ (i.e., it does not affect substrate binding) but decreases $V_{max}$ (i.e., inhibitor binding affects catalysis).

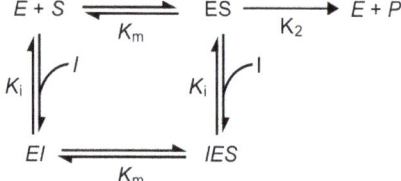

where $K_i$ is the dissociation constant for either the EI complex or the IES complex. Neither of these complexes can react to form $E + P$.

The Michaelis–Menten equation for non-competitive inhibition is:

$$V = \frac{V_{max}[S]}{([S]+K_m)\left(1+\frac{[I]}{K_i}\right)}$$

The Lineweaver–Burk equation for non-competitive inhibition is:

$$\frac{1}{V} = \frac{K_m}{V_{max}} \frac{1}{[S]}\left(1+\frac{[I]}{K_i}\right) + \frac{1}{V_{max}}\left(1+\frac{[I]}{K_i}\right)$$

## Uncompetitive Inhibition

It occurs when the inhibitor binds only to the enzyme–substrate complex, not to the free enzyme; the EIS complex is catalytically inactive. Inhibitor binds to ES complex at locations other than the catalytic site. This mode of inhibition is rare and causes a decrease in both $V_{max}$ and the $K_m$ value **(Fig. 2.13)**.

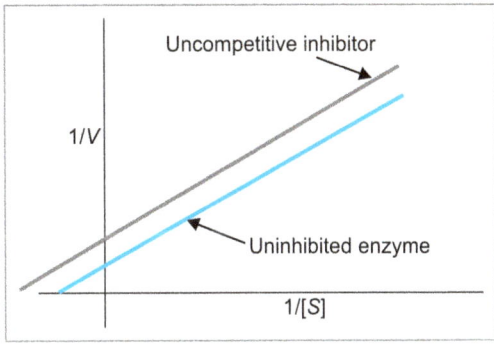

**Fig. 2.13:** Uncompetitive inhibition.

## Substrate and Product Inhibition

*Substrate and product inhibition* is where either the substrate or product of an enzyme reaction inhibits the enzyme's activity. This inhibition may follow the competitive, uncompetitive, or mixed patterns. In substrate inhibition, there is a progressive decrease in activity at high substrate concentrations. This may indicate the existence of two substrate-binding sites in the enzyme. At low substrate, the high-affinity site is occupied and normal kinetics is followed. However, at higher concentrations, the second inhibitory site becomes occupied inhibiting the enzyme. Product inhibition is often a regulatory feature in metabolism and can be a form of negative feedback. *Example*: Hexokinase inhibition by glucose-6-phosphate and inhibition of HMG CoA reductase by cholesterol.

**What are allosteric enzymes? Explain with and example.**

*Allosteric enzymes:* These enzymes have more than one subunit with a catalytic and regulatory site. Allosteric activator or inhibitor binds to the regulatory site and regulate the activity of the enzyme, e.g., HMG CoA reductase enzyme is a regulatory enzyme of cholesterol biosynthesis.

ADP and glucose-6-phosphate are the allosteric activator and inhibitor of hexokinase, respectively.

**What are isoenzymes? Briefly explain with examples.**

### Isoenzymes

They are defined as the different forms of a single enzyme and exist in the same species, which have same catalytic activity but differ structurally, physically, electrophoretically, and chemically.

*For example:* Lactate dehydrogenase (LDH)—LDH (has five different forms) and creatine phosphokinase—CK (has three different forms).

*LDH:* LDH has five different forms and each consists of four subunits (polypeptide chains). It is made up of two types of subunits (H and M) and contains four of them in different proportions as $LDH_1$, $LDH_2$, $LDH_3$, $LDH_4$, and $LDH_5$.

*CK:* It is a dimeric enzyme having two types of subunits (B and M). There are three isoenzyme forms of CK [$CK_1$ (BB), $CK_2$ (MB), and $CK_3$ (MM)].

**What are diagnostic enzymes and list them with the clinical importance.**

## Diagnostic Enzymes

The cells produce enzymes and they remain within the cells. Very small amount of the enzymes are released into the bloodstream, due to the normal breakdown of the cells. Hence, the enzymes are present even in the blood in very small amounts under normal conditions. The levels of these enzymes are greatly increased in blood under certain diseased conditions, which leads to breakdown of cells. Estimation of these enzyme levels in blood or plasma is useful in the diagnosis of various diseases. These enzymes indicate the organ from which they are released and based on this it is easy to find out which organ is affected **(Table 2.5)**.

The diagnostic enzymes are grouped according to the organ they belong. Important groups are as follows:
1. Liver enzymes: AST, alanine transaminase, ALP, and gamma-glutamyl transferase (GGT)
2. Cardiac enzymes: LDH, $LD_1$, CK, creatinine kinase myocardial bond (CKMB), and AST
3. Muscle enzymes: CK, LDH, and AST
4. Pancreatic enzymes: Amylase and lipase
5. Bone enzymes: ALP and ACP.

## Lactate Dehydrogenase

LDH is present in almost all the tissues of the body. Among different forms of LDH, which are known as isoenzymes, it is one of the best examples for isoenzymes.

**Table 2.5:** Diagnostic importance of certain serum enzymes.

| Serum enzymes | Diagnostic significance |
| --- | --- |
| 1. Acid phosphatase | Increases in carcinoma of prostate |
| 2. Alkaline phosphatase | Increases in obstructive jaundice and bone disorder such as rickets, Paget's disease, and hyperthyroidism |
| 3. Amylase | Increases in acute pancreatitis, intestinal obstruction, decreases in acute liver disease |
| 4. Creatine phosphokinase | |
|     CPK 1 (BB) | Brain disorder |
|     CPK 2 (MB) | Myocardial infarction (within 4 hours of onset) |
|     CPK 3 (MM) | Muscular dystrophy |
| 5. Ceruloplasmin | Increases in liver cirrhosis, decreases in Wilson's disease |
| 6. Choline esterase | Increases in nephrotic syndrome and decreases in acute liver disease and organophosphorus poisoning |
| 7. Glutamate oxaloacetate transaminase | Increases in myocardial infarction, toxic liver cell necrosis |
| 8. AST and ALT | Increases in viral hepatitis and other liver diseases |
| 9. Lactate dehydrogenase | |
|     $LDH_1$, $LDH_2$ | Myocardial infarction |
|     $LDH_4$, $LDH_5$ | Acute viral hepatitis |
| 10. Lipase | Increases in acute pancreatitis |
| 11. 5 Nucleotidase | Increases in liver disease and obstructive jaundice |
| 12. γ-Glutamyl transpeptidase | Alcoholic liver disease |

(ALT: alanine transaminase; AST: aspartate aminotransferase; GPT: glutamate pyruvate transaminase).

| Isoenzyme | Subunits | Source |
|---|---|---|
| $LD_1$ | HHHH | Heart, RBC |
| $LD_2$ | HHHM | RBC, heart |
| $LD_3$ | HHMM | Liver, lung, and spleen |
| $LD_4$ | HMMM | Liver, lung, and spleen |
| $LD_5$ | MMMM | Skeletal muscle |

Since LDH present in almost all the tissues, its increase in the serum is nonspecific. LDH level mainly increases in the following conditions:
* Myocardial infarction ($LD_1$ and $LD_2$ increased)
* Skeletal muscle diseases ($LD_5$ increased)
* Liver diseases ($LD_3$ and $LD_4$ increased)
* Cancer of lung, liver, and many other organ diseases ($LD_3$ and $LD_4$ increased).

## Cardiac Enzymes in Myocardial Infarction

The enzymes such as CKMB, LDH, $LDH_1$, and AST are included under cardiac enzymes. Estimation of these may help in the diagnosis, assessment, and prognosis of the heart diseases **(Fig. 2.14)**.

The increase and decrease in the levels of cardiac enzymes follow a particular pattern in myocardial infarction (MI), which is as follows:

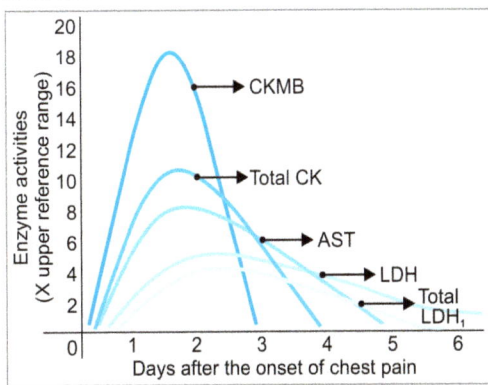

**Fig. 2.14:** Pattern of cardiac enzymes following myocardial infarction.
(CKMB: creatinine kinase myocardial band; CK: creatinine kinase; AST: aspartate aminotransferase; LDL: lactate dehydrogenase).

## Creatinine Kinase and Cratinine Kinase Myocardial Band

Following myocardial infarction (MI), the first enzyme to increase is CKMB. Immediately after the heart attack, the CKMB levels in serum start increasing. It goes on increasing and reaches a maximum level by the end of the first day. After reaching the peak level, CKMB decreases and reaches the normal level by the third day. Total CK also follows the same pattern (normally CKMB is about 6% of the total CK value). In myocardial infarction, CKMB form may go up to 10–30% of total CK.

## Aspartate Aminotransferase

AST levels in plasma increase 6–8 hours after the onset of chest pain and it reaches the peak value by the second day but comes to normal by the fourth or fifth day.

## Lactate Dehydrogenase and Lactate Dehydrogenase-1

Total LDH and $LDH_1$ begin to increase 8–12 hours after the onset of chest pain. It goes on increasing and reaches the maximum value by the third day and slowly comes to normal by about the seventh day.

The level of these enzymes in serum is related to the severe damage to heart muscle. So in severe MI these enzymes are elevated.

CKMB and $LD_1$ are the most sensitive and specific markers for the diagnosis of MI.

## Phosphatases

These are enzymes, which catalyze the removal of $PO^{2-}$ group from organic monophosphoric esters. Two types of phosphatases present normally are ALP, which has maximum activity at pH 10, and acid phosphatase with maximum activity at acidic pH 5.0.

## Alkaline Phosphatase

The ALP is present in all tissues of the body.
Its level is high in liver, bone, intestine, kidney, and placenta. Each of these organs contains a specific isoenzyme of ALP.

There are totally five isoenzyme forms of ALP. Normal adult serum contains ALP, which is mainly from liver and bile duct.

The source of serum ALP mainly in children is from bone.

Placenta ALP is found in pregnancy only.

The functions of ALP in the body are the transport of phosphate across the cell membranes and addition of phosphates during mineralization of the bone.

*Normal range:* 40–200 U/L (35–140 U/L).

## Acid Phosphatases

The prostate gland is the richest source for ACP. Other sources are red blood cells, platelets, bone, etc.
1. Serum ACP is increased in prostate gland enlargement (benign prostate hypertrophy) and carcinoma of the prostate gland.
2. The elevation of ACP is also seen in bone diseases.

## Gamma-glutamyl Transferase

*Source*: Liver and bile duct are the main sources of plasma GGT. Pancreas, prostate gland, and kidneys also contain this enzyme.

### Clinical Significance

GGT levels in serum are increased in:
1. Obstructive jaundice
2. Hepatitis
3. Alcoholic cirrhosis.

Plasma GGT level is a very sensitive indicator to diagnose alcoholic cirrhosis.

*Normal value*: 5–40 U/L.

## Amylase

Amylase helps in the digestion of starch in the small intestine. Amylase breaks $\alpha$-1,4-glucoside linkages of starch into maltose. Serum amylase originates from pancreas and salivary gland.

### Clinical Significance

Amylase level in serum is increased in acute pancreatitis, pancreas injury, and carcinoma of pancreas, tumors of lung, mumps, and other salivary lesions.

*Normal range*: 80–240 U/L.

## Lipase

It is the enzyme present in the intestine, which hydrolyzes triglycerides (fat) of the diet and finally helps to digest the fat. Bile salts are essential for the action of lipase.

*Source:* Pancreas is the major source for lipase in the serum.

Serum lipase is increased in chronic pancreatitis.

Serum amylase is increased in mumps pancreatic diseases or due to some other cause, whereas lipase is increased only in pancreatitis. Therefore, the determination of both amylase and lipase together helps in the diagnosis of acute pancreatitis.

*Normal range*: 40–200 U/L.

## Cholinesterase

Two types have been distinguished from true cholinesterase (acetylcholine hydrolase and acetylcholinesterase) present in nerve tissue and RBC, which are responsible for the hydrolysis of acetylcholine at synapses and the neuromuscular junction.

Serum cholinesterase level is an important indicator of insecticide poisoning. Its level markedly decreased in persons who have consumed insecticides, which are organophosphorous compounds.

*Normal levels*: 4,000–12,000 U/L.

## Glucose-6-$PO_4$ Dehydrogenase

Glucose-6-$PO_4$ dehydrogenase (G-6-PD) is present within the RBC. Deficiency of G-6-PD is inborn and it is prevalent throughout the world. The deficiency is of the mild type in most people. Deficiency is also observed in some rare cases and it is observed in childhood itself.

G-6-PD is the enzyme required in Hexose monophosphate pathway of carbohydrate metabolism. The enzyme catalyzes the reaction, with the production of NADPH.

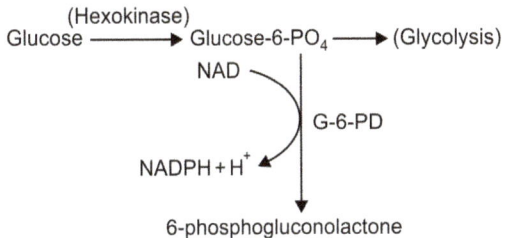

NADPH is essential for the stability of RBC membranes (NADPH is required to maintain reduced glutathione range which maintains the stability of RBCs). In case of G-6-PD deficiency, NADPH production will be decreased leading to breakdown of RBC and anemia. In the case of mild deficiency, a person will be healthy when he is treated with certain drugs such as primaquine and sulfonamides causing severe hemolysis. The NADPH supply is not sufficient to maintain the stability of RBC when these drugs are given. Hence, hemolysis takes place and may lead to anemia and death.

G-6-PDH estimation in blood is required in the following conditions:
1. When the patient is suffering from severe hemolytic anemia.
2. While treating a patient with malarial drugs.

*Reference*: 8–18 U/g Hb.

## SUMMARY

Enzymes are biological catalysts produced by the living cells and they catalyze several reactions in the body. They are proteins in nature and specific in action. The enzymes mainly catalyze the metabolic pathways in the human body. The deficiency of the enzyme results in metabolic errors. Most of the enzymes are of intracellular enzymes excluding some extracellular enzymes. The enzyme binds with its specific substrate to form enzyme–substrate complex. The enzymes have an active site where substrate binds. Many of enzymes of our body require coenzymes for the reaction to catalyze. These coenzymes are small organic molecules, which transport chemical groups from one enzyme to another. The factors that affect enzyme activity are pH, temperature, and concentration of substrate and enzyme. Enzymes are classified into six classes depending on their functions. The phenomenon of the decrease in the rate of enzymatic reaction brought about by the addition of a chemical substance is called enzyme inhibition. The substances, which inhibit the enzyme, are inhibitors. The inhibition is of competitive and noncompetitive type. The competitive inhibition is utilized in the drug therapy. Most of the enzymes are regulated by allosteric regulation to control the metabolic reactions.

## SELF-ASSESSMENT QUESTIONS

1. What are enzymes?
2. What are extracellular and intracellular enzymes? Explain with examples.
3. Briefly discuss the factors affecting enzyme activity.
4. Classify enzymes with an example for each class.
5. What is inhibitor? Give three examples.
6. What are the antimetabolites? Mention any two importance of it.

7. Can competitive inhibition be reversed by increasing substrate concentration?
8. How do you explain the competitive type of inhibition? Mention some of the uses of competitive inhibitors in drug therapy.
9. How the noncompetitive inhibition differs from competitive type of inhibition?
10. What are proenzymes? Give an example.
11. How is trypsinogen converted to trypsin?
12. Briefly discuss the isoenzymes with some examples.
13. Mention the clinical importance of diagnostic enzymes.
14. Add a note on the specificity of enzymes.
15. Give the formula for Michaelis–Menten constant.
16. Give the normal serum value for LDH and alkaline phosphatase.
17. Mention the importance of G-6-P dehydrogenase and which pathway needs this enzyme?
18. How many isoenzyme forms of lactate dehydrogenase are possible?
19. Mention the five organs which release alkaline phosphatase.
20. Derive the Michaelis–Menten equation.
21. Give the clinical significance of GGT estimation.
22. Write the different forms of CK.
23. Which form of LDH increases in MI?
24. Which form of LDH moves fast on electrophoresis?
25. Give the cardiac enzyme panel.

## MULTIPLE CHOICE QUESTIONS

1. **Most of the enzymes of glycolysis are:**
   - (a) Intracellular
   - (b) Extracellular
   - (c) Intermediate
   - (d) Neutral
2. **All the following statements regarding the coenzymes are correct, *except*:**
   - (a) Dialyzable and thermostable
   - (b) Organic substances
   - (c) NADH is the coenzyme for lactate dehydrogenase
   - (d) Does not bind to the enzyme
3. **One of the following factor does not affect the enzyme activity:**
   - (a) pH
   - (b) Temperature
   - (c) Isoenzyme concentration
   - (d) Substrate concentration
4. **Amylase is a:**
   - (a) Hydrolase class of enzyme
   - (b) Lyase class of enzyme
   - (c) Oxidoreductase class of enzyme
   - (d) Ligase class of enzyme
5. **Optimum pH for alkaline phosphatase is:**
   - (a) 5.0
   - (b) 7.0
   - (c) 9.0
   - (d) 2.0
6. **The enzyme that inhibits xanthine oxidase is:**
   - (a) Malonate
   - (b) Succinate
   - (c) Allopurinol
   - (d) Methotrexate
7. **Aminopterin or amethopterin competitively inhibits:**
   - (a) Folate reductase
   - (b) Glutathione reductase
   - (c) Lactate dehydrogenase
   - (d) Xanthine oxidase

8. The enzyme that elevates in prostate cancer is:
   (a) Alkaline phosphatase
   (b) Acid phosphatase
   (c) Lactate dehydrogenase
   (d) Amylase
9. The isoenzyme form of lactate dehydrogenase increases in skeletal muscle disease is:
   (a) LD5
   (b) LD1
   (c) LD3
   (d) LD4
10. Following myocardial infarction, the first enzyme to increase is:
    (a) CKMB
    (b) LDH
    (c) AST
    (d) None of the above
11. Concerning alkaline phosphates, one of the following statement is incorrect:
    (a) It has more than 5 isoenzyme forms
    (b) It is not present in placenta and kidney
    (c) It elevates in bone disorder
    (d) It elevates in obstructive jaundice
12. The enzyme that elevates in alcoholic cirrhosis is:
    (a) GGT
    (b) ACP
    (c) CK
    (d) LDH
13. Enzymes used to breakdown proteins in biological washing powders belong to the group:
    (a) Lactases
    (b) Lipases
    (c) Proteases
    (d) Hydrolases
14. Enzymes act as biological:
    (a) Inhibitors
    (b) Substrates
    (c) Solvents
    (d) Catalysts
15. Enzymes speed up biochemical reactions by:
    (a) Increasing the activation energy of the reaction
    (b) Lowering the activation energy of the reaction
    (c) Increasing the temperature of the reaction
    (d) Lowering the temperature of the reaction
16. The diagram shows a typical relationship between enzyme activity and:
    (a) pH
    (b) Enzyme concentration
    (c) Substrate concentration
    (d) Temperature

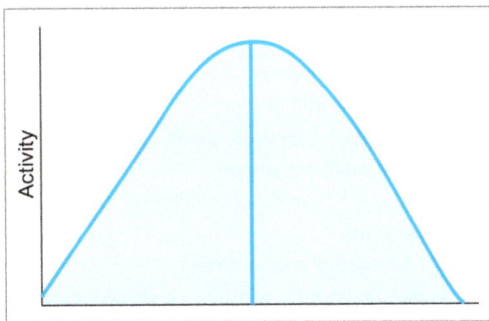

17. Chemicals (other than the substrate) that affect enzyme activity are called:
    (a) Exhibitors
    (b) Activators
    (c) Inhibitors
    (d) Inactivators

18. **Enzymes belong to which group of chemicals:**
    (a) Proteins
    (b) Polysaccharides
    (c) Lipids
    (d) Phospholipids
19. **The diagram shows a typical relationship between enzyme activity and:**
    (a) pH
    (b) Enzyme concentration
    (c) Substrate concentration
    (d) Temperature

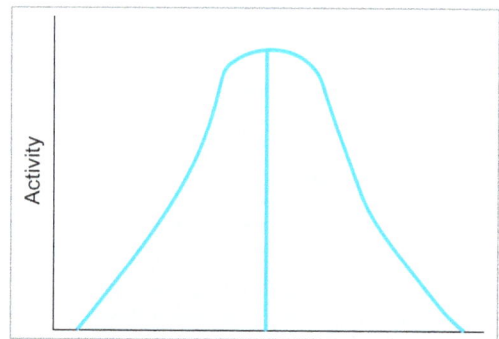

20. **Allosteric enzymes have:**
    (a) Single subunit
    (b) Obey Michaelis–Menten kinetics
    (c) Catalytic and a regulatory site
    (d) Affinity toward inhibitors only
21. **Concerning the allosteric enzymes, one of the following statements is incorrect:**
    (a) The inhibitor can bind to the enzyme at the same time as the enzyme's substrate
    (b) Binding of inhibitor to allosteric site changes the enzyme conformation
    (c) They contain many subunits and catalyze the committed step in a pathway
    (d) They do not obey Michaelis–Menten kinetics
22. **To confirm the Koshland mechanism, an enzyme must:**
    (a) Have more than one subunit
    (b) Exhibit allosteric behavior
    (c) Demonstrate negative cooperativity
    (d) Have more than one binding site
23. **All of the following about the MCW enzyme model are true, *except*:**
    (a) The enzyme exists in two states only
    (b) The T-state has greater affinity for substrate
    (c) In the absence of substrate, there is little R-state
    (d) This model cannot account for negative cooperativity
24. **Concerning the cooperativity, all are true, *except*:**
    (a) Positive cooperativity occurs when binding of the first substrate molecule increases the affinity of the other active sites for substrate
    (b) Phosphofructokinase shows negative cooperativity
    (c) Negative cooperativity makes enzymes insensitive to small changes in [S]
    (d) Hill equation is often used to describe the degree of cooperativity quantitatively in non-Michaelis–Menten kinetics
25. **The disorder of a system is measured by its:**
    (a) Activation energy
    (b) Heat of reaction
    (c) Entropy
    (d) Energy

26. The optimum pH of most human enzymes is:
    (a) 2.0
    (b) 6.0
    (c) 8.0
    (d) 7.1
27. The "lock and key" model of enzyme action illustrates that a particular enzyme molecule:
    (a) Forms a permanent enzyme–substrate complex
    (b) Denatured and renatured several time
    (c) Interacts with a specific type of substrate molecule
    (d) Reacts at identical rates under all conditions
28. An enzyme–substrate complex may result from the interaction of molecules of:
    (a) Fructose and lipase
    (b) Fat and amylase
    (c) Sucrose and maltase
    (d) Protein and protease
29. The place of the enzyme molecule into which the substrate fits is:
    (a) Active site
    (b) Coenzyme
    (c) Peptide
    (d) Key part
30. One of the following variables is least likely to affect an enzyme's rate of reaction is:
    (a) Temperature
    (b) Enzyme concentration
    (c) $CO_2$ concentration
    (d) Hydrogen bonds
31. Which of the following is characteristic of enzymes?
    (a) They lower the energy of activation of a reaction by binding the substrate
    (b) They raise the energy of activation of a reaction by binding the substrate
    (c) They lower the amount of energy present in the substrate
    (d) They raise the number of molecules moving quickly
32. An allosteric site on an enzyme is:
    (a) Similar to active site
    (b) Nonprotein in nature
    (c) Where ATP attaches and gives up its energy
    (d) Involved in feedback inhibition
33. In noncompetitive inhibition, the allosteric inhibitor:
    (a) Attaches to the active site, preventing the substrate from attaching there
    (b) Attaches to the substrate, preventing it from attaching to the active site
    (c) Changes the pH of the environment, thus preventing enzyme–substrate complex formation
    (d) Attaches to the enzyme at a site away from the active site, altering the shape of the enzyme
34. The minimum amount of energy needed for a process to occur is called the:
    (a) Minimal energy theory
    (b) Process energy
    (c) Kinetic energy
    (d) Activation energy
35. An inhibitor that changes the overall shape and chemistry of an enzyme is known as:
    (a) Allosteric inhibitor
    (b) Competitive inhibitor
    (c) Noncompetitive inhibitor
    (d) Active inhibitor
36. Inactive precursors of some enzymes that are activated through hydrolysis reactions are called:
    (a) Allosteric enzymes
    (b) Apoenzymes
    (c) Prosthetic groups
    (d) Zymogens
37. l-Amino acid dehydrogenase is an enzyme that can catalyze the oxidation of different l-amino acids. It cannot catalyze the oxidation of d-amino acids. Based on these characteristics of this enzyme, one can say that it shows:
    (a) Allosteric regulation
    (b) Absolute specificity over substrate
    (c) Relative specificity over substrate
    (d) Specific inhibition

38. These enzymes have different structure but the same catalytic function. Frequently they are oligomers made from different polypeptide chains. These enzymes are called:
    (a) Isozymes
    (b) Allosteric enzymes
    (c) Proenzymes
    (d) Zymogens
39. The model that explains that the active site is flexible and the catalytic group of the enzyme is brought into proper alignment by the substrate is called:
    (a) Concerted model
    (b) Induced fit model
    (c) Lock and key model
    (d) Sigmoid model

## ANSWERS

| | | | | | | | | |
|---|---|---|---|---|---|---|---|---|
| 1. a | 2. d | 3. c | 4. a | 5. c | 6. c | 7. a | 8. b |
| 9. a | 10. a | 11. c | 12. a | 13. c | 14. d | 15. b | 16. d |
| 17. c | 18. a | 19. a | 20. c | 21. d | 22. c | 23. d | 24. b |
| 25. d | 26. c | 27. c | 28. d | 29. a | 30. c | 31. a | 32. d |
| 33. d | 34. d | 35. c | 36. d | 37. b | 38. a | 39. b | |

# Chapter 3

# Chemistry of Carbohydrates

## LEARNING OBJECTIVES

*At the end of this chapter students should be able to:*
- Classify the carbohydrates with examples
- Explain the structure and function of starch and glycogen
- Understand the isomerism property of carbohydrates

## Introduction

Carbohydrates are organic substances containing C, H, and O usually in the ratio of 1:2:1. They are polyhydroxy aldehyde or ketone derivatives.

**Classify the carbohydrates and explain each class with specific examples.**

## Classification

They are classified into four major groups:

1. *Monosaccharides*: These are simple sugars and cannot be hydrolyzed further into simpler forms.
   Monosaccharides are further classified on the basis of number of carbon atoms present as well as on the presence of functional groups **(Table 3.1)**.

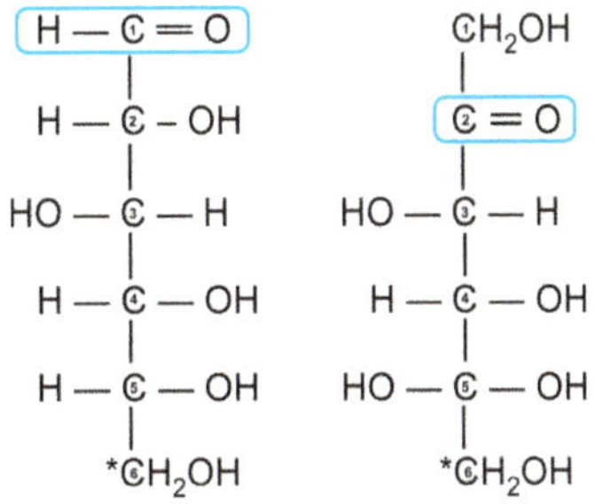

2. *Disaccharides*: They contain two molecules of same or different monosaccharide units. On hydrolysis, they yield two monosaccharide units. Two monosaccharide units are joined by glycosidic bond **(Table 3.2)**.

3. *Oligosaccharides*: They contain three to six molecules of monosaccharide units, for

D-Glucose

D-Fructose

**Table 3.1:** Classification of monosaccharides.

| Number of carbon atoms | Examples | Functional groups present |
|---|---|---|
| Trioses (three carbons) | Glyceraldehyde | Aldehyde (aldotriose) |
|  | Dihydroxyacetone | Ketone (ketotriose) |
| Tetroses (four carbons) | Erythrose | Aldehyde (aldotetrose) |
| Pentoses (five carbons) | Ribose | Aldehyde (aldopentose) |
|  | Xylose | Aldehyde (aldopentose) |
|  | Xylulose | Ketone (ketopentose) |
| Hexoses (six carbons) | Glucose | Aldehyde (aldohexose) |
|  | Galactose | Aldehyde (aldohexose) |
|  | Fructose | Ketone (ketohexose) |

**Table 3.2:** Examples of disaccharides.

| Examples | Product formed upon hydrolysis | Glycosidic linkage | Sources |
|---|---|---|---|
| Maltose | Glucose + glucose | α-1–4 | Malt |
| Lactose | Galactose + glucose | β-1–4 | Milk |
| Sucrose | Glucose + fructose | α-1–2 | Sugarcane |
| Isomaltose | Glucose + glucose | α-1–6 | Digestion of amylopectin |

example, maltotriose (glucose + glucose + glucose).

4. *Polysaccharides:* They contain more than six molecules of monosaccharide units.

They are further classified into homopolysaccharides and heteropolysaccharides.

## Homopolysaccharides

They are polymer of same monosaccharide units **(Table 3.3)**.

**Table 3.3:** Examples for homopolysaccharides.

| Examples | Monosaccharide unit | Sources |
|---|---|---|
| Starch | Glucose | Plant, rice |
| Dextrin | Glucose | From starch hydrolysis |
| Glycogen | Glucose | Liver, muscle |
| Cellulose | Glucose | Plant fibers |
| Inulin | Fructose | Dahlia roots |
| Chitin | N-acetyl glucosamine | Shells of arthropod |

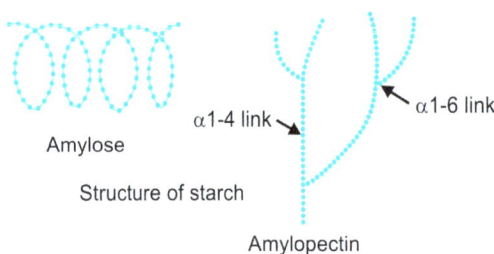

Structure of starch

**What are homopolysaccharides? Explain with specific examples.**

### Starch

Starch is a mixture of two polysaccharides such as amylose and amylopectin.

**How do you differentiate amylose from amylopectin?**

The major differences between amylose and amylopectin are in **Table 3.4**.

*Glycogen*
- Glycogen is stored in liver and muscle.
- It is a polymer of glucose units.
- It is also called animal starch.
- It is similar to the amylopectin component of starch, but it has more branches than starch.
- There are 11–18 glucose residues between any branch points.

*Dextrin*
These are partially hydrolyzed product of starch.

*Cellulose*
It is made up of β-D-glucose joined by β-1-4-glycosidic bonds. Cellulose is digested by cellulase enzyme, which is not present in the human body. But cellulose acts as dietary fiber, adds bulk to the food, and helps in peristalsis.

*Inulin*
Inulin consists of a small number of β-D-fructose joined by β-2-1-glycosidic linkages. It is used to measure the glomerular filtration rate, a test to assess the function of kidney.

**What are heteropolysaccharides? Explain with examples including their biomedical importance.**

## Heteropolysaccharide

They are polymer of different monosaccharide units or their derivatives, for example, mucopolysaccharides (MPSs) and blood group substances.

# CHAPTER 3: Chemistry of Carbohydrates

Table 3.4: Differences between amylose and amylopectin.

| Characteristics | Amylose | Amylopectin |
|---|---|---|
| 1. Amount present in starch | 15–20% | 80–85% |
| 2. Structure | Unbranched, linear | Highly branched. Branch point appears after every 24–30 glucose in straight chain form |
| 3. Molecular weight | 60 kDa | 500 kDa |
| 4. Linkage | 250–300 glucose residues are joined by α-1–4 glycosidic link | Mainly formed by α-1–4 linkages between glucose residues. Branch point occurs by forming α-1–6 glycosidic link |
| 5. Reaction with iodine solution | Blue color forms because the iodine molecules are trapped inside the helical structure. Color disappears upon heating. Reappears upon cooling | Reddish violet color |

MPSs are:
- Hyaluronic acid
- Chondroitin sulfate
- Heparin and keratan sulfate
- Heparan sulfate
- Dermatan sulfate.

MPSs are heteropolysaccharides (proteoglycan – protein = MPSs).

MPSs are also known as glycosaminoglycans.

## Biomedical Importance of MPSs

The biomedical importance of MPSs is as follows:
- MPSs are acidic in nature because of their polyanionic property. They are the components of ground substances throughout the extracellular space. They are attached to proteins and form proteoglycans.
- Hyaluronic acid acts as a barrier in tissues against the penetration of bacteria. Hyaluronidase present in bacteria can digest hyaluronic acid and acts as "spreading factor." Hyaluronidase present in testicular secretions can help in fertilization by favoring the entry of spermatozoa into the ovum **(Table 3.5)**.

## Isomerism in Carbohydrates

The presence of asymmetric carbon atoms (a carbon atom to which four different atoms

Table 3.5: Different mucopolysaccharides and their occurrence.

| Mucopolysaccharide | Composition | Occurrence |
|---|---|---|
| Chondroitin sulfate | Glucuronic acid + N-acetyl galactosamine | Cartilage |
| Dermatan sulfate | Glucuronic acid or iduronic acid and N-acetyl galactosamine | Animal tissue |
| Keratan sulfate | Galactose and N-acetyl glucosamine | Cornea and helps in corneal transparency |
| Heparin (highly sulfated) | Glucuronic acid and N-acetyl glucosamine | Liver, lungs, arterial wall, and blood anticoagulant |
| Hyaluronic acid (sulfate free) | Glucuronic acid + N-acetyl galactosamine | Synovial fluid of joint, vitreous humor of eye, umbilical cord, cell membrane, and skin |

or groups attached is known as asymmetric carbon) in a compound produces the following effects:

- Formation of the stereoisomerism of the compound.
- Confers optical activity to the compound.

**Discuss the optical activity carbohydrates including the enantiomers, anomerism, and epimerism with specific examples.**

## Stereoisomerism

Such compounds that are identical in composition and structural formula but differ in spatial configuration are called stereoisomers. These include:

A. *Enantiomer*: D- and L-sugars are referred to as enantiomers. Their structures are the mirror images of each other. Only D-glucose or D-sugars are utilized by humans. D- and L-glucose are termed D and L form depending on the arrangement of H and OH on the penultimate carbon atom. When the sugar has OH group on the right side, this form is D-isomer (see figure below). If OH group is on the left side, then it is L-isomer.

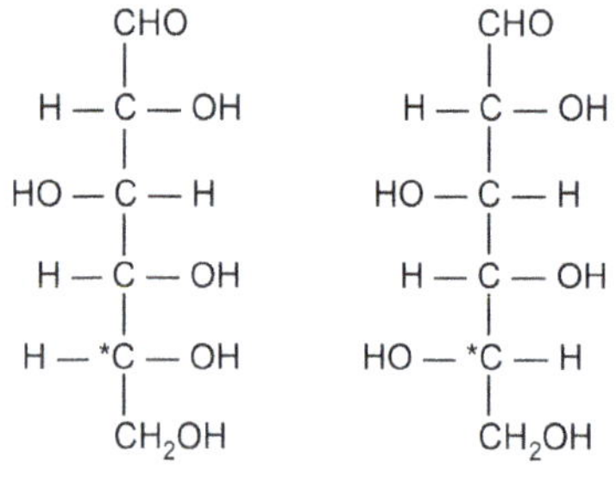
CHO
H — C — OH
HO — C — H
H — C — OH
H — *C — OH
$CH_2OH$
CHO
H — C — OH
HO — C — H
H — C — OH
HO — *C — H
$CH_2OH$

D-Glucose L-Glucose

B. *Anomerism*: Sugars in solution exist in ring form and not in straight chain form. Aldosugar forms mainly pyranose ring and ketosugar forms furanose ring structure.
Carbon 1 after ring formation becomes asymmetric and is called anomeric carbon atom.

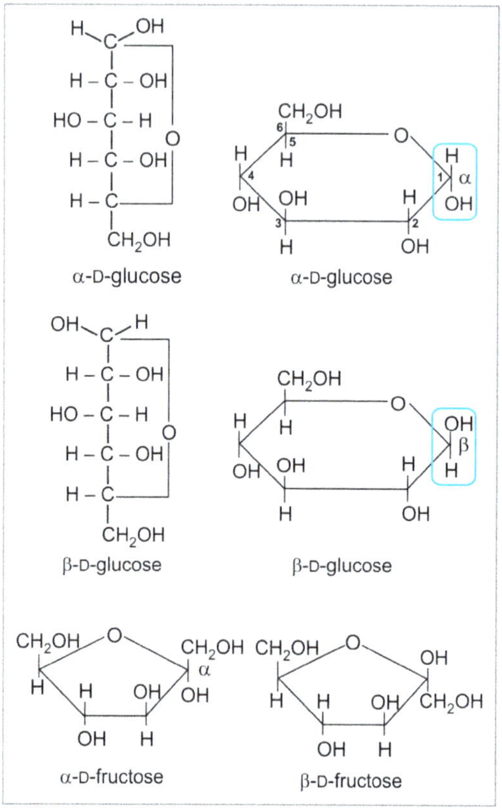
α-D-glucose
α-D-glucose
β-D-glucose
β-D-glucose
α-D-fructose
β-D-fructose

**Fig. 3.1:** Anomers.

The two sugars that differ in the configuration at only C1 in the case of aldoses and C2 in ketoses are known as anomers and represented as alpha and beta sugars, for example, (1) α-**D**-glucose and β-**D**-glucose and (2) α-D-fructose and β-**D**-fructose **(Fig. 3.1)**.

C. *Epimerism*: The isomers formed due to variations in the configuration of -H and -OH around a single carbon atom in a sugar molecule are called epimers.
Mannose is 2-epimer of glucose because these two have different configurations only around C2.
Similarly galactose is 4-epimer of glucose because these two have different configurations only around at C4 **(Fig. 3.2)**.
Ribose and xylose are epimers differing in configuration of groups around carbon 3.

# CHAPTER 3: Chemistry of Carbohydrates

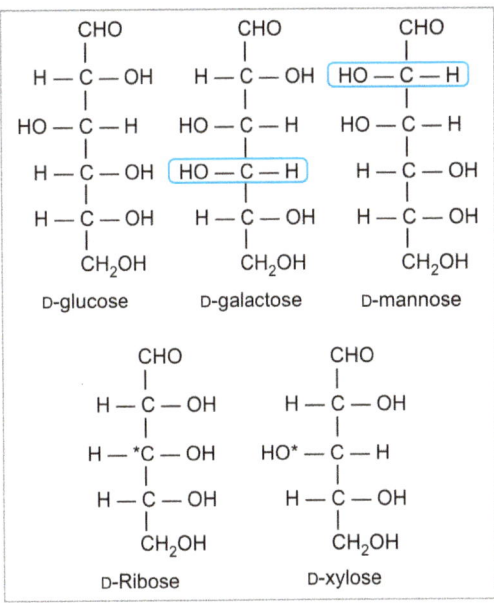

Fig. 3.2: Epimers.

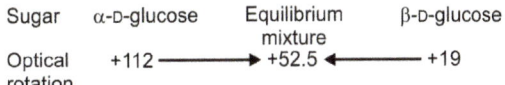

## What is invert sugar? Explain briefly with example.

### Inversion

- Sucrose shows this phenomenon.
- Sucrose is dextrorotatory in nature.
- After hydrolysis, it gives mixture of glucose and fructose.
- The hydrolyzed mixture shows levorotatory activity.
- This phenomenon is called inversion.
- This is because optical activity of fructose is −92° and glucose is 52.5°. The sum is negative.
- The enzyme that digests sucrose is sucrase, it is also known as *invertase*.
- The sucrose is the example for invert sugar.

### Glycosidic Bond

It is the linkage formed between OH group of anomeric carbon of one sugar with any OH group of another sugar (or alcohol) resulting in the loss of a water molecule. This linkage is involved in the formation of disaccharide and polysaccharides.

### Reduction Tests

Due to the presence of a free aldehyde or keto group, carbohydrates are readily oxidized and behave as reducing agents. These sugars have the capacity to reduce cupric ion ($Cu^{2+}$) to cuprous ion ($Cu^+$). Therefore, only the reducing sugars such as sucrose will give positive reactions, whereas nonreducing sugars such as sucrose will respond to these tests provided it is first hydrolyzed into its reducing components glucose and fructose.

### Benedict's Test

When 0.5 mL solution containing reducing sugar is boiled with 5.0 mL Benedict's reagent (blue color) for 5 minutes, brick red- or

## Optical Activity

The optically active compounds having asymmetric carbon atoms can rotate the beam of plane polarized light and which rotate the light to the right is called dextrorotatory, which can be designated as (D) or +, for example, D-(D)-glucose or it is also known as dextrose.

The isomer that rotates the plane of polarized light to left is known as levorotatory and is identified as (L) or (−), for example, D-(L) fructose.

A compound with D− configuration can be dextrorotatory (D+) or levorotatory (D−), for example, D+ glucose and D− fructose.

*Mutarotation*: Ordinary crystalline glucose (which is α form) is first dissolved in water, then the plane polarized light passes through this solution. The optical rotation of plane polarized light gradually changes to constant fixed rotation. This change in rotation is called mutarotation. The mechanism behind this is slow change of the form of sugar to its form to an equilibrium mixture.

green- or yellow-colored precipitate appears. This indicates the presence of reducing sugar in the given sample. This test is used for the detection of reducing sugars in urine in the case of diabetes and galactosemia (Benedict's reagent contains sodium citrate, sodium carbonate, and copper sulfate.)

## Special Carbohydrates

- *Amino sugars*: Sugars containing an $NH_2$ group in their structure are called amino sugars, e.g., D-glucosamine. *N*-acetyl derivative of D-glucosamine and D-galactosamine occurs as a constituent of MPSs. It is also present in some antibiotics.
- *Glycosides*: Glycosides are compounds containing a carbohydrate and a non-carbohydrate part, aglycone. Carbon 1 of carbohydrate is attached to aglycone part, e.g., cardiac glycosides, used in cardiac insufficiency and ouabain, a sodium pump inhibitor.
- *Sialic acid*: Sialic acid is *N*-acetyl neuraminic acid. It is present in MPS and glycolipid, ganglioside.
- *Deoxy sugar*: It lacks one O atom in II or III carbon atom of a carbohydrate, e.g., deoxyribose. It is present in nucleic acid DNA. 6-deoxy-L-galactose or fucose. It is present on the cell membrane.

## Glycoproteins and Proteoglycans

### Glycoproteins

They are proteins to which carbohydrates are covalently attached, for example, immunoglobulin and egg albumin.

### Proteoglycans

They are also proteins to which carbohydrates are covalently attached, but the carbohydrates differ chemically from those attached to glycoproteins. The carbohydrates may be glucosamine or galactosamine and/or their acetyl derivatives, uronic acids and sulfate groups.

## SUMMARY

Carbohydrates are organic substances of polyhydroxy aldehyde or ketone derivatives. They are classified into monosaccharide (glucose), disaccharides (sucrose), oligosaccharides (maltotriose), and polysaccharides. Polysaccharides are of homopolysaccharides (starch, glycogen, cellulose, and inulin) and heteropolysaccharides (hyaluronic acid, dermatan sulfate, keratin sulfate, and heparin). Carbohydrates form stereoisomers such as d- and l-sugars, which we call them as enantiomers (mirror images of each other). Carbon 1 of sugars is an anomeric carbon atom at which any special change in the group leads to the formation of α-d-glucose and β-d-glucose). The isomers formed due to variations in the configuration of –H and –OH around a single carbon atom in a sugar molecule is called epimers (mannose and galactose are two and four epimers of glucose, respectively). Sucrose is a nonreducing and also called invert sugar, and this will not answer Benedict's test.

## SELF-ASSESSMENT QUESTIONS

1. Define carbohydrates.
2. Classify the carbohydrates with a suitable example for each class.
3. Explain the stereoisomerism of carbohydrates.
4. How monosaccharides are further classified?
5. What are the two types of polysaccharides?
6. Define the asymmetric carbon atom.

# CHAPTER 3: Chemistry of Carbohydrates

7. Explain the term mutarotation.
8. What are disaccharides? Give example and composition.
9. What are proteoglycans and mucopolysaccharides?
10. Briefly explain the mucopolysaccharides and write their biomedical importance.
11. Discuss the structure of starch and glycogen.
12. Differentiate between amylose and amylopectin.
13. If the two monosaccharides differ in the configuration around a single carbon atom, are called what?
14. Name the nonreducing disaccharide.
15. What do you call for the α and β cyclic form of D-glucose?
16. Name the noncarbohydrate moiety present in glycoside.
17. Give an example for a glycoside.
18. Name the polysaccharide employed for the assessment of kidney function tests.
19. Mention the glycosaminoglycan that serves as a lubricant and shock absorbent of joints.

## MULTIPLE CHOICE QUESTIONS

1. **Which of the following is not an aldose sugar?**
   - (a) Glucose
   - (b) Galactose
   - (c) Mannose
   - (d) Fructose
2. **Which one of the following serves as an anticoagulant?**
   - (a) Heparin
   - (b) Hyaluronic acid
   - (c) Chondroitin sulfate
   - (d) Keratan sulfate
3. **The polysaccharide containing β-glycosidic linkage is:**
   - (a) Starch
   - (b) Glycogen
   - (c) Dextrin
   - (d) Cellulose
4. **In general the carbon atoms involved in reducing action are:**
   - (a) 1 and 2
   - (b) 2 and 3
   - (c) 3 and 4
   - (d) 5 and 6
5. **Concerning glucose, all of the following statements are true, *except*:**
   - (a) It is an aldohexose
   - (b) It is a reducing sugar
   - (c) It is present in starch and cellulose
   - (d) It is an epimer of fructose
6. **The glycosaminoglycan which does not contain uronic acid is:**
   - (a) Heparin
   - (b) Hyaluronic acid
   - (c) Chondroitin sulfate
   - (d) Keratan sulfate
7. **Which of the following is a deoxy sugar?**
   - (a) Ribose
   - (b) Fucose
   - (c) Glucosamine
   - (d) Xylulose
8. **___ is not found in glycosaminoglycan.**
   - (a) l-iduronic acid
   - (b) d-glucuronic acid
   - (c) Ribose
   - (d) N-acetyl galactosamine
9. **___ is a heteropolysaccharide.**
   - (a) Dextrin
   - (b) Chitin
   - (c) Inulin
   - (d) Heparin
10. **Concerning starch, one of the following statement is incorrect:**
    - (a) Starch is made of both linear and branched polysaccharide
    - (b) Starch gives red color with I2 reactions
    - (c) Starch can be hydrolyzed to glucose in the body
    - (d) Glycogen is known as animal starch

11. **One of the following is an example for invert sugar:**
    (a) Glucose
    (b) Fructose
    (c) Sucrose
    (d) Maltose
12. **All the following are the examples for monosaccharide, *except*:**
    (a) Glucose
    (b) Fructose
    (c) Sucrose
    (d) Galactose
13. **The bond that links the monosaccharide units is:**
    (a) Ester bond
    (b) Phosphate bond
    (c) Disulfide bond
    (d) Glycosidic bond
14. **All of the following polysaccharides contain glucose as the monosaccharide units, *except*:**
    (a) Starch
    (b) Inulin
    (c) Glycogen
    (d) Dextrin
15. **Regarding amylopectin component of starch the following statements are true, *except*:**
    (a) It is highly branched
    (b) It is unbranched
    (c) It gives reddish violet color with iodine
    (d) Its amount present in starch is 80–85%
16. **Concerning glycogen, one of the following statements is incorrect:**
    (a) A polymer of glucose
    (b) Stored in liver and muscle
    (c) Stored in liver and brain
    (d) Having 11–18 glucose residues between any branching points
17. **Concerning cellulose, one of the following statements is incorrect:**
    (a) Contains β-d-glucose β-1–4 glycosidic bonds
    (b) Digested by sucrase enzyme
    (c) Acts as dietary fiber
    (d) Digested by cellulase enzyme
18. **Regarding the heteropolysaccharides the following statements are correct, *except*:**
    (a) Polymer of different monosaccharide units
    (b) Heparin and chondroitin sulfate are the examples
    (c) Components of ground substances throughout the extracellular space
    (d) Glycogen is and starch are the examples
19. **All the following are the functions of heteropolysaccharides, *except*:**
    (a) Hyaluronic acid acts as a barrier in tissues against the penetration of bacteria
    (b) Hyaluronidase present in testicular secretions helps in fertilization by favoring the entry of spermatozoa into the ovum
    (c) Chondroitin sulfate acts anticoagulant
    (d) Heparin acts as anticoagulant in vitro as well as in vivo. It inhibits thrombin
20. **Concerning stereoisomerism of carbohydrates, all the following statements are true, *except*:**
    (a) D- and l-sugars are referred to as enantiomers
    (b) D-sugars are utilized by humans
    (c) When the sugar has OH group on right, it is D isomer
    (d) When the sugar has OH group on left, it is D isomer
21. **Anomerism means:**
    (a) Carbon 1, after ring formation becomes asymmetric and it is called anomeric carbon atom
    (b) Carbon 6, after ring formation becomes asymmetric and it is called anomeric carbon atom
    (c) Carbon 2, after ring formation becomes asymmetric and it is called anomeric carbon atom
    (d) Mirror images

22. **Regarding epimerism all of the following statements are true, *except*:**
    (a) The isomers formed due to variations in the configuration of –H and –OH around a single carbon atom in a sugar molecule is called epimers
    (b) Mannose is 2-epimer of glucose
    (c) Galactose is 4-epimer of glucose
    (d) Fructose is α-4-epimer of glucose
23. **One of the following is not a reducing sugar:**
    (a) Glucose
    (b) Sucrose
    (c) Fructose
    (d) Mannose
24. **Concerning carbohydrates, one of the following statements is incorrect:**
    (a) Are most abundant dietary source of energy for all organisms
    (b) Are precursors for many organic compounds like fats and amino acids
    (c) Participate in the structure of cell membrane and cellular functions
    (d) Build the muscle mass
25. **The monosaccharide that is present in DNA is:**
    (a) Glucose
    (b) Ribose
    (c) Fructose
    (d) Mannose
26. **The 2-epimer of glucose is:**
    (a) Mannose
    (b) Galactose
    (c) Ribose
    (d) Gibulose
27. **Glucose is an:**
    (a) Ketohexose
    (b) Aldohexose
    (c) Aldotriose
    (d) Aldopentose
28. **Polysaccharide that has fructose as their monosaccharide units is:**
    (a) Starch
    (b) Dextrin
    (c) Inulin
    (d) Cellulose
29. **Concerning the structure of starch, one of the following statements is false:**
    (a) It has 85% of amylopectin
    (b) Amylose is highly branched
    (c) Blue color appears when amylose reacts with iodine
    (d) The glucose units in amylose held by α-1,4-glycosidic linkage
30. **Concerning cellulose, all the following statements are true, *except*:**
    (a) It has β-d-glucose joined by β-1,4-glycosidic bonds
    (b) It is digested by cellulase enzyme in the humans
    (c) It acts as dietary fiber
    (d) It acts as storage form of glucose
31. **One of the following is not a heteropolysaccharide:**
    (a) Hyaluronic acid
    (b) Heparin
    (c) Dextrin
    (d) Chondroitin sulfate
32. **4-epimer of glucose is:**
    (a) Galactose
    (b) Mannose
    (c) Fructose
    (d) Maltose
33. **All the following answers Benedict's test, *except*:**
    (a) Glucose
    (b) Ascorbic acid
    (c) Sucrose
    (d) Fructose

34. Concerning stereoisomerism, all the following statements are true, *except*:
    (a) D- and L-sugars are referred to as enantiomers
    (b) Sugars in solution exist in ring form and not in the straight chain form
    (c) Carbon 1 in aldosugars is the anomeric carbon atom
    (d) Ketosugar forms pyranose ring

35. A 16-year-old male patient complains that lately, after the ingestion of dairy products, he experiences bloating, cramps and flatulence, and sometimes diarrhea. Therefore, the patient is intolerant to:
    (a) Lactose
    (b) Mannose
    (c) Sucrose
    (d) Maltose

36. This heteropolysaccharide has multiple uses in medicine that include its use in blood transfusions to prevent the blood from coagulating before administration, as anticoagulant therapy in prophylaxis and treatment of venous thrombosis and its extension, in pulmonary embolisms and in other similar situations:
    (a) Hyaluronic acid
    (b) Chondroitin sulfate
    (c) Heparin
    (d) Dermatan sulfate

37. Human beings do not have the enzymes necessary for the hydrolysis of the β-1,4-O-glycosidic linkages between molecules of glucose. That is why humans cannot digest this compound and it is part of some laxatives:
    (a) Glycogen
    (b) Cellulose
    (c) Amylopectin
    (d) Sucrose

## ANSWERS

| | | | | | | | | |
|---|---|---|---|---|---|---|---|---|
| 1. d | 2. a | 3. d | 4. a | 5. d | 6. d | 7. b | 8. c |
| 9. d | 10. b | 11. c | 12. c | 13. d | 14. b | 15. b | 16. c |
| 17. b | 18. d | 19. c | 20. d | 21. a | 22. d | 23. b | 24. d |
| 25. b | 26. a | 27. b | 28. b | 29. b | 30. c | 31. c | 32. a |
| 33. c | 34. d | 35. a | 36. c | 37. b | | | |

# Chapter 4

# Metabolism of Carbohydrates

## LEARNING OBJECTIVES

*After reading this chapter, one should be able to:*
- Understand the digestion and absorption of carbohydrates
- Explain the process of various metabolism including their regulation and significance
- Describe the blood glucose regulation
- Explain diabetes and the criteria to diagnose
- Know about various disorders of carbohydrate metabolism including lactose intolerance

## Digestion and Absorption of Carbohydrates

### Introduction

Digestion is the process of hydrolysis of naturally occurring foodstuffs into simpler forms.

The saliva of mouth contains salivary amylase and its action on foodstuffs is very limited.

Enzymes of gastrointestinal tract are shown in **Table 4.1**.

List the enzymes of gastrointestinal tract and briefly discuss how the carbohydrates our diet gets digested and absorbed.

### Digestion of Carbohydrates (Fig. 4.1)

- The diet of human beings contains carbohydrates, fat and proteins, which are of high molecular weight complex compounds.

**Table 4.1:** Enzymes of GI tract.

| Gastric juice | Pancreatic juice | Intestinal |
|---|---|---|
| 1. Pepsinogen (inactive form of the enzyme pepsin, which is secreted by chief cells of stomach) | 1. Trypsinogen (inactive form of trypsin) | 1. Aminopeptidase |
| 2. HCl (secreted by parietal cells) | 2. Chymotrypsinogen (inactive form of chymotrypsin) | 2. Dipeptidase |
| 3. Intrinsic factor (parietal cells) | 3. Procarboxypeptidase (inactive form of carboxypeptidase) | 3. Nucleotidase |
| 4. Mucin (mucus cells) | 4. Amylase | 4. Maltase |
| | 5. Lipase | 5. Sucrase |
| | 6. Ribonuclease | 6. Lactase |
| | | 7. Isomaltase |

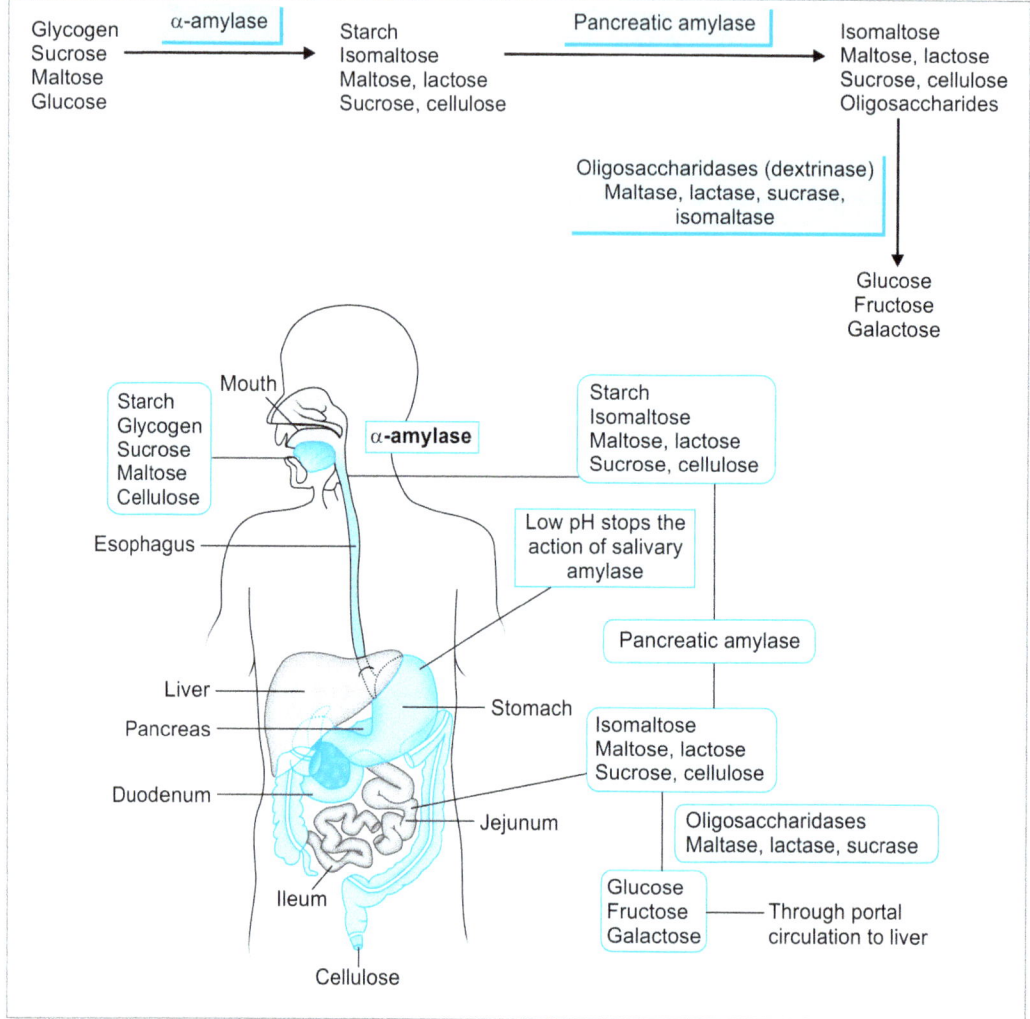

**Fig. 4.1:** Digestion of important food products.

- They are absorbed only when they are hydrolyzed to simpler forms.
- The major carbohydrates of our diet are starch and glycogen, are the polysaccharides.
- Sucrose and lactose are the disaccharides.
- Glucose and fructose are the monosaccharides and which need no digestion before they are absorbed because they are simpler sugars.
- The polysaccharides are hydrolyzed to maltose and glucose by the action of number of enzymes.
- The digestion of carbohydrates starts in the mouth.
- Salivary amylase hydrolyses $\alpha$-1,4-glycosidic linkages randomly within the polysaccharide chain and produce disaccharides and monosaccharides.
- The further digestion takes place in the small intestine by the intestinal enzymes, which hydrolyze terminal $\alpha$-1, 4-glycosidic linkage.
- When acidic contents of stomach reach small intestine, they stimulate mucosal cells of the duodenum to release secretin

and cholecystokinin. These are two local hormones that stimulate the exocrine pancreas to release pancreatic juice into the intestinal lumen. This secretin stimulates the release of bicarbonate to neutralize the acidic chime from the stomach and the cholecystokinin stimulates the release of digestive enzymes including pancreatic amylase.
- After the food reaches the duodenum, pancreatic amylase also helps in the digestion of polysaccharides. This results in maltose, isomaltose and a limit dextrin. The α-limit dextrins are smaller oligosaccharides containing 3–5 glucose units.
- At the same time disaccharidases like *maltase*, *lactase* and *sucrase* digest disaccharides like maltose, lactose and sucrose respectively into their respective monosaccharide units.
- Cellulose is not digested further it helps in easy peristalsis and provides bulk to the faeces.
- Cellulose is not digested further because humans do not produce and secrete 1, 4-endoglycosidase in digestive juice.
- Lactase deficiency leads to lactose intolerance.

## Absorption of Monosaccharides

- Monosaccharides formed are almost completely absorbed from the intestinal lumen through the mucosal epithelial cells into the bloodstream of the portal venous system.
- The galactose and glucose are absorbed very rapidly by the active process, which is linked to the transport of sodium and requires energy in the form of hydrolysis of high-energy phosphate bond ATP.
- Glucose cannot diffuse through lipid bilayer of the cell membrane because of its polar nature.
- Absorption from intestinal lumen into intestinal cell is by co-transport mechanism called sodium dependent glucose transporter **(Fig. 4.2)**.
- It occurs against the concentration gradient and requires a carrier protein.
- Oubain, indirectly inhibits glucose absorption.

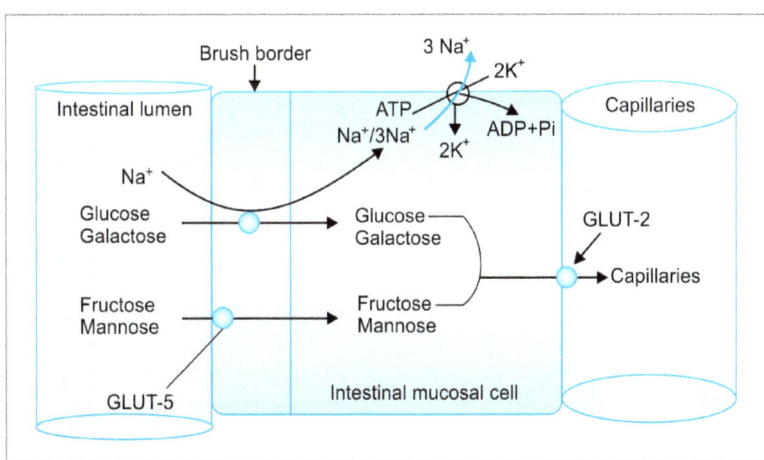

**Fig. 4.2:** Absorption of carbohydrates.
(ATP: adenosine triphosphate; GLUT-5: glucose transporter type 5; GLUT-2: glucose transporter type 2; ADP: adenosine diphosphate).

- Fructose and mannose are absorbed by a Na+ independent facilitative diffusion, which requires a carrier protein but not energy and occurs across the concentration gradient through portal circulation to liver.
- Sodium independent transporter GLUT-2 facilitates transport of sugars out of the mucosal cells, thereby entering the portal circulation to reach the liver.

## Metabolism of Carbohydrates

Glucose is the main source of energy to our body. Oxidation of glucose results in the formation of free energy which is converted into energy in the form of ATP. ATP is the energy currency of our body. If the glucose is oxidized without trapping the free energy, then much of the energy will be wasted. Hence the body preserves the energy in the form of ATP just like a battery cells.

In our body glucose can be obtained from:
- The digestion of dietary carbohydrates
- Glycogen breakdown
- Gluconeogenesis (synthesis of glucose from noncarbohydrate sources).

Different pathways, which involve glucose, are given in **Figure 4.3**:

*Glycolysis*: It is a process of oxidation of glucose either to pyruvate or lactate.

*Glycogenesis*: The synthesis of glycogen from glucose in liver or muscle for the purpose of storing glucose for energy is called glycogenesis.

*Glycogenolysis*: The formation of glucose or glucose-1-phosphate by breaking glycogen in liver or muscle respectively is called glycogenolysis.

*Gluconeogenesis*: Synthesis of glucose in liver and kidney using non-carbohydrate sources like pyruvate, lactate, glycerol, propionic acid

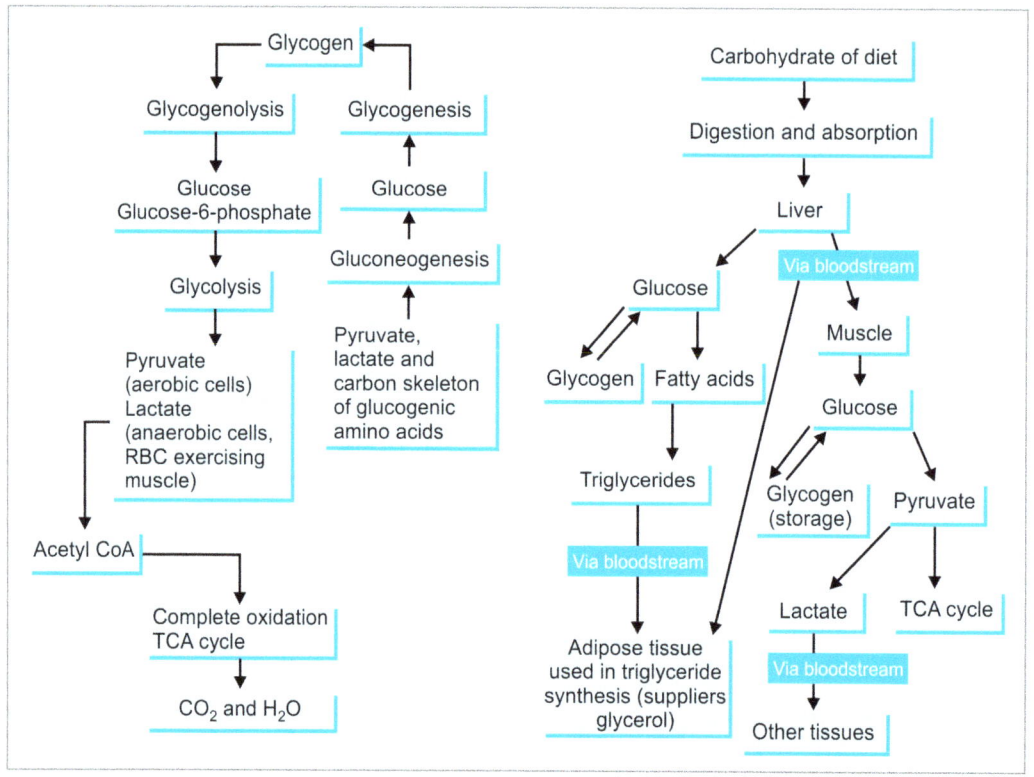

**Fig. 4.3:** Different pathways involving glucose.

or from the carbon skeleton of glucogenic amino acids like alanine, aspartic acid, etc. Other pathways, which involve glucose are:
- Hexose monophosphate shunt
- Uronic acid pathway
- Interconversion of glucose, galactose and fructose.

# Glycolysis

- The pathway involves the oxidation of glucose to yield energy is called as glycolysis.
- This pathway occurs in all types of living cells.
- It is the source of energy in erythrocytes.
- Anaerobic glycolysis forms the major source of energy for muscle during strenuous exercise.
- Provide carbon skeletons for the synthesis of nonessential amino acids.
- Most of the reactions of glycolysis are reversible.
- The entry of glucose from extracellular fluid to (ECF) to cell is under the control of insulin.
- Glycolysis occurrence is essential for the aerobic oxidation of carbohydrates.
- Aerobic oxidation takes place in cells possessing mitochondria.
- It is the major pathway for ATP synthesis in tissues lacking mitochondria (erythrocytes, cornea, lens, etc).

There are two types of glycolysis:
1. Aerobic glycolysis
   - This occurs in cells function in the presence of oxygen.
   - They are cells containing mitochondria actively using oxygen.
   - Here glucose is broken down to 2 molecules of pyruvate with 7 ATP.
2. Anaerobic glycolysis:
   - Occurs in cells under hypoxic conditions.
   - During severe exercise there will be depletion of oxygen in the tissues.
- Also RBC get its energy by anaerobic glycolysis.
- Two molecules of lactate are formed as the end product.
- In this type only 2 molecules of ATP are formed.

**Discuss the glycolysis including the energetics.**

## Aerobic Glycolysis

*Site of occurrence*: Cytosol
*Reactions of aerobic glycolysis* (**Figs. 4.4A and B**):
- In the first step, the glucose is irreversibly activated to glucose-6-phosphate in the cell. This step is catalyzed by *hexokinase* enzyme using $Mg^{2+}$ and ATP. In liver *glucokinase* the specific enzyme also catalyses this reaction at higher concentration of glucose (**Table 4.2**).

*Glucose-6-Phosphate*: Impermeable to the cell membrane. Central molecule with a variety of metabolic fates; glycolysis, glycogenesis, gluconeogenesis and HMP shunt.
- In the next step glucose-6-phosphate is isomerized to fructose-6-phosphate by *phosphohexose isomerase* enzyme.
- Fructose-6-phosphate is then irreversibly phosphorylated by phosphofructokinase enzyme to fructose-1,6-bisphosphate. Fructose-1,6-bisphosphate contains two phosphoric acid groups at C1 and C6 of fructose via phosphate ester bond.
- Later fructose-1,6-bisphosphate molecule (6 carbon sugar) is cleaved by aldolase enzyme to yield glyceraldehyde 3-phosphate and dihydroxy acetone phosphate (two 3 carbon sugars–trioses).
- Dihydroxy acetone phosphate formed in the above step can be converted back to glyceraldehyde 3-phosphate by *phosphotriose isomerase* enzyme.
- Now, we have two molecules of glyceraldehyde 3-phosphate molecules, which gets oxidized to 1,3-bisphosphoglycerate by the action of *glyceraldehyde 3-phosphate*

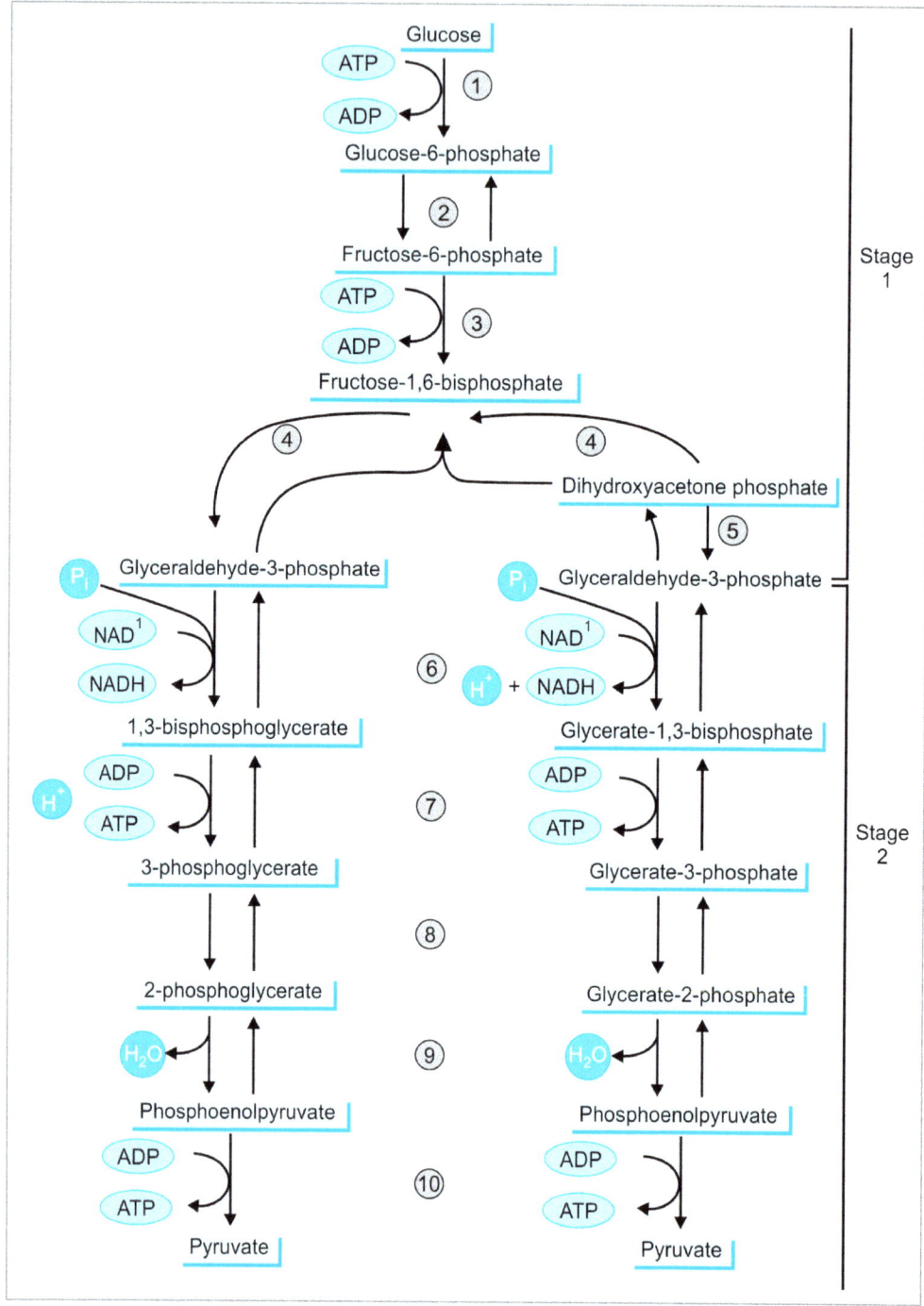

**Fig. 4.4A:** Reactions of glycolysis (aerobic).
(ATP: adenosine triphosphate; ADP: adenosine diphosphate; NAD: nicotinamide adenine dinucleotide; NADH: nicotinamide adenine dinucleotide hydrogen).

# CHAPTER 4: Metabolism of Carbohydrates

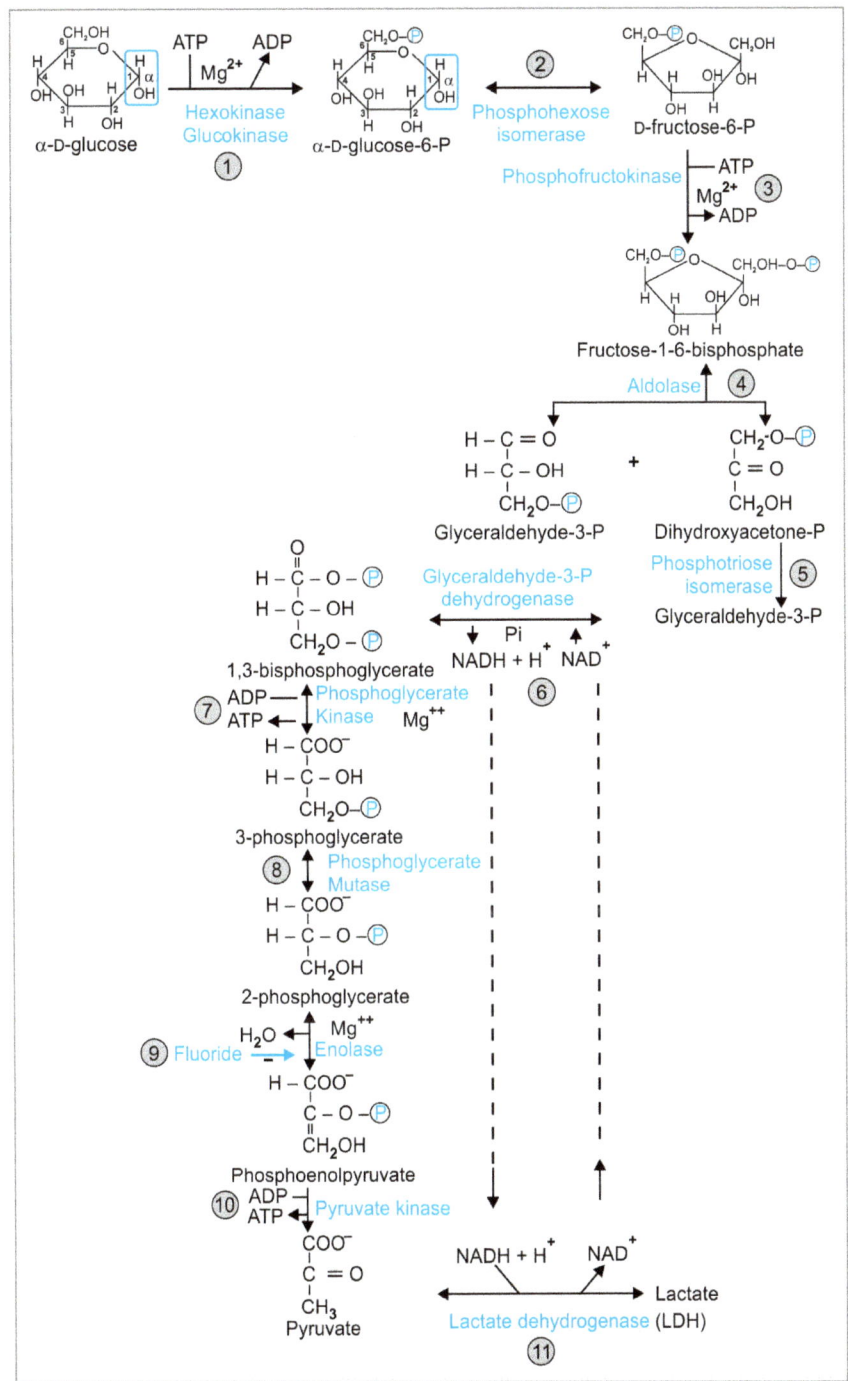

**Fig. 4.4B:** Reactions of glycolysis (reactions showing aerobic and anaerobic steps).
(ADP: adenosine diphosphate; ATP: adenosine triphosphate; NAD: nicotinamide adenine dinucleotide; NADH: nicotinamide adenine dinucleotide hydrogen).

## How do you differentiate glucokinase from hexokinase?

**Table 4.2:** Features of glucokinase and hexokinase.

| Glucokinase | Muscle hexokinase |
|---|---|
| Present in liver and pancreas | Present in all tissues |
| Low affinity for glucose (high $K_m$) | High affinity for its substrate glucose (low $K_m$) |
| Specific for glucose | Catalyze the phosphorylation of other hexoses |
| Not inhibited by glucose-6-P | Inhibited by glucose-6-P |
| Increases its synthesis in response to insulin | Not affected by insulin |
| It functions to remove glucose from the blood, when blood glucose increases | Function to ensure enough supply of glucose from the blood for the tissues irrespective of the blood glucose concentration |

*dehydrogenase* enzyme. This step utilizes inorganic phosphate (pi) to convert glyceraldehydes 3-phosphate into 1, 3-bisphosphoglycerate. In 1,3-bisphosphoglycerate the phosphate group at carbon atom number 1 is high-energy group. During oxidation of glyceraldehyde 3-phosphate the reducing equivalents are transferred to the acceptor NAD⁺ (nicotinamide adenine dinucleotide). The reduced NADH under aerobic conditions enters into mitochondria and produces 2.5 molecules of ATP through its passage into electron transport chain or respiratory chain. This type of formation of energy currency ATP through respiratory chain is called as oxidative phosphorylation.

❖ In the next step, the high-energy compound 1,3-bisphosphoglycerate transfers its high energy to ADP to form ATP resulting in the formation of 3-phosphoglycerate. This reaction is catalyzed by phosphoglycerate kinase enzyme. This type of formation of energy currency (ATP) by high-energy substrate is called as substrate level phosphorylation.

❖ 3-phosphoglycerate is then isomerized to 2-phosphoglycerate by *phosphoglycerate mutase* enzyme.

❖ 2-phosphoglycerate is then converted into one more high-energy compound called as phosphoenolpyruvate. This reaction is catalyzed by *enolase* enzyme. The activity of this enzyme is completely inhibited by fluoride. Hence, fluoride is used during blood collection for glucose estimation. This prevents the utilization of glucose by RBC.

❖ Later phosphoenolpyruvate is converted to pyruvate by pyruvate *kinase* enzyme. In this step one molecule of ATP is formed by substrate level phosphorylation.

Under aerobic conditions pyruvate is the end product of glycolysis.

Hence, pyruvate is then converted into acetyl CoA or oxaloacetate in the mitochondria.

Fructose is more rapidly oxidized by the liver than glucose, because it bypasses the step in glucose oxidation catalyzed by phosphofructokinase.

## Anaerobic Glycolysis

If anaerobic conditions prevail, the re-oxidation of NADH (formed in step 6) by transfer of reducing equivalents through the respiratory chain to oxygen is prevented and gets reoxidized by conversion of pyruvate to lactate by lactate *dehydrogenase* enzyme. Thus, the number of ATP produced will be less in anaerobic condition.

Steps 6 and 11 are linked to operate the pathway in anaerobic condition:
❖ Glycolysis is the only major source of energy in anaerobiosis.
❖ For smooth operation of the pathway NADH is to be converted to NAD⁺.

- The formation of lactate allows the regeneration of NAD⁺.
- NAD⁺ reused by glyceraldehyde 3-phosphate dehydrogenase and so that glycolysis proceeds even in the absence of oxygen to supply ATP.
- Fate of pyruvate depends on the presence or absence oxygen in the cells.
- The occurrence of uninterrupted glycolysis is very important in skeletal muscle during strenuous exercise.
- Brain, retina, renal medulla and GI tract derive energy from glycolysis.
- Glycolysis in the erythrocytes leads to lactate production, since the mitochondria, the centers for oxidation are absent.

## Energetics of Aerobic Glycolysis Per Glucose Molecule

- Energy consuming steps of glycolysis are:
  - Step 1 and step 3 → 2 ATP
- Energy-yielding steps of glycolysis are:
  - Oxidative phosphorylation
    Step 6 → NADH × 2 → 2.5 ATP × 2 = 5 ATP
  - Substrate level phosphorylation
    Step 7 and step 10 → 2 ATP × 2 = 4 ATP
    Total ATP produced = 9 ATP
    Net ATP production (9 – 2) = 7 ATP

## Energetics of Anaerobic Glycolysis Per Glucose Molecule

- Energy consuming steps of glycolysis are:
  - Step 1 and step 2 → 2 ATP
- Energy-yielding steps of anaerobic glycolysis are:
  - Substrate level phosphorylation
    Step 7 and step 10 → 2 ATP × 2 = 4 ATP
    Total ATP produced = 4 ATP
    Net ATP production (4 – 2) = 2 ATP

## Shuttle Pathways

If the cytosolic NADH uses malate-aspartate shuttle, 2.5 ATP is produced. If it uses glycerol phosphate shuttle produces 2 ATP.

**Explain how the glucose oxidation is regaled to maintain our blood glucose level.**

## Regulation of Glycolysis

Insulin favors glycolysis by activating key glycolytic enzymes like *glucokinase, phosphofructokinase* (PFK-1) and pyruvate kinase.

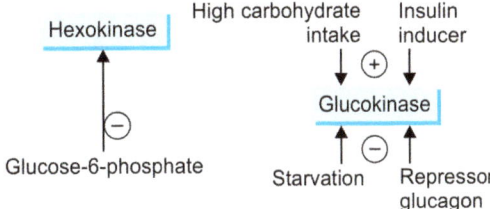

PFK-1 is the most important regulatory enzyme.
- ATP, citrate and H⁺ ions are the important allosteric inhibitors

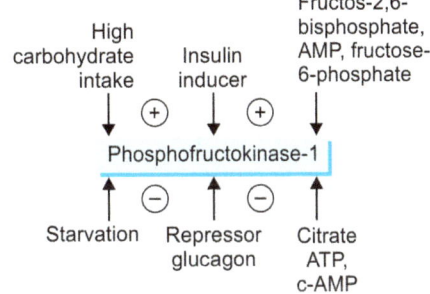

- Fructose-2,6-bisphosphate, AMP and Pi are the allosteric activators of PFK-1.
- Pyruvate kinase is an inducible enzyme that increases its synthesis in response to insulin and decreases in response to glucagon.
- Glucocorticoid inhibit glycolysis and favors gluconeogenesis.
- Glucose-6-phosphate inhibits hexokinase and the enzyme prevents the accumulation of glucose-6-phosphate.

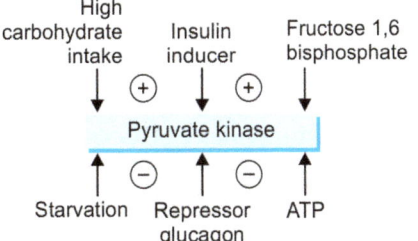

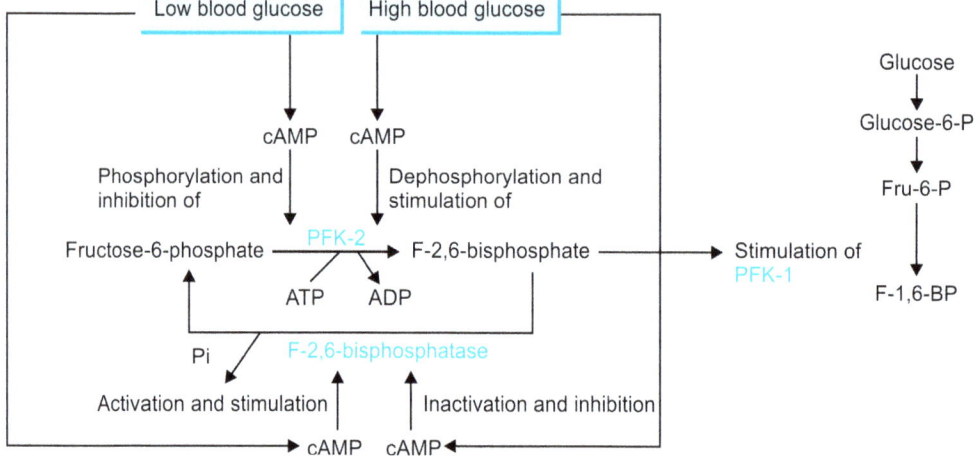

Fig. 4.5: Role of fructose 2,6-bisphosphate in the regulation of blood glucose.

Explain the role of fructose-2,6-bisphosphate and phosphofructokinase in the regulation blood glucose.

## Role of Fructose-2,6-Bisphosphate and PFK-2

It is the most regulatory factor for controlling PFK and ultimately glycolysis in the liver.

The function of synthesis and degradation of F-2,6-BP is brought out by a single enzyme (with two active sites), which is referred to as bifunctional or "Tandem enzyme". The activity of these enzymes is controlled by covalent modification, which in turn regulated by cyclic AMP. The cAMP brings about the phosphorylation of the tandem enzyme, resulting in inactivation of active site of the enzyme which is responsible for the synthesis of fructose-2,6-bisphosphate (F-2,6-BP) but the activation of the active site of the enzyme hydrolyse fructose-2,6-bisphosphate **(Fig. 4.5)**.

There is no stimulation when fructose-2,6-bisphosphate decreases, with low blood glucose the PFK-1 remains inactive.

## Rapoport–Luebering Cycle (2,3-Bisphosphoglycerate Shunt)

❖ It is the side reaction of the glycolytic pathway, occurring in erythrocytes **(Fig. 4.6)**.

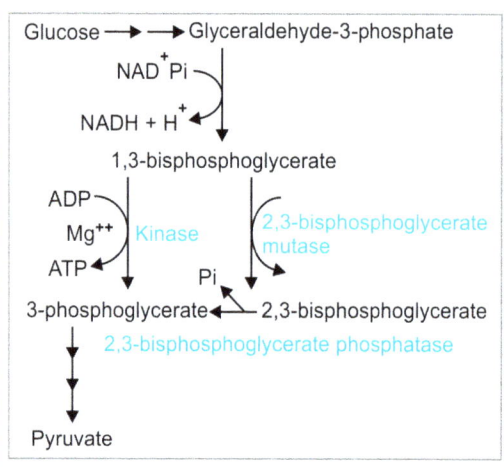

Fig. 4.6: Rapoport–Luebering cycle.

❖ Kinase reaction of glycolysis is bypassed in the erythrocytes.
❖ No energy is trapped from 2,3-BPG
❖ BPG when combines with Hb, reduces the affinity of Hb towards oxygen. In the presence of 2,3-BPG oxyhemoglobin will unload oxygen more easily in tissues. The reason for increased 2,3-BPG in hypoxic condition.
❖ 15–25% of the lactate formed goes through this pathway.
❖ In hexokinase deficiency phosphorylation does not takes place further. So 2,3-BPG decreases. Then affinity to Hb increases.

**List the compounds formed from pyruvate.**

## Compounds Formed from Pyruvate

Under aerobic conditions pyruvate is transported into mitochondria via pyruvate transporter. Then it is dehydrogenated to acetyl CoA by pyruvate dehydrogenase complex enzyme. This enzyme requires five coenzymes derived from water soluble vitamin [(they are TPP (thiamine pyrophosphate), CoASH (coenzyme A), $NAD^+$, FAD (flavin adenine dinucleotide)] and lipoic acid **(Fig. 4.7)**.

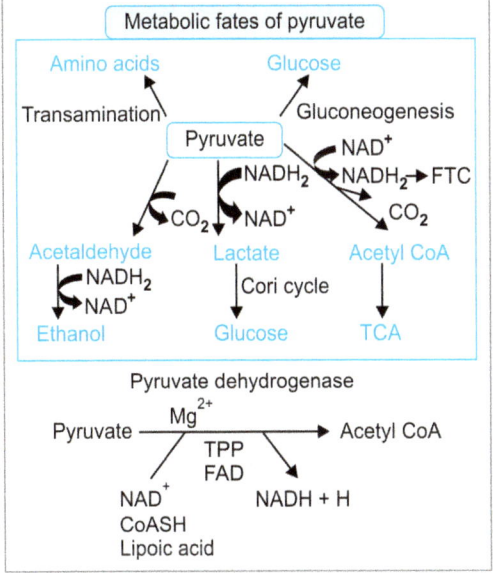

**Fig. 4.7:** Compounds formed from pyruvate.

**What happens if pyruvate dehydrogenase is inhibited and what is the significance of lactate determination? Explain why anaerobic glycolysis takes place in cancer cells.**

- The arsenic and mercuric ions react with the –SH groups of lipoic acid and inhibit pyruvate dehydrogenase, as does a dietary deficiency of thiamine, allowing pyruvate to accumulate. Alcoholics are thiamine-deficient and may develop pyruvic and lactic acidosis. Patients with inherited pyruvate dehydrogenase deficiency develop lactic acidosis after a glucose load.
- The determination of blood lactate is very useful in assessing the presence and severity of shock and to monitor the patient recovery.
- The lactate determination also helps in the early detection of oxygen debt (excess oxygen required to recover from the anoxic episodes) in various disorders.
- In cancer, the cancer cells stimulate the glucose uptake and glycolysis. As the cancer cells grow rapidly, blood vessels are unable to supply desired oxygen. Therefore, the metabolic adoption will occur for the survival of cancer cells and they continue to grow in the absence of oxygen. In this condition the glucose is oxidized anaerobically to lactic acid to supply ATP for tumor cells.
- Alcoholics develop thiamine deficiency due to the inhibition of transport of thiamine through intestinal mucosal cells. Lack of TPP a coenzyme form of thiamine inhibits the pyruvate dehydrogenase, which results in the conversion of pyruvate to lactate which leads to lactic acidosis and neurological disorders.

**What are compounds formed from acetyl CoA and list them.**

## Metabolic Fates of Acetyl CoA

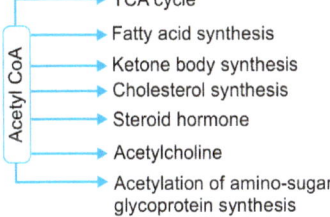

**Discuss the TCA cycle including the energy formation.**

## Tricarboxylic Acid Cycle (TCA Cycle) (Kreb's Cyclce)

- It takes place in mitochondria.
- Citric acid cycle is also called tricarboxylic acid cycle because of the presence of 3 COOH group in the citric acid.
- These reactions occur in a cyclic manner and generate large amounts of ATP since the enzymes of this cycle are located in mitochondria facilitating the transfer of reducing equivalents from Kreb's cycle to the respiratory chain, the enzymes of which are also located in the inner mitochondrial membrane **(Figs. 4.8A and B)**.

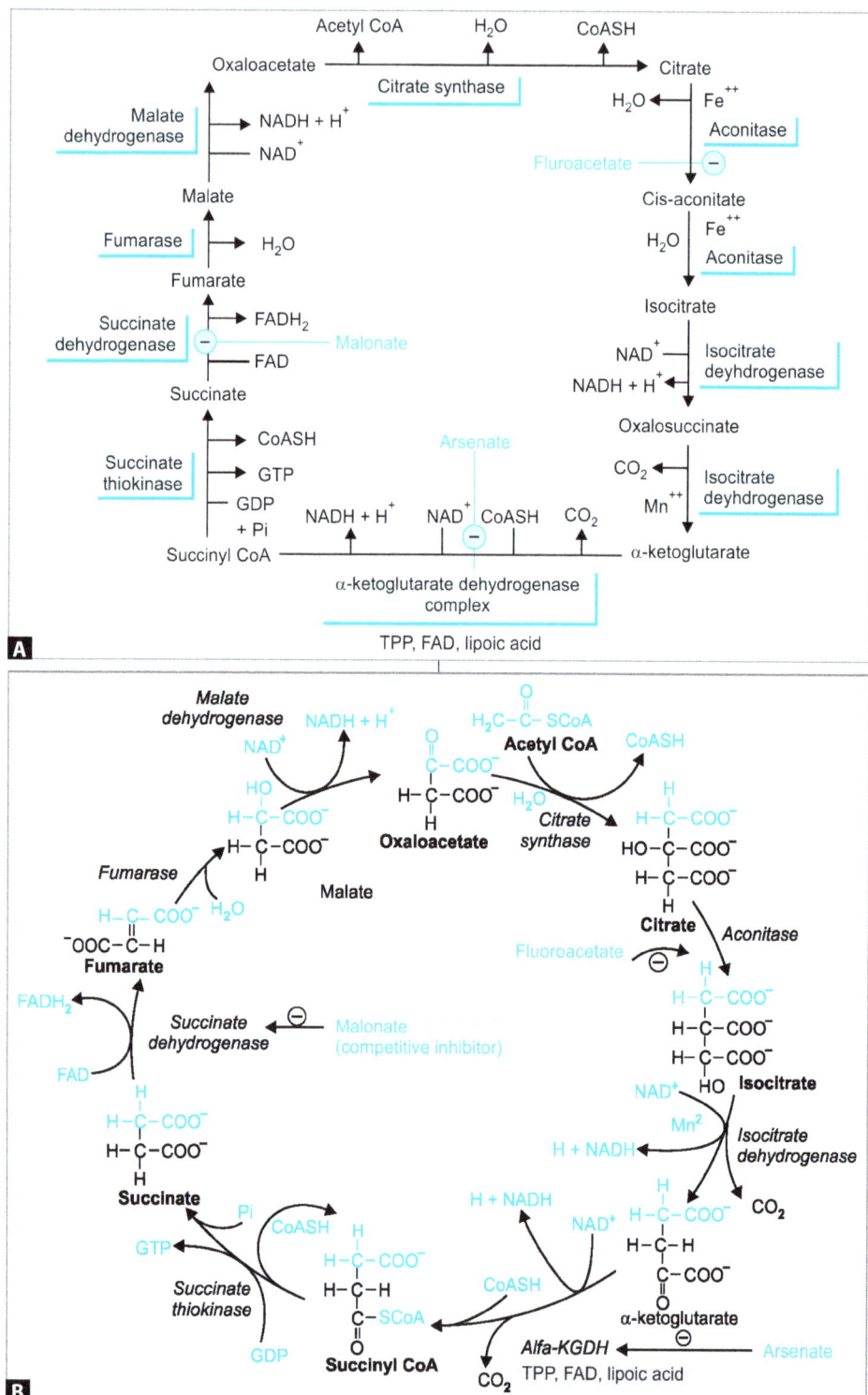

**Figs. 4.8A and B:** (A) Reactions of tricarboxylic acid (TCA) cycle without structure; (B) Reactions of TCA cycle.

- In the first step of Kreb's citric acid cycle, acetyl CoA formed from pyruvate under aerobic condition and also by fatty acid oxidation combines with oxaloacetic acid and forms citric acid (a tricarboxylic acid). The reaction is catalyzed by a condensing enzyme *citrate synthase*.
- In the second step, citrate is converted into isocitrate through the action of *aconitase* enzyme. Isocitrate undergoes dehydrogenation by the *isocitrate dehydrogenase* enzyme in the third step to form oxalosuccinate. Molecule of NADH formed here enters into electron transport chain and forms 3 ATPs.
- Next step will be decarboxylation to form alpha-ketoglutarate with the help of *isocitrate dehydrogenase* enzyme.
- Then the alpha-ketoglutarate undergoes decarboxylation to form succinyl CoA in a manner similar to the conversion of pyruvate to acetyl CoA. This is catalyzed by *a-ketoglutarate dehydrogenase enzyme*. One molecule of NADH formed here enters into electron transport chain and forms 3 ATPs.
- Succinyl CoA is then converted into succinate by the enzyme *succinate thiokinase*. In this step a high-energy phosphate is produced as GTP by substrate level phosphorylation.
- In the next step the dehydrogenation of succinate is catalyzed by mitochondrial inner membrane enzyme *succinate dehydrogenase*. This step produces 2 ATPs because of production of one molecule of $FADH_2$.
- *Fumarase* catalyzes the addition of water molecule to fumarate and forms malate. Malate is converted into oxaloacetate by *malate dehydrogenase* enzyme with production of one molecule of NADH, which is equivalent to three ATPs (step 8). *Cis*-acontitate is a transient one with very short half-life. Immediate $H_2O$ is added to it and forms isocitrate.

Isocitrate $\leftrightarrow$ Oxalosuccinate $\xrightarrow{CO_2}$ α-ketoglutarate.

- *It is an oxidative decarboxylation*: Oxalosuccinate is unstable so it undergoes spontaneous decarboxylation to from α-ketoglutarate.

*Twelve ATPs are formed per turn of TCA cycle:*
Steps 3, 4, 8 (3 $NADH^+$) → 3 × 2.5 ATP = 7.5 ATP
Step 6 (1 $FADH_2$) → 1.5 ATP = 1.5 ATP
Step 5 (1 ATP) → 1 ATP = 1 ATP
                                            10 ATP

Total number of ATPs formed by the complete oxidation of glucose is = 32 ATP.
From aerobic glycolysis                = 7 ATP
Action of pyruvate dehydrogenase (2.5 × 2)
                                              = 5 ATP
TCA cycle (2 mol pyruvate) 10 ATP × 2
                                        = $\frac{20\ ATP}{32\ ATP}$
                                Total = 32 ATP

*Inhibitors that inhibit the enzymes of TCA cycle are:*
Aconitase ← Fluoroacetate
α-ketoglutarate dehydrogenase ← Arsenate
{Succinate dehydrogenase ← Malonate} – Competitive

**Explain the regulation of TCA cycle including its importance.**

## Regulation of TCA Cycle

TCA cycle is controlled by respiratory rate, which is proportional to the energy consumption. The level of $NAD^+$ also stimulates the TCA cycle.
- *Citrate synthase*: Inhibited by ATP, NADH, acyl CoA and succinyl CoA.
- *Isocitrate dehydrogenase*: Inhibited by ATP and NADH and activated by ADP.
- α-KG inhibited by NADH and succinyl CoA.
  - The availability of ADP is important to proceeding the TCA cycle if not oxidation of NADH and $FADH_2$ through electron chain stops. Accumulation of NADH and FADH2, inhibit the enzymes of TCA cycle.

## Role of TCA Cycle

- It is the energy producing final pathway for the oxidation of glucose and acetyl CoA formed from fatty acid breakdown and from the product of breakdown of amino acids.
- It also provides citrate for fatty acid synthesis.
- The intermediates of TCA cycle are used for the synthesis of amino acids, glucose by gluconeogenesis.
- Since citric acid cycle is involved in the synthesis as well as breakdown of biological compounds, it is called as amphibolic pathway (anabolic and catabolic). TCA cycle takes part in gluconeogenesis, transamination, deamination and synthesis of fatty acids.

**Briefly explain the amphibolic role TCA cycle.**

## Anabolic Role of TCA Cycle

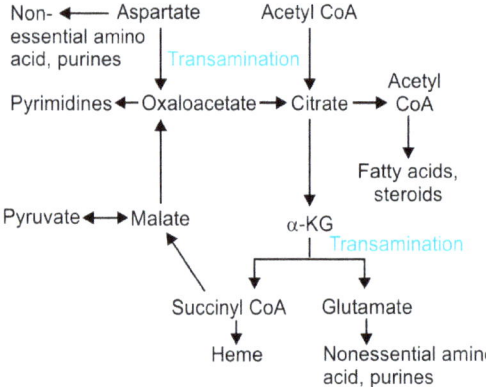

**What are anaplerotic reactions? Explain with examples.**

## Anaplerotic Reactions

- The reactions concerned to replenish the intermediates of TCA cycle are called anaplerotic reactions or anaplerosis.
- The intermediates of TCA cycle ($\alpha$-ketoglutarate, succinate and oxaloacetate) can be removed from the TCA cycle to

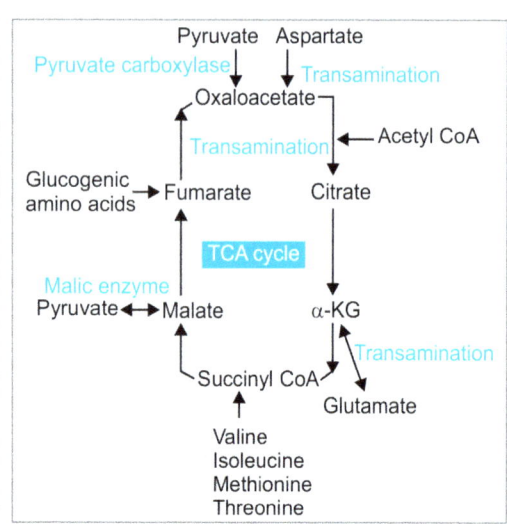

**Fig. 4.9:** Anapleurotic reactions.

synthesize many compounds required by the human body **(Fig. 4.9)**.

- For example, succinate and $\alpha$-ketoglutarate are removed to synthesize heme and gamma-amino butyrate respectively. Like this many of the intermediates of the TCA cycle are removed to synthesize the compounds. If this continues, the rate of TCA cycle may decrease. However, the intermediates of the TCA cycle can be replenished again by the action of certain enzymes.
  - Pyruvate+$CO_2$+AT $\xrightarrow{\text{Pyruvate carboxylase}}$ oxaloacetate+ADP+Pi
  - Pyruvate+$CO_2$+NADPH+$H^+$ $\xrightarrow{\text{Malic enzyme}}$ Malate

## Glyoxylate Cycle

- It is a modification of the TCA cycle which occurs in plants and some microorganisms.
- This will not occur in animals due to absence of enzymes *isocitrate lyase* and *malate synthase*.
- In plants glyoxylate cycle occurs in cytoplasmic organelles and glyoxysomes.
- In each turn of the glyoxylate cycle two molecules of acetate and one molecule of succinate is formed, which is used for the synthesis of glucose.

❖ Acetyl CoA condenses with oxaloacetate to form citrate, which is then isomerized to isocitrate. Isocitrate cleaved by lyase into succinate and glyoxylate. This glyoxylate combines with another molecule of acetyl CoA to form malate by malate synthase. Malate finally oxidized to oxaloacetate.

**Explain the process of gluconeogenesis and state its importance in regulating the blood glucose.**

## Gluconeogenesis (Fig. 4.10)

Gluconeogenesis is the process of formation of glucose from the various noncarbohydrate sources such as the glucogenic amino acids (*refer Chemistry of Amino Acids*), lactate, pyruvate, glycerol or and propionate.

Gluconeogenesis occurs in the fasting state or on a low carbohydrate diet particularly in liver and some other tissues, which are solely dependent on glucose for their energy

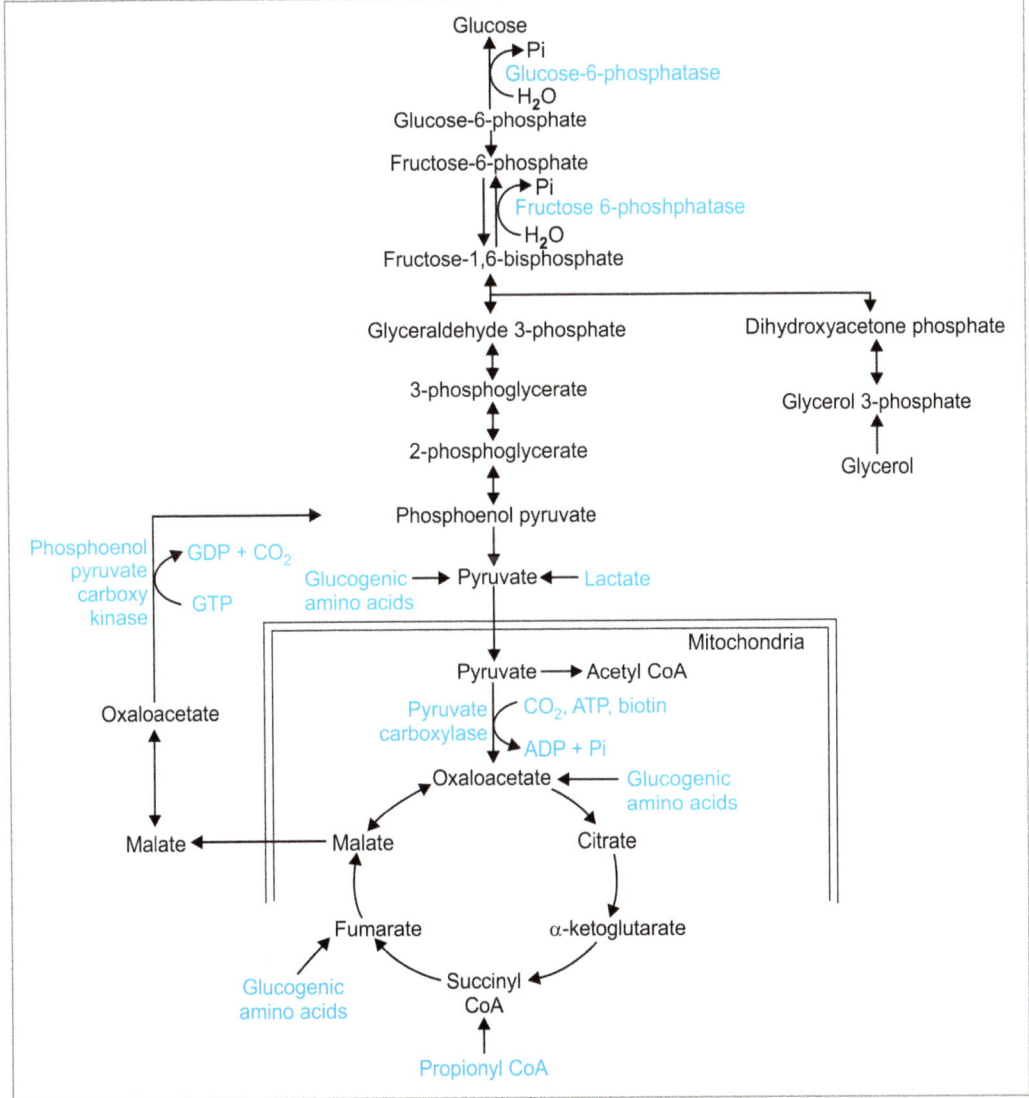

**Fig. 4.10:** Gluconeogenesis.

demand. The major metabolic significance of gluconeogenesis is to maintain the blood glucose level and to supply glucose for brain and cardiac muscle.

Glycolysis is the breakdown of glucose, whereas gluconeogenesis is the synthesis of glucose from noncarbohydrate sources.

But both these process are not exactly reciprocal each other. This is because three reactions in glycolysis are of irreversible nature.
* Mainly occurs in cytosol
* Some precursors are produced in mitochondria
* Takes place in liver and kidney
* Synthesis of glucose or glycogen from non-carbohydrates like pyruvate, lactate glucogenic amino acids, glycerol and propionic acid.
* Pathway involves steps of TCA cycle and reversal of glycolysis.
* The "3" irreversible steps of glycolysis are catalyzed by hexokinase, phosphofructokinase and pyruvate kinase.
* These three stages are bypassed by alternate enzymes specific to gluconeogenesis and they are called as key enzymes of gluconeogenesis.
    - Pyruvate carboxylase
    - Phosphoenolpyruvate carboxykinase (PEPCK)
    - Fructose-1,6-bisphosphatase
    - Glucose-6-phosphatase.
* The pathway meets the needs of the body for glucose.
* Continuous supply of glucose as a source of energy for the CNS, brain, RBC and skeletal muscle during starvation.

## Regulation of Gluconeogenesis

* The hormone glucagon and the availability of substrates mainly regulate gluconeogenesis (Fig. 4.11).
* Glucagon and glucocorticoid increases gluconeogenesis.
* Insulin inhibits gluconeogenesis
* Glucagon inactivates pyruvate kinase (which converts phosphoenol pyruvate

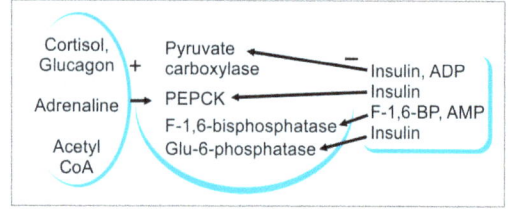

Fig. 4.11: Regulation of gluconeogenesis.

to pyruvate) through cAMP dependent phosphorylation.
* Glucagon reduces the concentration of fructose-2,6-bisphosphate so that PFK-1 remains inactive and activates fructose-1,6-bisphosphatase that increases gluconeogenesis
* Glucogenic amino acids have stimulating effect on key gluconeogenic enzymes.
* Acetyl CoA promotes gluconeogenesis.
* Starvation results in excessive lipolysis in adipose tissues. The fatty acids released are oxidized and the acetyl CoA accumulates in the liver. This acetyl CoA stimulates the gluconeogenic enzymes.

## Substrates for Gluconeogenesis (Fig. 4.12)

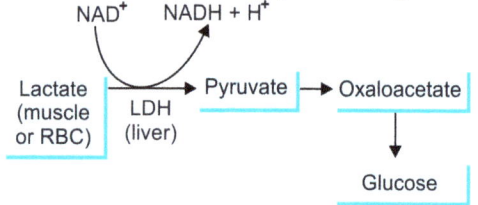

* *Synthesis of glucose from glycerol and propionic acid* (Fig. 4.13A): Lactate and glucogenic amino acids are the most important substrates.
* *Glucose-alanine cycle*: Alanine is the major amino acid released from muscle to liver during fasting by glucose alanine cycle. Some of the pyruvate resulting from glycolysis in skeletal muscle is transaminated to alanine and transported to liver, where it is converted back to pyruvate. This pyruvate in the liver is used to synthesize glucose and this glucose is returned to muscle. This is one of the processes also used to maintain nitrogen balance (Fig. 4.13B).

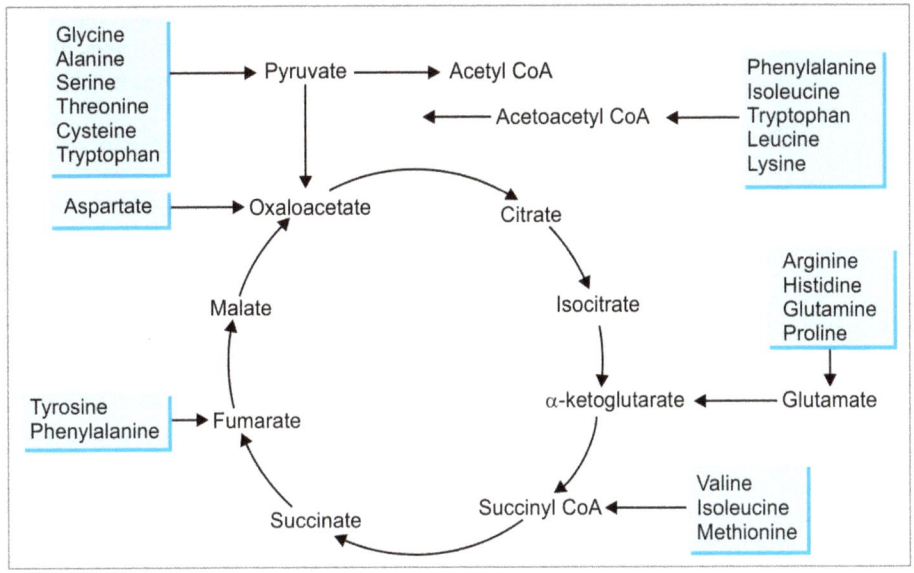

**Fig. 4.12:** Substrates for gluconeogenesis.

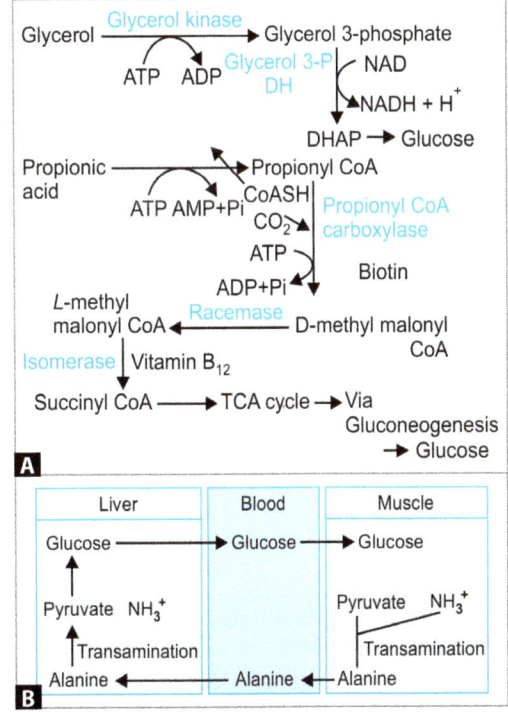

**Figs. 4.13A and B:** (A) Synthesis of glucose from glycerol and propionic acid; (B) Glucose-alanine cycle.

**Explain Cori's cycle including its clinical importance.**

## Cori's Cycle

Glucose/glycogen is converted to lactate in the muscle and this lactate is converted back to glucose in the liver **(Fig. 4.14)**.

During active muscle contraction, the glycogen breaks down and glucose-6-phosphate formed enters anaerobic glycolysis to generate lactate.

This lactate enters → Blood to → Liver (gluconeogenesis to form glucose) → Glucose → Blood → Back to tissues. This whole process is called Cori's cycle.

Acetyl CoA is not converted to glucose in humans due to:

- Irreversible reaction catalyzed by pyruvate dehydrogenase prevents the direct conversion of acetyl CoA to pyruvate.
- There is no net conversion of acetyl CoA to oxaloacetate via TCA cycle. Only one molecule is regenerated, which is used during the TCA cycle.

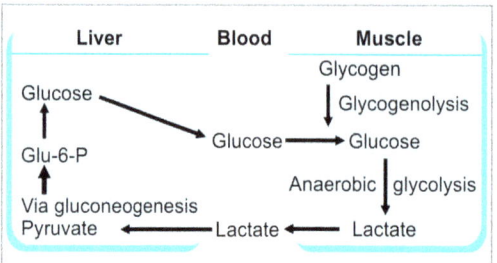

**Fig. 4.14:** Cori's cycle.

## Metabolism of Glycogen

Glycogen is the storage form of glucose in our body. It is mainly stored in muscle and liver. This stored glycogen of liver is used for maintaining blood glucose level during hypoglycemia. The muscle glycogen is used for providing energy during exercise.

## Glycogenesis

The synthesis of glycogen from glucose is called glycogenesis **(Figs. 4.15A and B)**.

It takes place in several tissues but liver and muscle are the main organs for the synthesis of glycogen.

**Briefly discuss the synthesis of glycogen from glucose.**

❖ For its conversion to glycogen, glucose is phosphorylated to form glucose-6-phosphate by the enzyme *hexokinase*, which also requires ATP and $Mg^{2+}$. In the fed state another enzyme *glucokinase*, present in the liver, converts most of the glucose into glycogen.

❖ Glucose-6-phosphate is then epimerized to form glucose-1-phosphate by *phosphoglucomutase* enzyme.

❖ Glucose-1-phosphate reacts with UTP and is converted to uridine diphosphate glucose (UDP-glucose). This reaction is catalyzed by *UDP-glucose pyrophosphorylase* enzyme. Pyrophosphate released during this process is hydrolyzed to inorganic phosphate

❖ From UDP-glucose, glucose is transferred to pre-existing glycogen molecule called glycogen primer. The incoming glucose is linked to the precursor glycogen by $\alpha$ 1,4 glycosidic linkage resulting in the elongation of pre-existing branches.

❖ When the chain length is increased by 10–12 glucose molecules, a minimum length of 6 glucose molecules, is transferred from this by the branching enzyme onto the neighboring chain in such a way that

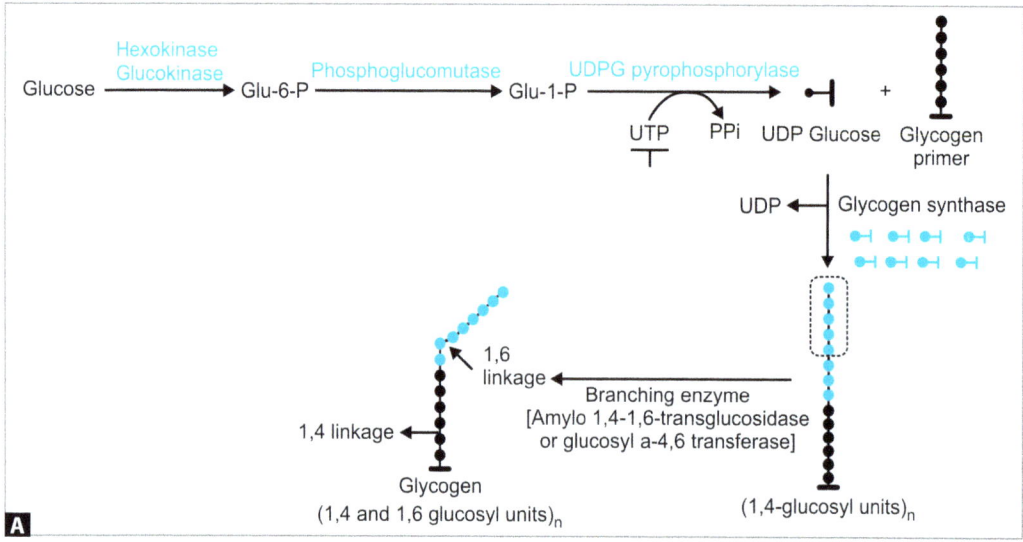

**Fig. 4.15A**

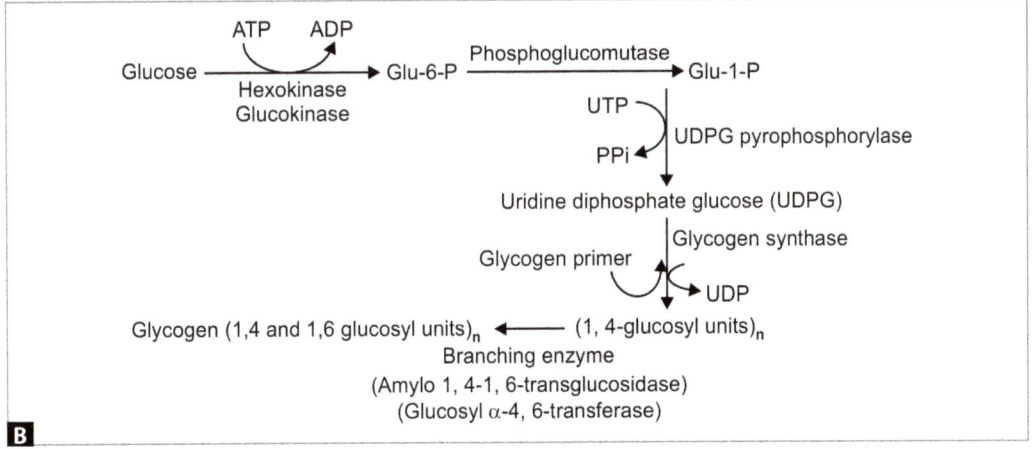

Fig. 4.15B

**Figs. 4.15A and B:** (A) Glycogen synthesis; (B) Glycogen synthesis.

it forms a new branching point (α 1-6 linkage).
- The branch again grows by the addition of the glucose molecules at the α 1–4 linkage. With the further branching it results in the formation of a highly branched polymer of glucose called glycogen.
- UDPG is the carrier of glucose
- Glucose from UDPG is attached at the non-reducing end of glucose molecules of glycogen primer.
- Branching enzyme (Amylo 1,4 –1,6 transglucosidase) transfers 6 glucose residue portion from one chain to a neighboring chain to form a α-1,6-linkage.

## Glycogenolysis

**What is glycogenolysis and explain briefly how glucose is generated from glycogen breakdown.**

Glycogenolysis is the process of breakdown of glycogen either to glucose-6-phosphate in muscle or to free glucose in liver **(Fig. 4.16)**.
- In the first step, glucose molecules are sequentially removed as glucose-1-phosphate. This reaction is rate controlling step and is catalyzed by glycogen phosphorylase enzyme. It removes glucose from the glycogen molecule until nearly four glucose residues are left on the outermost chain.
- Glucan transferase enzyme transfers a trisaccharide unit out of the four molecules of glucose left on the outer branch to the neighboring exposed branch point.
- Debranching enzyme removes the glucose molecule present at the branch point as free glucose.
- Thus with the combined action of glycogen phosphorylase, *glucantransferase* and debranching enzyme; the glycogen molecule is hydrolyzed to glucose-1-phosphate and free glucose.
- Glucose-1-phosphate formed is converted into glucose-6-phosphate by *phosphoglucomutase* enzyme.
- In liver and kidney, glucose-6-phosphate further hydrolyzed to glucose by the action of glucose-6-phosphatase enzyme. This enzyme is absent in muscle. Hence muscle glycogen cannot be converted to glucose. Liver glycogen is mainly used to maintain the level of blood glucose.
- Phosphorylase phosphorolytically splits α-1,4 glucoside bonds from the outermost chains of glycogen until 4 residues remain on either side of α-1,6 branch point (limit dextrin).
- α-1,4 glucan transferase transfers 3 glucose residue portion from one side chain to the other exposing a-1,6 branch points.
- *Amylo 1,6 glucosidase* splits the 1,6 linkages.

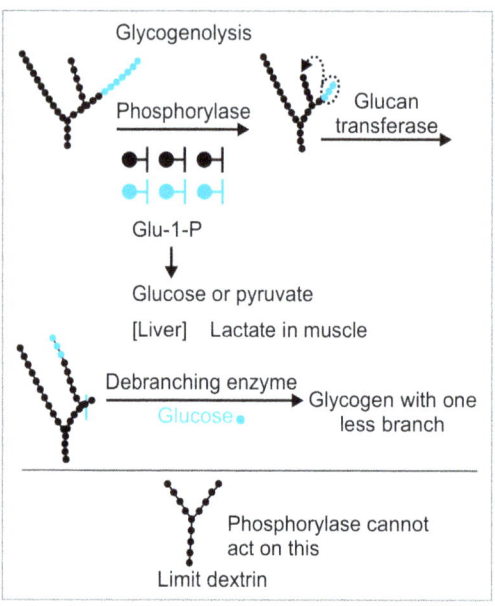

**Fig. 4.16:** Glycogenolysis.

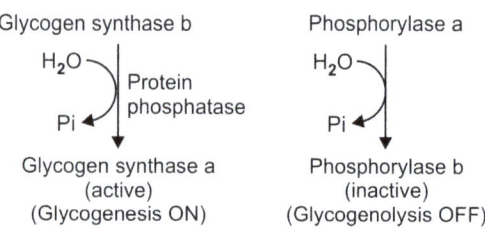

## Muscle Glycogenolysis

Glycogen → Glu-1-P → Glu-6-P → glycolysis → lactate.

### Lysosomal Degradation of Glycogen

A small amount of glycogen is degraded by lysosomal enzyme α-*1, 4 glucosidase* (acid maltase).

**Explain with a schematic diagram to show the regulation glycogenesis and glycogenolysis.**

## Regulation of Glycogenesis and Glycogenolysis (Fig. 4.17)

- The glycogen synthase and phosphorylase exist in active and inactive forms.
- The dephosphorylated form of glycogen synthase is active.
- Phosphorylated form of phosphorylase is active.
- The activation of phosphorylase depends on high cAMP level. At the same time high cAMP level inactivates glycogen synthase.

**List the compounds which regulate the glycogen metabolism.**

## Allosteric Regulation

- In a well fed state glucose-6-phosphate level is high which activates glycogen synthase.
- On the other hand, glucose-6-phosphate and ATP allosterically inhibit phosphorylase.
- Free glucose also acts as inhibitor to phosphorylase.

**Briefly explain the allosteric regulation of glycogenolysis by calcium.**

## Effect of Calcium

Calcium ($Ca^{2+}$) allosterically activates phosphorylase kinase and it is independent of cAMP and phosphorylation. When muscle contracts $Ca^{2+}$ ions are released from the sarcoplasmic reticulum. $Ca^{2+}$ binds allosterically to calmodulin, a subunit of phosphorylase kinase, and activates the enzyme without the need for its phosphorylation and allows glycogenolysis. When muscle relaxes $Ca^{2+}$ returns to the sarcoplasmic reticulum and phosphorylase kinase becomes inactive.

## Glycogen Storage Diseases

- Genetic diseases (may be inherited)
- Deposition of abnormal type or abnormal quantity of glycogen in the tissues is shown as in **Table 4.3**.

**Discuss the different types of glycogen storage disorders including the causes and features.**

*Location*: The enzymes of pathway are located in cytosol. This pathway found in all cells such as liver, adipose tissue, adrenal gland, RBC, testes, ovaries and lactating mammary gland are highly active in HMP shunt. These

# CHAPTER 4: Metabolism of Carbohydrates

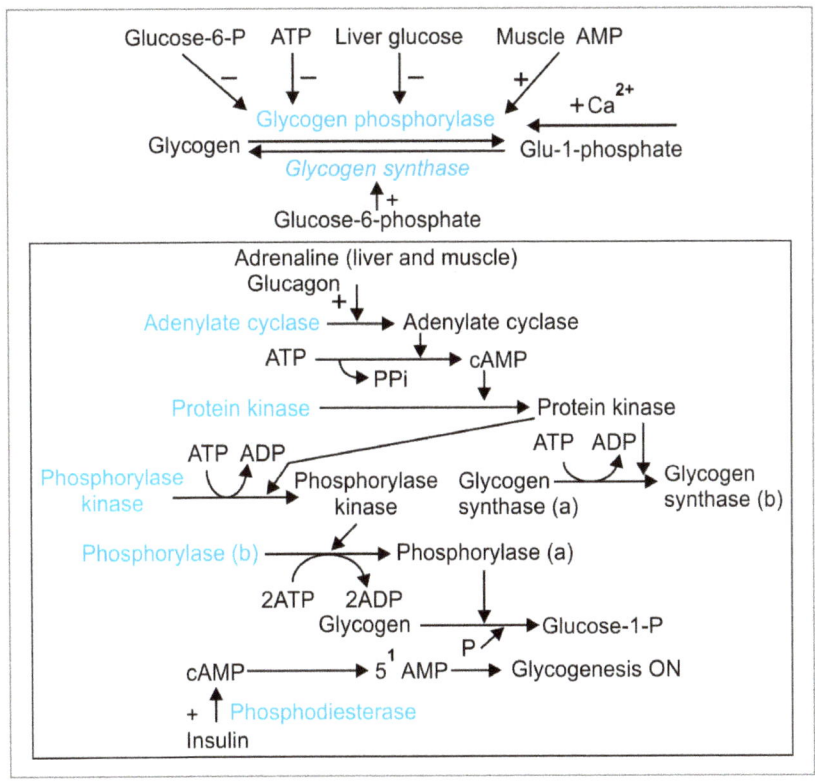

**Fig. 4.17:** Glycogen metabolism regulation.

**Table 4.3:** Deposition of abnormal type or abnormal quantity of glycogen in the tissues.

| Diseases | Causes and features |
|---|---|
| Type I: von Gierke's disease | • Glucose-6-phosphatase (liver)<br>• Fasting hypoglycemia<br>• *Lactic acidemia*: Glucose is not synthesized from the lactate produced in muscle and liver. Lactate level increases and pH decreases<br>• *Hyperlipidemia*: Block in gluconeogenesis leads to mobilization fat to meet energy requirement. So, this increases free plasma fatty acid and ketone bodies<br>• *Hyperuricemia*: Accumulated glucose-6-P diverted to HMP pathway, leading to increased synthesis of ribose and nucleotides, this enhances catabolism of purine nucleotides to uric acid<br>• Massive liver enlargement leads to cirrhosis. Children fail to grow<br>  – Food should be given in small quantity at frequent intervals |
| | Accumulation of glycogen in the liver |
| | Hypoglycemia and lactic acidemia |
| Type II: Pompe's disease | Lysosomal α-1,4-glucosidase |

*Contd...*

Contd...

| Diseases | Causes and features |
|---|---|
| | Glycogen accumulates in lysosomes in all tissues |
| | Enlarged liver and heart |
| Type III: Limit dextrinosis (Cori's disease) | Debranching enzyme (amylo-α-1,6-glucosidase) |
| | Accumulation of polysaccharide (limit dextrin) in liver, heart, and muscle |
| Type IV: Amylopectinosis or Andersen's disease | Branching enzyme (glucosyl-4,6-transferase) |
| | Accumulation of polysaccharide with few branch points. Cirrhosis of liver |
| Type V: McArdle's disease | Muscle glycogen phosphorylase |
| | Glycogen accumulates in the muscle |
| | Diminished tolerance to exercise |
| Type VI: Hers' disease | Liver glycogen phosphorylase |

tissues have high amount of pentose pathway enzymes for their determined functions which depends on NADPH.

## MP Shunt or Pentose Phosphate Pathway or Phosphogluconate Pathway

An alternative pathway to glycolysis and TCA cycle for the oxidation of glucose **(Fig. 4.18)**.

**Discuss the oxidative and nonoxidative phases hexose monophosphate pathway and state its importance.**

Adrenal gland → Steroid synthesis
Testes → Steroid synthesis
Ovaries → Steroid synthesis
Adipose tissue → Fatty acid synthesis
Mammary gland → Fatty acid synthesis
Liver → Fatty acid, bile acid, and cholesterol synthesis
RBCs → Maintenance of reduced glutathione (GSH).

*The reactions of the pathway are divided into two phases:* oxidative irreversible phase and nonoxidative reversible phase.

### Oxidative Irreversible Phase

❖ The reactions start with 3 molecules of glucose-6-phosphate.
❖ Glucose-6-phosphate is converted to:
- 6-phosphogluconolactone by glucose
- 6-phosphate dehydrogenase which is NADP dependent. This reaction produces first molecule of NADPH.
❖ 6-phosphogluconolactone is then converted to 6-phosphogluconate by 6-phosphogluconolactone hydrolase.
❖ 6-phosphogluconate undergoes decarboxylation step which is catalyzed by 6-phosphogluconate dehydrogenase. This reaction is NADP dependent and produces ribulose 5-phosphate, $CO_2$ and a second molecule of NADPH.

### Nonoxidative Irreversible Phase

❖ Ribulose 5-phosphate formed is converted back to glucose-6-phosphate by a series of reactions. Ribulose 5-phosphate serves as substrate for two different enzymes:
  1. Ribulose 5-phosphate epimerase forming two molecules of xylulose 5-phosphate (ketopentose) from two molecules of ribose 5-phosphate
  2. Ribose 5-phosphate keto-isomerase converts a molecule of xylulose-5-phosphate to ribose 5-phosphate, which is a precursor for ribose residues required for the synthesis of nucleotide and nucleic acids.

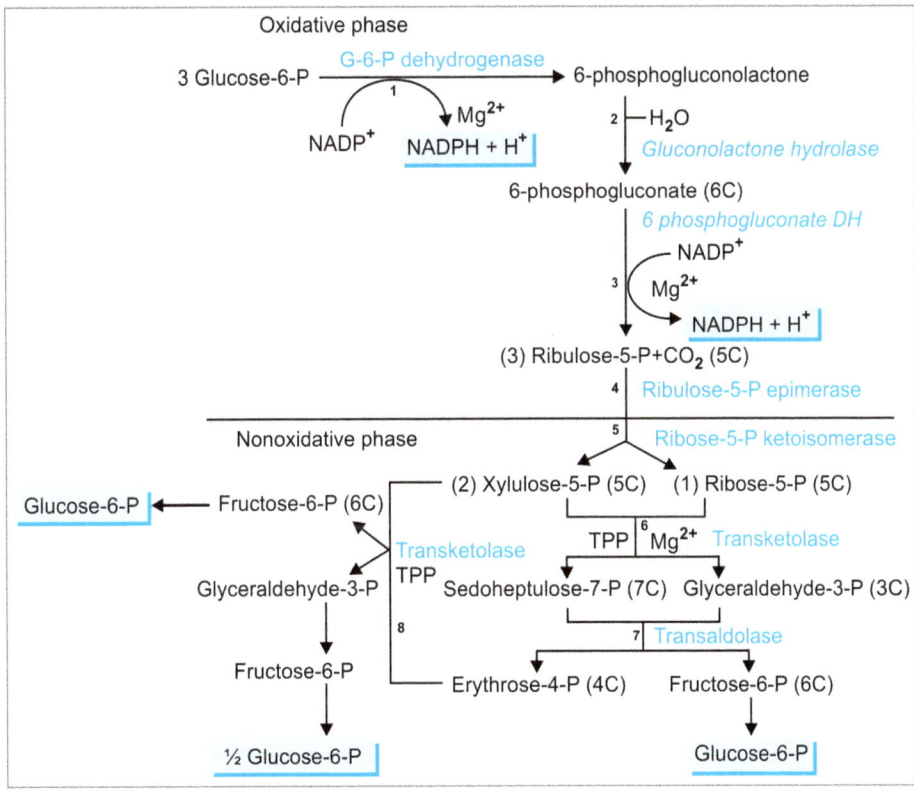

**Fig. 4.18:** Reactions of hexose monophosphate (HMP) shunt.

- Transketolase transfers two carbons from a molecule of xylulose 5-phosphate (ketose) to ribose 5-phosphate (aldopentose) forming sedoheptulose 7-phosphate (with two carbon more). The xylulose 5-phosphate after losing two carbon forms glyceraldehyde 3-phosphate.
- In the next reaction the transaldolase transfers three carbon dihydroxyacetone group from sedoheptulose 7-phosphate to the glyceraldehyde 3-phosphate to form fructose 6-phosphate and 4 carbon, erythrose 4-phosphate.
- Transketolase transfers two carbon units from remaining molecule of xylulose 5-phosphate to erythrose 4-phosphate forming fructose-6-phosphate and glyceraldehyde 3-phosphate.
- In order to oxidize glucose completely to $CO_2$ via HMP shunt, it is important to convert glyceraldehyde 3-phosphate to glucose-6-phosphate. This involves the enzymes of the glycolysis and gluconeogenesis (fructose-1,6-bisphosphatase).

## Summary

3 glucose 6-phosphate + $H_2O$ + 6 NADP$^+$ → 3 ribulose 5-phosphate + $CO_2$ + 6NADPH + 6 H$^+$.

## Significance of HMP Shunt

- Generating pentoses and NADPH
- The pentoses or its derivatives (Ribose 5-P) are useful for the synthesis of nucleic acids and nucleotides like ATP, NAD$^+$, FAD.
- NADPH is required for the biosynthesis of fatty acids, steroids and synthesis of glutamic acid.
- The continuous production of $H_2O_2$ in living cells can chemically damage unsaturated lipids, proteins. This is prevented through

antioxidant reactions involving NADPH that is through glutathione mediated reduction of $H_2O_2$. NADPH is necessary for the regeneration of reduced glutathione.
* In RBC, RBC has a high concentration of reduced form of glutathione (GSH), which protects RBC from oxidative damage by $H_2O_2$. In the GSH decomposition of $H_2O_2$ the oxidized form of GSH (GS-SG) is formed. The GS-SG is reduced back to GSH by NADPH formed in HMP shunt.

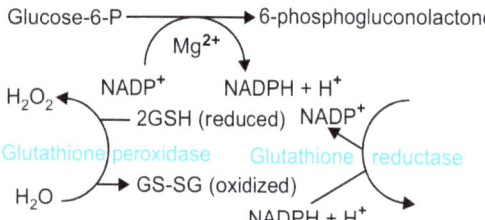

**What causes the deficiency of G6PD and state its diagnostic importance.**

## Glucose 6-Phosphate Dehydrogenase Deficiency

* It is an inborn genetic disease.
* RBC does not have active HMP shunt to provide enough NADPH to maintain high GSH concentration.
* Increased susceptibility of RBC to hemolysis.
* Babies with G6PD deficiency are very sensitive to antimalarial drugs like primaquine.
* Primaquine necessitates high GSH level and G6PD deficiency attenuates oxidation stress.
* When the drugs given, RBCs tend to hemolyze.
* Drugs like aspirin and sulpha drugs also cause hemolysis of RBCs.
* The G6PD estimation is useful when:
  * The patient is suffering from severe hemolytic anemia
  * Treating the patient with antimalarial drugs.

## Regulation of the HMP Shunt

The first regulatory step in the pathway is catalyzed by glucose-6-phosphate dehydrogenase, the rate limiting step. The activity of this enzyme dependent on the concentration of NADPH (it is a competitive inhibitor).

Under well-fed state the ratio of $NADPH/NADP^+$ decreases and the pathway is stimulated. Insulin also enhances the pathway by inducing glucose-6-phosphate dehydrogenase and 6-phosphogluconolactone dehydrogenase.

In starvation and diabetes, the ratio $NADPH/NADP^+$ is high and inhibits the pathway.

## Galactose Metabolism

Galactose is required for the formation of glycolipids, glycoproteins and lactose during lactation **(Fig. 4.19)**. In the liver galactose is readily converted to glucose.

**What causes galactosemia and list the signs and symptoms of it.**

## Galactosemia

* *Cause*: Deficiency of galactose-1-phosphate uridyl-transferase.
* It is a rare congenital disease in infants.
* Galactose accumulated → galactosemia (blood) → galactosuria (urine).
* High level of galactose in blood is reduced by aldose reductase in the eye to galacitol, which accumulated causing cataract.
* The accumulation of galactose-1-phosphate and galacitol in tissues like liver, nervous tissue, lens and kidney leads to impaired functions.
* *Symptoms*: Weight loss in infants, hepatosplenomegaly, jaundice, mental

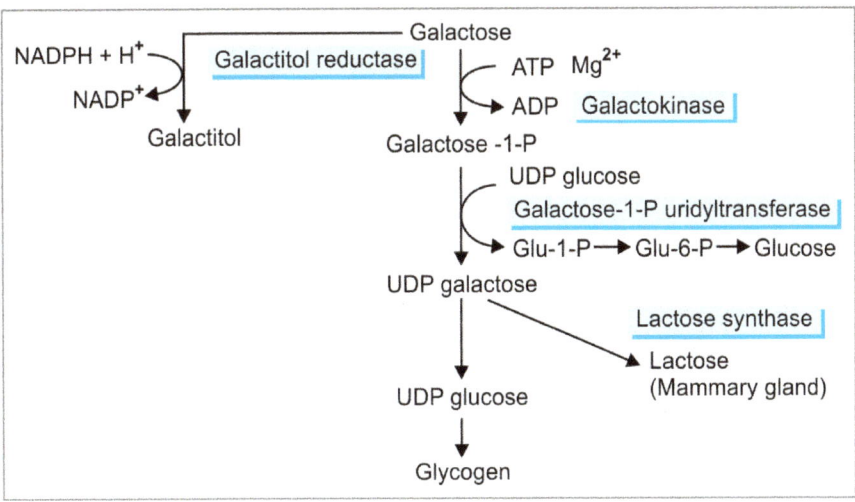

**Fig. 4.19:** Galactose metabolism.

retardation, etc. In severe conditions, cataract aminoaciduria and albuminuria are observed.

* *Treatment*: Withdrawal of the diet containing galactose and lactose.

## Fate of Galactose

* In liver most of the galactose is converted into UDP-galactose and then to liver glycogen.
* It is also used for the synthesis of glycolipid in brain and nervous tissue.
* In lactating mammary gland galactose is converted into lactose by synthase enzyme.

**Briefly explain with a diagram to fructose metabolism.**

## Fructose Metabolism

Liver is the major site of fructose metabolism (Fig. 6.20).

*Fructose intolerance*: It is an inborn error of metabolism. Aldolase B absent in this case.

*Essential fructosuria*: Fructokinase absent in this condition.

**Discuss the sorbitol pathway including its clinical significance.**

## Sorbitol Pathway (Polyol Pathway)

Mainly occurs in human lens.

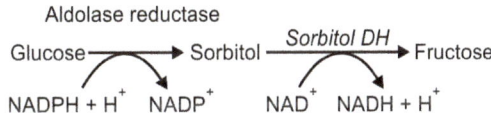

The enzyme *aldolase* reductase reduces glucose to sorbitol (glucitol) in the presence of NADPH. The enzyme *sorbitol dehydrogenase* oxidizes sorbitol to fructose.

### Aldolase

* Absent in liver
* Present in lens, retina kidney, nerve cells, RBC and seminal vesicles.

### Sorbitol Dehydrogenase

Present in liver, seminal vesicles, spleen and ovaries.

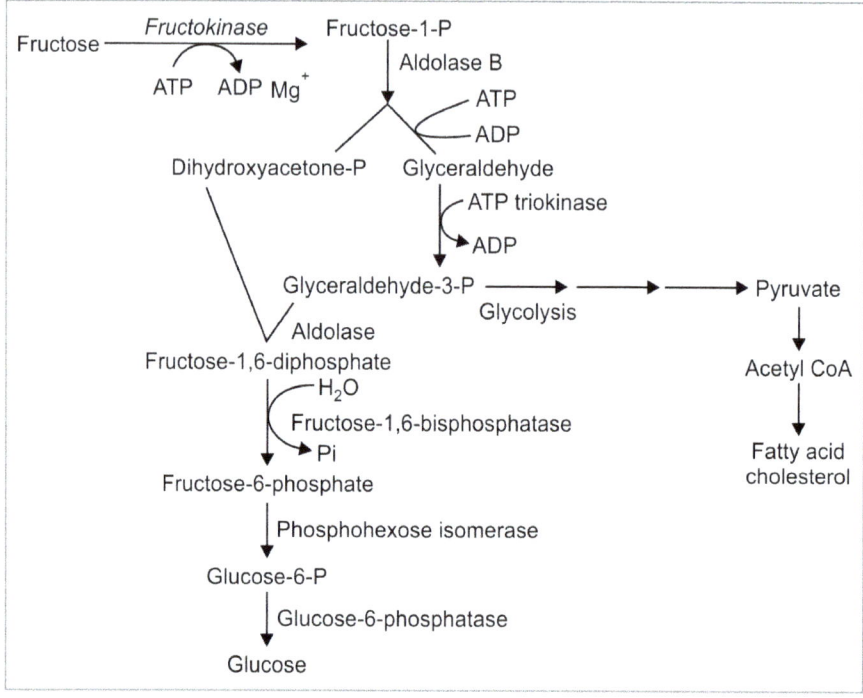

**Fig. 4.20:** Fructose metabolism.

In uncontrolled diabetes large amounts of glucose enters the cells which are not dependent on insulin. Significant increase in intracellular glucose takes place in diabetes; in cells (lens, retina, nerve cells and kidney) possess high activity of *aldolase reductase* and sufficient supply of NADPH. This results in a rapid and efficient conversion of glucose to sorbitol. The decreased or absence of *sorbitol dehydrogenase* level causes sorbitol to accumulated instead of converting to fructose and this sorbitol gets accumulated in the cells. Thus, involved in pathogenesis of diabetic cataract.

**Explain how high fructose is responsible for atherosclerosis.**

## High Content of Fructose is Linked to Atherosclerosis

Fructose undergoes glycosylation more rapidly by the liver than glucose due to bypassed step in the glucose metabolism catalyzed by phosphofructokinase (metabolic control is exerted at this step). This allows fructose to flood the pathways in the liver with more production acetyl CoA which is deviated to synthesize fatty acid and cholesterol. In the same way the glyceraldehyde part is reduced to glycerol and then to glycerol 3-phosphate which forms triacylglycerol after combining with fatty acid molecules. At the end this will leads to the increased production of VLDL and LDL.

**What is the cause for lactose intolerance? Explain with signs and symptoms of lactose intolerance.**

## Lactose Intolerance

*Cause*: A deficiency of the brush border enzyme lactase gives rise to a condition named lactose intolerance.

❖ Found frequently in people of East Asian descent past their infant age. If lactose is

# CHAPTER 4: Metabolism of Carbohydrates

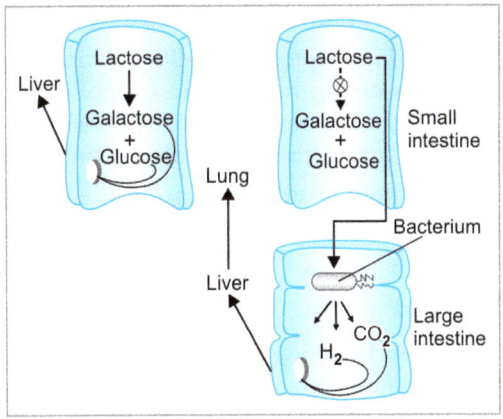

**Fig. 4.21:** Lactose intolerance.

not cleaved, it cannot be absorbed, so it makes its way 'down the drain' from the small into the large intestine. Many of the bacteria found there have the capacity to metabolize lactose, which they convert to acids and gas. This leads to abdominal discomfort and diarrhea.

❖ Since the environment in the large intestine lacks oxygen, hydrogen ($H_2$) generated in the bacterial fermentation is not oxidized but instead released as such, and in part is exhaled (**Fig. 4.21**).
❖ An increase in exhaled hydrogen upon ingestion of lactose can be used to diagnose the condition.
❖ Treatment consists in omission of lactose in the diet.
❖ Milk can be pretreated with purified bacterial α-galactosidase, rendering it suitable for consumption by lactose-intolerant individuals. Fermented milk products such as yoghurt and cheese are depleted of lactose by bacterial fermentation and therefore do not pose a problem for lactose intolerant individuals.

*Lactosuria*: Second common reducing sugar found in the urine.
❖ Observed in the urine of normal women during 3rd trimester of pregnancy and lactation.
❖ Also seen in neonates.

## Regulation of Blood Glucose

The concentration of glucose in the blood is regulated by several metabolic pathways which are mainly modulated by several hormones. The major metabolic pathways are glycogenesis, glycogenolysis, gluconeogenesis, glycolysis, TCA cycle, HMP shunt, lipogenesis, lipolysis and protein synthesis.

During a brief fast the decrease in the blood glucose level is avoided by breakdown of glycogen stored in the liver. After a meal the absorbed glucose is converted to glycogen or fat.

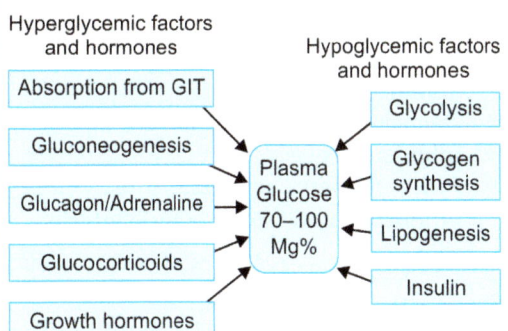

## Postprandial Blood Sugar Regulation

After the meal, absorption of glucose from the intestine increases the glucose level in the blood. The increased blood glucose stimulates the cells of pancreas to secrete insulin.

## Fasting Blood Sugar Regulation

In normal conditions after 4–5 hours of a meal, blood glucose level decreases near to fasting levels. Further decrease in the blood glucose is prevented by the hyperglycemic hormones.

## Normal Levels

*Fasting*: After 12 hours of fasting, the sugar estimated 70–100 mg/100 mL.

*Postprandial blood sugar (PPBS)*: After 2 hours of normal breakfast or lunch, the sugar estimated 90–140 mg/100 mL.

*Random blood sugar (RBS)*: At any time, sugar estimated 90–150 mg/100 mL.

**Explain the role of hormones in regulating the blood glucose.**

## Regulation by Hormones

*Insulin (Hypoglycemic Hormone)*
- Insulin lowers blood glucose
- Favors glycogen synthesis
- Promotes glycolysis
- Inhibits gluconeogenesis

*Glucagon*
- Promotes gluconeogenesis
- Enhances glycogenolysis
- Decreases glycogen synthesis
- Inhibits glycolysis
- Promotes fatty acid oxidation, energy production and ketone body synthesis.

*Cortisol*
- Increases glycogenolysis
- Enhances release of amino acids by the muscle
- Induces the enzymes PEPCK, fructose-1, 6-bisphosphatase, glucose 6-phosphatase and amino transferase.

*Adrenaline*
- Promotes gluconeogenesis
- Increases glycogenolysis
- Favors release of glucose

*Growth Hormone*
- Decrease glycolysis (inhibit PFK)
- Mobilizes fatty acids from adipose tissues.

*Factors Stimulating Insulin Secretion*
- Amino acids
- Gastrointestinal hormones
- GH, cortisol and estrogens
- Glucose is the important stimulus for the insulin release.

*Factors Inhibiting Insulin Secretion*

Epinephrine suppresses insulin secretion and promotes energy metabolism by mobilizing energy yielding compounds like glucose from liver and fatty acids from adipose tissue.

**Explain how insulin regulating the blood glucose through its action on various metabolism.**

## Metabolic Effects of Insulin

*Effects on Carbohydrate Metabolism*

Normally half of the ingested glucose is utilized to meet the energy demands of the body (glycolysis) other 50% may be converted to fat or glycogen.
- Insulin stimulates the uptake of glucose by muscle, adipose tissue, leukocytes and mammary glands. About 80% of glucose uptake is not dependent on insulin.
  Tissues into which glucose can freely enter include brain, kidney, erythrocytes, retina, nerve, blood vessels and intestinal mucosa. The entry of glucose into hepatocytes does not depend on insulin. However, it stimulates the glucose utilization in liver and indirectly promotes its uptake.
- *Effect on glucose utilization*: Increases glycolysis in muscle and liver; stimulate:
  - Glucokinase
  - PFK
  - Pyruvate kinase
  - Glycogen synthetase
  - HMP shunt through G6PD
- *Effect on glucose production*:
  - Decreases gluconeogenesis by inactivating
  - Pyruvate carboxy kinase, glucose 6-phosphatase
  - Decreases glycogenolysis by inactivating glycogen phosphorylase.

*Effects on Lipid Metabolism*
- *Lipogenesis*: Favors TG synthesis (providing more glycerol-3-p and NADPH). Increase activity of acetyl CoA carboxylase, a key enzyme of fatty acid synthesis.

- *Lipolysis*: Decreases the activity of hormone—sensitive lipase.
- *Ketogenesis*: Decreases ketogenesis. Increases the utilization of acetyl CoA.
- *Lipoprotein metabolism*: Helps to utilize VLDL and LDL.

*Protein Metabolism*
- Increases protein synthesis
- Decreases protein breakdown

**Discuss the mechanism of action of insulin in regulating the blood glucose.**

## Mechanism of Action of Insulin

Insulin binds to specific plasma membrane receptors present on the target tissues (muscle and adipose tissue) this result in a series of reaction ultimately leading to the biological action. There are three mechanisms known.
1. Insulin receptor-mediated signal transduction
2. Insulin-mediated glucose transport
3. Insulin-mediated enzyme synthesis

*Insulin receptor:* This is a tetramer consisting of four subunits of two types (α2, β2) of glycosylated form, held together by disulfide linkages.

The α-subunit is extracellular and it contains insulin-binding site.

The β-subunit is a transmembrane protein, which is activated by insulin. The cytoplasmic domain of β-subunit has tyrosine kinase activity.

## Signal Transduction (Fig. 4.22)

Binding of insulin causes dimerization of the receptor. It is then internalized, so that the signal is transmitted. Then the tyrosine kinase phosphorylates tyrosine residues on the cytoplasmic side of insulin receptor. This in turn, phosphorylates insulin receptor substrates (IRS).

## Insulin-mediated Glucose Transport

The binding of insulin to insulin receptors signals the translocation of vesicles containing

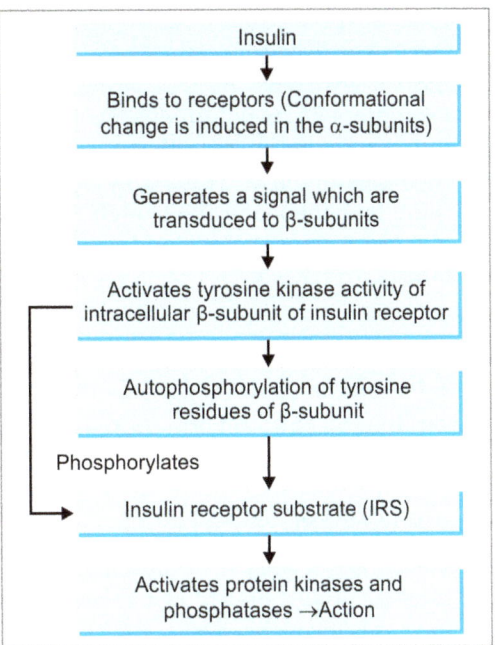

**Fig. 4.22:** Signal transduction.

glucose transporters from intracellular pool to the plasma membrane. The vesicles fuse with the membrane recruiting the glucose transporters. The glucose transporters are responsible for the insulin mediated glucose uptake by the cells. As the insulin level falls, the glucose transporters move away from the membrane to the intracellular pool for storage and recycle.

## Insulin-mediated Enzyme Synthesis

Insulin promotes the synthesis of enzymes such as glucokinase, phosphofructokinase, and pyruvate kinase, this is brought about by increased transcription (mRNA synthesis) followed by translocation.

**List the hyperglycemic hormones and explain their role in regulating the blood glucose when it goes down.**

## Glucagon

- Anti-insulin in nature
- Secreted from the alpha cells of pancreas
- Liver is the primary target for the glycogenolytic effect of glucagon.

- Promotes glycogenolysis, gluconeogenesis.
- Decreases glycogen synthesis
- Inhibits glycolysis
- Promoters FA oxidation energy production and ketone body synthesis.
- Increases amino acid uptake by liver, promote gluconeogenesis through PEPCK, glucose-6-phosphatase and fructose-1, 6-bisphosphatase.

## Mechanism of Action of Glucagon (Fig. 4.23)

Adrenaline or epinephrine increase liver glycogenolysis, increase lipolysis.

## Glucocorticoid

- The uptake of glucose by muscle
- Increase protein breakdown in muscle
- Increase gluconeogenesis

*Growth hormone*: Decrease uptake of glucose (releasing FA from adipose tissue).

*Thyroxine*: With the above functions increase absorption of glucose.

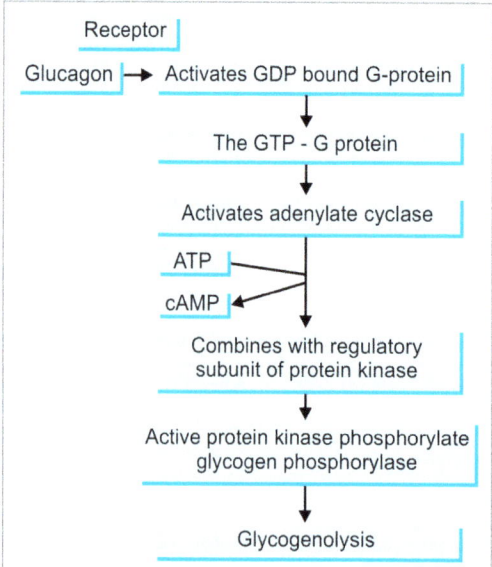

**Fig. 4.23:** Action of glucagon.

**What is diabetes and what are its major types?**

## Diabetes Mellitus

It is a group of metabolic diseases in which a person has high blood sugar (>126 mg/dL), either because the body does not produce enough insulin, or because cells do not respond to the insulin that is produced.

It is broadly divided into two types namely:
1. Type I insulin-dependent diabetes mellitus (IDDM).
2. Type II noninsulin-dependent diabetes mellitus (NIDDM).

**What are the signs and symptoms of diabetes mellitus?**

## Symptoms (Fig. 4.24)

- Frequent urination (polyuria)
- Excessive thirst (polydipsia)
- Extreme hunger or constant eating (polyphagia)
- Unexplained weight loss
- Presence of glucose in the urine
- Tiredness or fatigue
- Changes in vision
- Numbness or tingling in the extremities
- Slow-healing wounds or sores
- Abnormally high frequency of infection
- *Polyuria* (Large amount of glucose and water excretion).
- *Polydypsia*: Loss of fluid stimulates the thirst center. Person drinks more and more water.
- *Polyphagia*: Lipid and protein breakdown with weight loss. Person eats more frequently.
- Patient may show boils, abscesses, and cellulitis. Complications of this type are retinopathy, neuropathy and nephropathy.

## Type I or Insulin Dependent Diabetes Mellitus

Usually onset in childhood, early teenage years (12–15 years age).
- Genetic predisposition

# CHAPTER 4: Metabolism of Carbohydrates

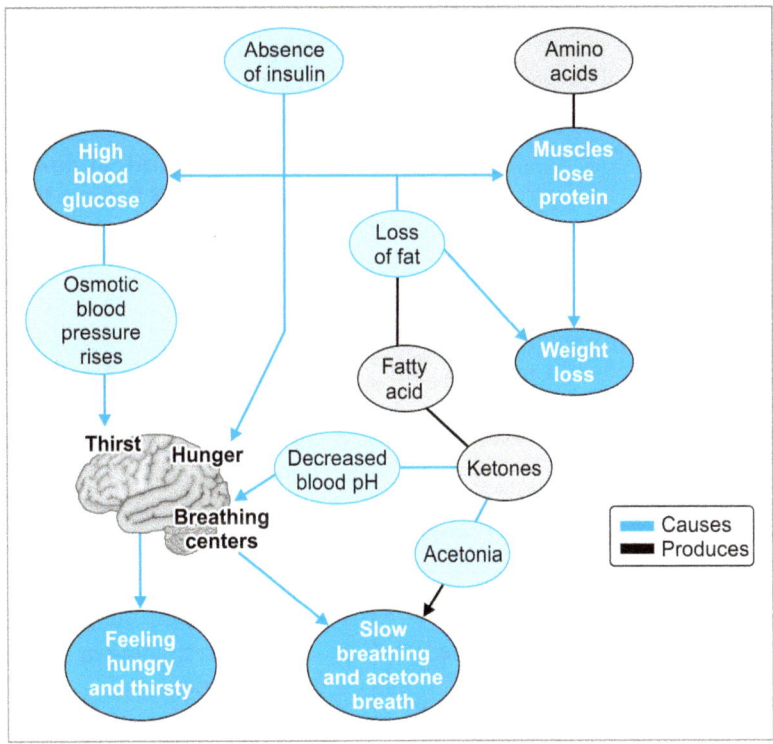

**Fig. 4.24:** Causes and symptoms of diabetes.

- Cause: Total deficiency of insulin due to destruction of β cells of pancreas.
- Clinical complications of this type are retinopathy, neuropathy and nephropathy.

## Type II or Noninsulin Dependent Diabetes Mellitus

This type comprises 90–95% of all diabetic population. The patients have minimum symptoms.
- Not dependent on insulin
- Obesity is common with NIDDM
- Usually occurs after the age of 40 years.
- Sometimes in young person also.

*Diagnosis*: Type I can be known by serious metabolic disturbances with increased blood glucose.

**List the criteria's used to diagnose the diabetes mellitus.**

## Criteria for the Diagnosis

- All adults older than 45 years of age should have a measurement of fasting blood glucose for every 3 months.
- Person with BMI of 27 kg/m$^2$
- Persons with family history of diabetes mellitus.
- Individual with history of gestational diabetes mellitus or delivery of large baby.
- With HDL <35 mg/dL
- Persons with impaired glucose tolerance
- Elevated fasting glucose on more than one occasion.

## Diabetes due to Secondary Causes

- Pancreatic disease

- Cushing's syndrome
- Acromegaly (– GH)
- Increased secretion of glucagon (tumor of pancreas)
- Hyperaldosteronism

## Metabolic Changes in Diabetes Mellitus

### Carbohydrate Metabolism

- Hyperglycemia ($\downarrow$ or impaired transport and uptake of glucose in muscles and adipose tissue).
- Key glycolytic enzymes decreases
- Increased gluconeogenesis
- Glycogen synthesis decreases
- Glycosylated hemoglobin increases in uncontrolled diabetes mellitus.
- *Sorbitol pathway*: Hyperglycemia → Glucose → Sorbitol.
- Increased breakdown of amino acids.

*Protein metabolism:* Protein synthesis decreases.

*Fat metabolism:* Fatty acid synthesis decreases.
- Lipid breakdown increases.
- FA → Acetyl CoA → Cholesterol synthesis or ketone body.

**What is gestational diabetes and what are its complications if not treated?**

## Gestational Diabetes Mellitus

If the carbohydrate intolerance is noticed for the first time during pregnancy in non-diabetic women it is referred to as gestational diabetes mellitus.
- Strong family history of diabetes mellitus, a history of stillbirth or neonatal death, a history of bearing a infant with congenital anomaly are the clues suggesting gestational diabetes mellitus.
- Delivery of large babies is one of the results of gestational diabetes.
- Symptoms of gestational diabetes are mild and it is not expressed in the mother. But it is associated with increased incidence of congenital malformations, increased risk of recurrence of diabetes after 10 years of parturition and prenatal mortality.

**What are the clinical complications of diabetes mellitus? Explain briefly.**

## Clinical Complications of Diabetes Mellitus

### Retinopathy

- Hyperglycemia leads to sorbitol formation
- This may lead to retinal microvascular abnormalities leads to retinopathy and blindness.

### Neuropathy

- A common complication
- Identified by symptoms like pain, numbness, tingling or burning sensation in extremities.

### Angiopathy

- Damage of basement membrane of blood vessels.
- It increases risk of stroke and coronary artery disease.
- It may cause atherosclerosis in medium sized cerebral arteries (leading to paralysis) coronary arteries (leading to myocardial infarction) or peripheral vessels (leading to gangrene of limbs).
- If small vesicles are affected it is called microangiopathy.
- Microangiopathy leads to diabetic retinopathy and nephropathy.

### Nephropathy

- Damage to the glomerulus of nephron of kidney and associated capillaries.
- This leads to decreased filtering capacity.
- Capillary damage is caused by angiopathy and urinary protein detection is useful in the diagnosis of nephropathy.

# CHAPTER 4: Metabolism of Carbohydrates

List the factors which increases the risk of atherosclerosis.

## Hyperlipidemia and Atherosclerosis
* Serum triglyceride, cholesterol and VLDL levels increases in type II.
* HDL decreases
* These factors increase the risk of atherosclerosis.

### Diabetic Ketoacidosis
Deficiency of insulin increases the lipid breakdown → Increased acetyl CoA → Increased cholesterol and ketone bodies. In this condition acetone smell of breath, ketonuria and ketonemia seen. Whole condition is called as ketosis. This leads to the decreased blood pH.

Metabolic acidosis seen due to diabetes, so it is called as diabetic ketoacidosis.

**What are the features of hyperglycemic hyperosmolar nonketotic coma (HHNC)?**

### Hyperglycemic Hyperosmolar Nonketotic Coma
* Characterized by glucose level above >600 mg%.
* Blood pH slightly decreases or normal. Serum osmolality >350 mOsm/kg. Osmotic diuresis due to glucosuria causes severe $H_2O$ and electrolyte depletion.
* Coma results from dehydration of cerebral cells.
* Hyperglycemic hyperosmolar nonketotic coma primarily seen in type II.

**What is glucose tolerance test and what are clinical significance of it?**

## Glucose Tolerance Tests
* Normal person should be able to remove a glucose load from his blood within a specified time. This is known as normal tolerance.
* If the person has elevated blood glucose concentration for longer than the normal time, the condition is called as reduced tolerance.
* If the glucose concentration becomes very low or normal very early than the normal time, then the condition is called as increased tolerance.
* The tests that are used to measure these changes in blood glucose after a glucose load are called glucose tolerance tests (GTT).

**What are the two types of glucose tolerance tests? Explain why and when OGT to be done.**

There are two types:
1. Oral
2. Intravenous GTT

They are mainly used in the detection of diabetes. Oral GTT is the one commonly used in all the laboratories. It is convenient to give glucose through oral route.

### Indications of GTT
* To know the family history of diabetes mellitus.
* Signs and symptoms comparable with diabetics without any complications.
* Glucosuric patients with normal fasting blood sugar.
* Border line of glucose in PPBS
* Reactive hypoglycemia for 3 hours or longer period after food intake.
* Pregnancy with history of abortions, stillbirth and large baby.

**Briefly describe the procedure for performing oral glucose tolerance test (OGTT).**

### Preparation of the Patients
* Patient should not be under fear or anxiety about the possibility of being a diabetic if so it leads to false positive results. So it is the duty of the technician to prepare the patient psychologically or mentally and convince the patients.
* Adequate carbohydrate intake. Before the test the patient should have been on a diet containing at least 150 g of carbohydrate per day with low fat for at least 3 days. An adequate deposit of glycogen in the liver and other tissues is essential for the production of a normal response. If

the subject is in a state of relatively low carbohydrate diet for some time before the test the rise in blood sugar levels following the ingestion of glucose will more pronounced and its fall to the normal level is delayed.
* It is desirable for the subject to fast for 10-12 hours before the test.
* The test patient must not have taken a cup of tea or coffee on the day of test.
* The patient should not have excess amount of exercise.
* If the patient is not well the test should be postponed.
* The patient should not receive any drugs at least for 3 days before the test.

## Factors Affecting GTT

* Factors associated with hyperglycemia, aldosterone, catecholamines, diphenyl-hydantoin (DPH), nicotin, oral contraceptives, thiazides, glucagon and growth hormone.
* Factors associated with hypoglycemia: Ethanol, INH, sulfonamide drugs.
* The glucose tolerance tends to become lower in old age. So age factor is also important.

## Method

* The test is usually carried out in the early morning after an overnight fasting.
* Fasting blood sample and urine is also collected. Then 75 g (or 100 g) of glucose dissolved in about 150–200 mL of water is given to drink.
* Venous blood for the estimation of blood glucose is collected at ½ hourly intervals for 2–2½ hour or hourly intervals for 3 hours after the ingestion of glucose. Urine specimens are also collected at the same time.
* Blood glucose is estimated in each samples and the urine is tested for the presence of the sugar.

## Comments

* Some prefer administration of 1.75 g/kg body weight of glucose. However, amount of glucose makes very little difference in the response of the test.
* It is preferable to give 100 mL of water after the ingestion of glucose which takes away the sweet taste and decreases the risk of vomiting.
* Plasma specimens are more satisfactory than whole blood for glucose analysis, because plasma gives more reliable results and it is independent of hematocrit values.
* Variation in hematocrit values can be accounted for differences in whole blood glucose values.

**Comment on the normal and abnormal glucose tolerance tests.**

## Normal Glucose Tolerance Curve (Fig. 4.25)

The normal curve has the following features:
* The fasting blood glucose in this category is usually within the range of 60–100 mg/dL.
* The blood glucose does not rise above 160 mg/dL.
* The blood glucose at 2 hours after the load is 110 mg/dL.
* The urine remains free of glucose throughout the test.
* The timing of the peak value is not defined as a part of the normal pattern of response but it is usually seen either in the 30 minutes or 60 minutes' blood sample.

| Sample No. | mg glucose/ 100 mL blood | Urine glucose |
| --- | --- | --- |
| Fasting | 90 | Negative |
| 30 minutes | 120 | Negative |
| 60 minutes | 150 | Negative |
| 90 minutes | 140 | Negative |
| 120 minutes | 90 | Negative |

CHAPTER 4: Metabolism of Carbohydrates

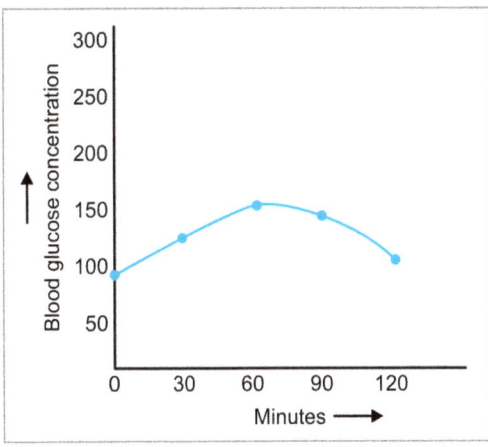

Fig. 4.25: Normal glucose tolerance test.

## Abnormal Glucose Tolerance (Fig. 4.26)

The main features are:
* The fasting level is above 120 mg
* The glucose level crosses 200 mg/100 mL in 30–60 minutes.
* The blood glucose level is more than 110 mg/dL even after 2 hours.

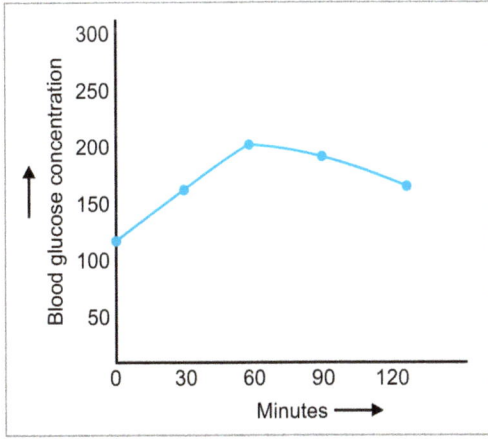

Fig. 4.26: Abnormal glucose tolerance test

* There may be glucose in at least two of the urine specimen.

| Sample No. | mg glucose/100 mL blood | Urine glucose |
|---|---|---|
| Fasting | 120 | Negative |
| 30 minutes | 160 | Positive |
| 60 minutes | 200 | Positive |
| 90 minutes | 180 | Positive |
| 120 minutes | 150 | Negative |

## Conditions Associated with Diminished Glucose Tolerance

* Due to lack of insulin there will be decreased tissue utilization of glucose, which is seen in diabetes mellitus.
* Increased glycogenolysis and gluconeogenesis. This is seen in glucocorticoid excess and hyperthyroidism.
* Increased rate of absorption which is seen in thyrotoxicosis.
* Decreased glycogen storage which is seen in severe hepatic diseases and glycogen storage diseases.

### Increased Glucose Tolerance

Increased glucose tolerance curve is characterized by a flat response.

Conditions associated with increased tolerance:
* Hypothyroidism
* Hypoadrenalism
* Hypopituitarism
* Malabsorption from the GIT
* Renal glycosuria
* *Hyperinsulinism*: This is also characterized by:
  * Fasting hypoglycemia
  * Slight increase in blood glucose following glucose ingestion.

## Intravenous Glucose Tolerance Test

### Preparation of Patient

Poor absorption of orally given glucose may result in a flat tolerance curve. Some patients are unable to tolerate a large amount of carbohydrate load. In these patients an intravenous glucose tolerance test may be performed to eliminate the factors related to the rate of the glucose absorption. This test is also used to monitor the first phase of insulin response in clinical studies.

The preparation of patient is as that of oral GTT. The dose of glucose is 0.5 g/kg body weight (25 g/dL solution). The dose is administered intravenously over 3 minutes through one hand and blood is collected at every 10 minutes from the opposite arm after the mid injection time for 1 hour and rate of glucose clearance is calculated.

**What is lactic acidosis and mention the cause for it.**

## Lactic Acidosis

*Cause:* Accumulation of lactic acid due to over production or underutilization.

If diabetic patients treated with hypoglycemic drugs (phenformes) lactic acidosis seen.
*Infection:* Susceptible to infection.
*Pregnancy:* Fetal abnormalities, premature birth, big babies, chances of absorption if they are not treated for diabetes.

## Hypoglycemia

### Fasting Hypoglycemia

Fasting hypoglycemia is a type of hypoglycemia, or low blood sugar, that occurs when the stomach is empty. Fasting hypoglycemia is diagnosed as a blood glucose level of less than 50 mg/dL. The signs and symptoms with prolonged hypoglycemia are: Headache, confusion, giddiness, lethargy to seizures and may lead to loss of consciousness and even death. These symptoms are also known as neuroglycopenia.

### Reactive Hypoglycemia

It is the general term for having a hypo after eating, which is when blood glucose levels become dangerously low following a meal. Also known as postprandial hypoglycemia, drops in blood sugar are usually recurrent and occur within 4 hours after eating.

### Neonatal Hypoglycemia

Plasma glucose level of less than 30 mg/dL in the first 24 hours of life and less than 45 mg/dL thereafter, is the most common metabolic problem in newborns.

## Glycosylated Hemoglobin

Hemoglobin to which glucose is bound. Glycation is one of the nonenzymatic processes where the addition of sugar residue to amino groups of proteins takes place.

Glycosylated hemoglobin is tested to monitor the long-term control of diabetes mellitus. The level of glycosylated hemoglobin is increased in the red blood cells of persons with poorly controlled diabetes mellitus.

The formation of glycated hemoglobin is an irreversible process, and the blood level depends on both the life span of the red blood cell and the blood glucose concentration.

Since the glucose stays attached to hemoglobin for the life of the red blood cell (normally about 120 days), the level of glycosylated hemoglobin reflects the average blood glucose level over the past 3 months.

The human adult usually consists of HbA1: 97%, HbA2: 2.5% and HbF: 0.5%.

The values of glycated hemoglobin are free of day-to-day glucose fluctuations and unaffected by exercise or food ingestion.

Glycated hemoglobin testing is recommended for both (a) checking blood sugar control in people who might be pre-diabetic and (b) monitoring blood sugar control in patients with more elevated levels, termed diabetes mellitus.

# CHAPTER 4: Metabolism of Carbohydrates

## SUMMARY

Carbohydrates are the essential component of diet. The pancreatic and intestinal enzymes hydrolyze the polysaccharides to simple monosaccharides. The galactose and glucose are absorbed very rapidly by the active process. Fructose and mannose are absorbed by a $Na^+$ independent facilitative diffusion. Glucose is the main source of energy to our body. Glucose undergoes glycolysis to generate the energy in the form of ATP. Pyruvate and lactate are the end products of aerobic and anerobic glycolysis respectively. Puruvate formed in aerobic glycolysis converted to acetyl CoA which enters TCA cycle to generate large number of ATPs. The acetyl CoA is also required to synthesize cholesterol, fatty acids, ketone bodies and steroid hormones. Insulin stimulates the glycogenesis through which excess glucose absorbed will be converted to glycogen and stored in muscle and liver. Hyperglycemic hormones stimulate the glycogen breakdown when glucose level goes down. Glycogenesis and glycogenolysis are regulated by glycogen synthase and glycogen phosphorylase respectively. Hyperglycemic hormones stimulate the gluconeogenesis to regulate the blood glucose level. Hexose monophosphate pathway generates large number of NADPH which is required to maintain the active reduced glutathione peroxidase and to synthesize fatty acids. Pathway also produces ribose sugars which is the essential component for the synthesis of nucleic acids. The insulin deficiency or defect in its mechanism of action results in diabetes mellitus which are of two types: insulin dependent diabetes mellitus and non-insulin dependent diabetes mellitus. The symptoms of diabetes are polyuria, polyphagia, polydipsia, numbness at the feet, infection and poor wound healing. The major complications of diabetes are retinopathy, nephropathy and neuropathy. The fasting blood glucose and HbA1c are used to detect and monitor diabetes. Oral glucose tolerance test is preferred to detect the diabetes mellitus during pregnancy and other conditions.

## SELF-ASSESSMENT QUESTIONS ON DIGESTION AND ABSORPTION

### Long Answer Questions

1. Briefly describe the process of digestion and absorption of carbohydrates.
2. Explain the process of sodium dependent glucose transport.
3. Mention the enzymes of gastrointestinal tract.

### Short Answer Questions

1. Add a brief note on absorption of glucose.
2. Mention the enzymes, which play a role in the digestion of carbohydrates.
3. Describe why cellulose is not digested. What is the importance of it in the diet?

## MULTIPLE CHOICE QUESTIONS

1. **All the following enzymes help in the digestion of carbohydrates, *except*:**
   (a) Amylase  (b) Lipase
   (c) Sucrase  (d) Maltase
2. **Following statements are true with the absorption of glucose, *except*:**
   (a) Occurs against the concentration gradient  (b) Requires a carrier protein
   (c) Does not require ATP  (d) Sodium dependent transport mechanism
3. **The qubain is the:**
   (a) Inhibitor of lipid absorption  (b) Carrier protein
   (c) Inhibitor of carbohydrate absorption  (d) Enzyme

| ANSWERS | | |
|---|---|---|
| 1. a | 2. c | 3. c |

## SELF-ASSESSMENT QUESTIONS ON METABOLISM OF CARBOHYDRATES

1. Outline the reactions of anaerobic glycolysis. Give its energetics.
2. Briefly discuss the aerobic glycolysis under the following headings:
   (a) Reactions
   (b) Energetics
   (c) Regulation.
3. Explain the steps involved in TCA cycle. Give the energetics.
4. Mention the importance of TCA cycle.
5. Describe how glycogen is formed and utilized in human body.
6. Discuss the metabolism which follows the strenuous exercise.
7. Explain the significance of HMP shunt.
8. Give the key reactions of gluconeogenesis.
9. How pyruvate is converted to acetyl CoA?
10. How the glycogenolysis operates in muscles to meet the energy demand?
11. Add a note on the pentose pathway and write its importance.
12. Briefly discuss the synthesis of glycogen from glucose and mention the condition it is active.
13. What are the two types of diabetes mellitus and discuss them briefly?
14. How the glycogenolysis operates in muscles to meet the energy demand?
15. How the hormones play a major role in the regulation of glucose?
16. Which pathway is referred to as amphibolic pathway?
17. Name the linkage present in glycogen at branching point.
18. Glucose-6-phosphatase deficiency leads what?
19. Which enzyme converts glucose to glucose-6- phosphate during fed state?
20. What do call if conversion of muscle lactates into liver glucose?
21. Which pathway helps in the detoxification of bilirubin?
22. Which enzyme deficiency leads to galactosemia?
23. Name the deficient enzyme of von Gierke's disease?
24. Which enzyme deficiency leads to McArdle's disease?
25. Name the enzyme, which is deficient in lactose intolerance?
26. Discuss the regulation of glycogenesis and glycogenolysis.

## MULTIPLE CHOICE QUESTIONS

1. **All of the following are inhibitors of the TCA cycle, *except*:**
   (a) Aconitase
   (b) Malonate
   (c) Fluoroacetate
   (d) Fluoride
2. **One of the following enzyme catalyzes substrate level phosphorylation:**
   (a) Hexokinase
   (b) Enolase
   (c) Phosphoglycerate kinase
   (d) Succinate dehydrogenase
3. **The noncompetitive inhibitor that inhibits glyceraldehyde-3-P dehydrogenase is:**
   (a) Fluoride
   (b) Bromohydroxy acetone-p
   (c) Malonate
   (d) Arsenite

## CHAPTER 4: Metabolism of Carbohydrates

4. The number of ATP molecules produced on complete oxidation of glucose under aerobic condition is:
   (a) 38 ATP
   (b) 10 ATP
   (c) 2 ATP
   (d) 8 ATP
5. All the following are the rate limiting enzymes of gluconeogenesis, *except*:
   (a) Pyruvate kinase
   (b) Glucose-6-phosphatase
   (c) Fructose-1,6-phosphatase
   (d) Phosphoenol pyruvate carboxykinase
6. All the following organs contain glucose-6-phosphatase, *except*:
   (a) Kidney
   (b) Liver
   (c) Muscle
   (d) Intestine
7. One of the following is not a symptom of von Gierke's disease:
   (a) Liver enlargement
   (b) Fasting hypoglycemia
   (c) Ketosis
   (d) Hypouricemia
8. The hexose monophosphate shunt is located in the:
   (a) Cytosol
   (b) Mitochondrion
   (c) Lysosome
   (d) Golgi apparatus
9. Hexokinase:
   (a) Present in all the tissues
   (b) Phosphorylates glucose only
   (c) Is not inhibited by glucose-6-phosphate
   (d) Has low affinity for substrates
10. The end-product of muscle glycolysis is:
    (a) Pyruvate
    (b) Fructose 6-P
    (c) Glyceraldehyde 3-phosphate
    (d) Lactate
11. Regarding 2,3 BPG, the following statements are true, *except*:
    (a) It binds to oxyhemoglobin and helps in unloading of oxygen
    (b) It reduces the affinity of hemoglobin to oxygen
    (c) It does not bind to hemoglobin
    (d) Its concentration increases in hypoxic conditions
12. All of the following enzymes catalyzes irreversible steps of glycolysis, *except*:
    (a) Pyruvate kinase
    (b) Hexokinase
    (c) Enolase
    (d) Phosphofructokinase
13. All of the following inhibits the enzyme glycogen phosphorylase, *except*:
    (a) Glucose-6-phosphate
    (b) ATP
    (c) AMP
    (d) Liver glucose
14. The pathway that predominantly produces NADPH is:
    (a) TCA Cycle
    (b) Glycolysis
    (c) HMP shunt
    (d) Gluconeogenesis
15. A classic example of exergonic reaction is the hydrolysis of:
    (a) ADP
    (b) GMP
    (c) ATP
    (d) GTP
16. The end product of anaerobic glycolysis is:
    (a) Pyruvate
    (b) Fructose-6-P
    (c) Glyceraldehyde-3-phosphate
    (d) Lactate
17. The glycolytic enzyme inhibited by fluoride is:
    (a) Pyruvate kinase
    (b) Enolase
    (c) Glyceraldehyde-3-phosphate dehydrogenase
    (d) Hexokinase

18. One of the following hormones inhibits gluconeogenesis:
    (a) Glucagon
    (b) Insulin
    (c) Adrenaline
    (d) Cortisol
19. One of the following is not a clinical complication of type II diabetes:
    (a) Nephropathy
    (b) Retinopathy
    (c) Neuropathy
    (d) Cardiomyopathy
20. The fate of pyruvate in aerobic condition is its conversion to:
    (a) Lactate
    (b) Cholesterol
    (c) Acetyl CoA
    (d) Ribose
21. The final and common pathway for the oxidation of carbohydrates, fats and proteins is:
    (a) Gluconeogenesis
    (b) Tricarboxylic acid cycle
    (c) Hexose monophosphate shunt
    (d) Glycogenesis
22. One molecule of glucose on complete oxidation in anaerobic condition generates:
    (a) 30 molecules of ATP
    (b) 24 molecules of ATP
    (c) 2 molecules of ATP
    (d) 38 molecules of ATP
23. Cori's cycle involves the conversion of:
    (a) Pyruvate to lactate in muscle
    (b) Muscle lactate to glucose in the liver
    (c) Pyruvate to glucose in the liver
    (d) Liver glucose to lactate
24. One of the following is not a coenzyme for pyruvate dehydrogenase:
    (a) TPP
    (b) NAD
    (c) PLP
    (d) CoASH
25. A hormone that stimulates the activation of glycogen phosphorylase is:
    (a) Glucagon
    (b) Insulin
    (c) Progesterone
    (d) Estrogen
26. McArdle's disease is due to the deficiency of:
    (a) Liver glycogen phosphorylase
    (b) Liver glycogen synthase
    (c) Lysosomal glucosidase
    (d) Muscle glycogen phosphorylase
27. Glucose-6-phosphate dehydrogenase catalyzes the conversion of glucose to:
    (a) Fructose 6-phosphate
    (b) 6-phosphogluconolactone
    (c) Xylulose 5-phosphate
    (d) Ribulose 5-phosphate
28. One of the following is not a significant function of the HMP shunt:
    (a) Pentose production
    (b) NADH production
    (c) NADPH production
    (d) Ribose-5-P production
29. All of the following inhibits the enzyme citrate synthase, *except*:
    (a) ATP
    (b) NADH
    (c) Acyl CoA
    (d) ADP
30. One of the following enzyme catalyzes substrate level phosphorylation of the TCA cycle:
    (a) Fumarase
    (b) Malate dehydrogenase
    (c) Succinate thiokinase
    (d) α-ketoglutarate dehydrogenase
31. All of the following stimulate the gluconeogenesis, *except*:
    (a) Glucagon
    (b) ADH
    (c) Acetyl CoA
    (d) Adrenaline
32. The complete oxidation of one molecule of acetyl CoA in the TCA cycle generates:
    (a) 12 ATP
    (b) 10 ATP
    (c) 38 ATP
    (d) 8 ATP

33. **Malonate is a competitive inhibitor of:**
    - (a) Aconitase
    - (b) α-ketoglutarate dehydrogenase
    - (c) Succinate dehydrogenase
    - (d) Fumarase
34. **All the following are the rate limiting enzymes of gluconeogenesis, *except*:**
    - (a) Pyruvate dehydrogenase
    - (b) Glucose-6-phosphatase
    - (c) Fructose-6-phosphatase
    - (d) Phosphoenolpyruvate carboxykinase
35. **During glycogenesis the α-1,6 linkage is introduced by:**
    - (a) Amylo-1, 4 α 1,6-transglucosidase
    - (b) 1,4-glucan transferase
    - (c) Phosphorylase
    - (d) Glycogen synthase
36. **Glucose-6-phosphatase is absent in:**
    - (a) Kidney
    - (b) Liver
    - (c) Muscle
    - (d) Intestine
37. **Von Gierke's disease is the result of a deficiency of:**
    - (a) Liver phosphorylase
    - (b) Liver glucose-6-phosphatase
    - (c) Glycogen synthase
    - (d) Muscle phosphorylase
38. **The TCA cycle is located in the:**
    - (a) Cytosol
    - (b) Mitochondrion
    - (c) Lysosome
    - (d) Golgi apparatus
39. **One of the following processes requires NADPH:**
    - (a) Synthesis of fatty acids
    - (b) Reduction of protein
    - (c) Synthesis of glycogen
    - (d) Synthesis of glucagon
40. **One of the following conditions supports the formation of fructose 2,6-bisphosphate:**
    - (a) High blood glucose
    - (b) Low blood glucose
    - (c) Normal blood glucose
    - (d) High blood cholesterol
41. **Regarding glucokinase, all of the following statements are true, *except*:**
    - (a) It is present in all the tissues
    - (b) It is present in liver
    - (c) It is not inhibited by glucose-6-phosphate
    - (d) It has high Km for glucose
42. **The synthesis of glucose from non-carbohydrate sources is called:**
    - (a) Gluconeogenesis
    - (b) Glycogenesis
    - (c) Glycolysis
    - (d) Glycogenolysis
43. **Hers' disease is due to the deficiency of:**
    - (a) Liver phosphorylase
    - (b) Liver glucose-6-phosphatase
    - (c) Glycogen synthase
    - (d) Muscle phosphorylase
44. **All of the following are the examples for noncompetitive inhibitors, *except*:**
    - (a) Iodoacetate
    - (b) Arsenite
    - (c) Malonate
    - (d) Fluoride
45. **total number of ATP formed during aerobic glycolysis is:**
    - (a) 10
    - (b) 8
    - (c) 4
    - (d) 2
46. **Net AtP formed during anaerobic glycolysis:**
    - (a) 8
    - (b) 4
    - (c) 2
    - (d) 10
47. **Hormone which stimulate glycolysis is:**
    - (a) Glucagon
    - (b) Insulin
    - (c) Thyroxine
    - (d) Cortisol

48. **Glycolysis cycle operates in:**
    (a) Cytosol
    (b) Mitochondria
    (c) Ribosomes
    (d) Nucleus
49. **Number of ATP formed in TCA cycle from acetyl CoA, is formed from a molecule of glucose is:**
    (a) 30
    (b) 32
    (c) 24
    (d) 40
50. **All the following are the examples for hyperglycemic hormones, *except*:**
    (a) Glucagon
    (b) Insulin
    (c) Epinephrine
    (d) Growth hormone
51. **Glutathione (GSH):**
    (a) Protects RBCs from oxidative damage
    (b) When oxidized decomposes $H_2O_2$
    (c) Once oxidized is converted back to reduced form by glutathione transferase
    (d) Is reduced by FADH and NADH
52. **Which of the following is inhibited by arsenate poisoning?**
    (a) Aconitase
    (b) Malonate dehydrogenase
    (c) α-ketoglutarate dehydrogenase
    (d) Succinate dehydrogenase
53. **One of the following is not a gluconeogenic substrate:**
    (a) Glycerol
    (b) Tryptophan
    (c) Lactate
    (d) Fructose
54. **A healthy 20-year-old boy ate a carbohydrate rich meal. After 2 hours the activities of the following enzymes would increase, *except*:**
    (a) Hexokinase
    (b) Phosphofructokinase
    (c) Glycogen synthase
    (d) Glycogen phosphorylase
55. **One of the following enzymes becomes active during strenuous exercise:**
    (a) Glycogen synthase
    (b) Glucose-6-phosphatase
    (c) Glycogen phosphorylase
    (d) Fructose-6-phosphatase
56. **Concerning glycogen metabolism, one of the following statements is incorrect:**
    (a) Glycogen synthesis takes place in liver and muscle
    (b) Glycogecn is stored in liver and muscle
    (c) Glucose-6-phosphatase is present in muscle
    (d) Muscle glycogen serves as a fuel reserve for the supply of ATP during muscle contraction
57. **Insulin activates the key enzymes of:**
    (a) Gluconeogenesis
    (b) Glycolysis
    (c) Glycogenolysis
    (d) None of the above
58. **The enzyme which is very active during hyperglycemia is:**
    (a) Pyruvate carboxykinase
    (b) Fructose-2,6-bisphosphatase
    (c) Fructose-1,6-bisphosphatase
    (d) Phosphofructokinase 2
59. **The conversion of pyruvate to acetyl CoA, requires all of the following, *except*:**
    (a) TPP
    (b) NAD
    (c) FAD
    (d) PLP
60. **A 12-year-old child was playing football for the first time. He immediately got tired and complained to his mother that he could not tolerate the exercise. the possible defect in this child may be the absence of:**
    (a) Liver glycogen synthase
    (b) Glucose-6-phosphatase
    (c) Amylo α-1,6-glucosidase
    (d) Muscle glycogen phosphorylase

## CHAPTER 4: Metabolism of Carbohydrates

61. One of the following blood parameter helps to know about the one month past history of blood glucose:
    (a) Insulin
    (b) C peptide
    (c) HbA1c
    (d) Cholesterol
62. All the following are necessary for glucose absorption:
    (a) $Na^+$
    (b) ATP
    (c) Carrier protein
    (d) $K^+$
63. One of the following is not a enzyme of pancreatic origin:
    (a) Amylase
    (b) Sucrase
    (c) Lipase
    (d) Ribonuclease
64. All the following are the criteria for the diagnosis of diabetes, *except*:
    (a) Persons family history of diabetes
    (b) Persons with BMI of 27 kg/m²
    (c) Persons with elevated creatinine
    (d) Persons with impaired glucose tolerance
65. One of the following enzyme deficiency leads to galactosemia is:
    (a) Galactose-1-phosphate dehydrogenase
    (b) Galactose-1-phosphate uridyl transferase
    (c) Galactose-1-phosphate kinase
    (d) Galactose-1-phosphate uridyl transpeptidase
66. One of the following enzymes is absent in humans:
    (a) Pepsin
    (b) Lipase
    (c) Cellulose
    (d) Carboxypeptidase
67. A 4-year-old child has massive liver enlargement and sever persistent hypoglycemia and ketosis. Which of the following disease classes should be suspected?
    (a) Diabetes
    (b) Glycogen storage disease
    (c) Glysosomal storage disorder
    (d) Mucopolysaccharidoses
68. For very high force contractions lasting 1–2 seconds, the initial energy source is from:
    (a) Glycolysis
    (b) Glycogenolysis
    (c) Phosphocreatine stores
    (d) ATP stores
69. The most rapid method to resynthesize ATP during exercise is through:
    (a) Glycolysis
    (b) Tricarboxylic acid cycle
    (c) Glycogenolysis
    (d) Phosphocreatine breakdown
70. Energy released from the breakdown of the high-energy phosphates, ATP and phosphocreatine, can sustain maximal exertion exercise for about:
    (a) 2–4 seconds
    (b) 5–10 seconds
    (c) 50–60 seconds
    (d) 100–220 seconds
71. The conversion of one molecule of glucose to two molecules of lactate results in the net formation of:
    (a) 6 molecules of water
    (b) 2 molecules of ATP
    (c) 8 molecules of ATP
    (d) 38 molecules of ATP
72. The enzymes of glycolysis are located in the:
    (a) Mitochondrion
    (b) Nucleus
    (c) Ribosomes
    (d) Cytoplasm
73. Glycogen breakdown in exercising muscle is activated by:
    (a) Insulin
    (b) Cortisol
    (c) Epinephrine
    (d) Hexokinase

74. **More hydrogen ions are formed when:**
    (a) Glycogen becomes reduced
    (b) Phosphocreatine catabolism occurs
    (c) Pyruvate is converted to lactate
    (d) Glycolysis is being used as a major means of resynthesizing ATP
75. **The net production of ATP via substrate level phosphorylation in glycolysis is:**
    (a) 8 from glucose and 10 from glycogen
    (b) 2 from glucose and 3 from glycogen
    (c) 3 from glucose and 4 from glycogen
    (d) 4 from glucose and 2 from glycogen
76. **Muscle lactate production increases when:**
    (a) Glycolysis is activated at the onset of exercise
    (b) Oxygen is readily available
    (c) Pyruvate cannot be formed from glucose breakdown
    (d) Muscle glycogen becomes depleted
77. **Embedded in the inner membrane of the mitochondrion are:**
    (a) The enzymes of the tricarboxylic acid cycle (Kreb's cycle)
    (b) Triacylglycerol molecules
    (c) GLUT2 molecules
    (d) The components of the electron transport chain
78. **Glucose enters muscle cells mostly by:**
    (a) Simple diffusion
    (b) Facilitated diffusion using a specific glucose transporter
    (c) Cotransport with sodium
    (d) Cotransport with amino acids
79. **Aerobic resynthesis of ATP occurs:**
    (a) In the mitochondria in a process called glycogenolysis
    (b) In the cytosol
    (c) In the mitochondria in a process called oxidative phosphorylation
    (d) In the sarcoplasmic reticulum
80. **The synthesis of glucose from lactate and amino acids is called:**
    (a) Gluconeogenesis
    (b) Glycogenolysis
    (c) Glycolysis
    (d) Glycogenesis
81. **The energy for all forms of muscle contraction is provided by:**
    (a) ADP
    (b) Phosphocreatine
    (c) GDP
    (d) ATP
82. **Liver glycogen breakdown is stimulated by:**
    (a) Insulin
    (b) Glucagon
    (c) Adrenaline
    (d) Both b and c
83. **The major source of carbohydrate in a typical Western diet is:**
    (a) Starch
    (b) Cellulose
    (c) Glycogen
    (d) Lactose
84. **Substrate-level phosphorylation differs from oxidative phosphorylation in that:**
    (a) Oxidative phosphorylation involves the transfer of electrons
    (b) Substrate level phosphorylation involves the transfer of electrons
    (c) Substrate level phosphorylation only occurs in the cytosol
    (d) Oxidative phosphorylation only occurs in the cytosol

85. Which of the following promotes glucose and amino acid uptake by muscle?
    (a) Adrenaline
    (b) Glucagon
    (c) Insulin
    (d) Cortisol
86. During prolonged exercise increased amounts of interleukin-6 are released from:
    (a) Exercising muscle and influence carbohydrate and fat metabolism
    (b) Macrophages and cause suppression of fibroblasts functions
    (c) Lymphocytes and inhibit macrophage function
    (d) All muscles in the body and influence carbohydrate metabolism
87. In the study of a 14-year-old male patient who suspect has a deficiency of muscle glycogen phosphorylase, indicate a test based in exercising his forearm by squeezing a rubber ball compared with the normal person performing the same exercise, this patient would exhibit which of the following?
    (a) Exercise for a longer time without fatigue
    (b) Increased glucose levels in blood drawn from his forearm
    (c) Decreased lactate levels in blood drawn from his forearm
    (d) Hyperglycemia
88. A 3-year-old male patient was transferred to hospital for further investigation of hepatomegaly. His parents were first cousins. It was learned that he was hospitalized for recurrent vomiting at 2 months of age, but no obvious cause was found and the symptoms then disappeared spontaneously. When he was 3 years old, his parents noticed his failure to thrive and hepatomegaly was noted on physical examination. Laboratory tests showed fructosemia and fructosuria. Other tests confirmed a hereditary fructose intolerance. Besides fructose, which of the following carbohydrates should be obviously forbidden in this patient diet?
    (a) Glucose
    (b) Starch
    (c) Lactose
    (d) Sucrose
89. A 20-month-old male patient presents convulsions after a history of frequent morning fatigue before feeding. RBS shows 25 mg% and the hypoglycemia is treated accordingly. At the physical examination it is found a liver span of 14 cm and a grade III systolic murmur. The patient is hospitalized for further study. ECG shows a left ventricular hypertrophy. While hospitalized, blood test shows normal RBS, but elevated ALT (alanine aminotransferase), AST (aspartate aminotransferase), GGT (gammaglutamyl transpeptidase) and creatine kinase. Given the history of the case a glycogen storage disease was suspected and specific test were indicated. The following results were obtained:

    During a fasting challenge the time to hypoglycemia was 3 hours

    Blood glucose increased after the administration of glucagon

    Liver biopsy showed fibrosis with glycogen filled hepatocytes.

    With this information, which of the following enzymes activity do you expect to find decreased in this patient hepatocytes?
    (a) Phosphoglucomutase
    (b) UDP-glucose uridyl transferase
    (c) Glycogen synthase
    (d) Debranching enzyme
90. A 69-year-old man with Alzheimer's disease and a 12 years' history of type 2 diabetes is brought to a family practice clinic by his elder son. The patient is unable to give a clear account of how carefully he controls his blood glucose. Which of the following laboratory parameters could be used to assess glycemic control over the past 3–4 months?
    (a) Fasting blood glucose
    (b) Blood insulin levels
    (c) Glycosylated hemoglobin (HbA1c)
    (d) Urinary glucose

**Answer is c.** The amount of glycosylated hemoglobin (HbA1c) is directly related to the level of glucose in the blood. Since HbA1c is a stable product, its concentration reflects glucose levels over the past 3–6 months. HbA1c forms as a result of nonenzymatic glycosylation, a fundamental biochemical abnormality that accounts for most of the histopathologic alterations in diabetes mellitus. At first, glucose forms reversible glycosylation products with proteins by formation of Schiff bases. Rearrangement of Schiff bases leads to more stable, but still reversible, Amadori products and subsequently to irreversible advanced glycosylation end products (AGE), of which HbA1c is an example. Blood ketones, blood glucose, urinary glucose, and blood insulin do not reflect long-standing metabolic abnormalities of diabetes mellitus and cannot be used to assess long-term glycemic control.

91. **Which one of the following statements is false?**
    (a) The enzymes of the tricarboxylic acid cycle (TCA) are located in the mitochondria
    (b) TCA cycle is of no metabolic significance for the oxidation of fatty acids or amino acids
    (c) TCA cycle is an oxidative process
    (d) The cycle functions irreversibly

92. **Gastric secretion is:**
    (a) Inhibited by cholecystokinin
    (b) Stimulated by gastric inhibitory peptide
    (c) Stimulated by sympathetic stimulation
    (d) Stimulated by nicotinic agonists

93. **Patient having McArdle's disease suffers from painful muscle cramping after brief exercise. The condition results from a deficiency of the following enzymes in glycogen breakdown:**
    (a) Muscle glycogen phosphorylase
    (b) Muscle amylo-1,6-glucosidase
    (c) Liver glycogen phosphorylase
    (d) Liver amylo-1,6-glucosidase activity

94. **A 30-year-old man with a history of insulin-dependent diabetes mellitus was treated for a urinary tract infection. Two weeks later, she presented with persistent flank pain. The examination showed that he was a moderately ill-appearing person who was afebrile with a heart rate of 100, respiratory rate of 16, and BP of 180/95 mm Hg. He did not appear to be dehydrated. There was costovertebral angle tenderness on the left and left lower quadrant tenderness with guarding, but without rebound tenderness. Laboratory results:**

    *Serum electrolytes*

    | | |
    |---|---|
    | Sodium | 127 mEq/l |
    | Potassium chloride | 5 |
    | Bicarbonate 17 | 92 |
    | Glucose | 640 mg/dL |
    | BUN | 32 |
    | Creatinine | 1.6 |

    *Urinalysis*

    | | |
    |---|---|
    | Appearance | Pink/cloudy |
    | Glucose | 3+ |
    | Ketones | 2+ |
    | Protein | 3+ |
    | Sediment | RBcs found plenty |
    | WBcs | Many |

    1. What is the probable cause of the patient's renal problem?
    2. How does the urinalysis support this diagnosis?
    3. What do you think the decreased bicarbonate value means?
    4. What do you think of the patient's BUN and creatinine values?

# CHAPTER 4: Metabolism of Carbohydrates

## ANSWERS

| | | | | | | | | |
|---|---|---|---|---|---|---|---|---|
| 1. d | 2. c | 3. b | 4. a | 5. a | 6. c | 7. d | 8. a |
| 9. b | 10. d | 11. c | 12. c | 13. c | 14. c | 15. c | 16. d |
| 17. b | 18. b | 19. d | 20. c | 21. b | 22. c | 23. b | 24. c |
| 25. a | 26. d | 27. b | 28. b | 29. d | 30. c | 31. b | 32. a |
| 33. c | 34. a | 35. a | 36. c | 37. b | 38. b | 39. a | 40. a |
| 41. a | 42. a | 43. a | 44. c | 45. b | 46. c | 47. b | 48. a |
| 49. c | 50. b | 51. a | 52. c | 53. d | 54. d | 55. c | 56. c |
| 57. b | 58. d | 59. d | 60. d | 61. c | 62. d | 63. b | 64. c |
| 65. b | 66. c | 67. b | 68. d | 69. d | 70. b | 71. d | 72. d |
| 73. c | 74. d | 75. b | 76. a | 77. d | 78. b | 79. c | 80. a |
| 81. d | 82. d | 83. a | 84. a | 85. c | 86. a | 87. b | 88. d |
| 89. c | 90. c | 91. b | 92. a | 93. a | | | |

*94. Acute Pyelonephritis*

Diabetic patients are generally susceptible to infections, and this patient has a potential source for a kidney infection in the previous UTI, which can ascend the ureters to reach the kidneys.

She has pain in her flank and appears ill, with an elevated white cell count and an increased number of immature white cell forms (bands). The physical examination reveals pain on palpation in the left lower back and abdomen. These signs point to a localized infection; back pain is suggestive of a retroperitoneal location. Patients with acute pyelonephritis will generally be febrile, but this patient has been treated for a UTI and may still be on oral antibiotics. This could be partially suppressing the infection.

The urinalysis is consistent with infection in the urinary tract: Pink urine is consistent with blood, the cloudiness is consistent with bacteria and/or tissue debris, more than 20 WBS/HPF confirms infection. Protein is commonly elevated in urinary tract and kidney infections and may be derived from the inflammatory response and tissue destruction.

The elevated glucose and ketones suggest that the patient's diabetes may not be in good control. This result is confirmed by the plasma glucose of 700 mg/dL.

This urinalysis could occur in a bladder infection, but is also consistent with a kidney infection. It would more strongly support a kidney infection if it contained casts, particularly white cell casts.

*Metabolic Acidosis*

Bicarbonate is reduced in metabolic acidosis or metabolic compensation of respiratory alkalosis. In this case, the serum glucose is markedly elevated and there are glucose and ketones in the urine. These findings in combination with the decreased bicarbonate suggest a mild diabetic ketoacidosis. Diabetic ketoacidosis is one of the forms of metabolic acidosis that produces an increased anion gap. If you calculate the anion gap for this patient, you will find that it is mildly elevated at 18, consistent with the hypothesis of a mild ketoacidosis.

The patient's creatinine is mildly elevated, suggesting some decrease in GFR. However, the BUN is disproportionately increased, leading to a BUN/creatinine ratio over 15. Part of this prerenal azotemia could be related to hypovolemia as a result of osmotic diuresis from elevated glucose (but the patient appears well-hydrated) or to increased urea production related to tissue destruction in the infected area.

# Chapter 5
# Chemistry of Amino Acids and Proteins

## LEARNING OBJECTIVES

*At the end of this chapter students should be able to:*
- Understand the classification of amino acids on the basis of their properties and functions
- Know about the biologically important peptides
- Define and classify proteins on the basis of their properties
- Explain the different structural organization of proteins
- Define the process of denaturation, causes and properties of the denatured proteins

## Introduction

Proteins are the group of organic compounds of carbon, hydrogen, oxygen, and nitrogen (sulfur and phosphorus may also be present). They are of prime importance to the living systems.

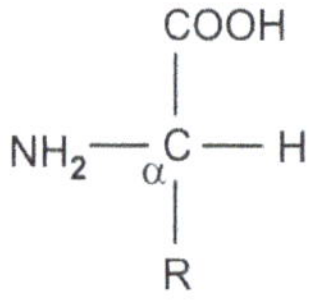

$$NH_2 - \underset{\alpha}{C} - H$$
with COOH above and R below

L-amino acid

All the biologically active proteins comprise nearly 22 different amino acids ($\alpha$-L-amino acids), which are called the building blocks of proteins.

## Definition of an $\alpha$-Amino Acid

Amino acids are organic compounds, which contain two functional groups—the basic $-NH_2$ group (amino group) and the $-COOH$ group or (carboxyl group).

The carbon atom attached with $-NH_2$ and $-COOH$ group is called $\alpha$-carbon.

Where R- is the side chain of amino acid and can be hydrogen or an aliphatic group, aromatic group, or heterocyclic group.

Following are the 20 different amino acids, which occur in the nature.

| Name | Abbreviation | Symbols | Structural formula |
|---|---|---|---|
| Alanine | Ala | A | $CH_3-CH(NH_2)-COOH$ 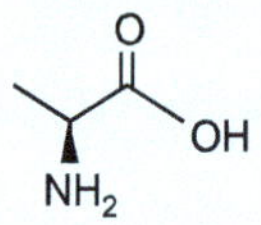 |
| | | | (structure with C=O, OH, $NH_2$) |
| Arginine | Arg | R | $HN=C(NH_2)-NH-(CH_2)_3-CH(NH_2)-COOH$ 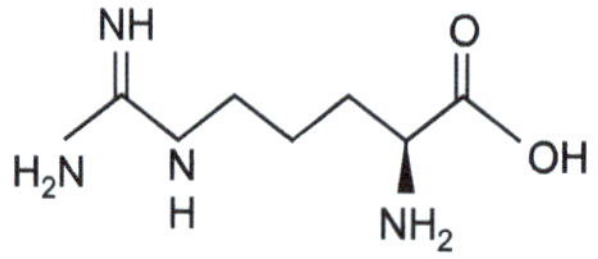 |
| | | | (structure with NH, $H_2N$, N, H, $NH_2$, OH) |

*Contd...*

*Contd...*

| | | | |
|---|---|---|---|
| Asparagine | Asn | N | $H_2N-CO-CH_2-CH(NH_2)-COOH$ 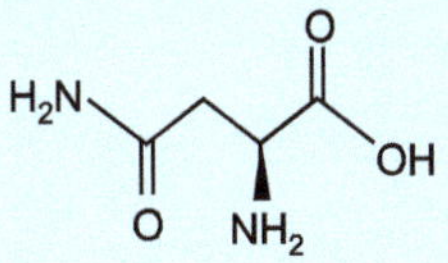 |
| Aspartic acid | Asp | D | $HOOC-CH_2-CH(NH_2)-COOH$ 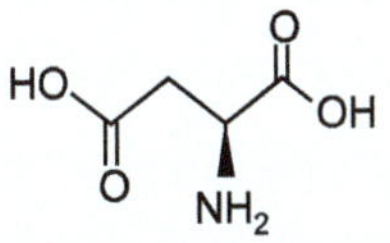 |
| Cysteine | Cys | C | $HS-CH_2-CH(NH_2)-COOH$ 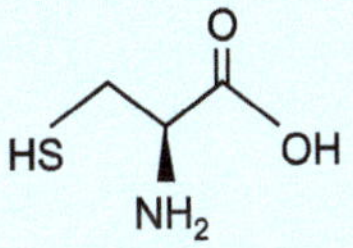 |
| Glutamine | Gln | Q | $H_2N-CO-(CH_2)_2-CH(NH_2)-COOH$ 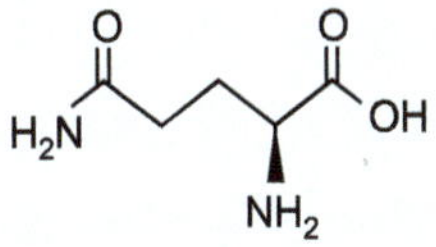 |
| Glutamic acid | Glu | E | $HOOC-(CH_2)_2-CH(NH_2)-COOH$ 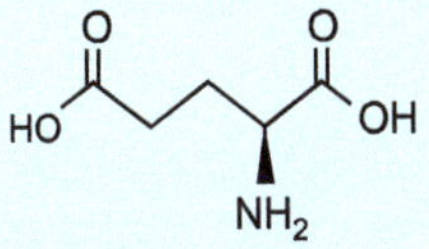 |
| Glycine | Gly | G | $NH_2-CH_2-COOH$ 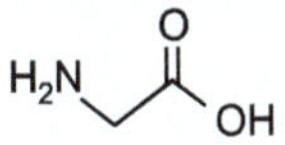 |
| Histidine | His | H | $HNH-CH=N-CH=C-CH_2-CH(NH_2)-COOH$ 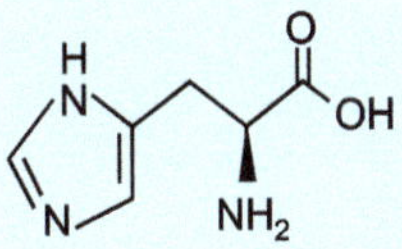 |
| Isoleucine | Ile | I | $CH_3-CH_2-CH(CH_3)-CH(NH_2)-COOH$ 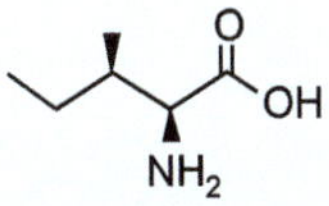 |
| Leucine | Leu | L | $(CH_3)_2-CH-CH_2-CH(NH_2)-COOH$ 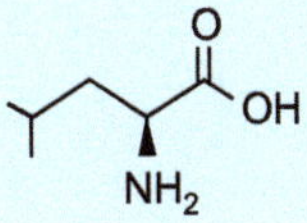 |

*Contd...*

Contd...

| Amino acid | Abbr. | Code | Structure |
|---|---|---|---|
| Lysine | Lys | K | $H_2N-(CH_2)_4-CH(NH_2)-COOH$ |
| Methionine | met | M | $CH_3-S-(CH_2)_2-CH(NH_2)-COOH$ |
| Phenylalanine | Phe | F | $Ph-CH_2-CH(NH_2)-COOH$ |
| Proline | Pro | P | $NH-(CH_2)_3-CH-COOH$ |
| Serine | Ser | S | $HO-CH_2-CH(NH_2)-COOH$ |
| Threonine | Thr | T | $CH_3-CH(OH)-CH(NH_2)-COOH$ |
| Tryptophan | Trp | W | $Ph-NH-CH=C-CH_2-CH(NH_2)-COOH$ |
| Tyrosine | Tyr | Y | $HO-Ph-CH_2-CH(NH_2)-COOH$ |
| Valine | Val | V | $(CH_3)_2-CH-CH(NH_2)-COOH$ |

# CHAPTER 5: Chemistry of Amino Acids and Proteins

## Classification of Amino Acids

Amino acids are mainly classified into three groups depending on their reaction in solution as neutral, acidic, and basic amino acids (**Fig. 5.1**).

They are also classified on the basis of charge they carry, as well as on their essentiality in the diet. Those that carry a net negative charge at pH 6.0 are called acidic amino acid and those that carry a net positive charge are called basic amino acid. Neutral amino acids carry no net charge at pH 6.0.

According to their chemical structure, they are also classified as aliphatic, aromatic, and heterocyclic amino acids.

**What are essential and nonessential amino acids? Explain with examples.**

Nutritionally amino acids are classified as essential and nonessential amino acids (**Table 5.1**).

**What are glucogenic and ketogenic amino acids? Explain with examples.**

## Glucogenic and Ketogenic Amino Acids

Refer **Table 5.2**.

## Chemical Properties of Amino Acids

The chemical properties of amino acids are due to their carboxyl group, amino group, and side chain R. All amino acids contain amino and carboxyl groups and undergoes chemical reactions that are characteristic for these groups.

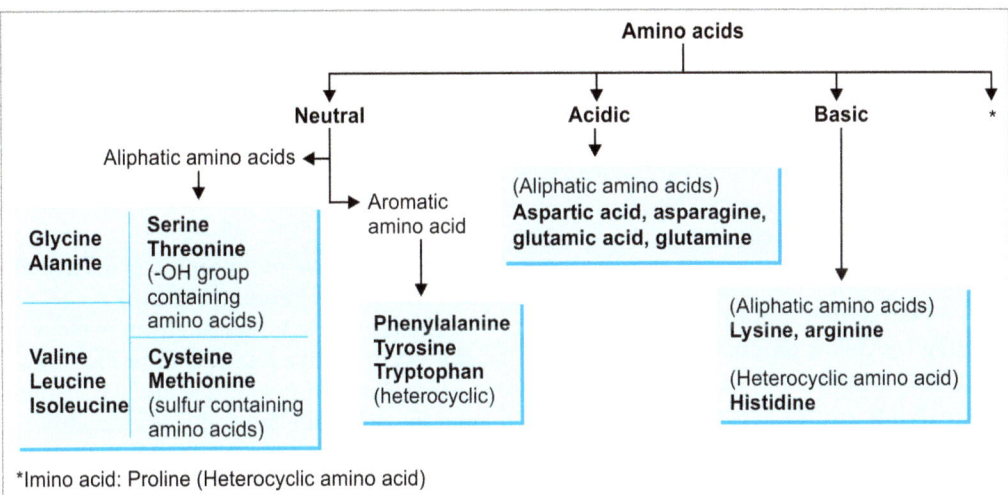

**Fig. 5.1:** Classification of amino acids.

| Table 5.1: Essential and nonessential amino acids. | | |
|---|---|---|
| | Definition | Examples |
| Essential amino acids | Are those 10 amino acids that our body cannot synthesize and should be supplied through diet | Methionine, arginine, threonine, tryptophan, valine, isoleucine, leucine, phenylalanine, histidine, and lysine. The code word to remember them is MATTVILPHLy |
| Nonessential amino acids | Are those 10 amino acids that our body can synthesize even if they are absent in our dietary proteins | Glycine, alanine, serine, cysteine, cystine, glutamine, glutamic acid, aspartic acid, and asparagine |

**Table 5.2:** Glucogenic and ketogenic amino acids.

| | Definition | Examples |
|---|---|---|
| Glucogenic amino acids | The carbon skeleton of amino acid can be converted into glucose in the body (after the removal of amino group of amino acid). Such amino acids are called glucogenic amino acids | Glycine, alanine, serine, threonine, valine, cysteine, cystine, proline, aspartic acid, glutamic acid, asparagine, glutamine, histidine, and arginine |
| Ketogenic amino acids | The carbon skeleton of amino acid is converted into ketone body (acetoacetic acid), such amino acids are called ketogenic amino acids | Leucine |
| Glucogenic and ketogenic amino acids | One part of the carbon skeleton is converted to glucose and other part is converted to ketone body, such amino acids are termed as both glucogenic and ketogenic amino acid | Lysine, isoleucine, phenylalanine, tyrosine, and tryptophan |

**Which reaction can be used to detect the amino acids with α-amino groups? Explain.**

## Ninhydrin Reaction

It is used to detect and quantify the amount of amino acid. When amino acids are heated with ninhydrin, the free α-amino groups react and give a purple-colored product.

Ninhydrin + α-Amino acid → Purple pigment.

Proline has imino group as α-amino group, which gives yellow product.

This ninhydrin reaction is used for quantifying amino acids by colorimetric method and to stain chromatographic plates. Fluorescamine reacts rapidly with amino acids, yielding highly fluorescent derivative that permits the detection of amino acid.

Dansyl chloride and 1-fluoro-2,4-dinitrobenzene (Sanger's reagent) give stable derivative. These derivatives absorb light and facilitate the detection and quantification of amino acid.

1-fluoro-2,4-dinitrobenzene + amino acid → 2,4-dinitrophenyl amino acid.

**What are peptides? Explain with naturally occurring peptides as examples.**

## Peptides and Peptide Bond

The proteins have many amino acids that are joined by peptide bonds **(Fig. 5.2)**.

The dipeptide formation from two amino acids occurs with a loss of a water molecule.

If amino acid 1 is glycine and 2 is alanine, then the dipeptide formed is glycylalanine. If the amino acids are interchanged, then the resulting peptide is alanylglycine. Always the amino group of the first amino acid in the peptide is free and the carboxyl group of the last amino acid is also free. The amino terminal of the peptide is always written on the left side and carboxyl terminal will be on the right side.

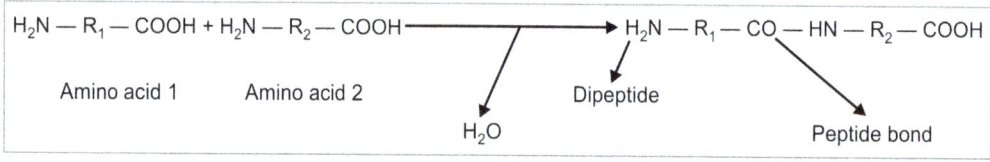

**Fig. 5.2:** Peptide bond formation between amino acids.

## Naturally Occurring Peptides

The naturally occurring peptides are as follows:
1. *Dipeptide*: Made up of two amino acids. For example,
   A. Carnosine
   B. Anserine.
   The two amino acids are β-alanine and histidine. Anserine is the derivative of carnosine. Both these peptides are found in muscle.
2. *Tripeptide*: Made up of three amino acids. For example,
   - Glutathione (GSH): The three amino acids present are glutamic acid, cysteine, and glycine. It contains –SH group [sulfhydryl group] from amino acid cysteine as active group. The oxidized form of GSH is represented as GS-SG.
     - GSH present in RBC in large amount.
     - It plays a major role in the oxidation–reduction reaction.
     - It protects the SH group of various other proteins.
     - It decomposes $H_2O_2$ and maintains the integrity of the cells and keeps hemoglobin in reduced state ($Fe^{2+}$ form) when it is oxidized to $Fe^{3+}$ form.

   ```
           SH
           |
   Glu–Cys–Gly  GSH
   ```

   - *Thyrotropin-releasing hormone (TRH)*: secreted from hypothalamus.
3. *Pentapeptide*: Made up of five amino acids. For example, enkephalins. They influence transmission in some parts of the brain.
4. *Nonapeptide*: Made up of nine amino acids. Oxytocin and vasopressin (antidiuretic hormone) secreted by posterior pituitary gland are the best examples for nonapeptides.
5. *Polypeptide*: They are made up of large number of amino acids.

For example, hemoglobin, myoglobin, and insulin. Hemoglobin is made up of four polypeptide chains, and each polypeptide chain contains several amino acids.

The insulin is the hormone secreted from cells of pancreas. It is made up of 51 amino acids. Insulin contains two polypeptide chains joined by disulfide bridge.

## Charge Properties of Amino Acids and Proteins

Each amino acid has at least two ionizable groups—the $-NH_2$ group and the –COOH group (in addition, charged groups present in the side group of amino acid if present).

In acidic medium, the $-NH_2$ group behaves as a base and accepts a proton and becomes positively charged (cationic form).

In basic medium, the –COOH group acts as proton donor and the amino acid becomes negatively charged (anionic form).

This property in which amino acids act as both acid and base is known as amphoteric nature of amino acids.

At specific pH, the amino acids carry both the charges in equal number and thus exist as dipolar ion or zwitterions. At this point, the net charge on the amino acid is zero. The number of positive charge is equal to number of negative charges at this condition.

The pH at which the amino acid or protein exists in zwitterionic form is called isoelectric pH (pI).

```
     COOH              COO⁻              COO⁻
      |                 |                 |
 ⁺H₃N–C–H          ⁺H₃N–C–H           H₂N–C–H
      |                 |                 |
      R                 R                 R
 1. Cation form   2. Zwitterion form   3. Anionic form
   at acidic pH    at isoelectric pH     at basic pH
```

Proteins are made up of amino acids and hence they also exhibit charged properties similar to amino acids.

For example, pI of:
- Albumin is 4.7

- Hemoglobin is 6.7
- Casein is 4.6

Proteins do not move under electrical field at their pI. Hence for the electrophoretic separation, the selection of pH of the medium should be different from the pI.

Proteins tend to aggregate and precipitate at their pI. As a result, they exhibit least solubility.

**Classify proteins with examples.**

## Classification of Proteins

There are several classifications of proteins:
1. Based on solubility: Different proteins of different soluble property **(Table 5.3)**.
2. Based on composition: They are classified into simple, conjugated, and derived proteins.
   - Simple proteins: Proteins made up of only amino acids are simple proteins, e.g., serum albumin, keratin, and lactalbumin.
   - Conjugated proteins: Proteins containing amino acid and an additional nonprotein part are called conjugated proteins. Nonprotein part is called prosthetic part. **Table 5.4** gives the examples of conjugated proteins and their composition.
   - Derived proteins: Proteins, which are formed by partial hydrolysis of high molecular weight proteins, are called derived proteins. Peptone and gelatin are the examples. Gelatin is formed from native protein collagen.
3. Based on the shape (conformation):
   - Globular proteins: These are spherical in shape, e.g., hemoglobin and albumin.
   - Fibrous proteins: They are long and fiber like, e.g., keratin, myosin, and collagen.

**List the important functions of proteins.**

## Biological Role of Proteins

### General Functions of Proteins

The general functions of proteins are as follows:
- Proteins play a central role in cell functions and cell structure. It constitutes 17% of body weight **(Table 5.5)**.
- Proteins form an essential part of the particular structure in the body. Membrane, muscle, connective tissues, and organs are the examples.
- Various proteins are enzymes in nature and catalyze biological reactions.
- Several proteins act as hormones and thus regulate various metabolic processes of the body.
- A number of proteins serve as carrier for the transport of various substances.

**Table 5.4:** Different conjugated proteins.

| Example for conjugated proteins | Nonporotein part + protein |
|---|---|
| 1. Hemoglobin (Hb) | Heme + globin |
| 2. Nucleoprotein | DNA + histone |
| 3. Lipoprotein | Lipids + apolipoprotein |
| 4. Phosphoprotein (casein) | Phosphate + protein |
| 5. Glycoprotein (egg albumin) | Carbohydrate + protein |
| 6. Rhodopsin | 11-cis-retinal + opsin (protein) |
| 7. Ferritin | Iron + apoferritin |

**Table 5.3:** Proteins of different soluble property.

| Class | Soluble in | Example |
|---|---|---|
| Albumins | Water | Serum albumin, egg albumin |
| Globulins | Dilute salt solutions | Serum globulins |
| Histones (basic proteins) | Dilute acids | Nucleoproteins, histones |
| Scleroproteins | Insoluble in $H_2O$ | Collagen, elastin |

## CHAPTER 5: Chemistry of Amino Acids and Proteins

**Table 5.5:** Biological importance of proteins with example.

| Biological role | Proteins | Function |
|---|---|---|
| 1. Structural proteins | Collagen, keratins | Bone and hair respectively |
| 2. Enzymes | Pepsin, amylase | Help in digestion of food |
| 3. Hormones | Insulin, prolactin | Regulate the metabolism |
| 4. Transport proteins | Hemoglobin (Hb) | Transport of oxygen |
| 5. Protein receptor | Hormone receptor | Insulin receptor on liver cell |
| 6. Storage proteins | Ferritin | Storage form of iron in liver |
| 7. Immune proteins | γ-globulins | Act against antigens |
| 8. Contractile proteins | Actin, myosin | Muscle contraction |
| 9. Buffering proteins | Plasma protein and Hb | Maintain the pH of blood |

- Some proteins act as receptor molecule for the transport of the compounds, across the cell membrane, such as hormone receptor.
- Various proteins bind to certain substances and store them in different tissues, acting as storage proteins.
- Some proteins such as γ-globulins act as antibodies and provide immunity.
- Proteins function as buffers to maintain pH of the cell.

**What are the different structural organizations of proteins? Explain with examples.**

## Structure of Proteins

Proteins are made up of one or more polypeptide chains. Four levels of structural organization recognized in proteins:
1. Primary structure
2. Secondary structure
3. Tertiary structure
4. Quaternary structure

## Primary Structure

Primary structure of proteins refers to the order and sequence of α-L-amino acids in a polypeptide chain in which these different amino acids are linked through the peptide linkage. It has an N-terminus (amino terminal) and a C-terminus (carboxyl terminal) **(Fig. 5.3)**.

## Secondary Structure

Folding or twisting the large polypeptide molecule possessing primary structure obtains secondary level of structure.

For the secondary level of protein structure, hydrogen bonds and disulfide linkages are involved.

*Hydrogen bonds:* Weak, low-energy noncovalent bond sharing single H between two electronegative atoms such as O and N. These occur between polar side chains of amino acids.

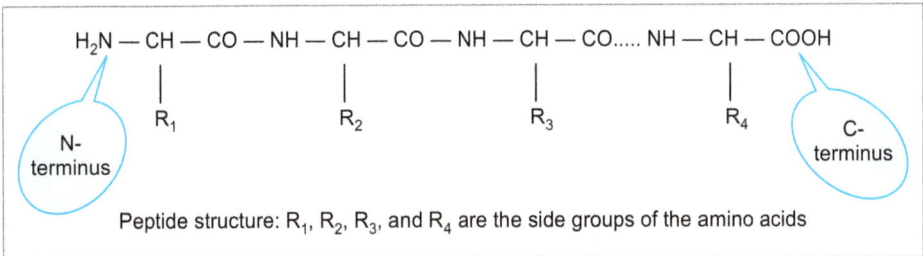

**Fig. 5.3:** Primary structure of protein.

*Disulfide linkages:* These occur between two cysteine residues. These are strong, high-energy covalent bonds. Cystine contains the disulfide (-S-S-) bridge formed by the oxidation of two cysteine molecules.

These forces cause indefinite number of configurations in protein structure. Hydrogen bond in secondary structure may form one or all of the following structure.
- α-helix (this is a coiling up like a Slinky or spring).
- β-pleated sheets (this is a fan-shaped bending).
- Random coils (this is when we cannot describe any real pattern to the folding).

*α-helix:* Hydrogen bonds may be formed between -CO and -NH groups within the same polypeptide chain (intrachain peptide linkage) resulting in its folding and forming a coil or helix **(Fig. 5.4)**.

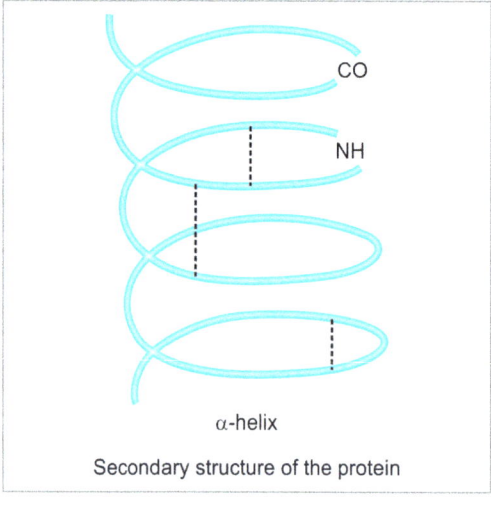

α-helix
Secondary structure of the protein

**Fig. 5.4:** α-Helix structure.

The right-handed folding, of protein chain, results in the formation of α-helix, for example, α-helix of many globular proteins such as myoglobin and hemoglobin.

*β-pleated sheets:* β-pleated sheets are formed by the formation of H bonds between -CO and -NH groups of different polypeptides (interchain peptide linkage).

Stretching, the helices of the polypeptide chains, results in β-pleated sheets **(Fig. 5.5)**, for example, β-pleated sheets of ribonuclease and fibroin protein of silk.

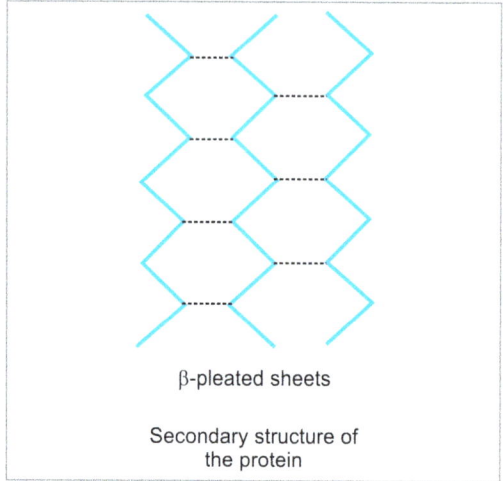

β-pleated sheets

Secondary structure of the protein

**Fig. 5.5:** β-pleated sheet.

## Tertiary Structure

Refolding of the polypeptide chain possessing secondary level of structure such as α-helix, β-pleated sheets, and random coils leads to the formation of tertiary structure **(Fig. 5.6)**.

The forces responsible for the interaction between different groups of amino acids are hydrogen bonds, hydrophobic interactions, ionic interactions, and van der Waals forces.

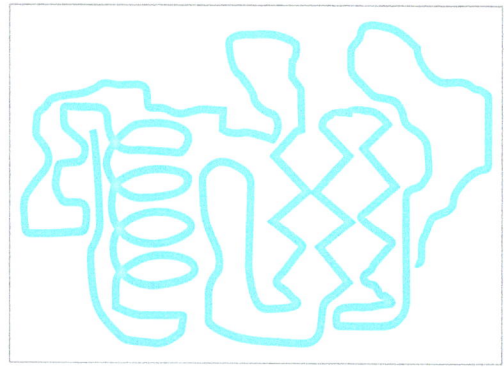

**Fig. 5.6:** Tertiary structure of protein.

*Hydrogen bonds:* It is formed between –CO and –NH groups of two different peptide bonds. It is also formed between –OH group of serine and –COOH groups of acidic amino acids.

*Hydrophobic interactions:* Hydrophobic interactions occur between nonpolar side chains of amino acids such as alanine and phenylalanine.

*Ionic interactions:* Ionic or electrostatic interactions occur between oppositely charged polar side groups of amino acids. They are lysine, arginine, histidine, and acidic amino acids.

*van der Waals forces:* These forces occur between nonpolar side chains of amino acids.

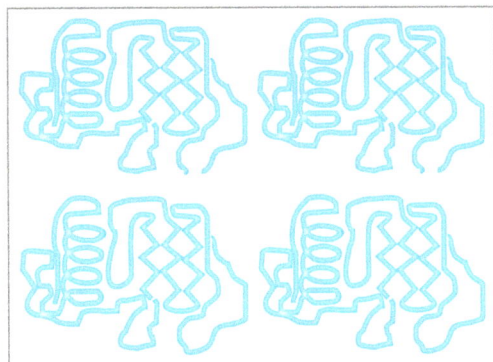

**Fig. 5.7:** Quaternary structure of hemoglobin.

## Quaternary Structure

Some proteins contain more than one polypeptide chain. They are known as oligomeric (multisubunit) proteins. Each subunit possesses primary, secondary, and tertiary level of structure as explained above.

When these subunits are held together by noncovalent interactions or by covalent crosslinks [(–S–S–) bridge], it is referred to as quaternary structure. Same weak bonds involved in the secondary and tertiary structure are also involved here. Disintegration of the quaternary structure leads to the loss of biologic activity of the proteins.

*For example,*
1. *Hemoglobin*: A tetramer having four polypeptide chains held together by noncovalent bonds. These polypeptide chains are called a1, a2, b1, and b2 chains **(Fig. 5.7)**.
2. *Lactate dehydrogenase*: It has four polypeptide chains.
3. *Creatine kinase*: It has two polypeptide chains.
4. *Immunoglobulins (Igs)*: They are also called antibodies. They are made up of two heavy and two light chains.
5. Collagen is a fibrous protein containing three helical polypeptide chains wound together. Glycine, proline, and lysine are

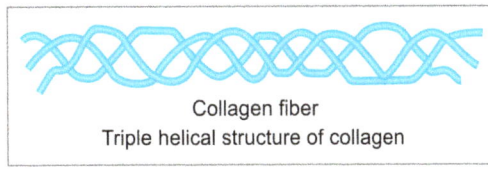

Collagen fiber
Triple helical structure of collagen

**Fig. 5.8:** Collagen.

the important amino acids present **(Fig. 5.8)**.

**What is denaturation? List the denaturing agents and what changes will happen with structure of protein after denaturation.**

## Denaturation of Proteins

❖ Denaturation of protein may be defined as a disruption of the secondary, tertiary, and wherever applicable quaternary organization of protein molecule due to cleavage of noncovalent bonds.
❖ Primary structure is not affected during this process.
❖ Peptide bonds are not broken.
❖ Various agents bring about denaturation of protein are:
   ▪ Physical agents: Heat, UV light, ultrasound, high pressure, and even violent shaking can cause denaturation.
   ▪ Chemical agents: Organic solvents, acids, alkalies, urea, and various detergents cause protein denaturation.

## Modification of Protein after Denaturation

Following are the modifications of protein after denaturation:
- Physical changes: Protein becomes more viscous and rate of diffusion decreases.
- Chemical changes: Decreased solubility at pI and floccules may occur. Many chemical groups become inactive (e.g., –SH group).
- Biological changes: Biologically enzymes and hormones become inactive.

**What are the different types of plasma proteins? Explain with examples.**

## Plasma Proteins

The major six plasma proteins are as follows:
1. Albumin
2. $\alpha 1$-Globulin
3. $\alpha 2$-Globulin
4. $\beta$-Globulin
5. Fibrinogen
6. $\gamma$-Globulin.

They are separated using electrophoresis technique and also by precipitation methods. Fibrinogen is absent in serum.

## Albumin

The name is derived from the white precipitate formed when egg is boiled (albus = white). It is present in high concentration that is about 60% of the total proteins is albumin. It has one polypeptide chain with about 585 amino acids and 17 disulfide bonds having a molecular weight of 69,000. Liver produces 12 g of albumin per day.

The decrease in serum albumin is called hypoalbuminemia. This is seen in cirrhosis, nephrotic syndrome, and malnutrition. In cirrhosis, the synthesis of albumin decreases and in nephritic syndrome, the damaged nephrons lead to the excretion of more albumin in the urine.

**Briefly explain the functions of albumin.**

Plasma albumin performs the following functions:

- Osmotic function
- Transport function
- Nutritive function
- Buffering functions

### Osmotic Function

Due to its high concentration and low molecular weight, albumin contributes to 80% of total plasma osmotic pressure (25 mm Hg). It plays a major role in maintaining blood volume and body fluid distribution. Decrease in plasma albumin level results in a fall in the osmotic pressure. This leads to enhanced fluid retention in tissue spaces leading to edema. Edema is seen in conditions where albumin level in blood is below 2 g/dL.

### Transport Function

Albumin is necessary for the transport of many hydrophobic substances such as:
- Bilirubin
- Free fatty acids
- Drugs (such as sulfa drugs, aspirin, salicylates, and phenytoin dicumarol)
- Steroid hormones
- Thyroxin
- Calcium
- Copper
- Heavy metals

### Nutritive Function

Albumin serves as a source of amino acids for tissue protein synthesis when it is broken down.

### Buffering Function

All proteins have buffering capacity. Since albumin is present in high concentration in blood, it shows the maximum buffering capacity. The large number of histidine residues present in the albumin is responsible for buffering action of albumin.

# CHAPTER 5: Chemistry of Amino Acids and Proteins

## Globulins

The different types of globulins present in plasma are $\alpha_1$, $\alpha_2$, $\beta_1$, $\beta_2$, and $\gamma$-globulins. These proteins are glycoproteins with the molecular weight range from 90,000 to 130,000. The $\alpha$- and $\beta$-globulins also function as transport proteins that transport hormones, vitamins, minerals, and lipids, etc. The $\gamma$-globulins are known as Igs and they provide mainly immunity against any infections.

## Fibrinogen

The fibrinogen is an acute-phase protein. It is an essential factor in blood coagulation. The conversion of fibrinogen to fibrin occurs by cleaving of Arg–Gly peptide bonds of fibrinogen. It is synthesized by the liver. The fibrin monomers aggregate and precipitate to form a clot.

Different types of plasma proteins and their concentration in the blood are shown in **Table 5.6**.

**Table 5.6:** Concentration of various plasma proteins.

| Plasma protein | g/dL | % |
| --- | --- | --- |
| Total protein | 6.5–8 | 100 |
| Albumin | 3.5–5 | 60 |
| Globulins | 1.8–3 | 40 |
| $\alpha_1$ |  | 3 |
| $\alpha_2$ |  | 11 |
| $\beta$ |  | 11 |
| $\gamma$ |  | 16 |
| Fibrinogen | 0.2–0.4 |  |

## Proteins Belong to Different Globulins

### $\alpha_1$-Globulin
- $\alpha_1$-Aantitrypsin
- $\alpha_1$-Acid glycoprotein
- $\alpha_1$-Lipoproteins
- Thyroxine-binding globulin.

### $\alpha_1$-Antitrypsin
- It is an acute-phase reactant (APR) and protease inhibitor present in the extracellular fluid throughout the body.
- The level of certain proteins in blood may increase up to 1,000 folds in several inflammatory and neoplastic conditions. Such proteins are called acute-phase proteins. It neutralizes the lysosomal elastase, which is released during phagocytosis of particles by polymorphonuclear leukocytes.
- Thus $\alpha_1$-antitrypsin has a protective role in the body.
- $\alpha_1$-Antitrypsin level is increased during any infection or inflammation because of this protective role. Hence, it is known as APR.
- $\alpha_1$-Antitrypsin inhibits activity of proteases particularly elastase, which degrades elastin.

**What is the relationship of excessive cigarette smoking and emphysema?**
Cigarette smoking inhibits the activity of $\alpha_1$-antitrypsin by oxidizing a specific methionine residue of $\alpha_1$-antitrypsin. Thus $\alpha_1$-antitrypsin loses the capacity of inhibiting elastase activity.

Cigarette smoking increases the number of neutrophils in the lung and therefore increases the amount of elastase (elastase is released from neutrophils in lungs). Elastase then causes the tissue breakdown and loss of elasticity in the lungs, i.e., emphysema.

### $\alpha_2$-Globulins
Important proteins under this group are:
- $\alpha_1$-Macroglobulins
  - This has protective role in the body.
  - It is synthesized by hepatocytes.
- Haptoglobins
  - The proteins, which bind with hemoglobin and help in the breakdown of hemoglobin to bilirubin.
- Ceruloplasmin
  - It is a copper-containing protein in the plasma.
  - It is known to have an antioxidant property.

- It is an acute-phase reactive protein.
- Its level is increased in the plasma in infections and malignant conditions, especially in Hodgkin's disease.
- Its levels are decreased in Wilson's disease and it is used in the diagnosis of this disease.

## Bence Jones Protein

- It is an abnormal protein, which occurs in blood and urine of multiple myeloma patients. It is a light chain of Ig.
- Simple heat test can detect its presence in urine. At 50–60°C, these proteins specifically precipitate and by further heating the precipitate dissolves. Reverse process occurs upon cooling.

**What are immunoglobulins? Explain the structure of these.**

## Immunoglobulin

The defense strategies of the body are collectively known as immunity.

Two types of immunity identified:
1. *Cellular immunity:* This is mediated by T-lymphocytes or T-cells (thymic origin).
2. *Humoral immunity:* Mediated by a specialized group of proteins known as Igs or antibodies.
   - The B-lymphocytes or B-cells (mature in bone) are responsible for the production of Igs.
   - The Igs are also known as γ-globulins.
   - Protective in function
   - Function as antibodies
   - Synthesized in response to a foreign substance called antigen.
   - Provide immunity
     - Five different types of Igs
     - They are IgA, IgG, IgM, IgD, and IgE [remember it as Government (IgG) MADE].

## Separation of Plasma Proteins

Chemical and immunological methods are available that can quantify the concentration of a specific plasma protein with a high degree of specificity. Less commonly electrophoresis is used to provide a semiquantitative estimate of the pattern of serum proteins. Plasma proteins can be separated by different techniques, which mainly depend on certain properties of proteins.

1. Charged groups that are present in the protein.
2. Molecular weight of the protein.
   *Gel filtration*: Columns that are packed with gel are used to separate the proteins. The proteins are separated depending on their molecular weight.
3. *Precipitation of proteins by salts (salt fractionation)*: Albumin is soluble in water, whereas globulins are less soluble in water. All proteins are soluble in dilute salt solutions. As the concentration of the salt increases proteins get precipitated from their solution. For example, when ammonium sulfate is added to a solution of protein until it completely saturate, the availability of water molecules for the protein is decreased causing the proteins to precipitate. This process is called salting out. Albumin is precipitated at full saturation with ammonium sulfate. Since albumin is having hydrophilic property, it requires higher concentration of salt to get precipitated. At full saturation, all the proteins are precipitated. Globulins are precipitated at half saturation with ammonium sulfate. Solutions of sodium sulfite (21–28%) are also used to precipitate globulins.
4. *Precipitation by organic solvents*: Organic solvents such as methanol, ethanol, and acetone are dehydrating agents, which cause the precipitation of proteins. These solvents reduce the amount of water required to keep protein in solution, this results in precipitation. The protein may get denatured in this process. Hence, this process is usually carried out at 0°C.

## Electrophoresis

Electrophoresis separates the proteins into five broad fractions—albumin and $\alpha_1$, $\alpha_2$, $\beta_1$, and $\beta_2$ globulins. Each of the globulin fractions consists of a mixture of several proteins. Electrophoresis is the migration of the charged molecule in an electric field. Negatively charged particles (anions) move toward anode (positively charged electrode), while positively charged particles (cations) move toward cathode (negatively charged electrode). Proteins in solution or plasma can be separated from one another by electrophoresis, because they are charged molecules. Proteins contain charges due to the presence of amino group ($NH_{3+}$) and carboxyl group (COO-). The presence of more number of negative charges depends on the number of COO- group. If a protein has more $NH_{3+}$ group, it will have more positive charges. At acidic pH, the proteins will have more positive charges so proteins will be positively charged and moves toward negative electrode in an electric field. At alkaline pH, the proteins have more negative charges. Hence, the protein will be negatively charged and moves toward positive electrode in an electric field **(Fig. 5.9)**.

## Protein Sequencing

Proteins are found in every cell and they are very essential for all the biological processes taking place inside the body.

It is very complex and determining its structure involves protein sequencing—determining the amino acid sequences of its constituent peptides and also what conformation it adopts and whether it is complexed with any nonpeptide molecules.

It is very important to know the structure and functions of proteins in living organisms

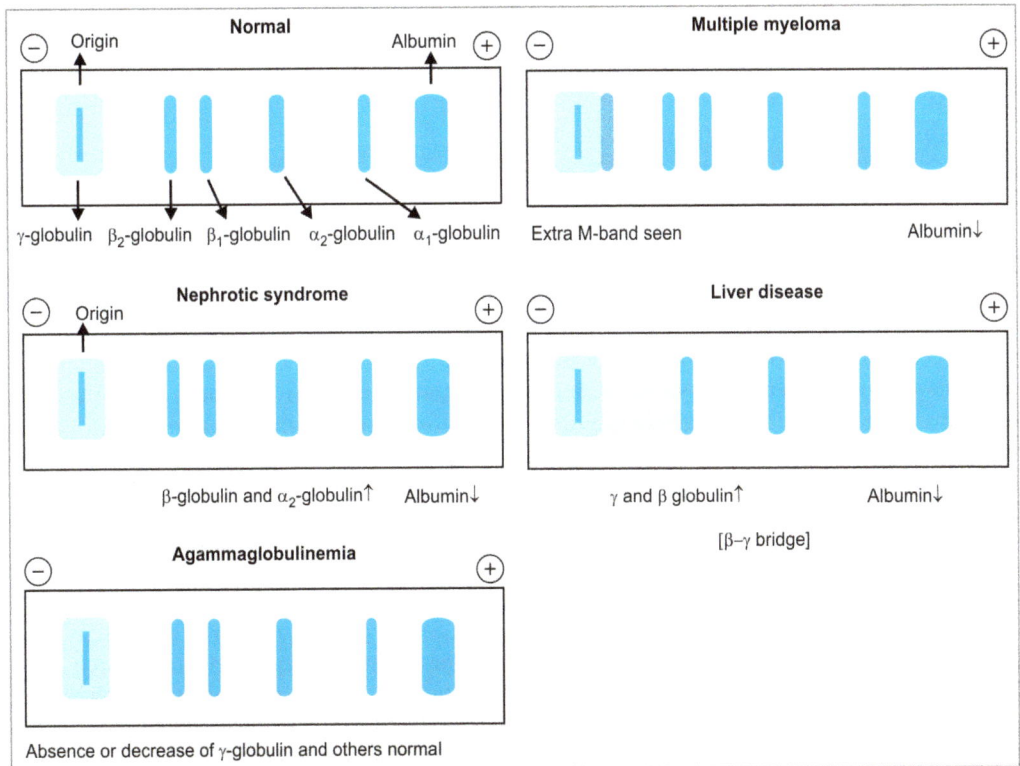

**Fig. 5.9:** Serum electrophoresis pattern of serum of normal and diseased conditions.

to understand cellular processes and allows drugs that target specific metabolic pathways to be invented more easily.

There are two major direct methods of protein sequencing such as mass spectrometry and the Edman degradation reaction. It is also possible to generate an amino acid sequence from the DNA or mRNA sequence encoding the protein, if this is known. There are a number of other reactions, which can be used to gain more information about protein sequences.

## Amino Acid Composition

It is often desirable to know the amino acid composition of a protein prior to attempting to find the ordered sequence, as this knowledge can be used to facilitate the discovery of errors in the sequencing process or to distinguish between ambiguous results. Knowledge of the frequency of certain amino acids may also be used to choose which protease to use for digestion of the protein. The steps are as follows:

1. Hydrolyze a known quantity of protein into its constituent amino acids. Hydrolysis is done by heating a sample of the protein in 6 M HCl at 100–110°C for about 24 hours.
2. Separate the amino acids in some way.

The amino acids can be separated by ion-exchange chromatography (sulfonated polystyrene as a matrix, adding the amino acids in acid solution and passing a buffer of steadily increasing pH through the column. Amino acids will be eluted when the pH reaches their respective isoelectric points). The other process is hydrophobic interaction chromatography or use of reversed-phase chromatography. Many commercially available C8 and C18 silica columns have demonstrated successful separation of amino acids.

## Chromatography

Chromatography is one of the most popular tools of biochemistry. This technique is used for the separation of a number of similar components in a mixture from each other so that these could be determined with a minimum of interference. These closely related compounds include proteins, peptides, amino acids, lipids, carbohydrates, vitamins, and drugs. This technique is working on the principle of adsorption, partition, and ion-exchange and exclusion properties.

## General Principle

Chromatography usually consists of a mobile phase and a stationary phase. The mobile phase refers to the mixture of substance to be separated in a liquid or a gas. The stationary phase is a porous solid matrix through which the sample contained in the mobile phase percolates. The interaction between the stationary phase and the mobile phase causes the separation of compounds from the mixture. These interactions include adsorption, partition, ion-exchange, and exclusion type of physiochemical properties **(Fig. 5.10)**.

## Quantitative Analysis

Once the amino acids have been separated, their respective quantities are determined by adding a reagent that will form a colored derivative. If the amounts of amino acids are in excess of 10 nmol, ninhydrin can be used for this—it gives a yellow color when reacted with proline, and a blue with other amino acids. The concentration of amino acid is proportional to the absorbance of the solution.

## N-Terminal Amino Acid Analysis

Determining the N-terminal amino acid of a peptide chain is useful for two reasons: to aid the ordering of individual peptide fragments' sequences into a whole chain and because the first round of Edman degradation is often contaminated by impurities and therefore does not give an accurate determination of the N-terminal amino acid.

The steps involved in the determination of N-terminal amino acid analysis are as follows:

# CHAPTER 5: Chemistry of Amino Acids and Proteins

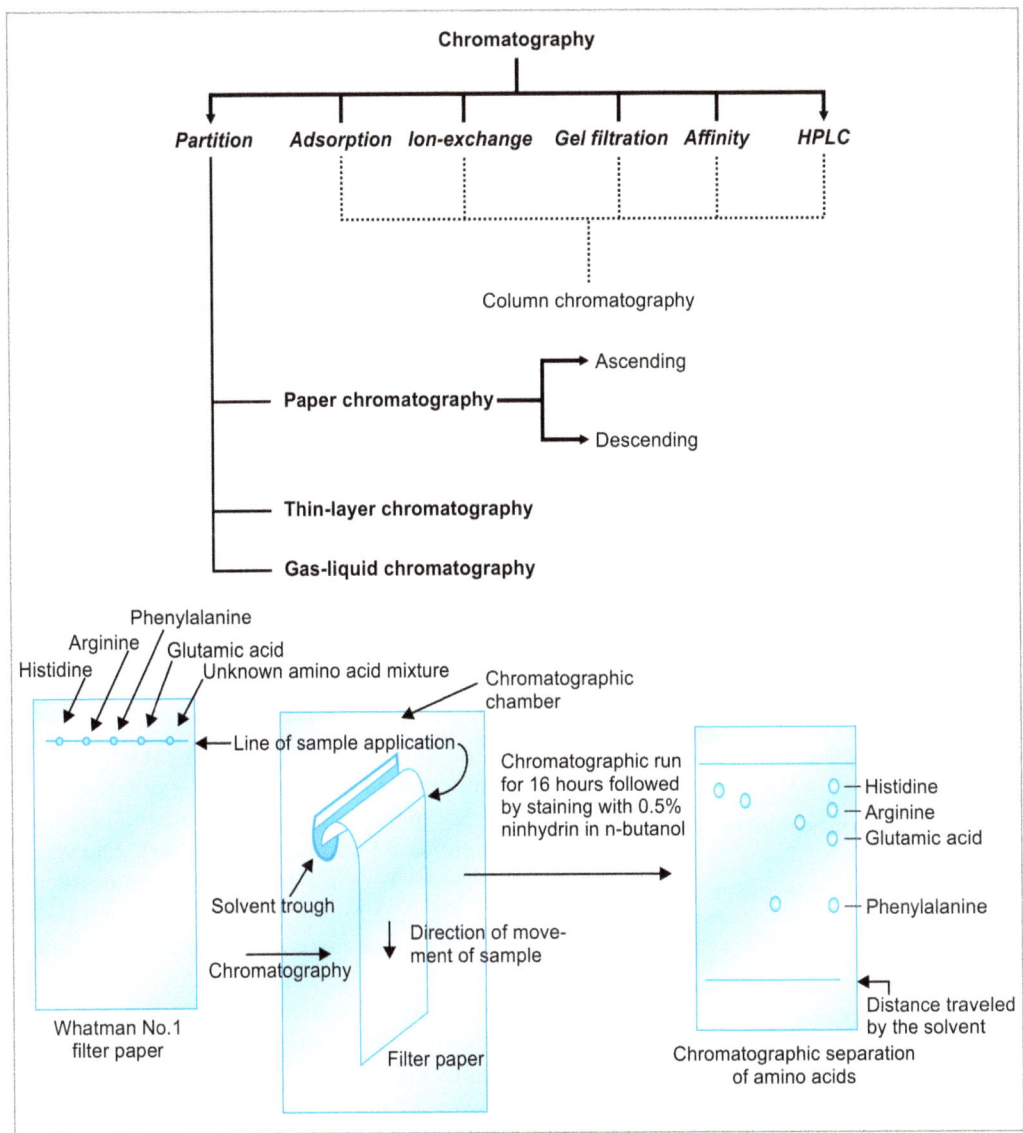

Fig. 5.10: Different types of chromatography and paper chromatography of amino acid.

1. Mix the peptide with a reagent that will selectively label the terminal amino acid. There are many different reagents that can be used to label terminal amino acids. They all react with amine groups and will therefore also bind to amine groups in the side chains of amino acids such as lysine—for this reason, it is necessary to be careful in interpreting chromatograms to ensure that the right spot is chosen.
Reagents used are Sanger's reagent: 1-fluoro-2,4-dinitrobenzene and dansyl chloride. Phenylisothiocyanate, the reagent for the Edman degradation, can also be used.

2. Hydrolyze the protein.

## C-Terminal Amino Acid Analysis

There are several methods available for C-terminal amino acid analysis. The most common method is to add carboxypeptidases to a solution of the protein, take samples at regular intervals, and determine the terminal amino acid by analyzing a plot of amino acid concentrations against time.

## Edman Degradation

It is a very important reaction for protein sequencing, because it allows the ordered amino acid composition of a protein to be discovered. Automated Edman sequencers are now in widespread use and are able to sequence peptides up to approximately 50 amino acids long. The reaction steps for sequencing a protein by the Edman degradation are as follows:

- Break any disulfide bridges in the protein by oxidizing with performic acid.
- Separate and purify the individual chains of the protein complex (if more than one chain).
- Determine the amino acid composition of each chain.
- Determine the terminal amino acids of each chain.
- Break each chain into fragments under 50 amino acids long.
- Separate and purify the fragments.
- Determine the sequence of each fragment.
- Repeat with a different pattern of cleavage.
- Construct the sequence of the overall protein.

*Digestion into peptide fragments:* Peptides longer than about 50–70 amino acids long cannot be sequenced reliably by the Edman degradation. Because of this, long protein chains need to be broken up into small fragments, which can then be sequenced individually.

Digestion is done either by endopeptidases such as trypsin or pepsin or by chemical reagents such as cyanogen bromide.

## The Edman Degradation Reaction

The peptide to be sequenced is adsorbed onto a solid surface—one common substrate is glass fiber coated with polybrene, a cationic polymer.

The Edman reagent, phenylisothiocyanate, is added to the adsorbed peptide, together with a basic buffer solution of 12% trimethylamine.

This reacts with the amine group of the N-terminal amino acid.

The terminal amino acid derivative can then be selectively detached by the addition of anhydrous acid.

The derivative then isomerizes to give a substituted phenylthiohydantoin, which can be washed off and identified by chromatography, and the cycle can be repeated.

The efficiency of each step is about 98%, which allows about 50 amino acids to be determined.

## Mass Spectrometry

The other major direct method by which the sequence of a protein can be determined is mass spectrometry. Peptides are also easier to prepare for mass spectrometry than whole proteins, because they are more soluble.

One method of delivering the peptides to the spectrometer is electrospray ionization.

The protein is digested by an endoprotease, and the resulting solution is passed through a high-pressure liquid chromatography column.

At the end of this column, the solution is sprayed out of a narrow nozzle charged to a high positive potential into the mass spectrometer.

The charge on the droplets causes them to fragment until only single ions remain.

The peptides are then fragmented and the mass–charge ratios of the fragments measured.

The mass spectrum is analyzed by computer and often compared against a database of previously sequenced proteins in order to determine the sequences of the fragments. This process is then repeated with a different digestion enzyme, and the overlaps in the sequences used to construct a sequence for the protein.

## Tests for Protein

*Biuret reaction*: Proteins and long peptides answer this test. In alkaline medium (NaOH), the nitrogen atoms of the peptide bonds react with cupric ion (from copper sulfate) and gives violet-colored complex. Exceptions are amino acids and dipeptide. They do not answer this test.

## SUMMARY

Amino acids are group of organic compounds which contains amino and carboxyl group. Proteins are the group of organic compounds of carbon, hydrogen, oxygen, and nitrogen. All the biologically active proteins comprise nearly 22 different amino acids, which are called the building blocks of proteins. Amino acids contain two functional groups such as amino ($NH_2$) and carboxyl (COOH) group. The carbon atom attached to $-NH_2$ group and –COOH group is called α-carbon and "R" is the side chain of amino acid and can be hydrogen or an aliphatic group, aromatic or heterocyclic group. Amino acids are classified mainly into three groups depending on their reaction in solution as neutral, acidic, and basic amino acids. Nutritionally amino acids are classified as essential and nonessential amino acids. Amino acids are of ketogenic (acetoacetic acid) and glucogenic (glucose from carbon skeleton). Amino acids are joined by peptide bonds to form peptides (proteins). Proteins play a central role in cell functions and cell structure. Proteins are made up of one or more polypeptide chains. Four levels of structural organization can be recognized such as primary, secondary, tertiary, and quaternary structure. Disruption of the secondary, tertiary, and wherever applicable quaternary without affecting the primary organization of protein molecule is denaturation. Human plasma has albumin and globulins. Globulins are classified into α, β, and gamma globulins. Plasma proteins can be separated using different types of electrophoresis.

Extracellular matrix (ECM) is a complex structural entity surrounding and supporting cells that are found within mammalian tissues and often referred to as the connective tissue. The ECM contains three major classes of biomolecules such as structural proteins (collagen, fibrillin, and elastin), specialized proteins (fibrillin, fibronectin, and laminin), and proteoglycans (composed of a protein core attached with long chains of repeating disaccharide units termed "glycosaminoglycans"). Collagen is the main protein of connective tissue in animals and the most abundant protein in mammals. There are 27 types of collagen in total. Glycosaminoglycans are the abundant heteropolysaccharides found in the body and are long unbranched polysaccharides with repeating disaccharide units.

## SELF-ASSESSMENT QUESTIONS

### Answer the Following Questions

1. How will you classify proteins? Give one example to each class.
2. How will you classify amino acids? Give one example to each class.
3. Define essential amino acids. Give examples.
4. Give important functions of proteins in the human body.
5. Explain the different levels of organization of protein structure.
6. What is denaturation of proteins? Give its consequences.
7. Name the proteins that belong to α-1-globulins and α-2-globulins.

## Short-Answer Questions

1. Which test is used as a general test for protein?
2. Which bond mainly stabilizes the primary structure of protein?
3. Give an example for a phosphoprotein.
4. Name the plasma protein, which provides immunity to our body.
5. Mention the important function of albumin.
6. How many polypeptide chains are present in hemoglobin molecule?
7. Give an example for tertiary structure of a protein.
8. Name the sulfur containing amino acids.
9. What is the isoelectric pH of casein?
10. Name the urine protein which helps in diagnosis of multiple myeloma.
11. Give an example for acute-phase proteins.
12. Give the reason for Wilson's disease.

## MULTIPLE CHOICE QUESTIONS

1. **All the following statements are true regarding the amino acids, *except*:**
    (a) They contain an amino group and a carboxyl groups
    (b) Proteins are made up of -l-amino acids
    (c) They form peptide bond with each other to form a polypeptide
    (d) They react in alkaline medium with copper to form violet color
2. **Which of the following is a neutral amino acid?**
    (a) Arginine
    (b) Aspartic acid
    (c) Lysine
    (d) Leucine
3. **Which of the following amino acids is both neutral and aromatic in nature?**
    (a) Alanine
    (b) Histidine
    (c) Phenylalanine
    (d) Proline
4. **Which of the following amino acid is called essential amino acid?**
    (a) Glycine
    (b) Glutamine
    (c) Phenylalanine
    (d) Proline
5. **All the following statements are true regarding a peptide, *except*:**
    (a) A peptide is formed by bond with a carboxyl group of an amino acid 1 with the amino group of the other amino acid 2
    (b) Glutathione is an example of dipeptide
    (c) Dipeptide reacts in Biuret reaction
    (d) Carboxy terminal of a peptide is written on the left side
6. **Following are the properties of proteins at isoelectric pH (pI), *except*:**
    (a) Proteins will have maximum solubility at pI
    (b) Protein possess equal number of positive and negative charges
    (c) Proteins exist in Zwitterionic form
    (d) Below the isoelectric point they possess net positive charge
7. **Which one of the following proteins is not a conjugated protein?**
    (a) Egg albumin
    (b) Hemoglobin
    (c) Serum albumin
    (d) Casein
8. **Which of the following statements is false regarding the structure of a protein?**
    (a) Immunoglobulin possess quaternary structure
    (b) Upon denaturation primary structure is broken
    (c) Protein lose their biological activity if their secondary, tertiary, and quaternary are damaged
    (d) Hydrogen bond is predominant force stabilizing the—helix and—pleated sheets

9. Which of the following proteins is absent in normal person's serum?
    (a) Albumin
    (b) γ-Globulin
    (c) Fibrinogen
    (d) $α_2$-Globulin
10. Following are the examples of globular proteins, *except*:
    (a) Hemoglobin
    (b) Collagen
    (c) Albumin
    (d) Myoglobin
11. The tripeptide that plays an important role in oxidation reduction reactions is:
    (a) Glutathione
    (b) Oxytocin
    (c) Carnosine
    (d) Vasopressin
12. Concerning amino acids one of the following statements about amino acids is false:
    (a) They all have at least two ionizable groups
    (b) Amino and carboxyl groups are attached to an α carbon
    (c) In acidic medium, the amino group is positively charged
    (d) In basic medium, the amino acid exists in Zwitterionic form
13. The carbon skeleton of the following amino acids can be converted to glucose as well as ketone bodies:
    i. Isoleucine
    ii. Tryptophan
    iii. Lysine
    iv. Leucine
    (a) i only
    (b) i and ii only
    (c) i, ii, and iii only
    (d) iii and iv only
14. The conjugated protein with a quaternary structure is:
    (a) Albumin
    (b) Insulin
    (c) Hemoglobin
    (d) Myoglobin
15. An amino acid has $pKa_1$, $pKa_2$, and $pKa_3$ values of 2.0, 3.9, and 10, respectively. Which of the following symbols best represents this amino acid?
    (a) K
    (b) M
    (c) D
    (d) F
16. One of the following is NOT an essential amino acid:
    (a) Valine
    (b) Phenylalanine
    (c) Lysine
    (d) Glutamine
17. Which of the following bonds is not affected when a protein is denatured?
    (a) Hydrogen bond
    (b) Ionic bond
    (c) Disulfide bond
    (d) Peptide bond
18. Which of the following is a basic amino acid?
    (a) Lysine
    (b) Asparagine
    (c) Glutamine
    (d) Alanine
19. A protein's ability to absorb ultraviolet radiation is based mainly on the presence of:
    (a) Cys
    (b) Asp
    (c) Trp
    (d) Val
20. All of the following proteins contain a quaternary structure, *except*:
    (a) Immunoglobulin
    (b) Myoglobin
    (c) Collagen
    (d) Lactate dehydrogenase

21. **Concerning pI of an amino acid, one of the following statement false:**
    (a) It is the pH at which the amino acid exists as a zwitterion
    (b) It is the same as the isoelectric pH of the amino acid
    (c) It is the pH at which the net charge on the amino acid is zero
    (d) It is the point at which amino acid has maximum solubility
22. **The α helix and β sheet represent the following level of structural organization of a protein.**
    (a) Primary level
    (b) Secondary level
    (c) Tertiary level
    (d) Quaternary level
23. **All of the following amino acids are polar, except:**
    (a) Phe
    (b) Asp
    (c) Tyr
    (d) His
24. **Which one of the following pairs contains only fibrous proteins?**
    (a) Collagen and myoglobin
    (b) Albumin and keratin
    (c) Hemoglobin and myosin
    (d) Collagen and keratin
25. **The immunoglobulin that crosses placenta is:**
    (a) IgG
    (b) IgM
    (c) IgE
    (d) IgA
26. **Collagen is the:**
    (a) Major protein of the ECF
    (b) Main protein of connective tissue in animals
    (c) Minor protein comprising the ECM
    (d) Nonfibrous protein
27. **Proteoglycans contain:**
    (a) Lipid core attached to protein
    (b) Carbohydrate attached to fatty acid and glycerol
    (c) Polyunsaturated fatty acid attached to a disaccharide unit
    (d) A protein core attached to repeating disaccharide units
28. **Concerning laminin, one of the following statements is incorrect:**
    (a) It anchors cell surfaces to the basal lamina
    (b) It has three chains wound together to form a crucifix shaped structure
    (c) It is tough and inextensible, with great tensile strength
    (d) It has multiple domains to bind cell surface receptors
29. **Hurler syndrome results from the reduced levels of:**
    (a) Glucosaminidase
    (b) Sulfatase
    (c) Acetyl transferase
    (d) l-Iduronidase
30. **The composition of hyaluronic acid is:**
    (a) Glucuronic acid and N-acetyl galactosamine
    (b) Glucuronic acid and N-acetyl glucosamine
    (c) Galactose and N-acetyl galactosamine
    (d) Iduronic acid and N-acetyl glucosamine
31. **Heparin:**
    (a) Is an excellent lubricator
    (b) Has glucuronic acid and galactosamine
    (c) Is highly sulfated
    (d) Is found in the synovial fluid of joints
32. **In the structure shown below:**
    (a) A represents chondroitin sulfate
    (b) B represents hyaluronic acid
    (c) C represents link protein
    (d) D represents collagen

# CHAPTER 5: Chemistry of Amino Acids and Proteins

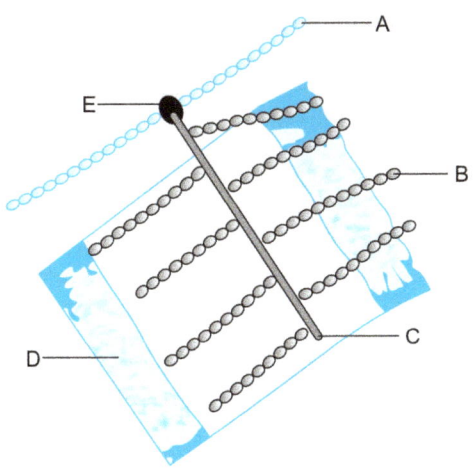

33. **Concerning fibronectin:**
    (a) It is the first collagen to be well characterized
    (b) It has single domain
    (c) It is a dimer with similar peptides
    (d) It attaches cells to all matrices except type IV
34. **Collagen synthesis depends on:**
    (a) Hydroxylysine and vitamin K
    (b) Glycine and fluoride
    (c) Epinephrine and vitamin C
    (d) Hydroxyproline and vitamin C
35. **Heparin is:**
    (a) Composed of glucuronic acid and N-acetyl glucosamine
    (b) Nonsulfated
    (c) Absent in liver
    (d) Found in synovial fluid
36. **Hurler syndrome presents with:**
    (a) Organomegaly and dwarfism
    (b) Bruised skin and magenta-colored tongue
    (c) Profuse bleeding and delayed clotting time
    (d) Skeletal and smooth muscle disorder
37. **Type III collagen is produced by:**
    (a) Fibroblasts after type I collagen formation
    (b) Young fibroblasts before tougher type I collagen is synthesized
    (c) Fibroblasts after the type IV collagen formation
    (d) Fibroblasts quickly after the tougher type collagen IX is synthesized
38. **Fibronectin:**
    (a) Contains six tightly folded domains
    (b) Does not attach cells to matrices
    (c) Attaches type IV collagen to matrices
    (d) Is a well-characterized adhesive protein
39. **The high viscosity and low compressibility of glycosaminoglycans make them ideal for:**
    (a) Binding tightly to bones
    (b) Hardening bones and teeth
    (c) Lubricating the joints
    (d) Attaching ligaments to bone
40. **Chondroitin sulfate consists of:**
    (a) Glucuronic acid and N-acetyl galactosamine
    (b) Glucuronic acid and N-acetyl glucosamine
    (c) Iduronic acid and N-acetyl galactosamine
    (d) Iduronic acid and galactosamine

41. **Concerning the proteoglycan shown below:**
    (a) A represents N-acetylated sugar
    (b) B represents galactose
    (c) D represents the glycoprotein
    (d) C represents tryptophan rings
42. **The most abundant collagen in the human body is type:**
    (a) II
    (b) I
    (c) IV
    (d) V

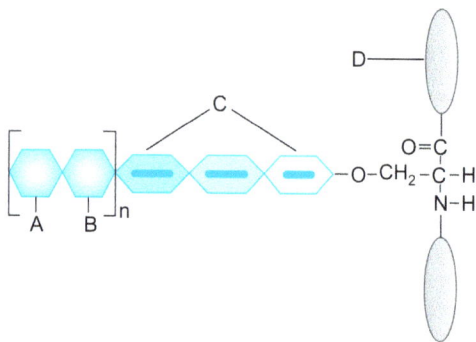

43. **Determination of hydroxyproline levels may be used to estimate the tissue levels of:**
    (a) Collagen
    (b) Fibronectin
    (c) Hyaluronic acid
    (d) Myosin
44. **Concerning collagen:**
    (a) It is the minor glycoprotein found in bone
    (b) Its degradation leads to wrinkles that accompany aging
    (c) It gives strength to ligaments
    (d) It is used in the treatment of ulcers
45. **The disorder that results from the defect in collagen synthesis is:**
    (a) Sanfilippo A
    (b) Ehlers–Danlos V
    (c) Hunter syndrome
    (d) Hurler syndrome
46. **Fibronectin:**
    (a) Has multiple domains
    (b) Attaches cells to collagen type II
    (c) Comprises monomers with a length of 70 nm
    (d) Has at least 20 peptide chains
47. **The cofactor essential for hydroxylation of proline is:**
    (a) Pantothenic acid
    (b) Vitamin $B_{12}$
    (c) Vitamin C
    (d) Folic acid
48. **Concerning glycosaminoglycans (GAGs):**
    (a) They are long branched polysaccharides
    (b) The disaccharide units contain N-acetylgalactosamine and N-acetylglucosamine
    (c) They are located primarily on the surface of cells and the ECM
    (d) They are positively charged molecules
49. **Concerning the hyaluronic acid, one of the following statements is false. It:**
    (a) Is composed of glucuronic acid and N-acetyl glucosamine
    (b) Is found in synovial fluid
    (c) Is found in the vitreous humor
    (d) Contains α-1,6 linkage

## CHAPTER 5: Chemistry of Amino Acids and Proteins

50. **Keratan sulfate contains:**
    (a) Galactose and N-acetyl glucosamine
    (b) Glucuronic acid and galactosamine
    (c) Glucuronic 2-sulfate and N-acetyl glucosamine
    (d) Galactose and N-acetyl galactosamine

### ANSWERS

| | | | | | | | | |
|---|---|---|---|---|---|---|---|---|
| 1. b | 2. d | 3. c | 4. d | 5. b | 6. c | 7. d | 8. d |
| 9. d | 10. a | 11. a | 12. b | 13. c | 14. c | 15. a | 16. a |
| 17. b | 18. a | 19. b | 20. b | 21. c | 22. c | 23. c | 24. d |
| 25. a | 26. d | 27. d | 28. c | 29. c | 30. b | 31. a | 32. c |
| 33. b | 34. c | 35. b | 36. a | 37. d | 38. c | 39. c | 40. c |
| 41. d | 42. d | 43. a | 44. c | 45. b | 46. d | 47. b | 48. a |
| 49. d | 50. a | | | | | | |

# Chapter 6

# Metabolism of Amino Acids

## LEARNING OBJECTIVES

*At the end of this chapter students should be able to:*
- Explain the process of digestion and absorption of proteins through our GI tract
- Understand the transamination, oxidative deamination and urea cycle
- Know the synthesis, catabolic products formed and inborn errors of different amino acids

## Digestion and Absorption of Proteins

The proteolytic enzymes act on proteins to convert them finally into amino acids. The amino acids are absorbed by active transport into the intestinal epithelial tissue.

**Briefly discuss the digestion and absorption of proteins in the gastrointestinal tract.**

### Digestion in the Stomach

- The protein does not undergo any digestion in the mouth.
- When protein enters the stomach, it stimulates the secretion of the hormone *gastrin,* from gastric mucosal cells.
- The gastrin stimulates the release of gastric juice, which contains hydrochloric acid (HCl) and pepsinogen (rennin in infants).
- The HCl that is secreted by parietal cells unfolds the proteins and activates the proteolytic enzyme pepsin. This is called **zymogen activation**.
- Pepsin secreted by chief cells as pepsinogen and later converted to pepsin by HCl. Pepsin converts protein polypeptides into tripeptides, dipeptides, and amino acids.

Rennin in infants is also called chymosin or rennet (it clots milk). The casein content of milk undergoes slight hydrolysis to produce paracasein, which coagulates in the presence of calcium ions, and results in an insoluble calcium paracaseinate (curd). Then this calcium paracaseinate is acted upon by pepsin. This is required to convert milk into solid form, which prevents rapid passage of milk from the stomach.

### Digestion in the Intestine

- When the acidic contents from the stomach pass into the small intestine, the low pH of the stomach constituents triggers the secretion of the hormones such as *cholecystokinin* and *secretin*.
- Secretin stimulates the release of bicarbonate and pancreatic juice from pancreas into the small intestine.
- Cholecystokinin stimulates the secretion of pancreatic endo and exopeptidases.
- Endopeptidases cleave the internal peptide bonds of proteins to convert them into smaller peptides. They are trypsin, chymotrypsin, and elastase.
- Trypsin hydrolyzes peptide bonds of proteins whose carboxyl groups are contributed by lysine and arginine residues.
- Chymotrypsin cleaves peptide bonds involving carboxyl group of aromatic amino acids and peptide linkages of leucine, methionine, asparagine, and histidine.
- Elastase hydrolyzes peptide bonds involving nonpolar amino acids such as alanine, serine, and glycine.

CHAPTER 6: Metabolism of Amino Acids

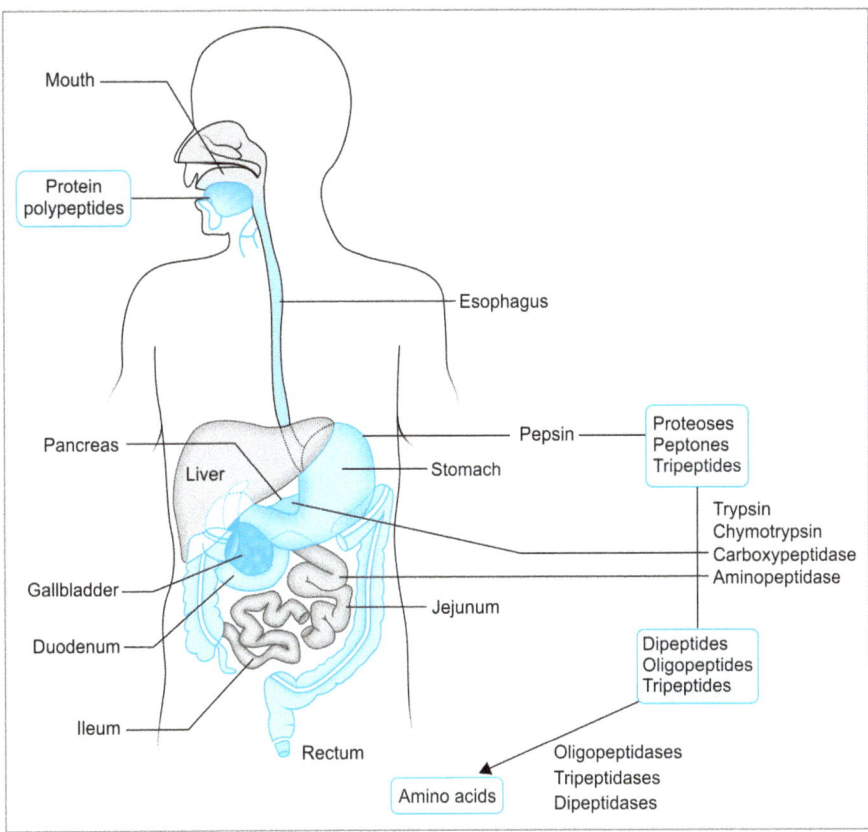

**Fig. 6.1:** Digestion of proteins.

- The exopeptidases such as carboxypeptidases and aminopeptidases are secreted in proenzyme forms and are converted to active forms by enteropeptidase or enterokinase.
- Carboxypeptidase removes amino acids from the carboxy terminal end of polypeptides and aminopeptidases removes amino acids from amino terminal end of polypeptide chain.
- The oligopeptidases act on the oligopeptides and convert them into tri- and dipeptides. The enzymes such as aminopeptidase, tripeptidase, and dipeptidase finally convert these peptides into amino acids **(Fig. 6.1)**.

## Absorption

The absorption of amino acids includes sodium-dependent active transport mechanism, which requires ATP as energy source. After the absorption, amino acids are utilized for the synthesis of protein but those and remaining excess amino acids are catabolized.

## Importance of Amino Acid in the Human Body

The amino acids, released by hydrolysis of dietary proteins, form an amino acid pool **(Fig. 6.2)**.

Amino acids are used for the synthesis of protein- and nitrogen-containing substances.

## ■ Catabolism of Amino Acids

**Explain the process of transamination and deamination of amino acids in detail.**

### Removal of Amino Groups

- The α-amino group of amino acids is removed as ammonia ($NH_3$).

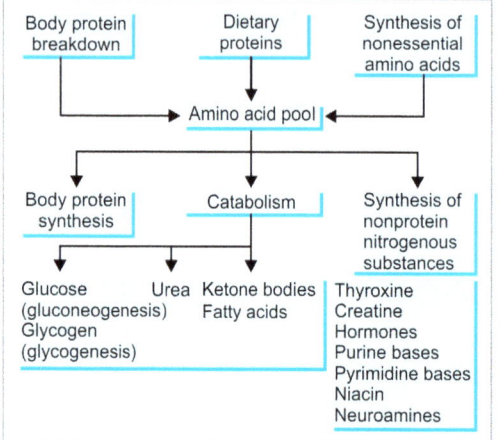

**Fig. 6.2:** Amino acid pool.

* The conversion of amino group to ammonia takes place in several tissues, but liver is the major site of removal of ammonia from amino acid.
* There are two major processes, which can remove the amino groups. These are transamination and deamination.

## Transamination

It is the process of transfer of α-amino group of an amino acid to a keto acid, forming a new amino acid and a keto acid. Enzymes, which catalyze the reversible set of reaction, are called transaminases or aminotransferases and they require vitamin $B_6$ as coenzyme.

α-amino acid 1 + α-keto acid 2 $\xrightarrow{\text{Transaminase (PLP)}}$ α-keto acid 1 + α-amino acid 2

Liver contains two most important transaminases; they are as follows:
1. Serum glutamate pyruvate transaminase (SGPT) or alanine transaminase (ALT).
   Alanine + α-ketoglutarate $\xrightarrow{\text{SGPT/ALT}}$ Pyruvate + glutamate
   *Diagnostic significance:* Enzyme increases in liver disease.
2. Serum glutamate oxaloacetate transaminase (SGOT) or aspartate transaminase (AST).
   Aspartate + α-ketoglutarate $\xrightarrow{\text{SGOT/AST}}$ oxaloacetate + glutamate

*Diagnostic significance:* This enzyme increases in cardiac disorders (myocardial infarction) as well as in liver diseases.

## Deamination

Since transamination involves only the transfer of an α-amino group from one amino acid to a keto acid and as such there is no net loss of the amino group, deamination is the actual process resulting in the removal of the α-amino group of an amino acid, which is released in the form of ammonia. Liver and kidney are the main organs involved in the deamination of an amino acid. There are two types of deamination reactions.
1. *Oxidative deamination:* L-Amino acid oxidase, D-amino acid oxidase, and glutamate dehydrogenase are the main enzymes involved in the deamination of amino acids. These enzymes remove electrons from the amino acids.

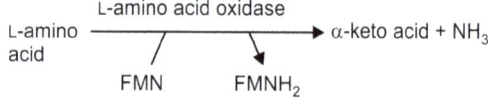

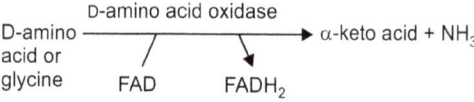

*Trans*-deamination using transaminase and glutamate dehydrogenase.

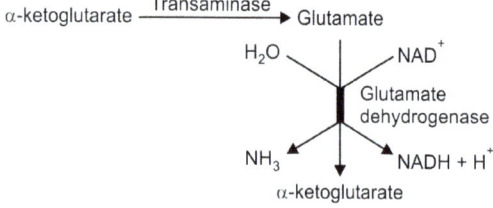

2. *Nonoxidative deamination:* Deamination of some of the amino acids such as serine, cysteine, and histidine is catalyzed by dehydratases, desulfhydrases, and histidase enzyme, respectively.

*Metabolic fate of ammonia:* In human beings and primates, the ammonia is converted to

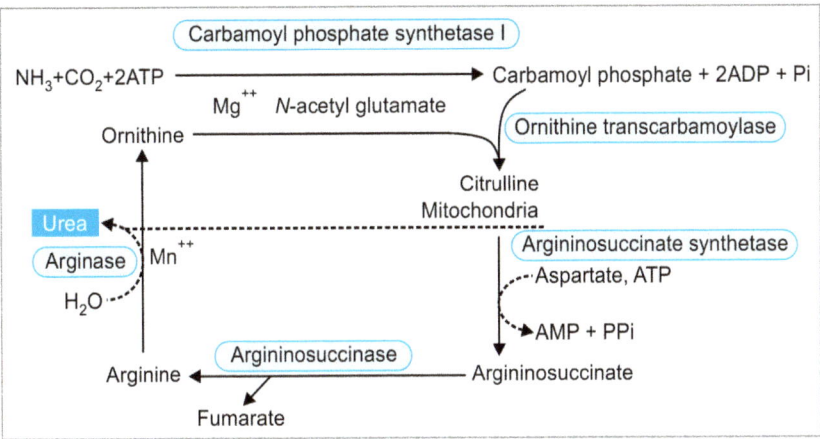

Fig. 6.3: Schematic view of urea cycle.

urea in the liver mainly through urea cycle and it is excreted as such. Therefore, human beings and primates are called ureotelic.

**State the significance of the urea cycle and how ammonia formed in the body converted urea.**

### Urea Cycle (Krebs–Henseleit Cycle)

It is the process where the highly toxic substance ammonia is converted to a less toxic excretory waste product urea ($NH_2$-CO-$NH_2$) in liver (Fig. 6.3).

- In the first step, ATP activates ammonia and it combines with $CO_2$ to form carbamoyl phosphate. This reaction is catalyzed by carbamoyl phosphate synthetase I enzyme, which requires *N*-acetyl glutamate as an activator.
- Ornithine transcarbamoylase transfers the carbamoyl group from carbamoyl phosphate to ornithine and produces citrulline.
- These first two reactions occur in the mitochondria. Other reactions proceed in cytosol.
- Citrulline combines with L-aspartate in the presence of argininosuccinate synthetase enzyme and ATP to form argininosuccinic acid.
- Argininosuccinic acid is hydrolyzed by argininosuccinase to form arginine and fumaric acid.
- In the last step, arginine is hydrolyzed by arginase to form ornithine and urea. Ornithine again enters the urea cycle.

**Briefly discuss the inborn errors of urea cycle and list the clinical symptoms of ammonia accumulation in the body.**

### The Inborn Errors of Urea Cycle

The decreased or absence of urea cycle enzymes results in urea cycle disorder and this in turn leads to many clinical symptoms such as vomiting, in infancy, lethargy, irritability, rejection of high-protein diet, and mental retardation **(Table 6.1)**.

**Table 6.1:** Inborn errors of urea cycle.

| Defective enzyme | Disorder |
| --- | --- |
| Carbamoyl phosphate synthetase I | Hyperammonemia type I |
| Ornithine transcarbamoylase | Hyperammonemia type II |
| Argininosuccinic acid synthetase | Citrullinemia |
| Argininosuccinase | Argininosuccinic aciduria |
| Arginase | Hyperarginemia |

### Ammonia Intoxication

*Accumulated ammonia results in the following symptoms:*
- Impaired brain function
- Ataxia

- Convulsions
- Lethargy
- Nausea
- Vomiting
- Slurred speech
- Blurred vision

*Treatment:* Low-protein diet and substitution of α-ketoanalogs for essential amino acids (carbon skeletons of essential amino acids are important and not their amino groups).

## Other Fates of Ammonia

Other fates of ammonia include the following:
- *Biosynthesis of nonessential amino acid:* Ammonia is used in the amination of α-keto acids derived from carbohydrates For example,

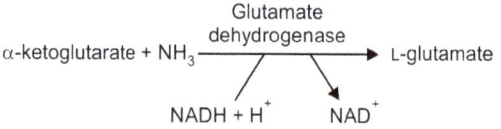

- *Formation of glutamine:* This is the main route of the disposal of ammonia from brain. Ammonia is converted into glutamine by glutamine synthetase. Glutamine is an important form for the transport of ammonia to kidney where glutaminase enzyme hydrolyzes glutamine to glutamic acid and ammonia.

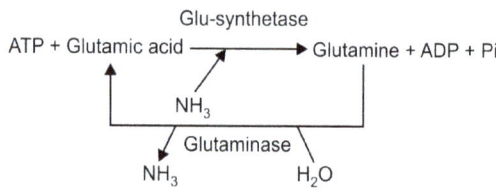

## Metabolism of Important Amino Acids

### Catabolism of Carbon Skeleton

After the removal of α-amino group as ammonia, the carbon skeletons of the amino acids form amphibolic intermediates, which are converted either into glucose or fats and ketone bodies (**Fig. 6.4**).

- Transamination of alanine, glutamate, and valine forms pyruvate, α-ketoglutarate, and

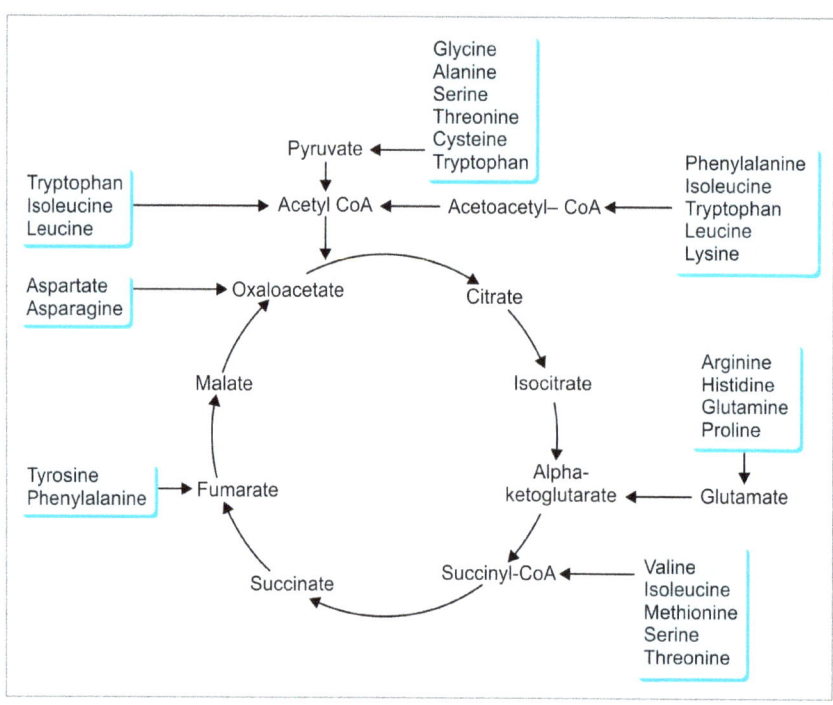

**Fig. 6.4:** Metabolic fates of carbon skeletons of amino acids.

# CHAPTER 6: Metabolism of Amino Acids

**Table 6.2:** End product of catabolism of different amino acids and their amphibolic role.

| Amino acids | End products |
|---|---|
| **Glucogenic amino acids** | |
| 1. Glycine, alanine, serine, threonine, cysteine, OH-proline | Pyruvate |
| 2. Glutamic acid, glutamine, proline, arginine, histidine | α-Ketoglutarate |
| 3. Valine, methionine | Succinyl CoA |
| **Both glucogenic and ketogenic amino acids** | |
| 1. Isoleucine | Succinyl CoA + acetyl CoA |
| 2. Phenylalanine, tyrosine | Fumarate + acetoacetyl CoA |
| 3. Tryptophan | Pyruvate |
| **Ketogenic amino acid** | |
| 1. Leucine | Acetyl CoA + acetoacetyl CoA |

succinyl CoA, respectively. These can be converted into glucose by gluconeogenesis. Such amino acids are called glucogenic amino acids.

❖ Catabolism of phenylalanine also forms acetyl CoA or acetoacetyl CoA, which are the precursors of ketone bodies. Phenylalanine also forms fumaric acid, which is glucogenic. Hence, phenylamine is grouped under both glucogenic and ketogenic amino acids.

❖ Leucine is the only amino acid whose end product of catabolism is acetoacetyl CoA. Hence, leucine is called ketogenic amino acid.

For end product of catabolism of different amino acids and their amphibolic role, are shown in **Table 6.2**.

**Discuss briefly the metabolism of glycine including the products formed from it.**

## Glycine

- Simplest amino acid
- Nonessential in the diet

*Synthesis:*

$$\text{Serine} + FH_4 \xrightarrow[\text{PLP}]{\text{Serine transhydroxy}} \text{Glycine} + N_5 \text{ (methylene } FH_4\text{)}$$

*Metabolic fate of glycine:* Biologically important compounds synthesized from glycine are as follows:

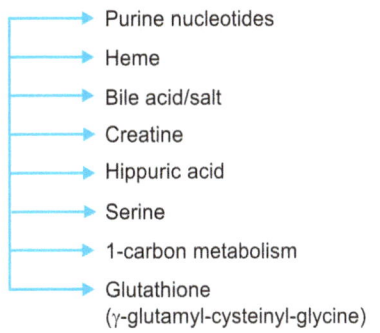

- Purine nucleotides
- Heme
- Bile acid/salt
- Creatine
- Hippuric acid
- Serine
- 1-carbon metabolism
- Glutathione (γ-glutamyl-cysteinyl-glycine)

❖ $C_4$, $C_5$, and $N_7$ of purine base present in adenine and guanine are contributed by glycine.

❖ Six glycine molecule combine with succinyl CoA totally form heme group of heme proteins (*viz*, hemoglobin).

❖ Bile acids (vizcholic acid) get conjugated with glycine and forms glycocholic acid.

❖ Glycine detoxifies benzoic acid in liver and forms hippuric acid.

❖ Creatine constitutes about 0.5% of total muscle weight. It is synthesized from three amino acids, glycine, arginine, and methionine.

❖ Creatine phosphate, the phosphorylated derivative of creatine found in muscle, is a high-energy compound that can reversibly donate a phosphate group to ADP to form ATP. This can be used to maintain the intracellular level of ATP during the first few minutes of intense muscular contraction.

$$\text{Creatine} + ATP \xrightarrow[\text{creatine kinase}]{\text{Phosphorylated}} \text{Creatine Phosphste} + ADP$$

$$\text{Arginine} + \text{glycine} \xrightarrow{\text{Arg-gly transminidase}} \text{Guanidoacetic acid} + \text{ornithine}$$

In kidney, the guanidoacetic acid is methylated by S-adenosyl methionine (SAM).

Guanidoacetic acid + SAM
↓
Creatine + S-adenosyl homocysteine (SAH)

## Glutamic Acid

- Nonessential amino acid
- It is synthesized by the action of glutamate dehydrogenase using

α-ketoglutarate and $NH_3$ amino acid + α-ketoglutarate

↓ Aminotransferase

α-ketoacid + glutamic acid.

**List the compounds formed from glutamate.**

## Metabolic Fate of Glutamate

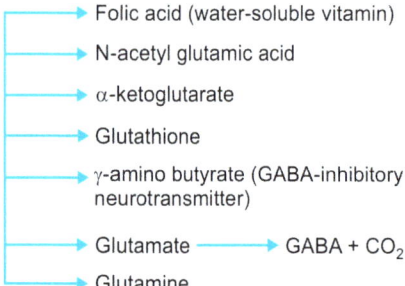

**Explain with a flow diagram showing the synthesis of tyrosine from phenylalanine.**

## Phenylalanine and Tyrosine

It is not synthesized in human body (essential amino acid) **(Fig. 6.5)**.

**Discuss the metabolism of tyrosine.**

## Catabolism of Tyrosine (Fig. 6.6)

*Normal condition*: Proteins and tyrosine are formed from phenylalanine. Formation of tyrosine from phenylalanine requires phenylalanine hydroxylase enzyme. Defect in phenylalanine hydroxylase leads to phenylketonuria. Mental retardation and convulsions are the signs. The metabolites of phenylalanine such as phenylpyruvate, phenyllactate, and phenylacetate are excreted in urine **(Fig. 6.7)**. The detection of these compounds helps in the diagnosis of phenylketonuria.

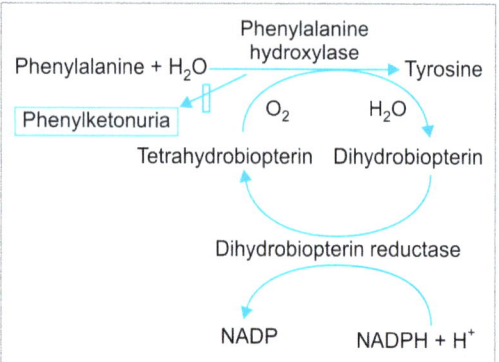

**Fig. 6.5:** Synthesis of tyrosine from phenylalanine.

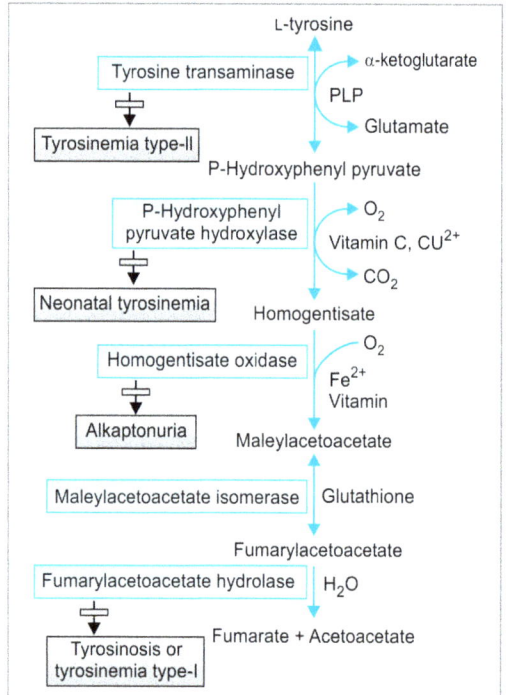

**Fig. 6.6:** Catabolism of tyrosine.

**What is phenylketonuria? Explain briefly.**

## Phenylketonuria

- *Cause*: Deficiency of *phenylalanine hydroxylase*.
- Because of the block due to enzyme deficiency the phenylalanine accumulates in the body.

- The accumulation leads to high level of phenylalanine in blood and excreted in urine.
- The accumulated phenylalanine is metabolized further by other route that normally does not take place in our body.
- Transamination of phenylalanine produces phenylpyruvate.
- The phenylpyruvate gives phenyllactate and phenylacetate by reduction and oxidative decarboxylation reactions, respectively (Fig. 6.7).
- The phenylacetate may conjugate with glutamine and excreted as phenylacetyl glutamine.
- So finally urine contains phenyllactate and phenylacetyl glutamine along with phenylalanine.

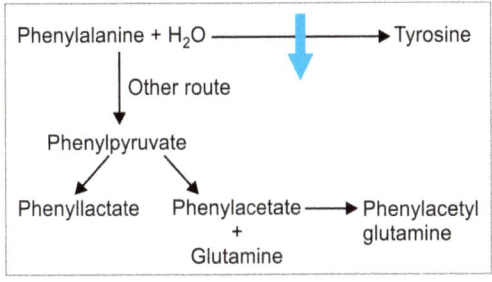

**Fig. 6.7:** Formation of phenyllactate and phenyl acetate from phenylpyruvate.

Phenylketonuria may be classified into three groups:
1. Classic phenylketonuria due to defect in phenylalanine hydroxylase. This is most common error.
2. Atypical phenylketonuria or hyperphenylalaninemia types II and III: defect in dihydrobiopterin reductase.
3. Hyperphenylalaninemia types IV and V: defect in dihydrobiopterin synthesis.

*Treatment:* Low phenylalanine diet.

## Tyrosinemia

This is a hereditary disease due to the lack of hepatic tyrosine transaminase enzyme **(Fig. 6.8)**.

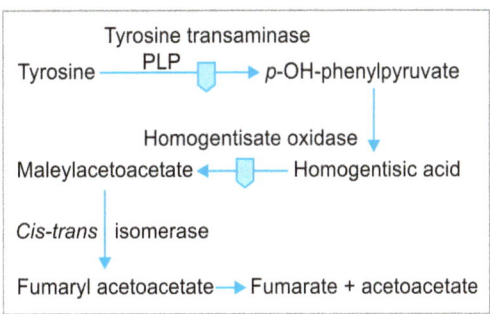

**Fig. 6.8:** Metabolic block in tyrosine catabolism.

**State the causes and clinical symptoms of alkaptonuria.**

## Alkaptonuria

Hereditary deficiency of *homogentisate oxidase* causes alkaptonuria. Homogentisic acid is excreted in urine. Urine turns black upon exposure to light. Black pigment is deposited in sclera, ear, nose, and cartilages.

Symptoms of PKU, alkaptonuria, and tyrosinemia are as follows:
- Mental retardation
- Children have low IQ
- Low serotonin levels in brain

**Synthesis of dopamine, epinephrine, and norepinephrine:**
- Epinephrine is produced in the adrenal medulla **(Fig. 6.9)**.
- Norepinephrine is a neurotransmitter produced in CNS and postganglionic sympathetic nerves **(Fig. 6.9)**.

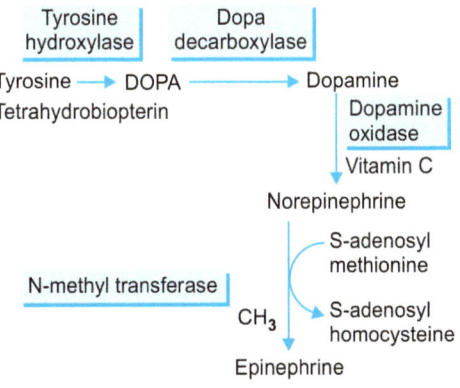

**Fig. 6.9:** Formation of catecholamines.

**List the metabolic products formed from tyrosine and explain briefly to show their formation.**

## Metabolic Fate of Tyrosine

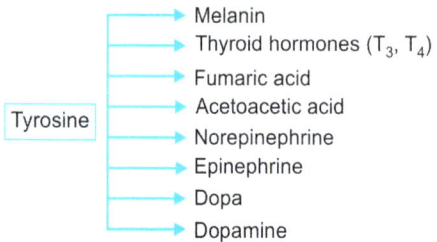

- Dopamine is present in localized regions of the brain and also functions in the peripheral organs.
- Both dopamine and norepinephrine are primary amines, whereas epinephrine is a secondary amine.
- Dopamine and norepinephrine functions as transmitters of nerve signals in the CNS.
- Epinephrine influences carbohydrate metabolism.
- These catecholamines have their characteristic physiological and pharmacological actions through the interaction with adrenergic or dopaminergic receptors that are located on the surface of target cells throughout the body.
- The overproduction of these catecholamines produces disorders.
- The α receptors interact with both epinephrine and norepinephrine, whereas β receptors interact with only epinephrine.
- Excess or reduced production of catecholamines is associated with many diseases such as thyroid hormone deficiency, congestive heart failure, and stress.
- Low levels of catecholamines are seen in idiopathic postural hypotension.
- Measurements of catecholamines are helpful in the diagnosis of catecholamine-secreting tumors such as pheochromocytomas, paraganglia, or neuroblastomas.
  - In Parkinson's disease, dopamine levels in the CNS are decreased due to a deficiency of cells that produce dopamine and depression is associated with low levels of serotonin.
  - The dephenyl is used treat this disease because this drug inhibits the action of monoamine oxidase.
  - Homovanillic acid is one of the catabolic products formed from epinephrine and norepinephrine.

## Melanin

- *Tyrosinase* deficiency leads to albinism.
- Melanin is a pigment that occurs in the eye, hair, and skin. In the epidermis, the pigment forming cells are called melanocytes. Here, the melanin is synthesized to protect the underlying cells from the harmful effects of sunlight.

$$\text{Tyrosine} \xrightarrow{\text{Tyrosinase}} \text{DOPA} \longrightarrow \longrightarrow \text{Melanin}$$

## Synthesis of $T_3$ and $T_4$

$$\text{Tyrosine} + I^+ \longrightarrow \text{Monoiodotyrosine (MIT)} \xrightarrow{\text{(MIT)}} \text{Diiodotyrosine (DIT)}$$

$$\text{MIT} + \text{DIT} \longrightarrow T_3 \text{ Triiodothyronine}$$

$$\text{DIT} + \text{DIT} \longrightarrow T_4 \text{ Tetraiodothyronine (thyroxine)}$$

**Discuss the tryptophan metabolism including its clinical significance.**

## Metabolism of Tryptophan

- It is an essential amino acid.
- It is mainly required for the synthesis of proteins, niacin, serotonin, and melatonin.

## Metabolic Fate of Tryptophan

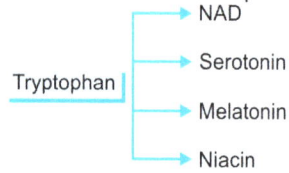

$NAD^+$ and $NADP^+$ are the acceptor of reducing equivalents ($H^+$) provided by various metabolic intermediates. About 60 mg of tryptophan forms 1 mg of niacin required for the formation of its coenzyme form NAD⁺ and NADP⁺.

## Synthesis of Serotonin

Serotonin is a vasoconstrictor and stimulator of smooth muscle contraction. The degradation product of serotonin is 5-hydroxy indole acetic acid.

Tryptophan ⟶ 5-OH-tryptophan ⟶ 5-OH-tryptamine (Serotonin)
                                    ↑
                                  $CO_2$

*Hartnup's disease:* This is caused by a defect in the intestinal absorption and renal reabsorption of tryptophan. Tryptophan and its catabolic products, high amount of indoleacetic acid, are excreted in the urine. Indoleacetic acetic acid excreted as indole acetyl glutamine after conjugation with glutamine.

*Malignant carcinoid (argentaffinoma):* This is characterized by serotonin-producing tumor cells in the argentaffin tissue of the abdominal cavity. Instead of 1%, the 60% of tryptophan is diverted to form serotonin. Pellagra-like symptoms may be seen. Urine contains large amounts of 5-hydroxy indole acetic acid.

**Briefly explain the histidine metabolism and state the importance of FIGLU excretion test.**

## Histidine Metabolism

❖ It is a basic essential genetically coded amino acid.

❖ Histidine is also a precursor of histamine, a compound released by immune system cells during an allergic reaction.

❖ It is needed for growth and for the repair of tissue, as well as the maintenance of the myelin sheaths that act as protector for nerve cells.

❖ It is further required for the manufacture of both red and white blood cells and helps to protect the body from damage caused by radiation and in removing heavy metals from the body.

❖ In the stomach, histidine is also helpful in producing gastric juice and people with a shortage of gastric juice or suffering from indigestion may also benefit from this nutrient.

Histidine $\xrightarrow[\text{PLP}]{\text{Decarboxylase}}$ Histamine + $CO_2$

❖ Histamine strongly stimulates the secretion of HCl by the parietal cells of the stomach.

## Catabolism of Histidine (Fig. 6.10)

### FIGLU Excretion Test

*Cause:* Folic acid deficiency leads to deficiency of $FH_4$, which is required for the conversion of N-formiminoglutamate (FIGLU) to glutamic

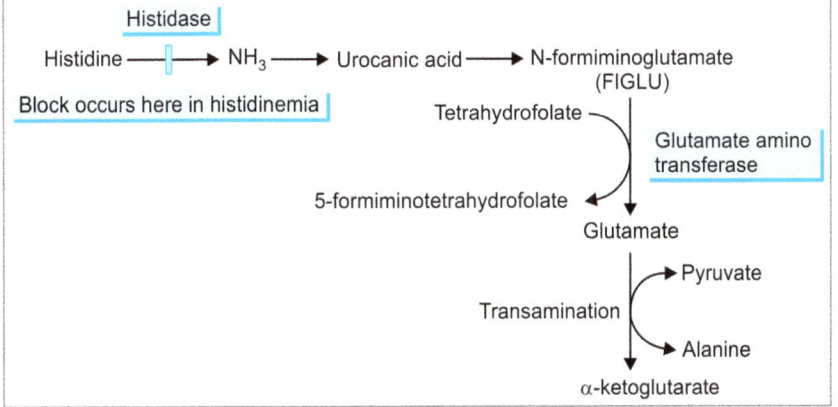

**Fig. 6.10:** Catabolism of histidine.

acid. Accumulation of FIGLU leads to excretion in the urine.
* Megaloblastic anemia occurs in the case of deficiency of both folic acid and vitamin $B_{12}$.
* To differentiate the anemia the FIGLU excretion test can be conducted.

**Discuss the metabolism of branched chain amino acids.**

## Metabolism of Branched Chain Amino Acids

Refer **Figure 6.11**.

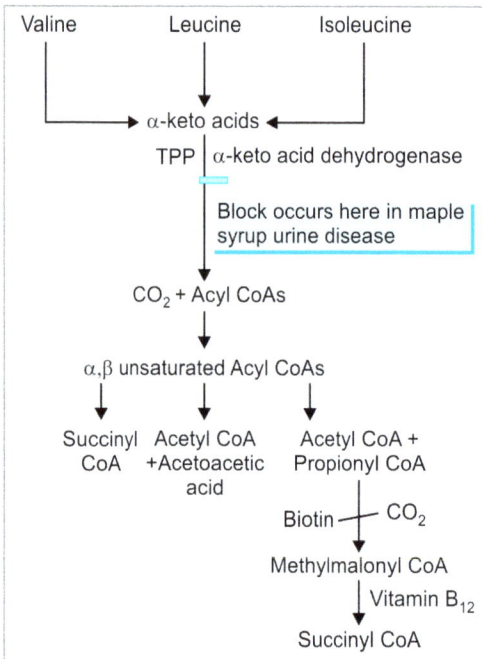

**Fig. 6.11:** Catabolism of branched chain amino acids.

## Maple Syrup Urine Disease

* It is an inborn error of branched chain amino acid metabolism.
  *Cause*: Deficiency or complete absence of α-keto acid dehydrogenase (**Fig. 6.11**).
* Accumulated α-keto acids excreted in the urine.
* These keto acids give a characteristic smell to the urine. It is similar to that of maple syrup.

*Symptoms*:
- Seizures
- Coma
- Mental retardation.

*Diagnosis*: Antenatal diagnosis may be done by measuring decarboxylase activity in cultured cells from amniotic fluid.
Analysis of urine with dinitrophenylhydrazine and measurement of plasma amino acid levels.

*Treatment*: Replacing dietary protein by mixture of amino acids that excludes leucine, isoleucine, and valine.

**State the importance of methionine and show the formation of S-adenosyl methionine.**

## Methionine

* Methionine is one of the essential amino acids (building blocks of protein), meaning that it cannot be produced by the body and must be provided by the diet.
* It supplies sulfur and other compounds required by the body for normal metabolism and growth.
* Methionine also belongs to a group of compounds called lipotropics, or chemicals that help the liver to process fats (lipids).
* Methionine and cysteine are the only sulfur-containing proteinogenic amino acids.
* The methionine derivative SAM serves as a methyl donor. Methionine plays a role in cystine, carnitine, and taurine synthesis by the transsulfuration pathway, lecithin production, the synthesis of phosphatidylcholine, and other phospholipids.
* Improper conversion of methionine can lead to atherosclerosis.

- Methionine is coded by a single codon (AUG) in the standard genetic code (tryptophan, encoded by UGG, is the other).

## S-Adenosyl Methionine

It is an enzymatic cofactor involved in methyl group transfers. It methylates targets, many of which are in the brain. It deactivates dopamine by methylating a hydroxy group on the catechol **(Table 6.3)**.

$$\text{Methionine} + \text{ATP} \xrightarrow{\text{Methionine adenosyltransferase}} \text{SAM} + \text{PPi} + \text{Pi}$$

**Table 6.3:** Special compounds formed from other amino acids.

| Amino acids | Special compounds |
| --- | --- |
| Histidine | Histamine, carnosine, anserine, formiminoglutamic acid (FIGLU) |
| Cysteine | Taurine, glutathione |
| Methionine | Cysteine, SAM one-carbon donor |

SAM: S-adenosyl methionine.

**What is formylmethionine and what is its importance in humans?**

## Formylmethionine

Formylmethionine (fMet) is a modified form of methionine in which a formyl group has been added to methionine's amino group. fMet is a starting residue in the synthesis of proteins in prokaryotes and, consequently, is located at the N-terminal of the polypeptide. fMet is delivered to the ribosome (30S)–mRNA complex by a specialized tRNA (tRNA. fMet) which has a 5′-CAU-3′ anticodon that capable of binding with the AUG start codon located on the mRNA.

The addition of the formyl group to methionine is catalyzed by the enzyme transformylase. Transformylase will catalyze the addition of the formyl group to methionine only if methionine has been loaded onto tRNA. fMet and not onto tRNA. Met.

**What is homocystinuria? Explain including the causes and clinical symptoms.**

## Methionine Catabolism

SAH undergoes hydrolysis to form homocysteine. Methionine without methyl group is homocysteine.

### Homocystinuria

It is an inherited disorder of methionine metabolism.

*Cause:* Deficiency or complete absence of cystathionine β-synthase in the liver which converts homocysteine and serine to cystathionine.

Another cause is deficiency of methyl tetrahydrofolate or methyl-$B_{12}$ due to inadequate intake folic acid or vitamin $B_{12}$ (or due to defective enzyme that joins methyl groups to THF, transferring methyl from methyl $B_{12}$ to homocysteine to form methionine).

There are four type of homocystinuria **(Fig. 6.12)**:
1. Homocystinuria-I (deficiency in cystathionine β-synthase).
2. Homocystinuria-II (defect in $N^5, N^{10}$-methylene THF reductase).
3. Homocystinuria-III (defect in homocysteinetransmethylase).
4. Homocystinuria-IV (defect in absorption from intestine).

*Signs and symptoms:* Myopia, glaucoma, retinal detachment, osteoporosis, thinning and lengthening of the long bones, and knock knee. The serious symptoms are caused by arterial and venous thrombosis.

*Treatment:* Therapy with pyridoxine to activate the enzyme cystathionine β-synthase is helpful. Those with complete enzyme deficiency should be treated with a diet low in methionine and supplemented with cystine. Vitamin $B_{12}$ can be given in its deficiency.

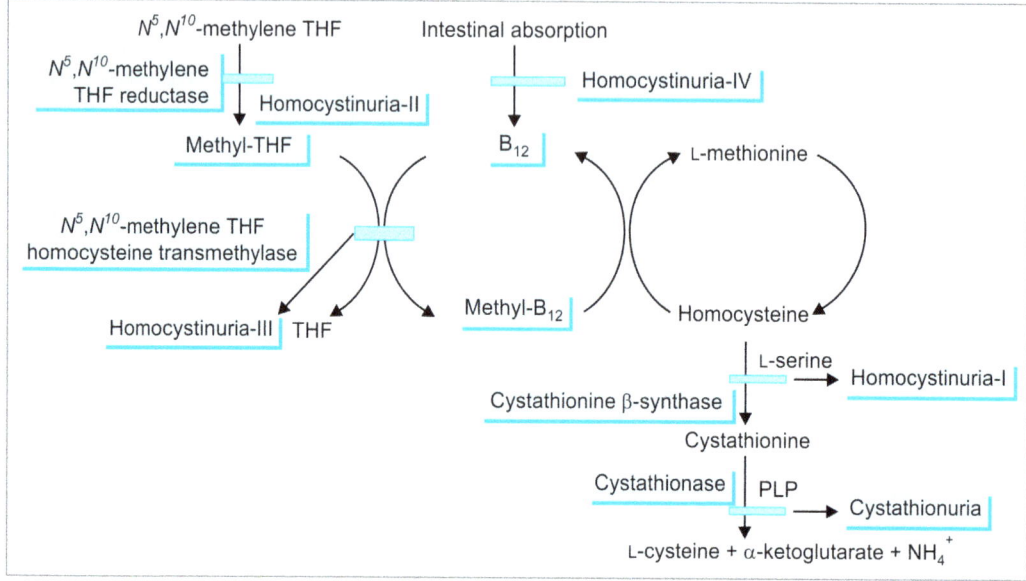

Fig. 6.12: Metabolic blocks in different types of homocystinuria.

Silver nitroprusside test is helpful in the diagnosis.

*Cystathionuria:* It is a genetic disorder due to cystathionase deficiency.

## Formation of Methionine from Homocysteine

For the conversion of methionine to homocysteine, the source of methyl group is $N^5$-methyl $FH_4$. It is transferred to vitamin $B_{12}$ to form methyl cobalamine, its coenzyme. The methyl group from this is transferred to homocysteine to form methionine.

## Synthesis of Creatine

Creatine is present in muscle, liver, and kidney. Synthesis takes place in kidney and liver using three amino acids glycine, arginine, and SAM (methyl donor).

Creatinine excretion in urine is always constant in normal person (1–1.5 g/day). It varies in kidney disease and muscle diseases.

## SUMMARY

Digestion of dietary proteins starts in the stomach. Secretion of HCl activates the formation of pepsin from pepsinogen, which hydrolyzes peptide bonds of dietary proteins to release aromatic amino acids. Similarly, in the small intestine digestion continues. Zymogens are activated for the breakdown of peptide bonds to release amino acids, which are absorbed into the small intestine through active transport mechanism. These absorbed amino acids are utilized to synthesize protein and undergo catabolism to generate nonprotein nitrogenous substances, urea, fatty acids, ketone bodies, and so on. The catabolism of amino acids results in the formation of ammonia, which is toxic to human body and therefore body will convert this to urea for excretion. Any defect with the urea cycle enzymes results in the accumulation ammonia or intermediates of urea cycle, which causes metabolic disorder. Glycine is the simplest amino acid responsible for the production of heme, glutathione, and purine nucleotides. Glutamate catabolism results in GABA and glutathione. Tyrosine can be synthesized by phenylalanine with the help of phenylalanine hydroxylase and the deficiency of this enzyme results in phenylketonuria. The tyrosine is responsible for the generation of DOPA, dopamine, melanin, epinephrine, and norepinephrine. Homogentisate oxidase deficiency results in alkaptonuria with a symptom of dark urine and mental retardation. Serotonin, melatonin, and niacin are the metabolic intermediates of tryptophan. The maple syrup urine disease is the clinical condition arises due to the deficiency of α-keto acid dehydrogenase enzyme of branched chain amino acid metabolism. Homocystinuria is an inherited disorder of methionine metabolism.

## SELF-ASSESSMENT QUESTIONS

1. Outline the urea cycle and note the site of synthesis.
2. What is the need for urea synthesis in our body?
3. Describe the process of removal of ammonia from amino acids.
4. Explain the specialized compounds formed from gly, phe, and trp.
5. Name the enzymes required for the following reactions:
   (a) $NH_3 + ATP + CO_2 \longrightarrow$ Carbamoyl phosphate
   (b) Phenylalanine $\longrightarrow$ Tyrosine
   (c) Creatine $\longrightarrow$ Creatine phosphate
   (d) Tyrosine $\longrightarrow$ DOPA
6. Describe the synthesis of creatine in our body.
7. Write a note on inborn errors of amino acid metabolism.
8. What are glucogenic, both glucogenic and ketogenic, and ketogenic amino acids?
9. Write the metabolic fate of tryptophan.
10. State the compounds formed from tyrosine.
11. How tyrosine is formed from phenylalanine?
12. Write the cause for the following inborn errors of metabolism:
    (a) Alkaptonuria
    (b) Phenylketonuria
    (c) Maple syrup urine disease
    (d) Albinism

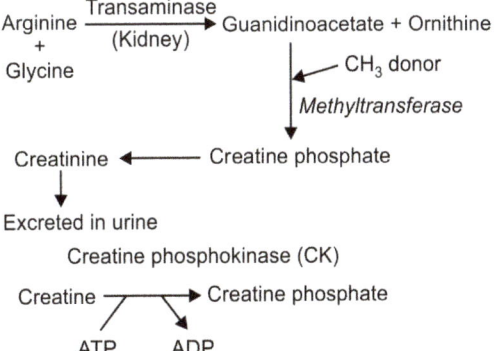

13. Write the flowchart to show the synthesis of serotonin from tryptophan.
14. Which amino acid is responsible for the synthesis of niacin in our body?
15. What is FIGLU excretion test and what is its significance?
16. Write the importance of glycine.

17. Name the compounds formed from glutamate.
18. Briefly discuss the transamination and oxidative deamination process.
19. What is the fate of ammonia?
20. Add a note on the inborn errors of urea cycle.

## MULTIPLE CHOICE QUESTIONS

1. **Pepsin is secreted in:**
   (a) Intestine
   (b) Liver
   (c) Stomach
   (d) Pancreas
2. **The coenzyme required for the catalytic activity of transaminase is:**
   (a) TPP
   (b) PLP
   (c) NAD
   (d) FAD
3. **Toxic ammonia produced in the body converted to:**
   (a) Uric acid
   (b) Citrulline
   (c) Purine
   (d) Urea
4. **Which of the following enzyme results in hyperammonemia type I?**
   (a) Carbamoyl phosphate synthetase 1
   (b) Arginase
   (c) Argininosuccinase
   (d) Argininosuccinic acid synthetase
5. **Which one of the following compounds is not synthesized from glycine?**
   (a) Heme
   (b) Creatine
   (c) Serine
   (d) Tyrosine
6. **Concerning glutamic acid, one of the following is not true:**
   (a) It is required for folic acid synthesis
   (b) It is a nonessential amino acid
   (c) Aspartate transaminase catalyzes its synthesis
   (d) It is a component of glutathione
7. **Phenylalanine:**
   (a) Is synthesized in the human body
   (b) Synthesis depends on phenylalanine hydroxylase
   (c) Synthesis defect results in alkaptonuria
   (d) Can synthesize tyrosine
8. **Concerning tyrosine metabolism, one of the following statements is incorrect:**
   (a) It is essential for thyroid hormone synthesis
   (b) It is required to synthesize DOPA and dopamine
   (c) Tyrosine transaminase deficiency results in phenylketonuria
   (d) Tyrosine-deficient children will have low IQ
9. **Concerning tryptophan, all of the following statements are true, *except*:**
   (a) It is required to synthesize serotonin
   (b) It is an essential amino acid
   (c) It can form niacin
   (d) It is essential to synthesize melanin
10. **Malignant carcinoid is a metabolic disorder of:**
    (a) Tyrosine
    (b) Tryptophan
    (c) Histidine
    (d) Glycine
11. **Concerning histidine one of the following statements is incorrect:**
    (a) It is an acidic essential amino acid
    (b) It is required for the manufacture of both red and white blood cells
    (c) It is also helpful in producing gastric juices
    (d) It is a precursor of histamine

12. **Maple syrup urine disease:**
    (a) Is an inborn error of glycine metabolism
    (b) Is the result of deficiency of α-keto acid dehydrogenase
    (c) Results in increased levels of amino acids in the urine
    (d) Does not results in mental retardation
13. **Concerning methionine, one of the following statements is incorrect:**
    (a) Methionine is the only sulfur-containing proteinogenic amino acids
    (b) It supplies sulfur and other compounds for metabolism and growth
    (c) Its derivative S-adenosyl methionine (SAM) serves as a methyl donor
    (d) It is coded by AUG
14. **Methionine without methyl group is:**
    (a) Homocysteine (b) Cysteine
    (c) Cystine (d) Formylmethionine
15. **All of the following are the steps in creatine metabolism, except:**
    (a) Arginine + glycine→Guanidoacetate (b) Creatine phosphate→Creatine
    (c) Creatine→Creatine phosphate (d) Ornithine→Creatine phosphate
16. **All of the special compounds are formed from histidine, except:**
    (a) Histamine (b) Carnosine
    (c) Taurine (d) Anserine
17. **Which of the following statements is correct?**
    (a) Urea is produced directly by the hydrolysis of ornithine
    (b) ATP is required for the reaction in which argininosuccinate is cleaved to form arginine
    (c) The urea cycle occurs exclusively in the cytosol
    (d) In humans, the major route of nitrogen metabolism from amino acids to urea is catalyzed by the combined actions of transaminase (aminotransferase) and glutamate dehydrogenase
18. **Which of the following statements concerning the synthesis of carbamoyl phosphate by carbamoyl phosphate synthetase I is incorrect?**
    (a) The enzyme catalyzes the rate-limiting reaction in the urea cycle
    (b) The reaction is allosterically activated by N-acetyl glutamate
    (c) The reaction is reversible
    (d) The reaction requires two high-energy phosphates for each carbamoyl phosphate molecule synthesized
19. **Tyrosine would be an essential amino acid in the diet of a child with:**
    (a) Lesch–Nyhan syndrome (b) Defective tyrosine aminotransferase
    (c) Deficiency of thiamine (d) Classical phenylketonuria
20. **One of the following amino acids give rise to α-keto acids that accumulate in the urine in maple syrup urine disease is:**
    (a) Phenylalanine (b) Valine
    (c) Lysine (d) Tyrosine
21. **The collagen defect present in scurvy is:**
    (a) Decreased protein stability due to decreased hydroxylation of proline and lysine residues
    (b) Substitution of valine for proline and lysine residues in the collagen sequence
    (c) Increased formation of Schiff base cross-links
    (d) Decreased protein stability due to increased glycosylation.

22. Smokers tend to develop emphysema more readily than nonsmokers. This is due to oxidation of a methionine residue in:
    (a) Elastin
    (b) Pulmonary collagen
    (c) Neutrophil elastate
    (d) Alpha 1-antitrypsin
23. Which amino acid serves as a carrier of ammonia from skeletal muscle to liver?
    (a) Alanine
    (b) Methionine
    (c) Arginine
    (d) Glutamine
24. Type of covalent bonds link the amino acid in a protein is:
    (a) Peptide bonds
    (b) Hydrogen bonds
    (c) Glycosidic bonds
    (d) Ester bonds
25. Which of the following statements is false?
    (a) After a resistance training session the rate of protein synthesis in the exercised muscles is increased
    (b) After a resistance training session the rate of protein breakdown in the exercised muscles is increased
    (c) Exercise increases the rate of secretion of growth
    (d) Protein cannot be used as a fuel for exercise
26. Which of the following is true?
    (a) Increasing the protein intake above 5 g/kg body mass/day will stimulate muscle growth and increase strength
    (b) Creatine supplements can increase muscle strength and power
    (c) Amino acid supplements can increase muscle strength and power
    (d) Muscle damage is induced by shortening contractions
27. When branched chain amino acids are deaminated in muscle, the ammonia produced is mostly:
    (a) Converted into glucose and released from the muscle
    (b) Converted into alanine and glutamine and released from the muscle
    (c) Converted into urea and released from the muscle
    (d) Used to synthesize purines and pyrimidines in the muscle
28. One of the following promotes glucose and amino acid uptake by muscle is:
    (a) Adrenaline
    (b) Insulin
    (c) Glucagon
    (d) Cortisol
29. Which amino acid is very important for optimal immune function and exhibits a reduced plasma concentration during heavy training?
    (a) Arginine
    (b) Glutamine
    (c) Phenylalanine
    (d) Isoleucine
30. Absorption of which one of the following amino acids is defective in Hartnup's disease?
    (a) Lysine
    (b) Leucine
    (c) Tyrosine
    (d) Tryptophan
31. Which one of the following deficiency results in homocystinuria?
    (a) Cystathionine β-synthase
    (b) Phenylalanine hydroxylase
    (c) Methyl transferase
    (d) Creatine phosphokinase
32. The cofactors involved in the regeneration of methionine from homocysteine are:
    (a) Retinoic acid
    (b) Tetrahydrofolic acid and vitamin $B_{12}$
    (c) TPP
    (d) Biotin and vitamin K

33. Amino acid that is both glucogenic and ketogenic is:
    (a) Phenylalanine
    (b) Alanine
    (c) Leucine
    (d) Lysine
34. The precursor for the synthesis of dopamine is:
    (a) Phenylalanine
    (b) Tryptophan
    (c) Lysine
    (d) Isoleucine
35. The rate-limiting step of urea cycle is:
    (a) Carbamoyl phosphate synthetase
    (b) Ornithine transcarbamoylase
    (c) Arginase
    (d) Argininosuccinase
36. Which of the following is not an essential amino acid?
    (a) Serine
    (b) Tyrosine
    (c) Isoleucine
    (d) Histidine
37. Phenylketonuria results from the deficiency of:
    (a) Keto acid decarboxylase
    (b) Arginase
    (c) Homogentisate oxidase
    (d) Phenylalanine hydroxylase
38. Excess lysine in the diet may impair the absorption of:
    (a) Arginine
    (b) Phenylalanine
    (c) Tyrosine
    (d) Tryptophan
39. The intermediate that links urea cycle directly with TCA cycle is:
    (a) Arginine
    (b) Fumarate
    (c) Glutamate
    (d) Pyruvate
40. The vitamin involved in carbon dioxide fixation reactions of amino acid metabolism is:
    (a) Niacin
    (b) Biotin C
    (c) Pyridoxine
    (d) Pantothenic acid
41. The major nonprotein nitrogenous substance present in urine is:
    (a) Creatinine
    (b) Uric acid
    (c) Urea
    (d) Amino acids
42. Catabolism of serine and alanine produces:
    (a) Pyruvate
    (b) Fumarate
    (c) Lactate
    (d) Succinate
43. All of the following are formed from amino acid precursors, *except*:
    (a) Parathyroid hormone
    (b) Thyroid hormones
    (c) Glucocorticoid hormone
    (d) Follicle-stimulating hormone
44. The site of urea synthesis is:
    (a) Liver
    (b) Kidney
    (c) Brain
    (d) Adrenal gland
45. The oxidative deamination of the amino acid alanine in muscle produces:
    (a) One molecule of pyruvic acid and a molecule of ammonia
    (b) One molecule of pyruvic acid and a molecule of carbon dioxide
    (c) One molecule of glutamic acid and another amino acid
    (d) One molecule of pyruvic acid and a molecule of urea

46. David, an 8-month-old male infant, emigrated with his parents from India to the Trinidad and Tobago a month ago. He was normal at birth but in the past several days a tremor in his extremities has appeared. Last night he presented gross twitching movements in his crib. When examined the patient noted a musty odor to the baby's wet diaper. Immediately ordered a screening test for PKU, which showed positive. Which of the following compounds can you expect that is elevated in this patient's urine?
    (a) Phenyllactate
    (b) Histidine
    (c) Methyl malonic acid
    (d) Homogentisate

47. **Multiple myeloma:**
    (a) Results from a polyclonal proliferation of lymph node plasma cells
    (b) Often presents with eye pain
    (c) Hypercalcemia develops in 50% of patients
    (d) Most patients have a serum alpha-proteinemia

## ANSWERS

| | | | | | | | | | |
|---|---|---|---|---|---|---|---|---|---|
| 1. c | 2. b | 3. d | 4. a | 5. d | 6. c | 7. b | 8. c |
| 9. d | 10. b | 11. a | 12. b | 13. a | 14. a | 15. c | 16. c |
| 17. d | 18. c | 19. d | 20. b | 21. a | 22. d | 23. a | 24. a |
| 25. d | 26. b | 27. b | 28. b | 29. b | 30. d | 31. a | 32. b |
| 33. a | 34. a | 35. a | 36. a | 37. d | 38. a | 39. b | 40. b |
| 41. c | 42. a | 43. d | 44. a | 45. a | 46. a | 47. c | |

# Chapter 7

# Chemistry of Lipids

## LEARNING OBJECTIVES

*At the end of this chapter students should be able to:*
- Classify the lipids with specific examples
- Explain the different phospholipids and glycolipids with their importance

## Introduction

Lipid or fat is characterized by their physical property with water, it says, "Touch me not" but it goes well into solution with organic solvents. To the tongue it is tasteful; within limits it is good for the life but makes it danger when it is in excess.

## Definition

Lipids are heterogeneous group of naturally occurring compounds, which are relatively insoluble in water but freely soluble in nonpolar organic solvents like, benzene, chloroform, ether and alcohol.
- Obtained from animals and plants
- Made up of long-chain hydrocarbon groups (carbon and hydrogen) but may also contain oxygen, phosphorus, nitrogen and sulfur.

## Functions of Lipids

Functions of lipids are as follows:
- Triglycerides are the major storage form of energy.
- They provide essential fatty acids; phospholipids, hormones (prostaglandins) and they form important constituents of cell membrane.
- Helps in the absorption of vitamin A, D, E and K.
- The basic unit of lipids, i.e., acetyl CoA is used for the synthesis of cholesterol and hence steroid hormones.
- The lipids maintain the membrane structure and integrity.
- Since lipids are **organic compounds with hydrocarbon chain**, its insulating effect has been utilized in the body for protecting internal organs from shock.
- They help in blood coagulation.
- Dipalmitoyl lecithin, a phospholipid act as surfactant and is required for the normal functioning of the lung alveoli.

**Classify the lipids with specific examples.**

## Classification of Lipids

Refer **Table 7.1**.

## Simple Lipids

They are esters of fatty acid with glycerol or higher alcohols.
Example: fats and waxes.

### Fats

Esters of fatty acids with glycerol. A fat in the liquid state is known as oil. Fat is also called as triglyceride or triacylglycerol.

*Triacylglycerol (Triglyceride)*
- Nearly all the commercially important fats and oils of animal and plant origin consist almost exclusively of the simple

**List the functions of lipids.**

**Table 7.1:** Classification of lipids.

| Simple lipids | Compound lipids | Derived lipids |
|---|---|---|
| They are esters of fatty acid with glycerol or higher alcohols<br>Examples: fats and waxes | They are esters of fatty acid with one of the various alcohols and in addition, they contain other groups (nonlipid component)<br>Examples: phospholipids:<br>• *Glycerophospholipids:* Lecithin, cephalin Phosphatidyl serine, phosphatidyl inositol Cardiolipins, plasmalogens<br>• *Sphingophospholipids:* Sphingomyelin<br>Glycolipids: cerebrosides and gangliosides<br>Lipoproteins: chylomicron, VDL, LDL, and HDL | Derived from simple or compound lipids<br>Examples: fatty acid, glycerol, alcohol, and cholesterol |

(HDL: high-density lipoprotein; LDL: low-density lipoprotein; VDL: very low-density lipoprotein).

lipid class triacylglycerols (often termed triglycerides).
* They consist of a glycerol moiety with each hydroxyl group esterified to a fatty acid. In nature, they are synthesized by enzyme systems, which determine that a center of asymmetry is created about carbon-2 of the glycerol backbone, so they exist in enantiomeric forms, i.e., with different fatty acids in each position.
* They are esters of fatty acid with the trihydric alcohol glycerol.
* Glycerol with one molecule of fatty acid is called monoacylglycerol.
* Glycerol with two molecule of fatty acid is called diacylglycerol.

$$\begin{array}{c} CH_2OH \\ | \\ R''COO-CH \\ | \\ CH_2OH \end{array}$$
2-monoacylglycerol

* Triglyceride = glycerol attached with three fatty acid.

$$\begin{array}{c} \alpha_{-1}CH_2\text{-}OH \\ | \\ \beta CH\text{-}OH \\ | \\ \alpha_{-2}CH_2\text{-}OH \end{array} \;\; +3 \text{ fatty acids} \longrightarrow \begin{array}{c} \alpha_1 CH_2\text{-}O\text{-}CO\text{-}R_1 \\ | \\ \beta CH\text{-}O\text{-}CO\text{-}R_2 \\ | \\ \alpha_2 CH_2\text{-}O\text{-}CO\text{-}R_3 \end{array}$$

Glycerol　　　　　　　　　　Triacylglycerol

$R_1$, $R_2$ and $R_3$ indicate the fatty acids. The fatty acids may be same or different type. Usually $R_2$ is an unsaturated fatty acid.

## Waxes

Esters of fatty acids with monohydric long chain alcohols.

In their most common form, wax esters consist of fatty acids esterified to long-chain alcohols with similar chain-lengths. The latter tend to be saturated or have one double bond only. Such compounds are found in animal, plant and microbial tissues and they have a variety of functions, such as acting as energy stores, waterproofing and lubrication.

$$\sim\!\sim\!\sim\!\sim\!\sim\!\sim\!\sim\!COO\!\sim\!\sim\!\sim\!\sim\!\sim\!\sim\!\sim$$

In some tissues, such as skin, avian preen glands or plant leaf surfaces, the wax components can be much more complicated in their structures and compositions. They can contain aliphatic diols, free alcohols, hydrocarbons (e.g., squalene), aldehydes and ketones.

## Compound Lipids

They are esters of fatty acid with one of the various alcohols and in addition, it contains other groups (non-lipid component). These are classified again on the basis of prosthetic group present in the lipid.
* Phospholipids (PLs)
* Glycolipids
* Lipoproteins (LPs).

# List the various types of phospholipids and state their importance.

## Phospholipid

Phospholipids are compound lipids containing alcohol, fatty acid, phosphoric acid and a nitrogenous base or other alcoholic group. Phospholipids may be classified on the basis of the type of alcohol present as:

1. *Glycerophospholipids*: The alcohol present in glycerophospholipids is glycerol.
   - Phosphatidyl choline (lecithin)
   - Phosphatidyl ethanolamine (cephalin)
   - Phosphatidyl serine
   - Phosphatidyl inositol
   - Cardiolipins
   - Plasmalogens
2. *Sphingophospholipids*: The alcohol present is sphingosine.

❖ **Glycerophospholipids:**
  - ***Phosphatidyl choline (lecithin)***: Contains alcohol, fatty acid, phosphoric acid and choline. The fatty acid part of $R_1$ is saturated fatty acid and $R_2$ at β position is an unsaturated fatty acid. Lecithin is present in brain, nervous tissue, and sperm and egg yolk. Lecithins are surface-active agent and help in emulsification of fats. Dipalmitoyl lecithin is a lung surfactant (lowers surface tension) prevents the collapse of lung alveoli. Absence of dipalmitoyl lecithin in premature infants may produce **respiratory distress syndrome or hyaline membrane disease.**

```
CH₂–O–CO–R₁              CH₂–O–CO–R₁
|                         |
CH–O–CO–R₂               CH–O–CO–R₂
|                         |
CH₂–O–phosphoric acid    CH₂–O–phosphoric acid—choline

Phosphatidic acid        Lecithin (phosphatidyl choline)
```

  - ***Phosphatidyl ethanolamine (cephalins)***: Contain alcohol, fatty acid, phosphoric acid and ethanolamine as a nitrogenous base instead of choline present in lecithin. Cephalins are present in brain, erythrocytes and many other tissues.
  - ***Phosphatidyl serine***: Contains alcohol, fatty acid, phosphoric acid and serine as a nitrogenous base.
  - ***Phosphatidyl inositol***: It is a phospholipid containing phosphatidic acid bound to the alcohol inositol instead of a nitrogenous base. They are important component of cell membrane. The action of certain hormones (e.g., oxytocin, vasopressin) is mediated through phosphatidyl inositol (PI). In response to hormonal action, PI is cleaved to diacyl glycerol (DAG) and inositol triphosphate (IP3). Both these compounds **act as second messenger for hormonal action.**

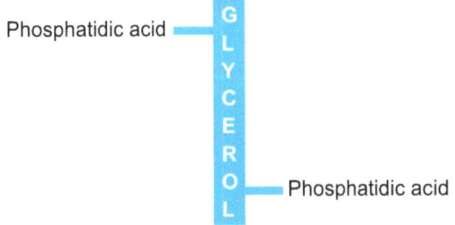

Phosphatidylinositol

  - ***Cardiolipin***: It is diphosphatidyl glycerol. It contains two molecules of phosphatidic acid held by glycerol. It is present in the inner mitochondrial membrane and has antigenic properties.

```
Phosphatidic acid —[GLYCEROL]— Phosphatidic acid
```

  - ***Plasmalogen***: They differ from lecithin or cephalin in α-1 position of glycerol where the fatty acid is replaced by a long chain unsaturated aliphatic aldehyde such as palmitic or stearic aldehyde. Plasmalogens are present in large quantities in the skeletal muscle, cardiac muscle and in semen.

❖ ***Sphingomyelin***: This is a sphingophospholipid. It does not contain glycerol but an unsaturated amino alcohol, i.e., sphingosine. They contain a molecule of choline, phosphoric acid and a fatty acid. Sphingomyelin makes up a large part of the myelin sheath. These are also present in brain, lungs, nerve and other tissues.

Deposition of sphingomyelin in liver, lymph nodes, bone marrow and central nervous system results in **Niemann–Pick disease**. It may be due to the deficiency of sphingomyelinase enzyme in these tissues.

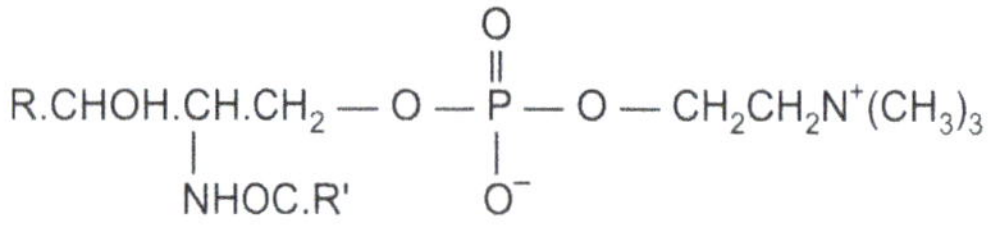

$$R.CHOH.CH.CH_2-O-\overset{\overset{O}{\|}}{\underset{O^-}{P}}-O-CH_2CH_2N^+(CH_3)_3$$
$$\underset{NHOC.R'}{|}$$

*Ceramide*: It is formed by the esterification of sphingosine (an amino alcohol) with a fatty acid of high molecular weight. Principally found in white matter of brain in myelin sheath and medullated nerves. Ceramide is common for all glycolipids and sphingomyelin.

## Glycolipids

They contain fatty acid, sphingosine (alcohol), carbohydrate or carbohydrate derivative.
1. *Cerebrosides*: They contain a molecule of fatty acid, an amino alcohol sphingosine and a sugar (usually galactose). They are present in white matter of brain and myelin sheath of nerves. Their level is increased in **Gaucher's disease** in tissues like reticuloendothelial cells of spleen, liver, lymph node and bone.
2. *Gangliosides*: They are designated as GM1, GM2, etc., and are found in gray matter of the brain and contain N-acetylneuraminic acid (sialic acid), fatty acid, alcohol sphingosine and three molecules of hexoses (such as glucose or galactose). In **Tay–Sachs disease** is characterized by elevated ganglioside level.

## Lipoproteins

### Structure and Function

Lipoproteins are conjugated proteins, composed of core and surface **(Fig. 7.1)**.
* LP core has
  - Triglycerides
  - Cholesterol esters
* LP surface has
  - Phospholipids
  - Proteins
  - Cholesterol
* Lipids are water insoluble
* Present in the blood in the form of lipoproteins which are water soluble.
* They have an outer polar surface, which makes them water soluble.

*Separation by ultracentrifugation*: Four distinct groups based on their density **(Figs. 7.2A and B)**.
* Chylomicron—transport of dietary triglyceride from intestine to extrahepatic tissues and liver.

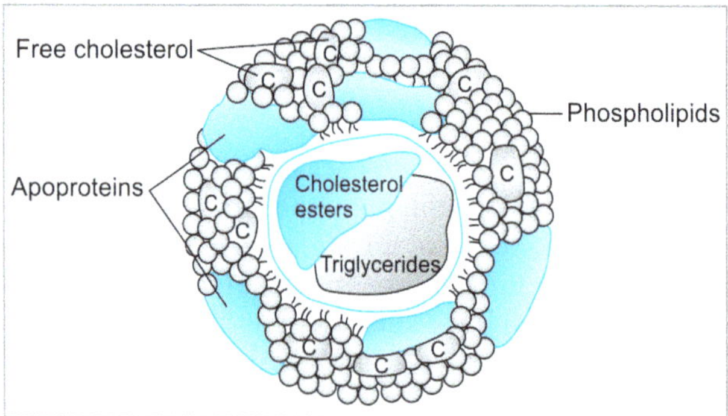

**Fig. 7.1:** Structure of lipoprotein.

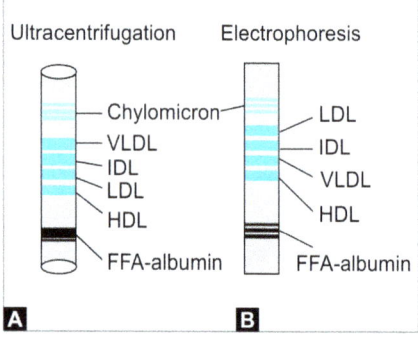

**Figs. 7.2A and B:** Separation of lipoproteins: (A) Ultracentrifugation; (B) Electrophoresis. (VLDL: very low-density lipoprotein; IDL: intermediate-density lipoprotein; LDL: low-density lipoprotein; HDL: high-density lipoprotein; FFA: free fatty acid)

- Very low-density lipoprotein (VLDL)—transport of endogenous triglyceride and cholesterol to extrahepatic tissues.
- Low-density lipoprotein (LDL)—transport of cholesterol from liver to extrahepatic tissues.
- High-density lipoprotein (HDL)—transport of cholesterol from extrahepatic tissues to liver.

## Derived Lipids

Substances derived from the above groups by hydrolysis, e.g., fatty acid, glycerol, alcohol and cholesterol.

### Fatty Acid

*Definition*: Fatty acids are aliphatic monocarboxylic organic acid with chain length usually ranging from C-4 to C-24 and it is a constituent of lipid. The fatty acids have the general formula R–CO–OH.

*Nomenclature*: Fatty acids are named after the name of the hydrocarbon with the same number of carbon atoms, with suffix—oic acid for saturated fatty acid and the suffix—enoic acid for the unsaturated fatty acid.

### Numbering of a Fatty Acid

- The carbon atoms of the fatty acids are numbered from the -COOH group (carboxyl group).
- Carboxyl group carbon is $C_1$, and then next carbon atom is $C_2$. The carbon atom adjacent to the –COOH group is also called as α-carbon atom; next carbon atom is β and so on. The last carbon atom or $CH_3$ group is designated as ω carbon. For example, oleic acid is written as 18:1; 9 or Δ9, 18:1

$$\underset{\omega}{CH_3}-(CH_2)_7-CH=CH-\underset{\underset{10\ \ 9}{}}{(CH_2)_5}-\underset{\underset{3\ \ 2\ \ 1}{\beta\ \ \alpha}}{CH_2-CH_2-COOH}$$

- Oleic acid (18:1; 9) or Δ9, 18:1 indicates fatty acid having 18 carbon with one double bond at carbon atom 9. The position of the double can also be indicated by the symbol Δ followed by the position of the double bond in superscript.
- The fatty acids are numbered from the ω carbon.
- The linoleic acid is called ω-6 series because of the presence of first double bond from ω-6 carbon at the 6th carbon.

$$\underset{\omega}{\overset{18\ \ 17}{CH_3}}-(CH_2)_4-\overset{13\ 12}{CH}=\overset{11}{CH}-\overset{10}{CH_2}-\overset{9}{CH}=\overset{8}{CH}-(CH_2)_7-\overset{1}{COOH}$$

- Likewise linolenic acid is ω-3 series.

$$\underset{\omega}{\overset{18}{CH_3}}-CH_2-CH=CH-CH_2-CH=CH-CH_2-CH=CH-(CH_2)_7-\overset{1}{COOH}$$

- Arachidonic acid is ω-6 series.

**What are saturated and unsaturated fatty acids? Explain with examples.**

## Classification of Fatty Acid

*Saturated Fatty Acid*
- No double bond present
- For example:
    - Acetic acid (two carbon atoms)
    - Butyric acid (four carbon atoms)
    - Palmitic acid (C16)
    - Stearic acid (C18)
    - Lignoceric acid (C24).

*Unsaturated Fatty Acids*
- The fatty acids, which have double bonds, are called unsaturated fatty acids. They are further classified into—monounsaturated fatty acid (MUFA): it contains one double bond, e.g., palmitoleic acid (C16, Δ9), oleic acid (C18, Δ9).

$$\underset{\omega}{\overset{20}{CH_3}}-(CH_2)_4-\overset{14}{CH}=CH-CH_2-\overset{11}{CH}=CH-CH_2-\overset{8}{CH}=CH$$
$$-\overset{5}{CH_2}-CH=CH-(CH_2)_3-COOH$$

- *Polyunsaturated fatty acid*: It contains more than one double bond (PUFA) For example:
    - Linoleic acid (C18, Δ9)
    - Linolenic acid (C18, Δ9, 12, 15)
    - Arachidonic acid (C20, Δ5, 8, 11, 14).

**Explain essential fatty acids with specific examples.**

## Essential Fatty Acids or PUFA

Fatty acids which are not synthesized in the body and should be supplied through diet are called essential fatty acids. They contain more than one double bond. Example: linoleic acid, linolenic acid and arachidonic acid (PUFA). These fatty acids are not synthesized in the human body because of lack of the desaturase enzyme, which introduces double bonds beyond 9th and 10th carbon atoms.

- Linoleic acid, represented as (18:2; 9, 12) or [$\Delta$9, 12; 18]. It means that this fatty acid contains 18 carbon atoms and two double bonds at position C9 and C12.
  $CH_3-(CH_2)_4-CH=CH-CH_2-CH=CH-(CH_2)_7-COOH$
- Linolenic acid, represented as (18:3; 9, 12, 15) or [$\Delta$9, 12, 15; 18]
  $CH_3-CH_2-CH=CH-CH_2-CH=CH-CH_2-CH=CH-(CH_2)_7-COOH$
- Arachidonic acid represented as (20:4; 5, 8, 11, 14,) or [$\Delta$5, 8, 11, 14; 20]
  $CH_3-(CH_2)_4-CH=CH-CH-CH=CH-CH_2-CH=CH-(CH_2)_3-COOH$.

## Functions of Fatty Acids

- Essential fatty acids are involved in the esterification of cholesterol and thus help in its transport and metabolism. So essential fatty acid lowers cholesterol level and hence decreases the risk of heart disease.
- Essential fatty acids are constituent of the cell membrane and membranes of cell organelle (e.g., mitochondria).
- They are essential for maintaining normal growth and health.
- Fatty acids are components of simple and compound lipids, which are present in various tissues like adipose tissue.
- They are responsible for the hydrophobic nature of the compounds contains them.
- They provide energy when they are oxidized in human body.
- Prostaglandins and leukotrienes are formed from PUFA (arachidonic acid). They act as local hormones.
- They protect the liver from accumulation of fat (prevent fatty liver).
- Essential fatty acids help to prevent skin disease.

## Cis versus Trans Fatty Acid

- *Cis*: Both H atoms are on the same side of the C = C double bond, which causes a bend in their structure.
- Most naturally occurring unsaturated fatty acids in food are *cis*.

- *Trans*: Both H atoms are on opposite sides of the C=C double bond.
  - Do not bend and have physical properties similar to saturated fatty acids.
  - Are not commonly found in nature.
- This form occurs in partially hydrogenated foods when hydrogen atoms shift around some double bonds and change the configuration from *cis* to *trans*.

- Major sources of *trans*—fatty acids:
  - Margarine
  - Cakes and cookies
  - Snack chips
  - Meat and dairy products
  - Peanut butter
  - Fried foods

## Chaulmoogric Acid

Chaulmoogric acid is a special type of fatty acid. It contains a cyclic ring and used in the treatment of leprosy.

## Glycerol

- It is a trihydric alcohol as it contains three hydroxyl groups.
- It is a gluconeogenic substance because on lipolysis of dietary lipid releases glycerol, which is converted into glucose in liver.

## Steroids and Cholesterol

Steroids are often found in association of lipids. They are compounds having special ring called cyclopentanoperhydrophenanthrene nucleus.

For example, steroid hormone, bile acid, vitamin D.

**Discuss the cholesterol including its functions.**

## Cholesterol

- It is one of the important steroids present in the body. It has 27 carbon, an –OH group, a double bond, two methyl groups at C10 and C13 and a side chain at C17.
- It is the precursor of various compounds such as vitamin $D_3$, bile acids and adrenocortical and sex hormones.
- Cholesterol is widely distributed in all cells of the body but nervous tissue is rich in cholesterol.
- Steroids containing one or more –OH groups are known as sterols **(Fig. 7.3)**.
- Normal fasting serum cholesterol level is 150–200 mg/dL.
- It is synthesized in our body using acetyl CoA as precursor (1 g/day).
- Cholesterol exists in free and ester form. Cholesterol gets esterified through esterase enzymes.
- Excess cholesterol is harmful to body in that it gets deposited in the intima of

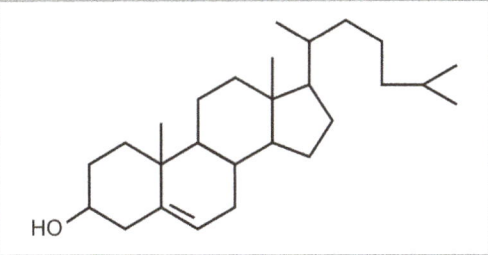

**Fig. 7.3:** Structure of cholesterol.

the arteries producing atherosclerosis. This can narrow the lumen of blood vessel impeding blood flow, which cause thrombosis.

## Functions of Cholesterol

Cholesterol if maintained in normal level has number of good effects. They are:
- It is a precursor for the synthesis of bile acids in liver.
- The steroid hormone in adrenal cortex and sex hormones in gonads are mainly synthesized from cholesterol.
- Cholesterol form 7 dehydrocholesterol in skin, it is converted to vitamin $D_3$ by UV rays
- Cholesterol is a poor conductor of heat and hence acts as an insulator.
- Cholesterol is a poor conductor of electricity. Cholesterol is abundant in brain and nervous tissue where it functions as an insulating covering for structure, which generates and transmits electrical impulse.

## Properties of Lipids

### Physical Properties

Oils and fats (lipids) are similar in nature. Oils and lipids are different only in their physical property. Triglycerides, which contain a higher proportion of unsaturated fatty acid or short chain fatty acid, are liquid at 20°C and are usually called as oils, e.g., vegetable oils.

On the other hand, fats are solid at room temperature and contain saturated long chain fatty acid, e.g., animal fat, and dalda.

## Amphipathic Nature of Lipids

The lipid that possess both hydrophobic (nonpolar) and hydrophilic (polar) groups is known as an amphipathic lipid. These include fatty acid, phospholipids (e.g., lecithin), sphingolipid and bile salts.

Phospholipids have a hydrophilic head (phosphate group) attached to choline or ethanolamine or inositol, etc., and a long hydrophobic tail. The general structure may be represented as polar head with a nonpolar tail.

$$\text{Triacylglycerol (Tripalmitin)} \xrightarrow[\text{(Sodium salt)}]{\text{Acid/Alkali/Lipase}} \text{Glycerol} + \text{3 palmitic acid}$$

When amphipathic lipids are mixed in water the polar heads faces towards aqueous phase while nonpolar tails face in opposite direction. This nature leads to the formation of a micelle. Amphipathic lipids are important constituents of the lipid bilayer of biological membranes (**Fig. 7.4**).

*Triglycerides (triacylglycerol):* Can be hydrolyzed by acids, alkali or enzymes like lipases.

## Saponification

It the hydrolysis of triglyceride by alkali which forms soap. Sodium and potassium soaps are soluble in water whereas magnesium and calcium soaps form insoluble soaps. Number of mg of KOH required to completely saponify 1 g of the oil or fat is called as saponification number. This is the measure of chain length of a fatty acid or average molecular size of the fatty acids present. The value is higher for fats containing short chain fatty acids.

$$\text{Triacylglycerol} + \text{Alkali (NaOH)} \longrightarrow \text{Glycerol} + \begin{matrix} R_1\text{–COO Na} \\ R_2\text{–COO Na} \\ R_3\text{–COO Na} \end{matrix}$$
[Soap formation]

## Iodine Number

It is a measure of the degree of unsaturation of a fat. It is defined as the number of grams of iodine that combines with 100 g of fat. High iodine numbers indicate higher degree of unsaturation. Iodine is incorporated into the double bonds present in the fatty acids. Determination of iodine number will help to know the degree of adulteration of given oil.

## Rancidity

Naturally occurring fats particularly from animal sources, on storage in the presence of moist air give unpleasant smell and develop a characteristic taste and odor. It is due to the partial hydrolysis of fats, which are further oxidized into aldehyde and ketones. This process is called rancidity. Bacteria and lipolytic enzymes cause hydrolytic rancidity. Presence of oxygen or intermediates like peroxides causes oxidative rancidity. Butter contains volatile (free) fatty acids and hence more prone to rancidity.

Antioxidants like vitamin E, vitamin C, butylatedhydroxy toluene (BHT) and butylatedhydroxy anisole (BHA) can prevent oxidation of fats and thus the development of rancidity.

## Peroxidation

Peroxidation (auto-oxidation) of lipids when exposed to oxygen is responsible not only for deterioration food but also for damage to tissues in vivo. Lipid peroxidation is a chain reaction continuously generating free radicals that initiate further peroxidation. To reduce this peroxidation humans make use

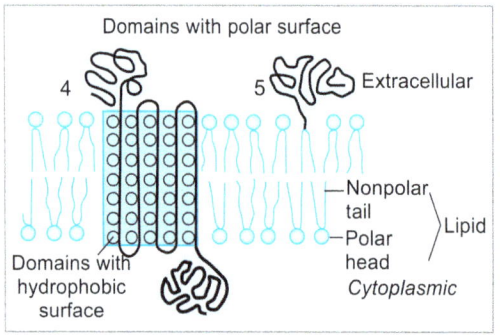

**Fig. 7.4:** Lipid bilayer of membrane.

of antioxidants which prevents the oxidative damage.

**What are prostaglandins and state their functions.**

## Prostaglandins and Related Compounds

* Prostaglandins (PGs) and their related compounds are prostacyclins (PGI) thromboxanes (TXA) and leukotrienes (LT) are collectively known as eicosanoids
* Eicosanoids are considered as locally acting hormones with a wide range of biochemical functions.
* Prostaglandins are derivatives of a hypothetical 20 carbon fatty acid namely prostanoic acid.
* The various prostanoids are:
  * Prostaglandins, e.g., $PGE_1$, $PGE_2$, $PGE_3$
  * Prostacyclins, e.g., $PGI_2$, $PGI_3$
  * Thromboxanes, e.g., $TXA_1$, $TXA_2$.
* Prostaglandins are named as PG plus a third letter (E, F, A, D), which corresponds to the type, and arrangement of functional group in the molecule and the subscript indicate number of double bonds ($PGE_1$).
* Prostaglandins are synthesized from arachidonic acid, which is released from membrane bound phospholipids.
* Corticosteroid and aspirin inhibit the prostaglandin synthesis.
* They act as local hormones and are involved in a wide range of biochemical function. In general prostaglandins are involved in the lowering of blood pressure, induction of inflammation, medical termination of pregnancy, induction of labor, inhibition of gastric HCl secretion, decrease in immune response and increase in glomerular filtration rate.

## Synthesis

Arachidonic acid is the precursor for most of the prostaglandins in humans.

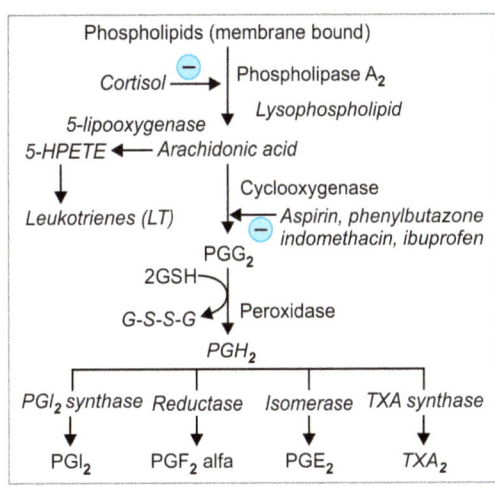

**Fig. 7.5:** Prostaglandin synthesis.

* Release of arachidonic acid from membrane bound phospholipids by phospholipase $A_2$—this is due to the stimuli by epinephrine or bradykinin.
* Oxidation and cyclization of arachidonic acid to $PGG_2$, which is then converted to $PGH_2$ by a reduced glutathione dependent peroxidase.
* $PGH_2$ serves as the immediate precursor for the synthesis of a number of prostaglandins, including prostacyclins and thromboxanes (Fig. 7.5).

## Inhibition of Prostacyclins Synthesis

* A number of structurally unrelated compounds can inhibit prostaglandin synthesis.
* Cortisol inhibit the enzyme phospholipase A2.
* Aspirin irreversibly inhibits the cyclooxygenase.

## Degradation

* Almost all the eicosanoids are metabolized rapidly.
* Lung and liver are the major sites of PG degradation.
* 15-β-hydroxy PG dehydrogenase and 13-PG reductase convert hydroxyl group at

C-15 to keto group and then to C-13 and C-14 dihydro derivative.

## Biochemical Actions of Prostaglandins

- Prostaglandins act as local hormones.
- They differ from the true hormones in many ways.
- They are produced in almost all the tissues.
- They are not stored and they are degraded to inactive products at the site of their production.
- They are produced in small amounts with low half-lives.

### Regulation of Blood Pressure

- PGs mediate (PGE, PGA and $PGI_2$) are vasodilator in function, this result in increase the blood flow and decreased peripheral resistance to lower the BP.
- Serve as agents in the treatment of hypertension.

### Inflammation

- The PGs ($PGE_1$ and $PGE_2$) induce the symptoms of inflammation (redness, swelling, edema, etc.) due to arteriolar vasodilation.
- Corticosteroids are usually used to treat inflammation which inhibits PG synthesis.

### Reproduction

$PGE_2$ and $PGF_2$ are used for the medical termination of pregnancy and induction of labor.

### Pain and Fever

- Pyrogens (fever producing agents) may promote PG synthesis leading to the formation of $PGE_2$ in the hypothalamus, the site of regulation of body temperature.
- $PGE_2$ along with histamine and bradykinin cause pain. The cause for migraine is increased $PGE_2$ level.
- Aspirin and other nonsteroidal drugs inhibit PG synthesis and thus control fever and pain.

### Prevention of Gastric Ulcer

*Effects on Respiratory Function*
PGE is a bronchodilator whereas PGF act as constrictor of smooth muscles. $PGE_1$ and $PGE_2$ are used in the treatment of asthma.

### Influence on Renal Function

- PGE increases GFR and promotes urine output.
- PGE increases the excretion of sodium and potassium.

### Metabolism

*PGE*
- Decreases lipolysis
- Increases glycogenesis
- Promotes mobilization of calcium from the bone.

### Platelet Aggregation and Thrombosis

- The prostaglandins, namely prostacyclins ($PGI_2$), inhibit platelet aggregation.
- Thromboxanes ($TXA_2$) and $PGE_2$ promote platelet aggregation and blood clotting that might lead to thrombosis.
- Thus they are antagonistic in their action.
- In the overall effect $PGI_2$ act as a vasodilator, while $TXA_2$ is a vasoconstrictor.
- Thromboxane ($TXA_2$) and prostaglandin ($PGE_1$) promote platelet aggregation and prostacyclin ($PGI_2$) inhibits the platelet aggregation.
- Inhibitors of prostaglandin synthesis (aspirin, ibuprofen) are used in controlling fever, pain, migraine and inflammation.
- Prostaglandins are found in seminal fluid, plasma and other tissues. They have pharmacological and biochemical action and act on smooth muscle, blood vessel and adipose tissue.

## Leukotrienes

- These are the mediators of allergic reactions and inflammation.
- They also cause bronchoconstriction, increase vascular permeability and mucus secretion (e.g., $LTA_3$, $LTA_4$).
- Certain fish foods contain an unsaturated fatty acid namely eicosapentanoic acid (EPA) (20 carbon atoms and 5 double bonds), which inhibit the synthesis of thromboxanes ($TXA_2$), thus decrease platelet aggregation and thrombosis and therefore lower the risk of myocardial complications as seen in the Eskimos.

## Lipotropic Factors

- These are substances, which facilitate mobilization of fat from liver.
- Various lipotropic factors (agents) are choline, betaine, methionine and inositol.
- They are required for the conversion of triglyceride (TG) to phospholipid (PL) and thus help in normal transport and utilization of lipids especially in liver.
- The deficiency of lipotropic factors leads to a condition known as fatty liver, i.e., increased accumulation of fat content in liver.

## SUMMARY

Lipids are heterogeneous group of naturally occurring compounds insoluble in water and soluble in nonpolar organic solvents. They are classified into simple, compound and derived lipids. Fats and waxes are simple lipids. Phospholipids, glycolipids and lipoproteins are the examples for compound lipids. Fatty acids and cholesterol are derived lipids. Lipids are the major form of energy, provide essential fatty acids, maintain membrane structure and integrity, act as lung surfactant and essential for the absorption of fat soluble vitamins. Compound lipids like lipoproteins are of different types like chylomicron, VLDL, LDL, and HDL. The protein part of the lipoprotein is called apo-protein. HDL is the good cholesterol which transports cholesterol from extrahepatic tissues to liver for metabolism. LDL is a bad cholesterol because it transports cholesterol from liver to extrahepatic tissues for deposition. Fatty acids are of saturated and unsaturated. The essential fatty acids are those which have to be supplied through diet and they are linoleic acid, linolenic acid and arachidonic acid. Nonessential fats acids are those which can be is synthesized in the body. Triglyceride is a simple lipid which is made of glycerol, one unsaturated and two saturated fatty acids. Lipids are amphipathic in nature. Cholesterol is formed from acetyl CoA which is required for steroid hormone synthesis.

## SELF-ASSESSMENT QUESTIONS

### Essay Type Questions

1. Write an account of classification of lipids with suitable example.
2. Define lipids. What are their biomedical importance?
3. Describe the structure, classification and functions of phospholipids.
4. Discuss the saturated and unsaturated fatty acids of biological importance.
5. Describe the structure of steroids. Add a note on functions of cholesterol.
6. What are lipoproteins? How are they separated? What is the significance of their level in blood?

## Briefly Explain the Following

1. Structure of triacylglycerol (TG).
2. Glycolipids.
3. Essential fatty acids.
4. Rancidity.
5. Saponification number.
6. Iodine number.
7. Lecithin.
8. Atherosclerosis.
9. Sphingomyelin.
10. Prostaglandins.
11. Lipoproteins.
12. Lipotropic factors.
13. Amphipathic nature of the lipids.

## Short Answer Questions

1. Which lipid serves as fuel reserve in animals?
2. The number of mg of KOH required to hydrolyze 1 g of fat or oil is known as what?
3. Name the phospholipids that produces second messenger in hormonal action is.
4. Name the glycolipid containing N-acetyl neuraminic acid.
5. What do you call it if the steroids contain a cyclic ring?
6. Give an example for an antioxidant.

## Explain the Following

1. Vegetable oil are liquid at room temperature whereas animal fat is solid.
2. Lecithin is amphipathic molecule.
3. Butter becomes rancid faster than ghee.
4. Saponification number decreases with increase in molecular weight of fat.

## MULTIPLE CHOICE QUESTIONS

1. **The nitrogenous base present in lecithin is:**
    (a) Ethanolamine  (b) Inositol
    (c) Serine  (d) Choline
2. **The number of double bonds present in arachidonic acid is:**
    (a) 1  (b) 2
    (c) 3  (d) 4
3. **Which of the following is an amphipathic lipid?**
    (a) Phospholipid  (b) Fatty acid
    (c) Bile salts  (d) All the three
4. **Name of the test employed to check the adulteration of butter:**
    (a) Iodine number  (b) Saponification number
    (c) Zak's method  (d) Reichert-Meissl number
5. **All the following alcohol are present in phospholipids, *except*:**
    (a) Sphingosine  (b) Inositol
    (c) Mannitol  (d) Glycerol

# CHAPTER 7: Chemistry of Lipids

6. Which of the following is not a phospholipid?
   - (a) Plasmalogen
   - (b) Lecithin
   - (c) Sphingomyelin
   - (d) Ganglioside
7. Which of the following is a essential fatty acid:
   - (a) Oleic acid
   - (b) Arachidic acid
   - (c) Linoleic acid
   - (d) Palmitic acid
8. Sphingomyelin contains which of the following component?
   - (a) Glycerol, phosphoric acid, 2 fatty acids and choline
   - (b) Sphingosine, phosphoric acid, 1 fatty acid and choline
   - (c) Sphingosine, phosphoric acid and 2 fatty acid
   - (d) Glycerol, phosphoric acid and 2 fatty acids
9. The plasma lipoprotein which is least dense:
   - (a) VLDL
   - (b) LDL
   - (c) HDL
   - (d) Chylomicron
10. The plasma lipoprotein which moves fast towards the anode during electrophoresis is:
    - (a) VLDL
    - (b) LDL
    - (c) HDL
    - (d) Chylomicron
11. The polyunsaturated fatty acids (PUFA) are richly present in:
    - (a) Sunflower oil
    - (b) Butter
    - (c) Ghee
    - (d) Coconut oil
12. Deficiency of which phospholipid causes respiratory distress syndrome:
    - (a) Cardiolipin
    - (b) Phosphatidic acid
    - (c) Dipalmitoyl lecithin
    - (d) Cephalin
13. Triglycerides have:
    - (a) One saturated and two unsaturated fatty acid
    - (b) Glycerol and three unsaturated fatty acid
    - (c) Three saturated fatty acid and glycerol as the backbone
    - (d) Two saturated and one unsaturated fatty acid
14. Phospholipids consist of:
    - (a) Glycerol and fatty acid esters
    - (b) Alcohol, cholesterol and phosphoric acid
    - (c) Alcohol, phosphoric acid, fatty acids and a nitrogenous base
    - (d) Alcohol, fatty acids and a nitrogenous base
15. Concerning lecithin all the following statements are true, *except*:
    - (a) It has both saturated and unsaturated fatty acids
    - (b) Dipalmitoyl lecithin is a lung surfactant
    - (c) Presence of dipalmitoyl lecithin in premature infants may produce respiratory distress syndrome
    - (d) Present in brain and nervous tissue
16. Phosphatidyl inositol:
    - (a) Is absent in cell membrane
    - (b) Consists of glycerol and phosphatidic acid
    - (c) Has antigenic properties
    - (d) Act as second messenger for hormonal action
17. All the following are the examples of compound lipids, *except*:
    - (a) Glycolipids
    - (b) Plasmalogen
    - (c) Cholesterol
    - (d) Lipoprotein

18. The structure shown below is:
    $CH_3-CH_2-CH=CH-CH_2-CH=CH-CH_2-CH=CH-(CH_2)_7-COOH$
    (a) Arachidonic acid
    (b) Linolenic acid
    (c) Linoleic acid
    (d) Oleic acid
19. Concerning lipoproteins, one of the following statements is false:
    (a) LDL cholesterol transports cholesterol from extrahepatic tissues to liver
    (b) It consists of triglyceride and cholesterol ester, proteins, phospholipid and free cholesterol
    (c) Chylomicron transports dietary triglyceride and cholesterol esters from intestine to peripheral tissues and liver
    (d) Separates into four different types on the basis of their density
20. One of the following is the nonessential fatty acid:
    (a) Arachidonic acid
    (b) Linolenic acid
    (c) Palmitic acid
    (d) Linoleic acid
21. The enzyme responsible for prostaglandin synthesis is:
    (a) 15-Hydroxy prostaglandin dehydrogenase
    (b) Cyclooxygenase
    (c) Oxidoreductase
    (d) Adenylcyclase
22. Phospholipase:
    (a) Is involved in the synthesis of prostaglandin
    (b) Is the key enzyme in the hormone action where $Ca^{++}$ is necessary
    (c) Activation of protein kinase
    (d) Is activated by adenylatecyclase
23. The physical property that allows lipids to form membranes:
    (a) Inherent flexibility
    (b) They are amphipathic and have hydrophobic tails and hydrophilic heads
    (c) Tight binding to proteins
    (d) High degree of reactivity
24. All the following compounds are esterified with membrane phospholipids, *except*:
    (a) Serine
    (b) Inositol
    (c) Ethanolamine
    (d) Ribose
25. According to the chemical and biological classifications of fatty acids, we can classify palmitic acid as:
    (a) Monounsaturated and essential
    (b) Monounsaturated and nonessential
    (c) Polyunsaturated and nonessential
    (d) Saturated and essential
26. Different compounds included in this classificatory group of lipids, can act as pulmonary surfactant, component of membranes and precursors of second messengers. This is the group of:
    (a) Steroids
    (b) Sphingolipids
    (c) Triacylglycerols
    (d) Fatty acids
    (e) Phosphoglycerides
27. A premature baby, shortly after birth, presents with rapid breathing, intercostal retractions, and grunting sounds while breathing. A blood gas analysis reveals low oxygen and acidosis. A diagnosis of respiratory distress syndrome is quickly made. This syndrome is seen in newborns with immature lungs whose pneumocytes do not synthesize enough:
    (a) Phosphatidyl inositol
    (b) Phosphatidyl choline
    (c) Sphingosin
    (d) Sphingomyelin

## CHAPTER 7: Chemistry of Lipids

28. **Polymers of polysaccharides, fats and proteins are all synthesized from monomers by:**
    (a) Connecting monosaccharides together
    (b) The addition of water to each monomer
    (c) The formation of disulfide bridges between monomers
    (d) Condensation or dehydration reaction

### ANSWERS

| | | | | | | | | |
|---|---|---|---|---|---|---|---|---|
| 1. d | 2. d | 3. a | 4. a | 5. c | 6. d | 7. a | 8. b |
| 9. a | 10. c | 11. a | 12. c | 13. d | 14. c | 15. c | 16. d |
| 17. c | 18. b | 19. a | 20. c | 21. b | 22. b | 23. d | 24. d |
| 25. c | 26. b | 27. b | 28. d | | | | |

# Chapter 8

# Metabolism of Lipids

## LEARNING OBJECTIVES

*At the end of this chapter students should be able to:*
- Explain the process of digestion and absorption of lipids
- Know about the beta-oxidation of fatty acids and its importance
- Explain the process of fatty acid synthesis and its regulation in post-absorptive and fasting conditions
- Explain the process of ketone body formation and their utilization
- Know about the metabolism of various lipoproteins including hyperlipoproteinemias

## ■ Introduction

The lipids of our diet gets digested with the help of pancreatic lipase and the enteric hormones secretin and cholecystokinin. The digested dietary lipids enter the liver as chylomicron. The absorbed lipids undergo metabolism which includes both catabolic as well as anabolic.

**Discuss in detail the digestion and absorption of lipids.**

## ■ Digestion and Absorption of Lipids

The process of lipid digestion is dependent on bile salts for the emulsification. Before fat digestion to occur, it must be converted into fine droplets as an emulsion, which facilitates the digestion of lipids.

- The lipids delay the rate of emptying the stomach, by way of the hormone enterogastrone, which inhibits gastric motility and retards the discharge of food from the stomach. Therefore, fats have the satiety value.
- The heat of the stomach is important in liquefying dietary lipids. The enzyme of stomach gastric lipase and lingual lipase present in the chyme are active only at neutral pH. In adults no digestion of fat takes place in stomach due to acidic pH. These enzymes may be active in infants and act on short and medium chain fatty acids due to the pH of the stomach content which is nearer to neutral pH. The hydrophilic short and medium chain fatty acids are absorbed via stomach wall and enter the portal vein. The longer chain fatty acids dissolve in the diet and pass on into the duodenum.
- Entry of acidic chyme from the stomach into the duodenum stimulates the secretion enteric hormones like **gastrin** and **cholecystokinin** by the mucosal cells of duodenum.
- Further **cholecystokinin** acts on the gallbladder, causing it to contract. Thus releasing bile salts into the small intestine.
- Cholecystokinin also acts on the exocrine cells of the pancreas, causing them to release digestive enzymes including lipase.
- The same cholecystokinin also decreases gastric motility, which results in a slow release of the gastric contents into small intestine.

## CHAPTER 8: Metabolism of Lipids

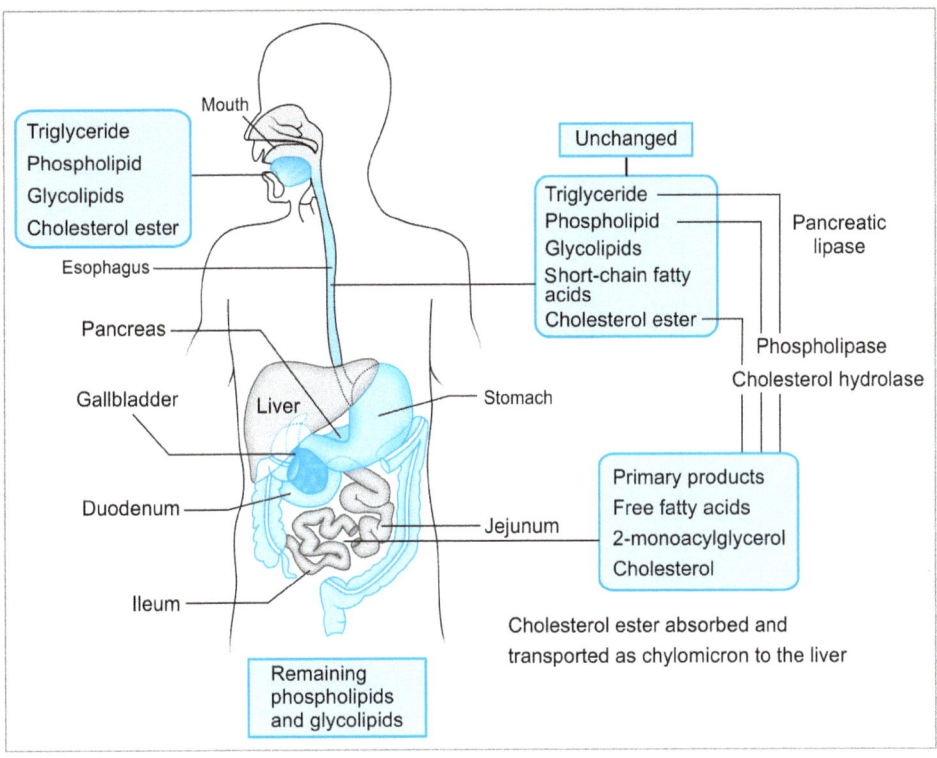

**Fig. 8.1:** Digestion of lipids.

- **Secretin** causes the pancreas to release a bicarbonate rich solution which neutralizes the acidic chyme and changes the pH to the alkaline side. The conversion to alkaline pH is very important for the action of lipase and intestinal enzymes. The bile (with bile salts and phosphatidylcholine) enters the duodenum and provides the emulsifying action. After emulsification, the lipolytic enzymes such as lipase, phospholipase $A_2$ and cholesterol esterase present in the pancreatic juice hydrolyze lipids.
- Dietary glycerophospholipids are digested by pancreatic phospholipase-$A_2$ **(Fig. 8.1)** which hydrolyses fatty acid residues at the 2nd position leaving lysophospholipids. This lysophospholipid enter the mucosal cell or degraded further by lysophospholipase enzyme (secreted by intestinal cells) to remove final fatty acid residue.
- Inside the mucosal cells fats are resynthesized and converted to chylomicron and transported to blood via lymphatic vessel **(Fig. 8.2)**.
- Fatty acids less than 10 carbon atoms along with glycerol are carried by portal blood to the liver.
- The long chain free fatty acids, free cholesterol, 2-monoglyceride and 1-monoglyceride and lysophospholipid together with bile salts form **mixed micelles**. The bile salts aggregate with their hydrophobic region placed internally and hydrophilic region facing the water medium and makes the micelle water soluble. The glycerides and long chain fatty acids in these micelles are transported into the intestinal mucosal cells leaving bile salts in the medium itself. The bile salts are reabsorbed in the intestine and returned to the liver by the portal vein for resecretion into the bile.

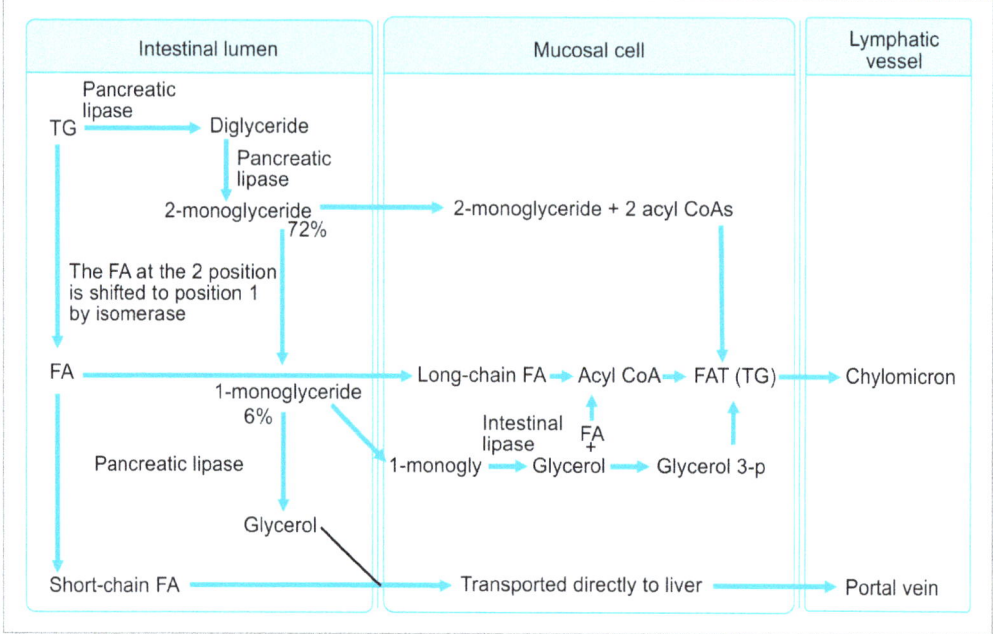

**Fig. 8.2:** Absorption of lipids.

This process is called enterohepatic circulation of bile salts.

* The short and medium chain fatty acids are absorbed directly into the intestinal epithelial cells and enter the portal blood to reach the liver.
* The 1-monoacylglycerol are further hydrolyzed in the intestinal mucosal cell by intestinal lipase.
* The 2-monoacylglycerol is reconverted to triglyceride as shown in the **Figure 8.2**. The utilization of fatty acids inside the mucosal cell for the re-synthesis of triacylglycerol needs the activation to acyl CoA by thiokinase enzyme.
* The absorbed lysophospholipids and cholesterol are also recycled with acyl CoA to regenerate phospholipids and cholesterol esters.
* The triacylglycerol, phospholipid, cholesterol ester synthesized in the intestinal mucosal cell and the absorbed fat soluble vitamins are transported from the mucosal cells into the lymph in the form of chylomicron.
* After absorption lipids are either oxidized mainly in the liver or stored in the depots (adipose tissue). For utilization by the body, triglycerides are first hydrolyzed by lipase to release glycerol and free fatty acids. Glycerol is converted into glucose by gluconeogenesis or enters into glycolysis. Fatty acids are oxidized to $CO_2$ and $H_2O$ with the liberation of large amount of energy.
* The abnormalities of fat absorption occur during the diseases affecting intestinal mucosa, inhibition of pancreatic lipase by low pH and decreased synthesis of bile salts in liver cirrhosis.

**Explain fate of triacylglycerol in the adipose tissue.**

## Fate of Triacylglycerol in Adipose Tissue

- In response to energy demands, the fatty acids of stored triacylglycerol can be mobilized for use by peripheral tissues.
- The release of metabolic energy, in the form of fatty acids, is controlled by a complex series of inter-related cascades that result in the activation of hormone-sensitive lipase.
- The stimulus to activate this cascade, in adipocytes, can be glucagon, epinephrine or α-corticotropin.
- These hormones bind to the cell-surface receptors that are coupled to the activation of adenylate cyclase upon ligand binding.
- The resultant increase in cAMP leads to activation of pyruvate kinase, which in turn phosphorylates and activates hormone-sensitive lipase.
- This enzyme hydrolyzes fatty acids from carbon atoms 1 or 3 of triacylglycerol.
- The resulting diacylglycerols are substrates for either hormone-sensitive lipase or for the non-inducible enzyme diacylglycerol lipase.
- Finally, the monoacylglycerols are substrates for monoacylglycerol lipase. The net result of the action of these enzymes is three moles of free fatty acid and one mole of glycerol.
- The free fatty acids diffuse from adipose cells, combine with albumin in the blood, and are thereby transported to other tissues, where they passively diffuse into cells.
- The glycerol released in adipose tissue, cannot be processed further by adipocytes because they lack glycerol kinase. Therefore, it is transported through the blood to the liver for phosphorylation.
- The glycerol phosphate formed can be used to form triacylglycerol in the liver or to be converted to dihydroxyacetone phosphate.

Model for the activation of hormone-sensitive lipase by epinephrine are shown Figure 8.3.

**Discuss the beta-oxidation of fatty acids including its energetics.**

## Oxidation of Fatty Acids

Oxidation of fatty acid takes place in mitochondria where the various enzymes for fatty acid oxidation are present close to the enzymes of

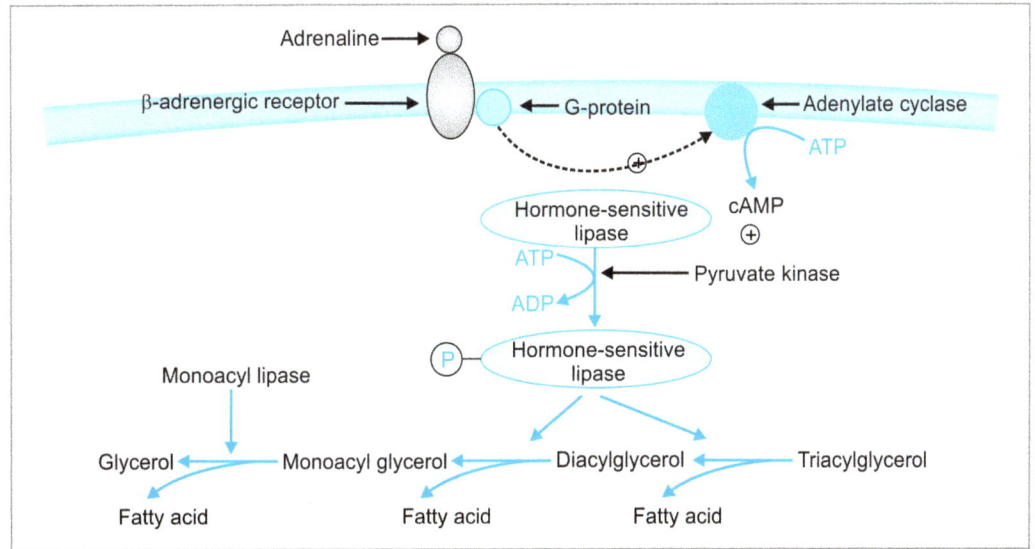

**Fig. 8.3:** Activation of hormone-sensitive lipase by epinephrine.

the electron transport chain. Most important theory of the oxidation of fatty acid is the β-oxidation of fatty acid.

The primary sources of fatty acids for oxidation are dietary and mobilization from cellular stores. Fatty acids from the diet are delivered from the gut to cells via transport in the blood. Fatty acids are stored in the form of triacylglycerol primarily within adipocytes of adipose tissue.

- Fatty acids are rich sources of energy.
- Energy is released when fatty acid undergoes β-oxidation.
- The β-carbon atom of fatty acid is oxidized.
- It is a cyclic process.
- Oxidation of fatty acid occurs at the β-carbon atom resulting in the elimination of two terminal carbon atoms as acetyl CoA leaving fatty acyl CoA which has 2 carbon atom less than the original fatty acid.
- Active form of fatty acid is called as fatty acyl CoA.
- If the starting fatty acid is palmitic acid, which has 16 carbon atoms, at a time 2 carbon atoms are removed as acetyl CoA, then 7 cycles of β-oxidation occurs to convert palmitic acid (16 c) into 8 acetyl CoA (2 c) molecules.
- First step in of fatty acid is the activation to its fatty acyl CoA form.

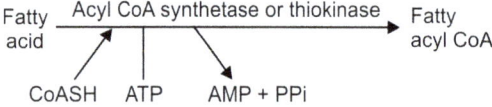

This reaction occurs outside the mitochondria.

**Write the flow diagram to show the entry of activated fatty acids into the inner mitochondrial membrane.**

Fatty acyl CoA formed inside the mitochondria cannot cross the inner mitochondrial membrane. "Carnitine", a carrier substance carries the acyl group into the mitochondrial membrane **(Fig. 8.4)**.

- Once the activated fatty acid enters the mitochondria, flavoprotein linked acyl

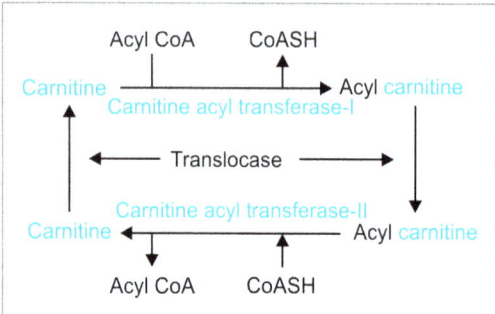

**Fig. 8.4:** Transport of acyl CoA carnitine.

CoA dehydrogenase (DH) removes two hydrogen atoms from fatty acyl CoA forming α, β-unsaturated fatty acyl CoA. This contains a double bond at α and β position **(Fig. 8.5)**.

- Enoyl CoA hydratase enzyme adds a molecule of water at the double bond position of α, β-unsaturated fatty acyl CoA forming β-hydroxyacyl CoA.
- In the presence NAD$^+$, β-hydroxyacyl CoA dehydrogenase enzyme oxidizes β-hydroxyacyl CoA to form β-ketoacyl CoA.
- Thiolase in the presence of CoASH cleaves β-ketoacyl CoA to yield acetyl CoA and fatty acyl CoA having 2-carbon atom less than the original fatty acid. Newly formed acyl CoA undergoes another 6 more cycles starting from step 1 and is finally degraded into acetyl CoA molecules.

## Energetics of Palmitic Acid Oxidation

- Palmitic acid when undergoes β-oxidation, it releases 8 molecules of acetyl CoA in seven cycles of the oxidative process.
- In each round of β oxidation one molecule of FADH2 and one molecule of NADH + H$^+$ are produced, which generates 1.5 and 2.5 molecules of ATP respectively through oxidative phosphorylation in an electron transport chain.
- The total number of ATPs produced in 7 rounds of oxidation process is 28.

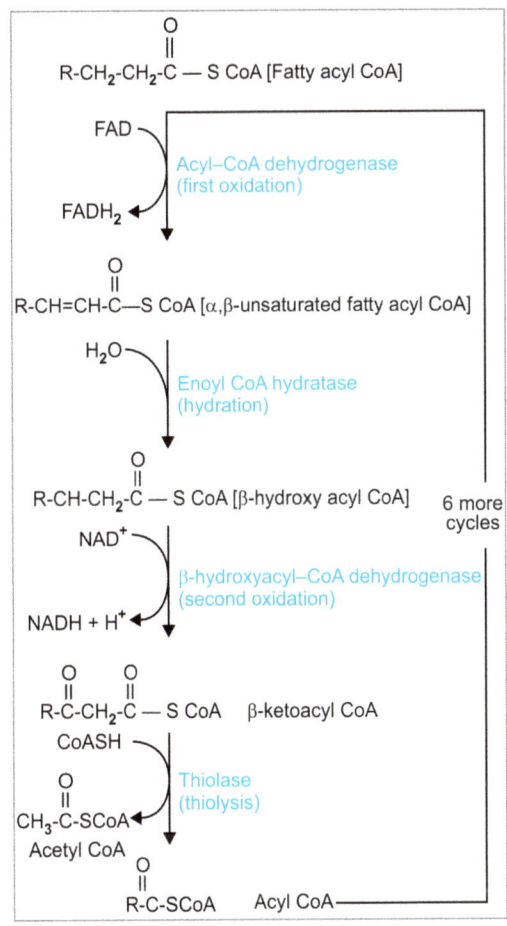

**Fig. 8.5:** Steps of β-oxidation of palmitic acid.

- In addition, when each acetyl CoA molecule oxidized in TCA cycle, 12 ATPs are generated.
  Per one cycle of β-oxidation
  Step I (FADH$_2$) → = 1.5 ATP
  Step III (NADH + H$^+$) → = $\dfrac{2.5\ \text{ATP}}{4.0\ \text{ATP}}$
  
  7 cycles of β-oxidation → = 28 ATP
  Number of ATPs produced in TCA cycle/acetyl CoA = 10 ATP
  Total number of acetyl CoA formed from palmitic acid = 8
  Total number of ATP produced by complete oxidation = (8 × 10) = 80 + 28 = 108 ATP

Number of ATPs utilized for activation of FA = 2 ATP
Net ATPs produced by complete oxidation of palmitic acid = 106 ATP
The standard free energy of palmitate
 = 2,340 Cal 106 × 7.3 Cal = 773.8 Cal
The efficiency of energy conservation by FA oxidation

$$= \dfrac{773.8 \times 100}{2{,}340} = 33\%$$

Fatty acids are predominantly oxidized by the process of β-oxidation in mitochondria.

**Briefly explain the regulation of fatty acid oxidation in a well-fed and fasting condition.**

## Regulation of β-oxidation

- The rate limiting step in the β-oxidation is the formation fatty acylcarnitine catalyzed by carnitine acyl transferase-1 (CAT-1). It is an allosteric enzyme and inhibited by malonyl CoA (first intermediate in the biosynthesis of fatty acid from acetyl CoA catalyzed by acetyl CoA carboxylase) **(Fig. 8.6)**.
- Malonyl CoA concentration increases in a well fed state, which inhibits CAT- 1 and leads to decrease in the fatty acid oxidation.
  - In starvation, due to decrease in the Insulin/glucagon ratio, acetyl CoA carboxylase is inhibited and concentration of malonyl CoA decreases, releasing the inhibition of CAT-1 and permitting more acetyl CoA for oxidation.

**State the cause for Jamaican vomiting sickness.**

## Jamaican Vomiting Sickness

It is characterized by:
- Severe hypoglycemia, vomiting, convulsions, coma and death.
- *Cause*: Eating unripe ackee fruit which contains unusual toxic amino acid, hypoglycine-A.

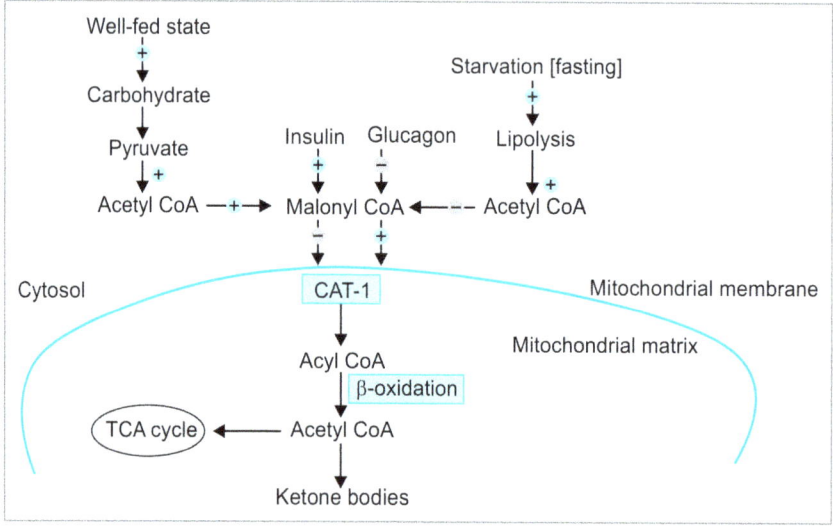

Fig. 8.6: Regulation of fatty acid metabolism.

- This inhibits the enzyme acyl CoA dehydrogenase and thus β-oxidation of FA is blocked, leading to various complications.

**What is peroxisomal fatty acid oxidation and what is importance.**

## Peroxisomal Fatty Acid Oxidation (Lipolysis)

- Peroxisomes are subcellular organelles found in all nucleated cells.
- Peroxisomes are able to conduct oxidation of long chain fatty acids. Oxidation of very long chain fatty acids (20–26 carbon atoms) begins in peroxisomes by a process similar to β-oxidation (completed in the mitochondria).
- The action of acyl CoA dehydrogenase differs; it produces $H_2O_2$ rather than $FADH_2$.
- Catalase located in peroxisomes converts this $H_2O_2$ to water and molecular oxygen. This process is not linked directly to phosphorylation and the generation of ATP. Once the long chain fatty acids reduced to octanoyl-CoA (with 8 carbons in its fatty acyl chain) leave the peroxisomes, it is transferred to carnitine through which it enters mitochondria, where they undergo β-oxidation.

## Clinical Importance

Clofibrate, a drug used to treat certain types of hyperlipoproteinemias, stimulates proliferation of peroxisomes and causes induction of the peroxisomal fatty acid oxidation.

## Zellweger's Syndrome

- Rare inborn error of peroxisomal oxidation of fatty acid oxidation.
- *Cause*: Inherited absence of functional peroxisomes in all tissues.
- The syndrome is caused by defect in the transport of enzymes into the peroxisomes, thus long chain fatty acids (with 26–38 carbons) are not oxidized and accumulate in tissues like brain, kidney and muscle.

## What is alpha-oxidation of fatty acids? Explain briefly.

### α-oxidation

* α-oxidation of fatty acid can also occur in human body mainly in liver and brain by removing one carbon from carboxyl end. There is no activation step.
* Hydroxylation occurs at α-carbon atom done by *mono-oxygenase* system and then oxidized to ketoacid.
* Ketoacid undergoes decarboxylation.
* Liberates a molecule of $CO_2$ and a fatty acid
* This process occurs in the endoplasmic reticulum.
* It does not require any CoA and it does not release energy.
* Defect in enzyme system leads to Refsum's disease.

## What causes Refsum's disease?

### Refsum's Disease

* Is a rare but severe neurological disorder.
* Patients with this disease accumulate large quantities of an unusual fatty acid, Phytanic acid derived from phytol, a constituent of chlorophyll.
* Also present in milk and animal fats.
* Phytanic acid cannot undergo β-oxidation due to the presence of a methyl group on carbon-3.
* This fatty acid undergoes initial α-oxidation to remove α-carbon and this is followed by β-oxidation.
* Refsum's disease is caused by a defect in the α-oxidation due to the deficiency of the enzyme phytanic acid oxidase.
* So phytanic acid cannot be converted to a compound that can be degraded by β-oxidation.
* In this condition the patients should avoid diet containing chlorophyll.

### ω-oxidation

* It is a minor pathway of oxidation of long chain fatty acid in microsomes.
* It occurs from both the ends of fatty acid chain.
* It needs hydroxylase enzymes with NADPH and cytochrome P-450.
* Dicarboxylic acids are produced during this process.
* It is important when β-oxidation is defective. The dicarboxylic acids are excreted in urine causing dicarboxylic aciduria.
* Unsaturated fatty acid can also be activated and transported across the inner mitochondrial membrane and undergo β-oxidation.

## List the compounds formed from acetyl CoA.

### Metabolic Fate of Acetyl CoA

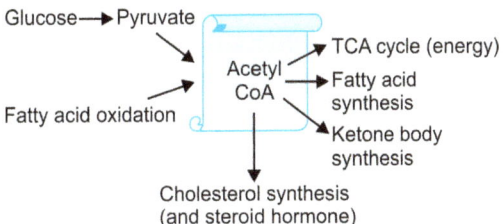

Acetyl CoA is produced by aerobic glycolysis of glucose, oxidation of fatty acid via β-oxidation. Acetyl CoA is mainly used in citric acid cycle.

## Discuss the fresh synthesis of fatty acid.

### Biosynthesis or *De Novo* Synthesis of Fatty Acid

The majority of the fatty acids required by the body is supplied by our diet. Fatty acids are synthesized whenever there is a caloric excess in our diet. This excess amount of carbohydrate and protein obtained from the diet can be converted to fatty acids which are stored as glycerol.

* Fatty acid synthesis involves the similar steps involved in β-oxidation of fatty acid but in a reverse way.
* Mammals can synthesize major portion of the saturated fatty acid as well as monounsaturated fatty acids.
* The system for the fresh synthesis of fatty acid is known as *de novo* synthesis of fatty

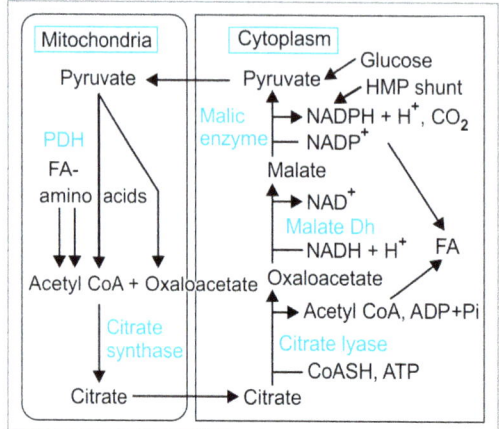

Fig. 8.7: Entry of acetyl CoA into cytoplasm.

acid, occurs in liver, adipose tissue, kidney and lactating mammary glands.
- The enzyme machinery is located in cytoplasm.
- It is referred to as extra mitochondrial or cytoplasmic fatty acid synthase system.
- Palmitic acid is the major fatty acid synthesized.
- All the 16 carbon atoms are from acetyl CoA.
- Acetyl CoA and NADPH are the pre-requisites for fatty acid synthesis.
- Acetyl CoA produced in the mitochondria cannot enter cytoplasm through inner mitochondrial membrane. So acetyl CoA condenses with oxaloacetate in mitochondria to form citrate. Citrate is freely transported to cytosol where it is cleaved by citrate lyase to liberate acetyl CoA and oxaloacetate (Fig. 8.7).
- For the synthesis of fatty acid, 8 acetyl CoA are transported from the mitochondria to cytosol, which is linked with the synthesis of 8 NADPH.
- As such 14 NADPH are needed to synthesize one molecule of palmitate.
- The remaining 6 NADPH are supplied from HMP shunt.

The first reaction is the synthesis of malonyl CoA from acetyl CoA by *acetyl CoA carboxylase*

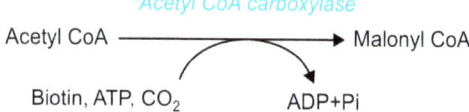

*Regulatory enzyme of FA synthesis

- The remaining reactions of FA synthesis are catalyzed by multifunctional enzyme known as fatty acid synthase complex (FAS) (Fig. 8.8).
- It is a dimer with two identical subunits.
- Each monomer possesses the activities of seven different enzymes and an acyl carrier protein (ACP) bound to 4'-phosphopantetheine-SH group.
- Two subunits lie in anti-parallel (head to tail) orientation.
- The SH group of phosphopantetheine of one subunit is in close proximity with the -SH of cysteine residue of the other subunit.
- Each monomer of FAS contains all the enzyme activities of fatty acid synthesis.
- But only the dimer form is functionally active.
- This is because the functional unit consists half of each subunit.
- Subunit interacts with the complimentary half of the other.

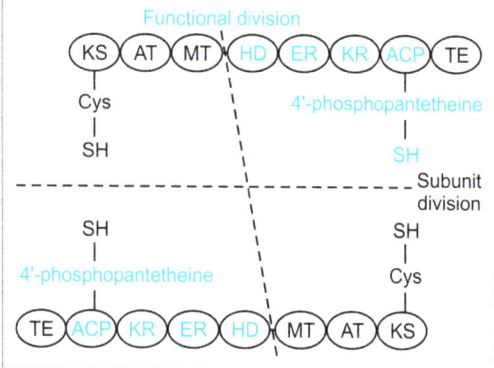

Fig. 8.8: Fatty acid synthase enzyme complex.

Components of fatty acid synthase complex are:
- Acetyl transferase (AT)
- Malonyltransferase (MT)
- β-keto acyl synthase (KS)
- β-keto acyl reductase (KR)
- β-hydroxy acyl dehydratase (HD)
- Enoylreductase (ER)
- Thioesterase (TE).
- Acyl carrier protein

❖ Fatty acid synthesis starts with the transfer of an acetyl CoA to cysteinyl SH group of Acyl carrier protein (ACP) **(Fig. 8.9)**.
❖ Malonyl CoA-ACP transferase transfers malonate from malonyl CoA to bind to ACP.
❖ The acetyl unit attached to cysteine is transferred to malonyl group attached to ACP. Malonyl moiety loses $CO_2$, which was added by acetyl CoA carboxylase and form β-ketoacyl enzyme.
❖ β-ketoacyl-enzyme is reduced to β-hydroxybutyryl enzyme complex using NADPH + $H^+$.
❖ Molecule of $H_2O$ is removed from β-OH butyryl enzyme to form α, β unsaturated acyl enzyme.
❖ The unsaturated bond in α, β unsaturated acyl enzyme is again reduced using NADPH + $H^+$ to form butyryl or acyl enzyme. The carbon chain attached to ACP is transferred to cysteine residue and the reactions 2–6 are repeated 6 more times and finally palmitic acid is synthesized.
❖ The completely synthesized fatty acid is released from the enzyme system by the action of thioesterase enzyme.
❖ Chain elongation of fatty acid occurs in the mitochondria and liver microsomes.
❖ Of the 16 carbons present in palmitate, only two come from acetyl CoA directly.

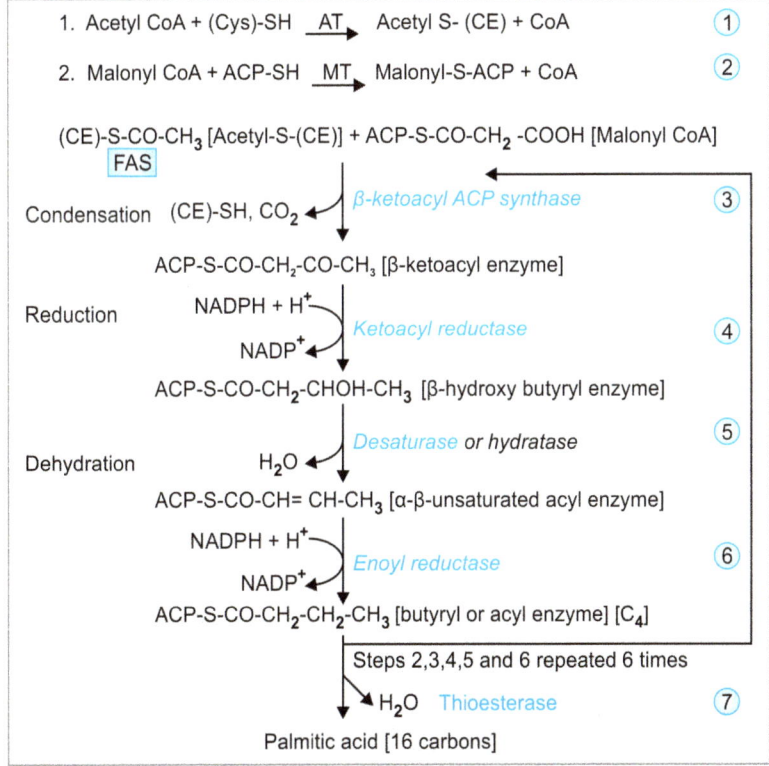

**Fig. 8.9:** Steps of fatty acid synthesis.

The remaining 14 are from malonyl CoA which, in turn, is produced by acetyl CoA.
- During elongation in microsomes palmitate is activated to palmitoyl CoA. Malonyl CoA serves as the donor of two carbons at a time in series of reactions.
- The major elongation reaction occurs in the body involves the formation of stearyl CoA [C18] from palmitoyl CoA [C16].
- Elongation of this stearyl CoA in brain increases during myelination to provide C22 and C24 fatty acids present in the sphingolipids.
- Mitochondrial elongation is less active and uses acetyl CoA as the source of two carbon units
- 8 Acetyl CoA + 7 ATP + 14 NADPH + 14 $H^+$ → Palmitate + 8 CoA + 7 ADP + 7 Pi + 6 HO + 14 $NADP^+$.

**Explain briefly the hormonal and dietary regulation of fatty acid.**

## Regulation

- Acetyl CoA carboxylase enzyme controls a committed step in fatty acid synthesis.
- This enzyme exists as an inactive protomer (monomer) or as an active polymer. Citrate promotes polymer formation, hence increases fatty acid synthesis. Palmitoyl CoA and malonyl CoA causes depolymerization of the enzyme and inhibits FA synthesis.
- *Hormonal influence*: Glucagon, epinephrine and norepinephrine inactivate the enzyme by cAMP dependent phosphorylation.
- Insulin dephosphorylates and activates the enzyme.
- Insulin promotes and glucagon inhibits fatty acid synthesis.
- *Dietary regulation*: High carbohydrate or fat free diet increases the synthesis of acetyl CoA carboxylase and fatty acid synthase, which promotes fatty acid synthesis.
- Fasting or high fat diet decreases fatty acid production.
- NADPH influences fatty acid synthesis.

**Briefly explain the synthesis and the importance of cholesterol.**

## Cholesterol Metabolism

- Cholesterol is a sterol, present in cell membrane, brain and lipoprotein.

- It is a precursor for all steroids.
- It is amphipathic in nature (hydrophilic and hydrophobic).
- About 1 g of cholesterol is synthesized/day in humans.
- 80% of the liver cholesterol converted to bile acids.
- Vitamin $D_3$ is formed from 7-dehydrocholesterol.
- All the steroids have cyclopentanoperhydrophenanthrene ring made up of three cyclohexane rings, A, B and C and a cyclopentane ring D.
- Normal blood level is 200 mg/dL.
- Hypercholesterolemia is seen in nephrosis, diabetes mellitus, hypothyroidism and obstructive jaundice.
- Increased cholesterol level leads to atherosclerosis.
- The OH group in the 3rd position can be get esterified with fatty acids to form cholesterol esters. This esterification occurs in the body by transfer of PUFA moiety by lecithin cholesterol acyl transferase. This step is important in the regulation of cholesterol level.
- It is a poor conductor of electricity.

## Synthesis (Fig. 8.10)

- *Site (extra mitochondrial):* The enzymes involved are found in cytosol and microsomal fractions of the cell.

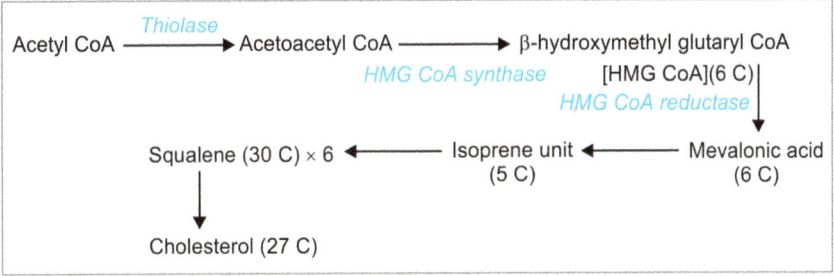

**Fig. 8.10:** Cholesterol synthesis.

- Synthesis takes place in liver, skin and intestine and also in adrenal cortex and testis.
- All the 27 carbon atoms are derived from acetyl CoA.
- 18 acetyl CoA are required.
- Acetyl CoA formed by the glycolysis and oxidation of fatty acid are the precursors for the cholesterol synthesis.

**Discuss in detail the regulation of cholesterol synthesis.**

## Regulation of Cholesterol Synthesis

Cholesterol biosynthesis is controlled by the rate limiting enzyme HMG CoA reductase (Fig. 8.11).

- *Feedback control*: The end product cholesterol controls its own synthesis of the enzyme by a feedback mechanism. Increase in the cellular concentration of cholesterol reduces the synthesis of the enzyme by decreasing the transcription of the gene responsible for the production of HMG CoA reductase.
- *Hormonal regulation*: The HMG CoA reductase exists in two interconvertible forms.
- The dephosphorylated form of the enzyme is more active, phosphorylated is less active. Hormones exert their influence through cAMP.
- *Inhibition by drugs*: The drugs compactin, lovastatin, mevastatin and simvastin drugs which inhibits HMG CoA reductase and which are used to decrease the cholesterol level.
- HMG CoA reductase is inhibited by bile acids.
- LDL transports cholesterol from the liver to peripheral tissues.

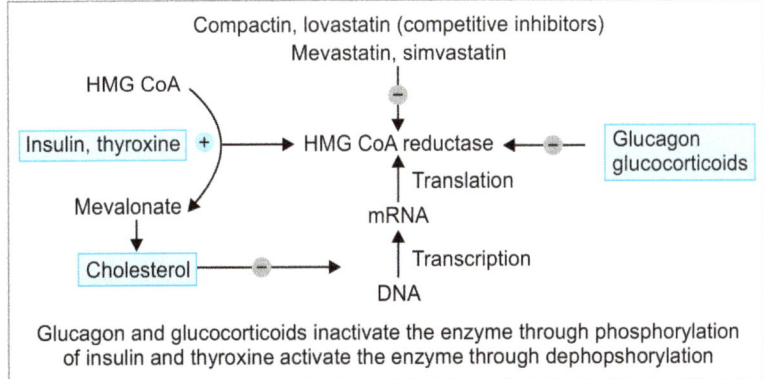

**Fig. 8.11:** Regulation of cholesterol synthesis.

- HDL transports cholesterol from peripheral tissues to the liver.

**What is lecithin-cholesterol acyl transferase and state its importance.**

## Role of LCAT

- High density lipoprotein (HDL) and the enzyme lecithin-cholesterol acyl transferase (LCAT) are responsible for the transport and elimination of cholesterol from the body.
- LCAT is a plasma enzyme, synthesized by the liver.
- LCAT catalyzes the transfer of fatty acid from the second position of phosphatidyl choline (lecithin) to the OH group of cholesterol.
- HDL cholesterol is the real substrate for LCAT and this reaction is freely reversible.
- LCAT activity is associated with Apo-A1 of HDL.

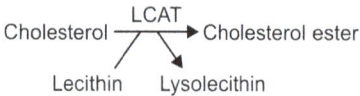

## Metabolic Fate of Cholesterol

Cholesterol is converted into following compounds as shown below **(Fig. 8.12)**.

Cholesterol is mainly excreted in the form of bile salts in stool.

Increased plasma cholesterol results in the accumulation of cholesterol under the tunica intima of the arteries causing atherosclerosis. The progression of the disease process leads to narrowing of the blood vessels. Dietary intake of polyunsaturated fatty acid (PUFA) helps in transport and metabolism of cholesterol and prevents atherosclerosis.

## Bile Acids Synthesis and Utilization

- The end products of cholesterol utilization are the bile acids, synthesized in the liver.
- Synthesis of bile acids is one of the predominant mechanisms for the excretion of

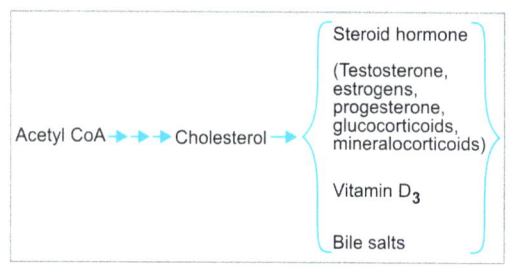

**Fig. 8.12:** Products formed from cholesterol.

excess cholesterol. However, the excretion of cholesterol in the form of bile acids is insufficient to compensate for an excess dietary intake of cholesterol.
- The most abundant bile acids in human bile are:
  - Chenodeoxycholic acid (45%)
  - Cholic acid (31%).

These two are referred to as the primary bile acids.
- Before secretion they will be conjugated with either glycine or taurine, which increases their polarity and water solubility.
- This mechanism of conjugation leads to the formation of four bile acids, within cholesterol.
  - Glycocholic acid (GCA)
  - Taurocholic acid (TCA)
  - Glycochenodeoxycholic acid (GCDCA)
  - Taurochenodeoxycholic acid (TCDCA).
- Within the intestines the primary bile acids are acted upon by bacteria and converted to the secondary bile acids, identified as deoxycholate (from cholate) and lithocholate (from chenodeoxycholate).
- Both primary and secondary bile acids are reabsorbed by the intestines and delivered back to the liver via the portal circulation.

## Clinical Significance of Bile Acid Synthesis

Bile acids perform four physiologically significant functions:
- Synthesis and subsequent excretion in the feces represent the significant mechanism for the elimination of excess cholesterol.

- Bile acids and phospholipids solubilize cholesterol in the bile, thereby preventing the precipitation of cholesterol in the gallbladder as gallstones.
- They facilitate the digestion of dietary triglycerides by acting as emulsifying agents that render fats accessible to pancreatic lipases.
- They facilitate the intestinal absorption of fat-soluble vitamins.

**What are ketone bodies and list the conditions in which they are formed.**

## Ketone Body Formation and Utilization

- Acetoacetate, β-hydroxy butyrate and acetone are collectively called as ketone bodies.
- The process of formation of ketone bodies in the liver is called as ketogenesis.
- Ketone body level in the blood is usually less than 2 mg% in well-fed state.
- The ketone body excretion in the urine is approximately around 100 mg/day.
- Increased production of ketone bodies is known as ketosis.
- High level of ketone bodies in blood are referred to as ketonemia.
- If the level of ketone bodies is high in the urine it is called as ketonuria.
- Lungs mainly eliminate acetone.
- The acetyl CoA formed in fatty acid oxidation enters into TCA cycle only if fat and carbohydrate degradation are appropriately balanced.

Conditions in which ketone body formation are:

### Prolonged Starvation
During starvation the carbohydrate level will be low. So the stored fat of the adipose tissue break down to free fatty acids. The free fatty acids formed enter the liver and undergoes α-oxidation to release acetyl CoA which cannot be utilized by the liver through TCA cycle due to lack of oxaloacetate.

In starvation TCA cycle is impaired due to the deficiency of oxaloacetate which is diverted to glucose synthesis (gluconeogenesis).

Therefore, acetyl CoA is converted to ketone bodies to meet the energy needs.

### Uncontrolled Diabetes Mellitus
- Because of the lack of insulin, the carbohydrate metabolism is impaired.
- The adipose tissue fat becomes the main source of energy and its degradation is generally accelerated.
- This results in the excessive production of acetyl CoA, leading to accumulation of acetyl CoA and its conversion to ketone bodies.

### Feeding High Fat Diet
- Excess breakdown of fatty acids in the liver takes place.
- The above condition results in the formation of more acetyl CoA.
- Once the acetyl CoA formation exceeds more than the requirement of the liver tissues it is converted to ketone bodies and exported to muscle, heart and kidney to meet the energy requirement.
- So the peripheral tissues switch over to utilize ketone bodies.

**Explain the synthesis and breakdown of ketone bodies.**

## Formation of Ketone Bodies (Fig. 8.13)

*Site*: Liver mitochondria.

Both acetoacetate and β-hydroxy butyrate are weak acids, which slowly deplete alkali reserves (bicarbonate) of the body and cause metabolic acidosis. This condition is known as ketoacidosis.

## Utilization of Ketone Bodies (Ketolysis)

- The liver cannot utilize ketone bodies because it lacks the enzyme thiophorase

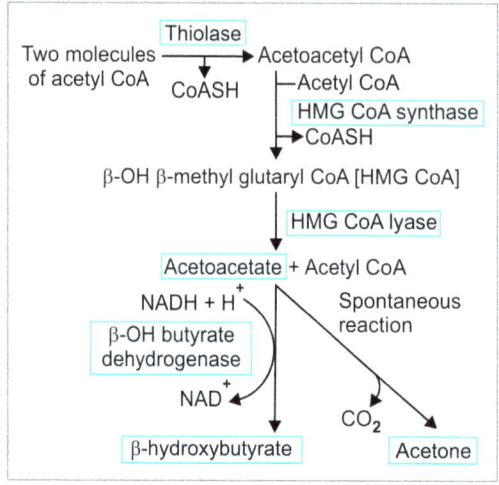

**Fig. 8.13:** Ketone body synthesis.

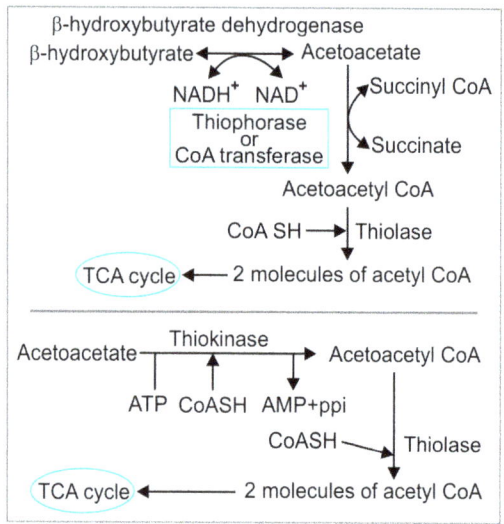

**Fig. 8.14:** Ketolysis.

or CoA transferase which is required for the activation of ketone bodies **(Fig. 8.14)**. Acetoacetate and β-hydroxybutyrate can be used as a source of energy in peripheral tissues (kidney, muscle).

* The β-hydroxybutyrate is reconverted to acetoacetate and the acetoacetate is then reactivated to acetoacetyl CoA.
* Acetoacetyl CoA, formed is cleaved by thiolase to yield two molecules of acetyl CoA which can be oxidized in the TCA cycle to $H_2O$ and $CO_2$.
* During prolonged starvation brain utilizes ketone bodies.
* Ketone bodies are water soluble and they are easily transported from the liver to various tissues.

## Regulation

* Glucagon stimulate ketogenesis
* Insulin inhibit ketogenesis
* The increased ratio of glucagon/insulin in diabetes mellitus promotes ketone body formation.

*Ketogenic substances*: Fatty acids, amino acids.
*Antiketogenic substances*: Glucose, glycerol and glucogenic amino acids (glycine, alanine, serine, glutamate, etc.).

## Biosynthesis of Triacylglycerol (Fig. 8.15)

**What is the fate of triacylglycerol in liver and adipose tissue? Explain.**

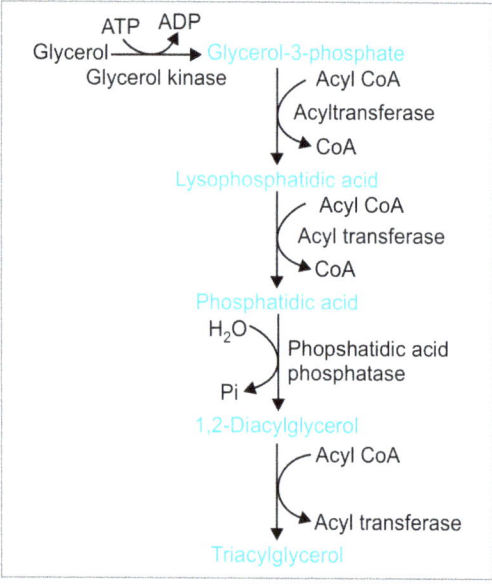

**Fig. 8.15:** Triacylglycerol synthesis.

## Fate of Triacylglycerol Formed in Liver and Adipose Tissue

In the liver very small amount of triacylglycerol is stored.

The most is packaged with cholesterol, phospholipids and proteins to form VLDL and released into the bloodstream. This triacylglycerol of VLDL is hydrolyzed by lipoprotein lipase, which is located in the walls of blood capillaries. This enzyme clears the triacylglycerol and glycerol.

In adipose tissue, triacylglycerol is stored in the cells and it serves as fat depot ready for mobilization when the body requires energy.

## Role of Liver in Lipid Metabolism

Lipids are mainly stored in adipose tissue but liver has a central role in lipid metabolism.

- Fatty acid synthesis (glucose →→ acetyl CoA →→ fatty acid)
- Cholesterol synthesis
- Plasma lipoproteins such as VLDL, LDL and HDL are synthesized in liver.
- Ketone bodies are synthesized in the liver.
- Fatty acid chain elongation (medium chain to long chain fatty acid).
- Synthesis of bile acid and bile salts
- β-oxidation of fatty acid

## Regulation of Lipid Metabolism

### Action of Insulin

- It stimulates HMP shunt and increases the supply of NADPH + H$^+$.
- It increases the peripheral utilization of glucose and depresses ketogenesis.
- Triglyceride synthesis is stimulated.

*Glucocorticoids*: These hormones increase the rate of release of fatty acid from adipose tissue which in turn leads to ketogenesis and increase cholesterol synthesis.

## ■ Alcohol Metabolism

Excess of alcohol produces cirrhosis in liver.
- It is readily absorbed from the gastrointestinal tract.
- It cannot be stored and the body must oxidize it to get rid of it.
- Alcohol can only be oxidized in the liver, where enzymes are found to initiate the process.
- Alcohol directly contributes to malnutrition.
- Ethanol does not have any minerals, vitamins, carbohydrates, fats or protein associated with it.
- It causes inflammation of the stomach, pancreas, and intestines which impairs the digestion of food and absorption into blood.
- The acetaldehyde (the oxidation product) can interfere with the activation of vitamins.
- The first step in the metabolism of alcohol is the oxidation of ethanol to acetaldehyde catalyzed by alcohol dehydrogenase and the coenzyme NAD$^+$.
- The acetaldehyde is further oxidized to acetic acid and finally to $CO_2$ and water (citric acid cycle).
- Metabolic effects from alcohol are directly linked to the production of an excess of both NADH and acetaldehyde.

## Metabolic Fates of NADH

### Pyruvic Acid to Lactic Acid

The conversion of pyruvic acid to lactic acid requires NADH.

Pyruvic Acid + NADH + H$^+$ → Lactic Acid + NAD$^+$

This pyruvic acid normally made by transamination of amino acids, is intended for conversion into glucose by gluconeogenesis. This pathway is inhibited by low concentrations of pyruvic acid, since it has been converted to lactic acid. The final result may be acidosis from lactic acid build-up and hypoglycemia from lack of glucose synthesis.

### Synthesis of Lipids

Excess NADH may be used as a reducing agent in two pathways—one to synthesize glycerol and the other to synthesize fatty acids. As a result, heavy drinkers may initially be overweight.

## Electron Transport Chain

The NADH may be used directly in the electron transport chain to synthesize ATP as a source of energy. This reaction has the direct effect of inhibiting the normal oxidation of fats in the fatty acid and citric acid cycle. Fats or acetyl CoA may accumulate resulting in production of ketone bodies. Accumulation of fat in the liver can be alleviated by secreting lipids into the bloodstream.

The higher lipid levels in the blood are responsible for heart attacks.

## Alcoholism Effects

A central role in the toxicity of alcohol may be played by acetaldehyde itself. Although the liver converts acetaldehyde into acetic acid, it reaches a saturation point where some of it escapes into the bloodstream. The accumulated acetaldehyde exerts its toxic effects by inhibiting the mitochondria reactions and functions. When the metabolism of acetaldehyde to acetic acid decreases, more acetaldehyde accumulates, and causes further liver damage—hepatitis and cirrhosis **(Fig. 8.16)**.

## Lipoproteins

### Structure and Function

Lipoproteins are conjugated proteins, composed of core and surface.
* LP core has
  - Triglycerides
  - Cholesterol esters
* LP surface has
  - Phospholipids
  - Proteins
  - Cholesterol
* Lipids are water insoluble
* Present in the blood in the form of lipoproteins which are water soluble.
* They have an outer polar surface, which makes them water soluble.

*Separation by Ultracentrifugation*: Four distinct groups based on their density **(Fig. 8.17A)**.

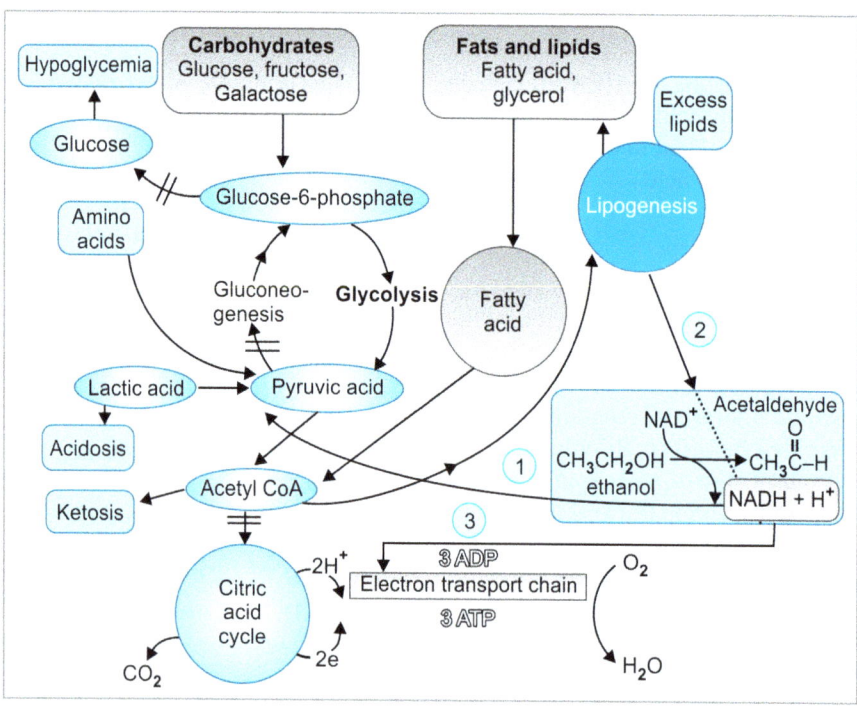

**Fig. 8.16:** Effects of alcohol.

# CHAPTER 8: Metabolism of Lipids

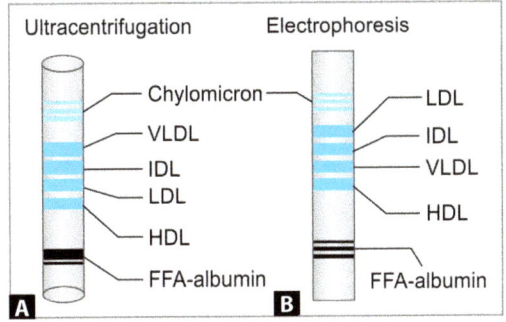

**Figs. 8.17A and B:** Separation of lipoproteins: (A) Ultracentrifugation; (B) Electrophoresis.

(VLDL: very low-density lipoprotein; IDL: intermediate-density lipoproteins; LDL: low-density lipoprotein; HDL: high-density lipoprotein)

- Chylomicron—transport of dietary triglyceride from intestine to extrahepatic tissues and liver.
- Very low-density lipoprotein (VLDL)—transport of endogenous triglyceride and cholesterol to extrahepatic tissues.
- Low-density lipoprotein (LDL)—transport of cholesterol from liver to extrahepatic tissues.
- High-density lipoprotein (HDL)—transport of cholesterol from extrahepatic tissues to liver.

## Separation by Electrophoresis

Based on difference in their mobilization in an electric field (**Fig. 8.17B**).

Composition and characteristics of lipoproteins are shown in **Table 8.1**.

## Plasma Lipoproteins Classes and Functions

**Briefly explain lipoprotein structure and function.**

## Chylomicron (Fig. 8.18)

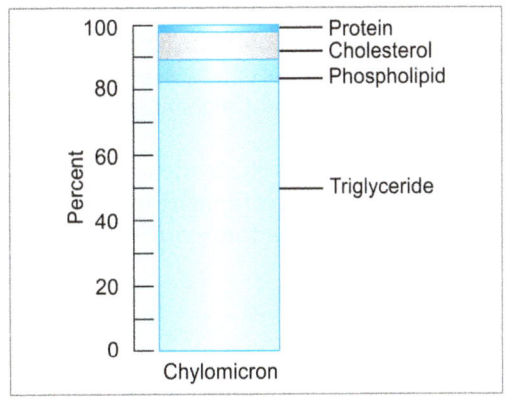

**Fig. 8.18:** Chylomicron composition.

- Synthesized in small intestine (mucosal cells)
- To mobilize dietary lipids
- Transport dietary lipids
- 98% lipid, large sized, lowest density
- Apo B-48: Receptor binding
- Apo C-II: Lipoprotein lipase activator
- Apo E: Remnant receptor binding
- Nascent chylomicron (Apo B-48, Apo A) before they enter circulation.
- Mature chylomicron (Apo C and Apo E in addition to Apo B-48, Apo A).

**Table 8.1:** Composition and Characteristics of lipoproteins

| Characteristics | Chylomicron | VLDL | LDL | HDL |
| --- | --- | --- | --- | --- |
| Density | <0.96 | d = 0.96 -1.006 | 1.006–1.063 | 0.063–1.21 |
| Electrophoretic mobility | Origin | Pre β | β | α |
| Protein | 2% | 10% | 22% | 40% |
| Cholesterol | 8% | 22% | 46% | 30% |
| TAG | 83% | 50% | 10% | 8% |
| PL | 7% | 18% | 22% | 22% |
| Apoproteins | A,B,C,E | BCE | B | AE |

(HDL: high-density lipoprotein; LDL: low-density lipoprotein; VLDL: very low-density lipoprotein)

- Lipoprotein lipase found on the surface of endothelial cells lining the capillaries in muscle and adipose tissues removes the fatty acids of triglycerides.
- Chylomicron remnant
  - Apo C removed
  - Removed in liver
- Substantial portion of the phospholipid, Apo A and Apo C are transferred to HDLs during the process of fatty acid removal.
- Chylomicron remnant containing primarily cholesterol.
- Apo E and Apo B-48 are then delivered to taken up by the liver though the interaction with the chylomicron remnant receptor (Fig. 8.19).

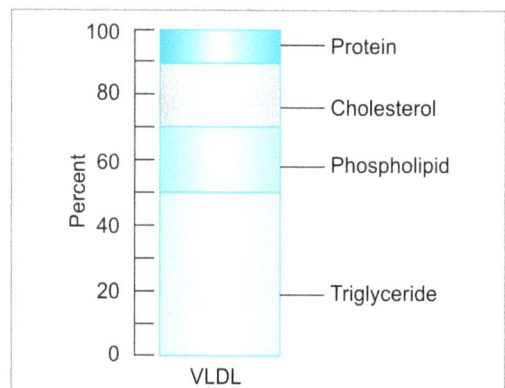

Fig. 8.20: Composition of very low-density lipoprotein (VLDL).

- Nascent VLDL (B-100) + HDL (Apo C and E) = VLDL.
- LPL hydrolyzes TG forming IDL: IDL loses Apo C-II (reduces affinity for LPL).
- 75% of IDL removed by liver: Apo E and Apo B mediated receptors.
- 25% of IDL converted to LDL by hepatic lipase: Loses apo E to HDL.
- The remnant is designated as IDL and contain less of triglycerides and more of cholesterol thus IDL contains Apo-B-100 and Apo-E: A small part of IDL is taken up by the liver, by receptor mediated endocytosis, helped by B-100 and Apo-E and converted to LDL (Fig. 8.21).

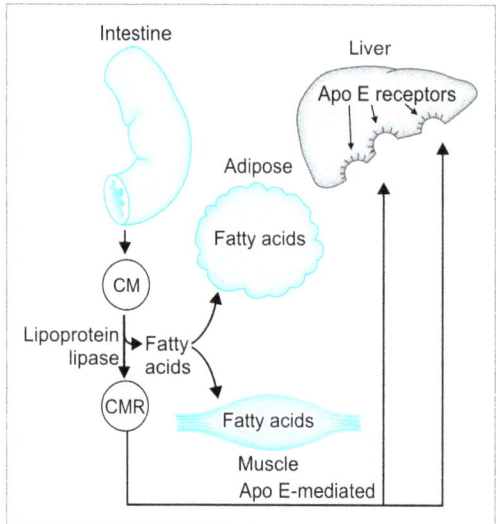

Fig. 8.19: Transport of chylomicron.

## Very Low-density Lipoprotein

- Synthesized in liver
- Transport endogenous triglycerides (liver to peripheral tissues
- 90% lipid, 10% protein (Fig. 8.20)
- Apo B-100: Receptor binding
- Apo C-II: LPL activator liberates free fatty acids that are taken up by the adipose tissue and muscle.
- Apo E: Remnant receptor binding

## Intermediate-density Lipoprotein

- Synthesized from VLDL during VLDL degradation.
- Triglyceride transport and precursor to LDL.
- Apo B-100: Receptor binding
- Apo C-II: LPL activator
- Apo E: Receptor binding

## Low-density Lipoprotein

- Synthesized from IDL
- Half-life of LDL in blood is 2 days
- Cholesterol transport liver to peripheral tissues.
- 75% of the plasma cholesterol is incorporated into the LDL particles are

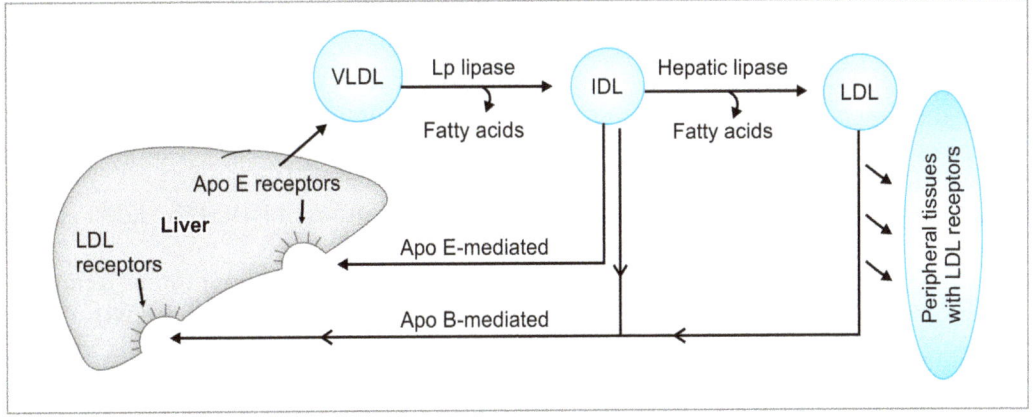

**Fig. 8.21:** Metabolism of VLDL.
(VLDL: very low-density lipoprotein; LDL: low-density lipoprotein; IDL: intermediate-density lipoprotein.)

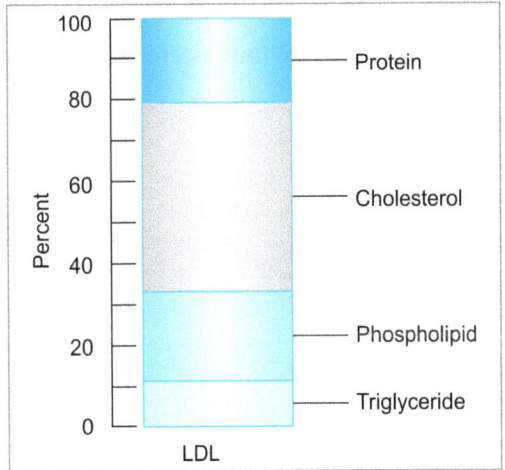

**Fig. 8.22:** Composition of low-density lipoprotein (LDL).

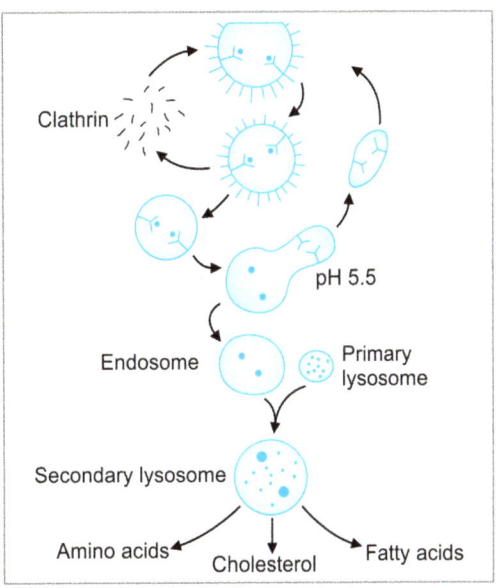

**Fig. 8.23:** Endocytosis.

derived from VLDL, a small part is directly released from liver.
- 78% lipid, 58% cholesterol and CE
- *Apo B-100* **(Fig. 8.22)**: Receptor binding: Interaction of LDL with LDL receptor.
- LDL receptor-mediated endocytosis
- About 75% of LDLs are taken up by the liver, adrenal and adipose tissue cells by LDL receptor mediated endocytosis **(Fig. 8.23)**.
- LDL receptors on 'coated pits'

*Clathrin*: A protein polymer that stabilizes pit.
- Endocytosis:
  - Loss of clathrin coating
  - Uncoupling of receptor, returns to surface.
- Fusing of endosome with lysosome: Frees cholesterol and amino acids.

## High-density Lipoprotein

- Synthesized in liver and intestine as protein rich discoid particles.
- Reservoir of Apo-proteins
- Reverse cholesterol transport
- 52% protein, 48% lipid, 35% C & CE (**Fig. 8.24**)

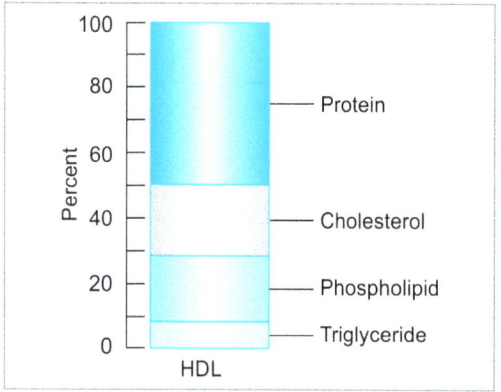

**Fig. 8.24:** Composition of high-density lipoprotein (HDL).

- Apo A: Activates lecithin-cholesterol acyltransferase (LCAT)
- Apo C: Activates LPL
- Apo E: Remnant receptor binding
- Apo-protein exchange: Provides Apo C and Apo E to/from VLDL and chylomicrons.

- Reverse cholesterol transport: Discoid HDLs are converted into spherical lipoprotein through the accumulation of cholesterol ester.
- Uptake of cholesterol from peripheral tissues (binding by apo A-I).
- Esterification of HDL-C by LCAT: LCAT activated by Apo A-1.
- Transfer of CE to lipoprotein remnants (IDL and CR) by CETP (**Fig. 8.25**).
- Removal of CE-rich remnants by liver, converted to bile acids and excreted.

The characteristic apoproteins present in chylomicron is Apo B 48 and in LDL and VLDL it is Apo B 100.

## Abnormal Form of Lipoprotein

**Explain the clinical importance of lipoprotein (a).**

*Lipoprotein (a) (LPa)*
- Lipoprotein (a) consists of an LDL-like particle and the specific apolipoprotein [apo (a)], which is covalently bound to the apo B of the LDL like particle.
- Normal human being contains very small amount of LP (a). The physiological function of LP (a) is still unknown.

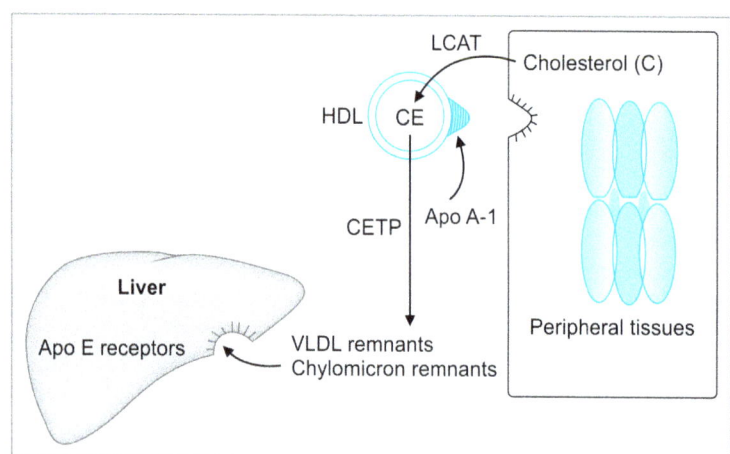

**Fig. 8.25:** Reverse cholesterol transport.
(LCAT: lecithin cholesterol acyltransferase; HDL: high-density lipoprotein; VLDL: very low-density lipoprotein; CE: cholesterol ester; CETP: cholesteryl ester transfer protein)

- They interfere with the action of plasminogen, impairing the process of clot resolution (fibrinolysis).
- Its structure is similar to plasminogen and TPA (tissue plasminogen activator) and it competes with plasminogen for its binding site, leading to reduced fibrinolysis. Also because Lp (a) stimulates secretion of PAI-1 it leads to thrombogenesis.
- In addition, because of LDL cholesterol content, Lp (a) contributes to atherosclerosis.
- High Lp (a) in blood is a risk factor for coronary heart disease (CHD), cerebrovascular disease (CVD), atherosclerosis, thrombosis, and stroke.
- Lipoprotein (a) levels
  - *Desirable*: <14 mg/dL
  - *Borderline risk*: 14–30 mg/dL
  - *High-risk*: 31–50 mg/dL
  - *Very high-risk*: >50 mg/dL.

### Hyperlipoproteinemias

The presence of excessive amounts of VLDL (excess TG), LDL (excess cholesterol) or chylomicron in plasma following 12–14 hours of fasting is collectively called hyperlipoproteinemia or hyperlipidemia. The elevation of lipids in plasma leads to deposition of cholesterol in the intima of the arterial walls leading to atherosclerosis.

The hyperlipidemias are of several types. They are:

*Hyperlipoproteinemia Type I*: Presence of chylomicron, high TG, VLDL and normal cholesterol.

*Hyperlipoproteinemia Type II a*: Normal TG, high LDL and therefore high cholesterol.

*Hyperlipoproteinemia Type II b*: High LDL, high VLDL, high cholesterol and high TG.

*Hyperlipoproteinemia Type IV*: High VLDL and therefore increased TG and normal cholesterol.

## Atherosclerosis and Coronary Heart Disease

- **Atherosclerosis** is the condition where LDL cholesterol deposited in the sub-intimal regions of arteries causing obstruction to the flow of blood (**Fig. 8.26**). This may lead to extra burden on the heart, which may be one of the reasons for hypertension. If this condition is neglected for long time may lead to cardiac diseases and ischemia.
- Atherosclerosis leads to coronary heart diseases (CHD) or coronary artery diseases

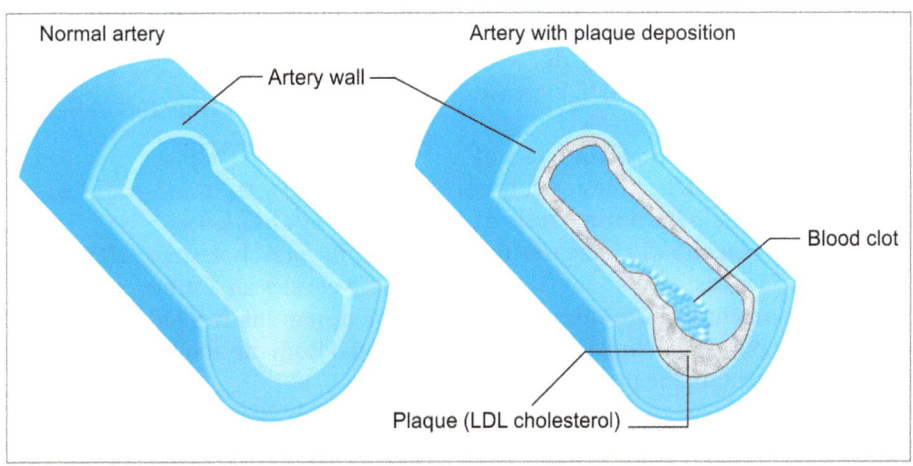

**Fig. 8.26:** Plaque formation.
(LDL: low-density lipoprotein)

(CAD) or (IHD). The deposited organic matter mainly composed of cholesterol and cholesterol ester. Hypercholesterolemia may be due to defects in transport, utilization and excretion.

## Risk Factors for Atherosclerosis

### Serum Cholesterol

- Values **above 250 mg/dL increase the risk** and the person needs active treatment.
- Values **around 220 mg/dL** indicate **moderate risk**.
- Values **below 200 mg/dL are safer**.

### LDL Cholesterol

- LDL cholesterol level is directly related to risk of atherosclerosis. So LDL is named as **bad cholesterol.**
- Values **above 190 mg/dL** indicate high-risk.
- Values **between 130–159 mg/dL** are in borderline risk.
- Values **below 130 mg/dL** are safer.

### HDL Cholesterol

- HDL cholesterol is inversely related to the risk of atherosclerosis. So it is named as **good cholesterol.**
- HDL cholesterol values **above 60 mg/dL** indicate very low-risk for atherosclerosis.
- HDL **below 35 mg/dL** increases the risk of atherosclerosis. Below 35 mg/dL, with every 1 mg/dL decrease in HDL increase the risk of atherosclerosis by 3%.
- It is very important to note the ratio of total cholesterol to HDL cholesterol. It is important to maintain the normal **ratio of below 4.5.** Increase in ratio increases the risk of atherosclerosis.
- It is also important to note the ratio of LDL cholesterol to HDL cholesterol. It is important to maintain the normal ratio of less than 3.
- Women have higher HDL (due to the presence of estrogens) and so they are less prone to heart diseases compared to men.

## Lipid Profile

Lipids are a group of fats and fat-like substances that are important constituents of cells and sources of energy. A lipid panel measures the level of specific lipids in the blood.

To assess your risk of developing cardiovascular disease (CVD); to monitor treatment of unhealthy lipid levels the following tests of lipid profile to be done:

- Total cholesterol
- Triglyceride
- LDL cholesterol
- HDL cholesterol
- VLDL
- Total cholesterol/HDL cholesterol ratio
- Lipoprotein electrophoresis

Maintaining healthy levels of these lipids is important in staying healthy. While the body produces the cholesterol needed to function properly, the source for some cholesterol is the diet. Eating too much of foods that are high in saturated fats and trans-unsaturated fats (trans-fats) or having an inherited predisposition can result in a high level of cholesterol in the blood. The extra cholesterol may be deposited in plaques on the walls of blood vessels. Plaques can narrow or eventually block the opening of blood vessels, leading to hardening of the arteries (atherosclerosis) and increasing the risk of numerous health problems, including heart disease and stroke.

### Specimen: Blood Collected in Red Top Tube, Fasting Sample

*Estimation of LDL Cholesterol and VLDL Cholesterol by Calculation*

Commonly total cholesterol, HDL cholesterol and triglycerides are estimated.

The remaining two (VLDL and LDL) are calculated from the above values as follows:

$$\text{VLDL cholesterol} = \frac{\text{Serum triglycerides}}{5}$$

LDL cholesterol = total cholesterol – (HDL cholesterol + VLDL cholesterol).

*Normal serum values:*
Total cholesterol = 150–200 mg/dL
Triglyceride = 40–160 mg/dL
HDL cholesterol:
Males = 28–61 mg/dL
Females = 38–75 mg/dL
LDL cholesterol = 60–130 mg/dL

*Clinical Significance of Cholesterol Estimation*
Increased levels of cholesterol in serum is called **hypercholesterolemia**. This is seen in:
* Nephrosis
* Nephrotic syndrome
* Obstructive jaundice
* Myxoedema
* Xanthochromatosis
* Coronary artery thrombosis and angina pectoris.

Decreased level is called hypocholesterolemia and seen in:
* Hyperthyroidism
* Pernicious and other anemia
* Malabsorption syndrome
* Hemolytic jaundice

**List the risk factors which causes cardiovascular diseases.**

## Risk Factors for Cardiovascular Disease

Cardiovascular diseases are the leading cause of illness and death in the world.

The majority of cases stem from atherosclerosis (a condition in which cholesterol, fat, and fibrous tissue build up in the walls of large and medium-sized arteries). In coronary heart disease (CHD), the arteries to the heart muscle (myocardium) are narrowed leads to reduced blood supply to the heart can result in chest pain (angina pectoris) or other symptoms, typically triggered by physical exertion. If a narrowed blood vessel is completely blocked by a blood clot, the area of the heart just beyond the blockage is denied oxygen and nourishment, resulting in a heart attack (myocardial infarction) **(Fig. 8.27)**.

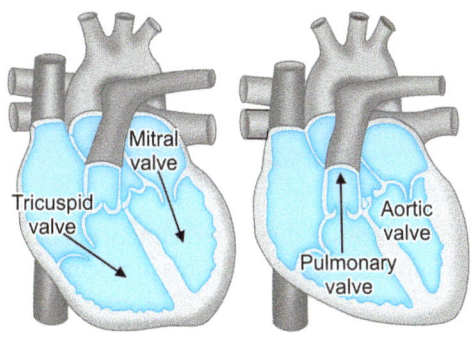

**Fig. 8.27:** Risk factors for cardiovascular disease.

The ten risk factors help to predict the likelihood of CHD are:
1. Heredity
2. Gender
3. Age
4. Cigarette smoking
5. High blood pressure
6. Diabetes
7. Obesity
8. Lack of physical activity
9. Abnormal blood cholesterol
10. Homocysteine levels

The more risk factors a person has, the greater the likelihood of developing heart disease. Heredity, gender and age cannot be modified, but the others can be influenced by the individual's behavior.

## Major Risk Factors (Cannot be Modified)

* *Age*: Over 83% of people who die of coronary heart disease are 65 or older.
* *Gender*: Men have a greater risk of heart attack than women do, and they have attacks earlier in life.
* *Heredity (including race)*: Children of parents with heart disease are more likely to develop it themselves. African Americans have more severe high blood pressure than Caucasians and a higher risk of heart disease. Heart disease risk is also higher among Mexican Americans, American Indians, native Hawaiians and some Asian Americans. This is partly due to

higher rates of obesity and diabetes. Most people with a strong family history of heart disease have one or more other risk factors.

## Major Risk Factors (Can be Modified)

Can be modified through treatment or control by changing lifestyle or taking medicine.

- *Tobacco smoke*: Smokers' risk of developing coronary heart disease is 2–4 times that of nonsmokers. Cigarette smoking is a powerful independent risk factor for sudden cardiac death in patients with coronary heart disease; smokers have about twice the risk of nonsmokers. Cigarette smoking also acts with other risk factors to greatly increase the risk for coronary heart disease. People who smoke cigars or pipes seem to have a higher risk of death.
- *High blood cholesterol*: As blood cholesterol rises, so does risk of coronary heart disease. When other risk factors (such as high blood pressure and tobacco smoke) are present, this risk increases even more. A person's cholesterol level is also affected by age, sex, heredity and diet.
  Total blood cholesterol is classified by levels:
  - *Desirable*: Under 200 mg/dL
  - *Borderline*: 200–239 mg/dL
  - *High risk*: 240 mg/dL and above
- *LDL cholesterol:*
  - *Optimal (ideal)*: Less than 100 mg/dL
  - *Near optimal/above optimal*: 100–129 mg/dL
  - *Borderline high*: 130–159 mg/dL
  - *High*: 160–189 mg/dL (high-risk)
  - *Very high*: 190 mg/dL and above (very high-risk).
- *HDL cholesterol*:
  - *Major heart disease risk factor*: Less than 40 mg/dL
  - *Protection against heart disease*: 60 mg/dL and above
- *High blood pressure*: High blood pressure increases the heart's workload, causing the heart to thicken and become stiffer. It also increases stroke, heart attack, kidney failure and congestive heart failure. When high blood pressure exists with obesity, smoking, high blood cholesterol levels or diabetes, the risk of heart attack or stroke increases several times.
  - Healthy adult (at rest) should have a systolic pressure below 120 and a diastolic pressure below 80.
- *Physical inactivity*: An inactive lifestyle is a risk factor for coronary heart disease. Regular, moderate-to-vigorous physical activity helps prevent heart and blood vessel disease. Physical activity can help control blood cholesterol, diabetes and obesity, as well as help lower blood pressure in some people.
- *Obesity and overweight*: People who have excess body fat especially at the waist— are more likely to develop heart disease and stroke even if they have no other risk factors. Excess weight increases the heart's work. It also raises blood pressure and blood cholesterol and triglyceride levels, and lowers HDL cholesterol levels. It can also make diabetes more likely to develop.
- *Diabetes mellitus*: Diabetes seriously increases your risk of developing cardiovascular disease. Even when glucose (blood sugar) levels are under control, diabetes increases the risk of heart disease and stroke, but the risks are even greater if blood sugar is not well controlled. About three-quarters of people with diabetes die of some form of heart or blood vessel disease. If you have diabetes, it is extremely important to work with your healthcare provider to manage it and control any other risk factors you can.

## Other Factors Contribute to Heart Disease

- Stress may be a contributing factor. For example, people under stress may overeat, start smoking or smoke more than they otherwise would.

- Too much alcohol can raise blood pressure, cause heart failure and lead to stroke.
  - It can contribute to high triglycerides. It contributes to obesity, alcoholism.
  - Experts say that moderate intake is an average of one to two drinks per day for men and one drink per day for women.
  - One drink is defined as 1½ fluid ounces (floz) of 80-proof spirits (such as Scotch, vodka, gin, etc.), 1 floz of 100-proof spirits, 4 floz of wine, or 12 floz of beer.

But drinking more than a moderate amount of alcohol can cause heart-related problems such as high blood pressure, stroke, irregular heartbeats, and cardiomyopathy (disease of the heart muscle).

## SUMMARY

The lipids are hydrolyzed to smaller and long chain fatty acids with the help of several enzymes. The hormone-sensitive lipase is the major enzyme which digests triacylglycerol. The short and medium chain fatty acids are absorbed directly into the intestinal epithelial cells and enters the portal blood to reach the liver. The long chain fatty acids form mixed micelle with bile salts and then absorbed. The absorbed fatty acids undergo beta-oxidation to generate energy and acetyl CoA. The beta-oxidation starts with an activation step and then transfer of activated fatty acyl CoA into the inner mitochondrial membrane through carnitine cycle. Carnitine acyltransferase-I is the regulatory enzyme in the beta-oxidation of fatty acids. The majority of the fatty acids required by the body are supplied through diet. Caloric excess of our diet results in the fatty acid synthesis. Acetyl CoA and NADPH are required for the *de novo* synthesis of fatty acids which takes place in cytoplasm. Fatty acid synthase complex enzyme, with two monomer units catalyzes the synthesis of fatty acids. The dimer form of the enzyme complex is active and each monomer has 7 different enzyme activities. Acetyl CoA carboxylase enzyme catalyzed step is a committed step in fatty acid synthesis regulation. Cholesterol synthesis requires acetyl CoA. HMG CoA reductase is the regulatory enzyme of cholesterol synthesis. Most of the statin drugs controls the cholesterol synthesis by inhibiting the HMG CoA reductase. Lecithin cholesterol acyl transferase is responsible for the transport and elimination of cholesterol from the body. Cholesterol metabolized to bile acids and bile salts in the liver. Uncontrolled diabetes mellitus and starvation are the two major conditions which results in the ketone body formation. Ketone bodies (acetoacetate, β-hydroxybutyrate and acetone) are produced in the liver but utilized by the extrahepatic tissues.

## SELF-ASSESSMENT QUESTIONS

1. Briefly discuss the digestion and absorption of lipids in the gastrointestinal tract.
2. Outline the β-oxidation of fatty acids.
3. How many ATPs are produced when one mole of palmitic acid is completely metabolized to acetyl CoA?
4. Explain the de novo synthesis of fatty acid. What is the source of NADPH?
5. Name the compounds formed from cholesterol?
6. Write a short note on atherosclerosis.
7. Name the ketone bodies and mention the conditions in which ketone bodies are formed.
8. Briefly discuss on the formation and utilization of ketone bodies.

9. Write short note on the following:
    a. Role of liver in lipid metabolism.
    b. Metabolic fate of acetyl CoA.
    c. Carnitine cycle.
    d. Ketoacidosis.
10. Explain the terms ketonemia, ketonuria and ketolysis.
11. Describe the pathway for the storage of glucose in the liver in the fed state? How is this pathway regulated?
12. What pathway provides for the production of pyruvate to be used for fatty acid synthesis in the fed state? How is this pathway regulated?
13. During the conversion of glucose to fatty acid, how is pyruvate, produced from glycolysis, converted to citrate in the cytosol? In which compartment does each reaction take place?
14. What are the sources of the reducing agent used for the reductive biosynthesis of fatty acids?
15. Which enzyme controls the pathway for the synthesis of fatty acids from acetyl CoA in the cytosol? How is this pathway regulated?
16. What keeps newly formed free fatty acid from entering the mitochondria in the fed state?
17. What happens to the product of the fatty acid synthase complex before it is foundin the blood?
18. Compare the $K_m$ for lipoprotein lipase in heart and adipose tissue. What implications dose this have for the usage of blood triacylglycerol in the fed and fasting state?
19. How does insulin affect the delivery of free fatty acid into adipose cells in the fed state?
20. What are the pathways for the synthesis of triacylglycerol in adipose from glucose and free fatty acids? How is the production of glycerol phosphate regulated?
21. What happens to the glycerol released in the lipoprotein lipase reaction in the fedstate?
22. What pathways provide blood glucose during fasting? Why are these pathways active?
23. Why glycogen is not made in the liver during fasting?
24. Glycolysis does not function when gluconeogenesis is functioning. What factors turn on gluconeogenesis and turn off glycolysis?
25. What is the control enzyme for the release of free fatty acids during a fast and how is this enzyme regulated?
26. Why are ketone bodies produced during a fast?
27. Besides providing ATP, how does increased beta-oxidation enable gluconeogenesis?
28. Explain how increased fatty acid oxidation and decreased insulin spares blood glucose by muscle in the fasting and resting state?
29. What is the effect of exercise upon the use of blood glucose by muscle in the fasting state? What is the mechanism?

## Fill in the Blanks

1. Net ATP produced during complete oxidation palmitic acid is_____.
2. _____compound is required for the transport of activated fatty acid inside the mitochondria.
3. _____enzyme digest triglycerides.
4. _____lipid absorption requires for emulsification.

## Match the Following

*Enzyme*

1. Thiokinase
2. Thiolase
3. HMG CoA reductase
4. HMG CoA synthase
5. β-OH butyrate DH
6. β-OH acyl CoA DH

*Actions*

1. Formation of HMG CoA
2. β-Ketoacyl CoA synthesis
3. Interconverts beta-OH butyrate and acetoacetate
4. Required for the activation of fatty acid
5. Synthesis of mevalonic acid
6. β-Ketoacyl CoA to acyl CoA and acetyl CoA

# CHAPTER 8: Metabolism of Lipids

## MULTIPLE CHOICE QUESTIONS

1. **Which of the following is an incorrect description for cholesterol?**
   (a) It is a low water soluble lipid found in blood
   (b) It exists in only one form in plasma
   (c) It is a major structural component of cell surfaces
   (d) It is esterified to some long chain fatty acids, which enhances its hydrophobicity

2. **Regarding cholesterol determination on serum, the following statements are true, *except*:**
   (a) It is determined by a modified method of Zak reaction.
   (b) The reddish brown color produced is due to the action of the $FeCl_3H_2SO_2$
   (c) The color is directly proportional to the concentration of the substance present and quantitated spectrophotometrically at 550 nm
   (d) The color is inversely proportional to the concentration of the substance present and quantitated spectro photometrically at 550 nm

3. **If 20 mg standard cholesterol dissolved in 100 mL absolute ethanol then concentration of cholesterol in 1.0 mL solution is:**
   (a) 0.02 mg
   (b) 0.8 mg
   (c) 0.2 mg
   (d) 2.0 mg

4. **All the following are synthesized from cholesterol, *except*:**
   (a) Bile acids
   (b) Vitamin C
   (c) Vitamin D
   (d) Steroid hormones

5. **In all the following clinical conditions we find high blood cholesterol, *except*:**
   (a) Pernicious anemia
   (b) Nephrosis
   (c) Obstructive jaundice
   (d) Diabetes mellitus

6. **Which of the following is an incorrect statement regarding the structure of cholesterol?**
   (a) It has a molecular formula of $C_{27}H_{46}O$
   (b) It has 5 rings
   (c) It has cyclopentanoperhydrophenanthrene ring
   (d) It has three cyclohexane and one cyclopentane rings

7. **Which of the following is an accurate description of cholesterol?**
   (a) Low density lipoprotein is responsible for the transport and elimination of cholesterol from the body
   (b) In healthy individuals the total plasma cholesterol is in the range of 90–150 mg%
   (c) Cholesterol is not found in animals
   (d) High density lipoproteins and lecithincholesterol acyltransferase are responsible for the transport and elimination of cholesterol from the body

8. **Which of the following is an accurate description of ketone bodies?**
   (a) Their synthesis is stimulated by insulin and inhibited by glucagon
   (b) They are a water-soluble form of acetyl units that are synthesized in the liver and used by many other tissues in the body as a fuel source
   (c) They are the major fuel source for the brain under basal metabolic conditions
   (d) They are not produced during starvation

9. **Which of the following accurately describes fatty acid synthesis in humans?**
   (a) Fatty acid synthase sequentially adds 2-carbon units from malonyl CoA until palmitate is made
   (b) Complex of seven enzymes makes $C_{16}$ palmitate directly from eight molecules of acetyl CoA

(c) Acetyl CoA is transported out of the mitochondrial matrix as the three-carbon activated molecule malonyl CoA
(d) Fatty acid synthesis generates large quantities of NADPH, which can be used by the electron transport chain and ATP synthase to generate ATP

10. Net amount of ATP formed when one molecule of palmitic acid undergoes beta-oxidation is:
    (a) 29
    (b) 140
    (c) 129
    (d) 130

11. The regulatory enzyme of cholesterol synthesis is:
    (a) Glucosyltransferase
    (b) HMG CoA reductase
    (c) HMG CoA synthase
    (d) Mevalonate kinase

12. One of the following is not a biochemical action of prostaglandin:
    (a) Regulation of blood pressure
    (b) Reproduction
    (c) Development of bone
    (d) Inflammation

13. Regarding fatty acid synthase complex, all the following statements are true, *except*:
    (a) Is a dimmer with identical subunits
    (b) Monomer form is functionally active
    (c) Monomer has seven different enzymes and an acyl carrier protein
    (d) Two subunits lie in antiparallel orientation

14. All of the following involve acetyl CoA, *except*:
    (a) Ketone body synthesis
    (b) Cholesterol synthesis
    (c) Nucleotide synthesis
    (d) Fatty acid synthesis

15. During prolonged starvation the brain mainly depends on one of the following for energy:
    (a) Glucose residues
    (b) Ketone bodies
    (c) Amino acids
    (d) Lactose molecules

16. For the synthesis of 16 carbon palmitic acid, number of acetyl CoA transported from mitochondria to cytosol is:
    (a) 10
    (b) 20
    (c) 2
    (d) 8

17. Net amount of ATP formed one cycle of β-oxidation of fatty acid is:
    (a) 29
    (b) 140
    (c) 5
    (d) 130

18. Reduced glutathione is required for the formation of:
    (a) $PGH_2$ from $PGG_2$
    (b) $PGI_2$ from $PGH_2$
    (c) $PGG_2$ from arachidonic acid
    (d) $PGE_2$ from $PGH_2$

19. The substance, which carries acyl CoA into the inner mitochondrial membrane for oxidation is:
    (a) β-carotene
    (b) Carnitine
    (c) Malate
    (d) Creatinine

20. The main regulatory enzyme of fatty acid synthesis is:
    (a) Acetyl CoA carboxylase
    (b) Hexokinase
    (c) Phosphofructokinase
    (d) Thioesterase

21. All the following are the biochemical actions of prostaglandins, *except*:
    (a) Regulation of blood pressure
    (b) Reproduction
    (c) Inhibition of platelet aggregation
    (d) Destruction of free radical

22. Regarding starvation, all the following statements are true, *except*:
    (a) Increased gluconeogenesis
    (b) Increased glycogen degradation
    (c) Decreased fatty acid oxidation
    (d) Increased fatty acid oxidation

23. All the following are the ketone bodies, *except*:
    (a) Acetoacetate
    (b) Beta hydroxyl butyrate
    (c) HMG CoA
    (d) Acetone
24. Ketosis occurs in all of the following conditions, *except*:
    (a) Starvation
    (b) In controlled diabetes mellitus
    (c) In the well fed state
    (d) Feeding high fat diet
25. In humans most of the prostaglandins are predominantly formed from:
    (a) Linoleic acid
    (b) Arachidonic acid
    (c) Palmitic acid
    (d) Stearic acid
26. All the following are the components of fatty acid synthase complex, *except*:
    (a) Acetyl transferase (AT)
    (b) Malonyltransferase (MT)
    (c) β-keto acyl synthase (KS)
    (d) Succinate dehydrogenase (SD)
27. Compound required for the transport of activated fatty acid inside the mitochondria is:
    (a) Lipoprotein
    (b) Apoprotein
    (c) Carnitine
    (d) β-carotene
28. One of the following enzymes mainly digests triglycerides:
    (a) Amylase
    (b) Lipase
    (c) Chymotrypsin
    (d) Pepsin
29. Micelle formation with bile salts is essential for:
    (a) Lipid absorption
    (b) Carbohydrate absorption
    (c) Lipid digestion
    (d) Protein transport
30. The enzyme which splits HMG CoA is:
    (a) Thiokinase
    (b) Thiolase
    (c) HMG CoA lyase
    (d) HMG CoA reductase
31. One of the following is an example for ketone bodies:
    (a) Acetoacetic acid
    (b) Lactic acid
    (c) Pyruvic acid
    (d) Gluconic acid
32. The enzyme which esterifies cholesterol is:
    (a) Acyl transferase
    (b) Acyl CoA dehydrogenase
    (c) Lecithin cholesterol acyl
    (d) Cephalin acyl transferase
33. The absorbed cholesterol transported as:
    (a) VLDL
    (b) HDL
    (c) Chylomicron
    (d) LDL
34. The enzyme which hydrolyzes phospholipids is:
    (a) Phospholipase
    (b) Cholesterol hydrolase
    (c) Pancreatic lipase
    (d) Amylase
35. Odd chain FA-oxidation ends up with:
    (a) Acyl CoA
    (b) Propionyl CoA
    (c) Malonyl CoA
    (d) Succinyl CoA
36. Hormone sensitive lipase acts on stored:
    (a) Liver fat
    (b) Adipose tissue fat
    (c) Kidney fat
    (d) Skin triacylglycerol
37. Insulin:
    (a) Reduces the release of free fatty acids from adipose tissue
    (b) Increases the release of triacylglycerol from adipose tissue
    (c) Increases the release of alanine from muscle
    (d) Reduces triglyceride synthesis

38. **After three weeks of starvation, the brain:**
    (a) Gets glucose through glycogenolysis
    (b) Completely depends on gluconeogenesis to generate ketone bodies
    (c) Depends on muscle proteins
    (d) Depends on acetyl CoA to generate ketone bodies
39. **Concerning insulin action, one of the following statements is incorrect, it:**
    (a) Activates pyruvate kinase
    (b) Stimulates glycerol phosphate acyltransferase
    (c) Increases HMG CoA reductase activity
    (d) Activates hormone sensitive lipase
40. **Lipase phosphatase is stimulated by:**
    (a) Insulin
    (b) Epinephrine
    (c) Prostaglandin
    (d) ACTH
41. **The enzyme responsible for prostaglandin synthesis is:**
    (a) 15-hydroxy prostaglandin dehydrogenase
    (b) Cyclo-oxygenase
    (c) Oxidoreductase
    (d) Adenylcyclase
42. **Before fats can be acted upon by the digestive enzymes, they must be:**
    (a) Neutralized
    (b) Esterified
    (c) Emulsified
    (d) Hydrolyzed
43. **In liver, the metabolism of acetyl-CoA can lead to all of the following, *except*:**
    (a) Cholesterol
    (b) β-hydroxybutyrate
    (c) Oxaloacetate.
    (d) Oleate
44. **Bile salts:**
    (a) Are synthesized from lipoprotein
    (b) Contain bilirubin
    (c) Increase the surface tension in fat particles in the small intestine
    (d) Form micelles with lipids in the small intestine
45. **A 40-year-old man patient with familial hypercholesterolemia undergoes a detailed serum lipid and lipoprotein analysis. Studies demonstrate elevated cholesterol in the form of increased LDL without elevation of triglyceride other lipids. This patient's hyperlipidemia is best classified as which of the following types?**
    (a) Type 1
    (b) Type 2a
    (c) Type 2b
    (d) Type IV
46. **The blood level of total cholesterol concentration recommended by the International diabetic association is:**
    (a) Less than 240 mg/dL
    (b) Less than 250 mg/dL
    (c) Less than 150 mg/dL
    (d) Less than 200 mg/dL
47. **Which of the following constituents is not usually found in bile?**
    (a) Cholic acid
    (b) Glycocholic acid
    (c) Deoxycholates
    (d) Phosphodeoxycholates
48. **If a patient has inadequate bile secretion, which of the following could contribute to the condition?**
    (a) Excessive steroid hormones
    (b) Excessive release of cholecystokinin
    (c) Excessive release of pepsin
    (d) Excessive release of secretin

## CHAPTER 8: Metabolism of Lipids

49. An 8-year-old male patient with type I diabetes mellitus feel nauseated and drowsy and have been vomiting for a few hours. Clinical examination shows mild signs of dehydration and low blood pressure. You request laboratory tests and the results show the following results:

| | | |
|---|---|---|
| Blood glucose | : | 380 mg/dL (above the reference range) |
| Hemoglobin A | : | 11.8 g/dL (reference range: 13.5–17.0 g/dL) |
| Hemoglobin A1c | : | 12% of total Hb (reference range: <6%) |
| Urine ketones | : | Positive |
| Urine glucose | : | Positive |
| Blood pH | : | 7.29 |
| Pa $CO_2$ | : | Below reference range |
| Serum bicarbonate | : | Below reference range |

Which of the following best indicates that this patient has had hyperglycemia over a period of weeks?
   (a) Ketonemia
   (b) Hemoglobin A1c
   (c) Glucosuria
   (d) Blood pH

50. Insulin facilitates energy storage in liver. Which enzymes of carbohydrate metabolism are coordinately regulated in liver in response to insulin signaling?
   (a) Glycogen synthase
   (b) Phosphofructokinase-2
   (c) Pyruvate kinase
   (d) All the above

51. One of the following enzymes of carbohydrate metabolism is not dephosphorylated in liver in response to insulin signaling?
   (a) Glycogen synthase
   (b) Glycogen phosphorylase
   (c) Phosphofructokinase-1
   (d) Pyruvate kinase

52. Enzymes like glycogen synthase, glycogen phosphorylase, the PFK-2/FBPase-2 and pyruvate kinase are phosphorylated by glucagon and/or epinephrine action. Which kinase is responsible for these phosphorylation events?
   (a) Protein kinase A
   (b) Calmodulin-dependent protein kinase
   (c) Protein kinase C
   (d) Receptor tyrosine kinase

53. The receptor to which epinephrine binds in order to stimulate phosphorylation of glycogen synthase and glycogen phosphorylase is:
   (a) α-1
   (b) α-2
   (c) b
   (d) g

54. Insulin regulates all of the following enzymes in liver. Which of these enzymes are also regulated by insulin in muscle?
   (a) Glycogen synthase
   (b) Glucokinase
   (c) Glycogen phosphorylase
   (d) a and c

55. The hormone that increases the rate of absorption of hexoses from intestine is:
   (a) Glucocorticoids
   (b) Thyroxine
   (c) Anterior pituitary hormones
   (d) Epinephrine

56. In a fasting state, glucocorticoids:
   (a) Decreases protein catabolism
   (b) Decreases hepatic uptake of amino acids
   (c) Stimulate the utilization of glucose in extrahepatic tissues
   (d) Increases the activity of aminotransferase

57. **Concerning insulin action, one of the following statements is incorrect, it:**
    (a) Activates pyruvate kinase
    (b) Stimulates glycerol phosphate acyltransferase
    (c) Increases HMG CoA reductase activity
    (d) Activates hormone sensitive lipase
58. **Starvation associated with:**
    (a) Increased insulin and decreased glucagon
    (b) Decreased epinephrine and increased insulin
    (c) Decreased insulin and increased glucagon
    (d) Decreased insulin and decreased glucocorticoids
59. **Lipase phosphatase is stimulated by:**
    (a) Insulin
    (b) Epinephrine
    (c) Prostaglandin
    (d) ACTH
60. **During starvation:**
    (a) Acetyl CoA carboxylase remains inactive
    (b) Hormone sensitive lipase becomes active
    (c) Fructose 1, 6-bisphosphatase becomes inactive
    (d) Glycogen phosphorylase becomes inactive through cAMP dependent phosphorylation

## ANSWERS

| | | | | | | | | | |
|---|---|---|---|---|---|---|---|---|---|
| 1. b | 2. d | 3. c | 4. b | 5. a | 6. b | 7. d | 8. b |
| 9. a | 10. c | 11. b | 12. c | 13. b | 14. c | 15. b | 16. d |
| 17. c | 18. a | 19. b | 20. a | 21. d | 22. c | 23. c | 24. c |
| 25. b | 26. d | 27. c | 28. b | 29. a | 30. c | 31. a | 32. c |
| 33. c | 34. a | 35. b | 36. b | 37. a | 38. d | 39. d | 40. a |
| 41. b | 42. a | 43. d | 44. d | 45. b | 46. d | 47. d | 48. a |
| 49. b | 50. d | 51. c | 52. a | 53. c | 54. d | 55. b | 56. d |
| 57. d | 58. c | 59. a | 60. b | | | | |

# Integration of Metabolism and Homeostasis

**Chapter 9**

## LEARNING OBJECTIVES

*At the end of this chapter students should be able to:*
- Understand how the metabolism integrated themselves during well fed and fasting conditions
- Explain the role of hormones in integrating the metabolism during well fed and fasting conditions
- Explain the role of adiponectin and leptin in hunger and satiety
- Know about the various artificial sweeteners and their metabolic effects

## ▍Introduction

All organisms possess their variable energy demands; hence the supply is also equally variable. The consumed metabolic fuel may be oxidized to carbon dioxide ($CO_2$) and water ($H_2O$) or stored to meet the energy requirements as per the body needs **(Fig. 9.1)**. Adenosine triphosphate (ATP) serves as the energy currency of the cell. Any deficiency or reduced action of insulin causes diabetes. Obesity is one of the major cause for developing diabetes. Artificial sweeteners used by diabetic and obese people mainly to control their weight. It is better to monitor cholesterol status of our body by performing lipid profile testing. High level of cholesterol as well as LDL cholesterol results in atherosclerosis and later myocardial infarction. Myocardial infarction can be diagnosed by analyzing blood levels of troponin T and cardiac enzymes.

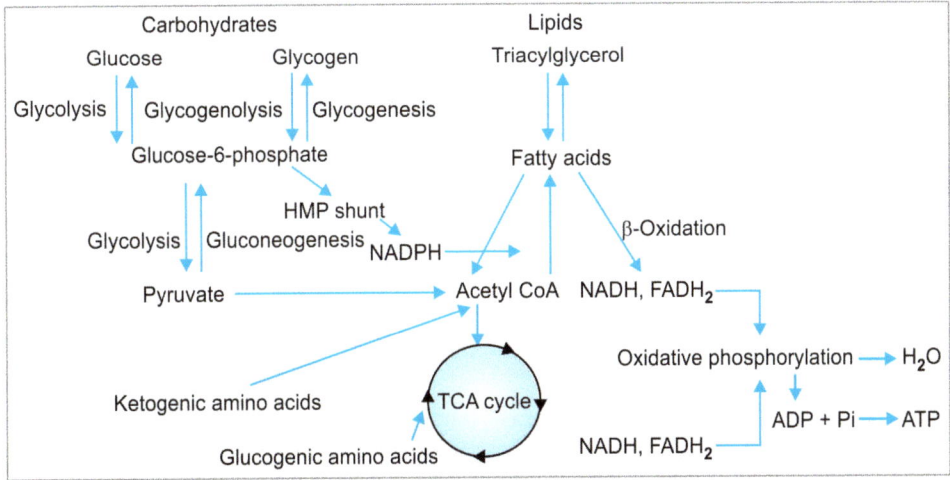

**Fig. 9.1:** Overview of metabolism.
(TCA: tricarboxylic acid; HMP: hexose monophosphate pathway; NADH: nicotinamide adenine dinucleotide; FADH: flavin adenine dinucleotide; ATP: adenosine triphosphate; ADP: adenosine diphosphate)

## Pathways of Metabolism

### Glycolysis

Degradation of glucose to pyruvate (lactate under anaerobic) generating ATP.

### Fatty Acid Oxidation

Fatty acid (FA) oxidizes to acetyl coenzyme A (acetyl-CoA). Energy is trapped in the form of nicotinamide adenine dinucleotide (NADH) and flavin adenine dinucleotide ($FADH_2$).

### Amino Acid Degradation

When amino acids consumed more than the required, are degraded to meet the fuel demands of the body. The glucogenic amino acids can serve as the precursor for the synthesis of glucose via pyruvate or intermediates of tricarboxylic acid (TCA) cycle.

The ketogenic amino acids form the precursor for acetyl-CoA.

**Briefly explain the role of different organs in integrating the metabolism in a well fed state (post-absorptive period).**
1. Briefly explain the role of different organs and tissues in integrating the metabolism after 2–4 hours of food intake.

**Or**

A 30-year-old man went to a marriage party and had a heavy lunch, which provided him enough carbohydrates, proteins, and fats. Explain how the various organs of his body work in a well-coordinated manner to meet his metabolic demands?

The various organs of the body work in a well-coordinated manner to meet its metabolic demands (usually 2–4 hours after food consumption) **(Fig. 9.2)**.

### Liver

Liver is specialized to serve as the body's central metabolic clearing house. After a meal, the liver takes up the carbohydrates, lipids and amino acids, processes them and routes to other tissues. The major metabolic functions of liver in absorptive state are:

* **Carbohydrate metabolism:** Increased glycolysis, glycogenesis and hexose monophosphate pathway (HMP) shunt, and decreased gluconeogenesis.
* **Lipid metabolism:** Increased FA and triacylglycerol (TG) synthesis.
* **Protein metabolism:** Increased degradation of amino acids and protein synthesis.

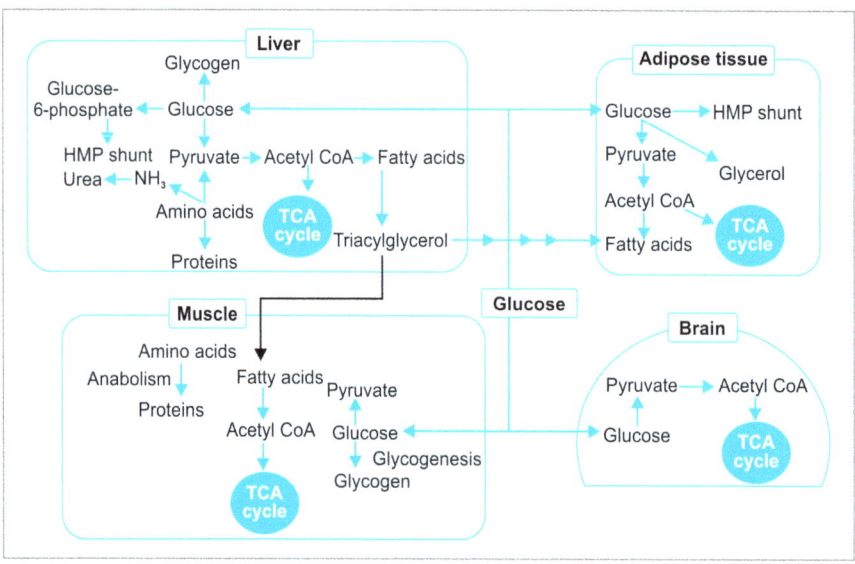

**Fig. 9.2:** Integration of metabolism during fed state.
(TCA: tricarboxylic acid; HMP: hexose monophosphate pathway)

## Adipose Tissue

Adipose tissue is regarded as the energy storage tissue:
- **Carbohydrate metabolism:** Increases uptake of glucose, glycolysis and HMP shunt.
- **Lipid metabolism:** FA and TG synthesis increases.
- Breakdown of TG inhibited.

## Skeletal Muscle

The major metabolic functions of skeletal muscle in absorptive state are:
- **Carbohydrate metabolism:** Uptake of glucose is higher and glycogenesis increased.
- **Lipid metabolism:** FA taken up from the circulation.
- **Protein metabolism:** Incorporation of amino acids into proteins is higher.

## Brain

- **Carbohydrate metabolism:** Glucose is the only source of fuel in an absorptive state, about 120 g of glucose is utilized per day.
- **Lipid metabolism:** Free FAs cannot cross the blood-brain barrier; hence their contribution for the supply of energy to the brain is insignificant.

2. **Briefly discuss the integration of metabolism during starvation.**

**Or**

Factory workers went on a hunger strike demanding a hike in their salary. The management did not respond to their demand and the workers decided to continue their hunger strike. Discuss the different organs and tissues that take part in integrating the metabolism during this condition to meet their energy requirement.

This part explains how all the metabolism is integrated in different organs and tissues of our body followed by starvation (Fig. 9.3):
- Starvation may be due to food scarcity or the desire to rapidly lose weight or during surgery and burns.
- It is metabolic stress, which imposes certain metabolic compulsions on the organism.

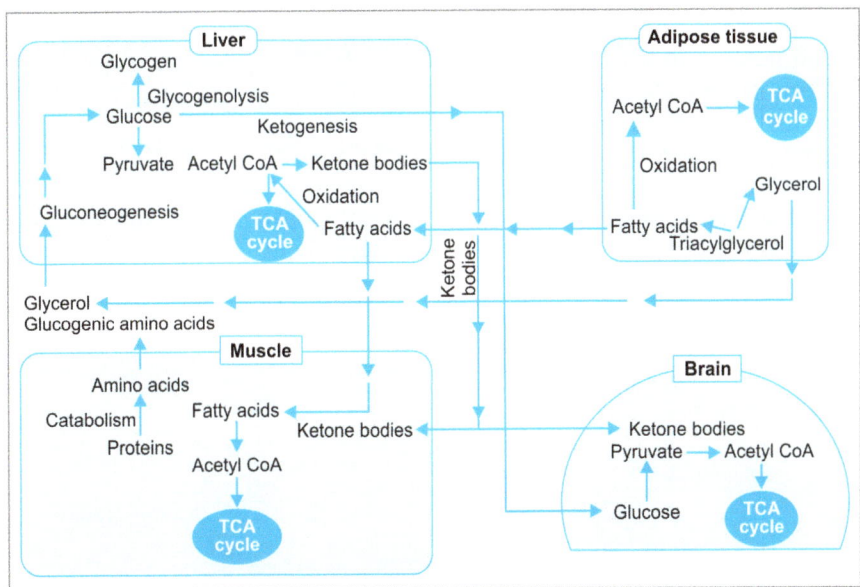

**Fig. 9.3:** Integration of metabolism during fasting condition.
(TCA: tricarboxylic acid)

- The metabolism is reorganized to meet the new demands of starvation.
- Glucose is the fuel of choice for brain and muscle. Unfortunately, the carbohydrate is not sufficient to meet the requirements.
- The TG of adipose tissue is the predominant energy reserve of the body. Protein can also meet the fuel demands of the body.
- Starvation associated with decreased insulin and increased glucagon.

### Liver in Starvation

- **Carbohydrate metabolism:** Increased gluconeogenesis and glycogen degradation.
- **Lipid metabolism:** FA oxidation increased. The TCA cycle cannot cope-up with the excess production of acetyl-CoA, so it is diverted for ketone body formation. The fuel demands of the brain are met by ketone bodies.

### Adipose Tissue in Starvation

- **Carbohydrate metabolism:** Glucose uptake and its metabolism are lowered.
- **Lipid metabolism:** Degradation of TG increased leading to increased release of FA from the adipose tissue, which serves as fuel for various tissues (brain is an exception). Glycerol liberated during lipolysis is used for glucose synthesis by the liver. FA and TG synthesis is completely stopped here.

### Skeletal Muscle in Starvation

- **Carbohydrate metabolism:** Glucose uptake and its metabolism are lowered.
- **Lipid metabolism:** FA and ketone bodies are utilized as fuel by the muscle. Prolonged starvation adopted to utilize FA.
- **Protein metabolism:** Muscle proteins are degraded and the amino acids are utilized for glucose synthesis by liver. Protein breakdown is reduced, if the starvation is prolonged.

### Brain in Starvation

In the early 2 weeks of starvation, the brain depends on glucose, supplied by liver gluconeogenesis. This, in turn, depends on the amino acids released from the muscle protein breakdown. Starvation beyond 3 weeks results in increased plasma ketone bodies and the brain adopts itself to depend on ketone bodies for the energy.

## Hormonal Regulation of Metabolism During Well-fed State (Fig. 9.4)

### Hormonal Regulation of Carbohydrate Metabolism

- In the regulation of blood glucose the liver, extrahepatic tissues and hormones play a major role.

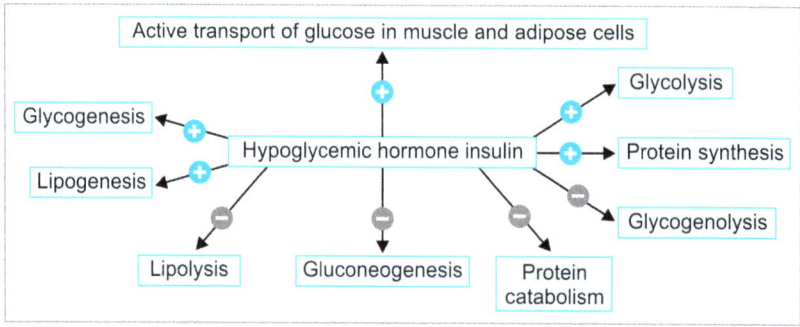

**Fig. 9.4:** Hormonal regulation metabolism during well-fed state.

- Increased level of circulating glucose releases insulin and this hormone reduces the blood glucose level in many ways.
- Insulin stimulates glucose transporter type 4 (GLUT-4) to increase the active transport of glucose across membranes of muscle and adipose tissue. Glucose is rapidly taken up into liver via GLUT-2 transporter.
- In the liver, insulin increases the use of glycolysis by inducing the glycolytic enzymes such as glucokinase, phosphofructokinase and pyruvate kinase.
- Glucokinase is important in regulating blood glucose after meal.
- In the liver and muscle, insulin stimulates glycogenesis by stimulating glycogen synthase by reducing the elevated cyclic adenosine monophosphate (cAMP) levels and thereby leading to suppression of glycogenolysis **(Fig. 9.5)**.
- Insulin inhibits gluconeogenesis by suppressing the action of key enzymes of gluconeogenesis, i.e., pyruvate carboxylase, phosphoenolpyruvate carboxykinase (PEPCK), fructose-1,6-bisphosphatase and glucose-6-phosphatase.
- In adipose tissue, glucose is converted to the glycerol-3-phosphate, needed for the formation of TG and inhibits the lipolysis by inhibiting hormone-sensitive lipase.
- Insulin increases protein synthesis and decreases protein catabolism, thereby decreasing releasing of amino acids for gluconeogenesis.

## Hormonal Regulation of Fat Metabolism

Insulin inhibits the activity of hormone sensitive lipase and reduces the release of free FAs, and glycerol from the adipose tissue, this result in fall in the circulating plasma-free FAs.

## Insulin Enhances TG Synthesis

Insulin enhances lipogenesis both in liver and adipose tissue by stimulating pyruvate dehydrogenase, acetyl-CoA carboxylase, and glycerol phosphate acyltransferase.

## Hormonal Regulation of Metabolism During Fasting/Starvation

## Regulation of Carbohydrate Metabolism in Fasting State

### Glucagon

- In the liver, it stimulates glycogenolysis by activating glycogen phosphorylase and inhibits glycogen synthase. It exerts its action on metabolic processes through the generation of cAMP.
- It enhances gluconeogenesis from amino acids and lactate.
- Alanine is the predominant amino acid released from muscle to liver by glucose alanine cycle.

### Epinephrine

Epinephrine favors glycogenolysis in liver and muscle through cAMP-dependent activation of adenylyl cyclase, which converts ATP to cAMP (stimulates phosphorylase) **(Fig. 9.6)**.

### Glucocorticoids

Increases:
- Gluconeogenesis
- Protein catabolism to provide amino acids for gluconeogenesis

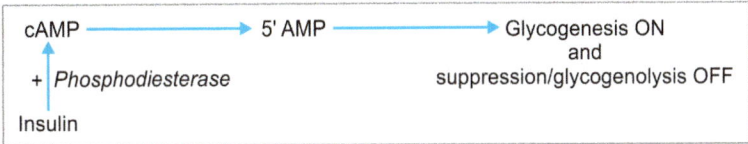

**Fig. 9.5:** Control of glycogen metabolism by insulin.
(AMP: adenosine monophosphate; cAMP: cyclic adenosine monophosphate)

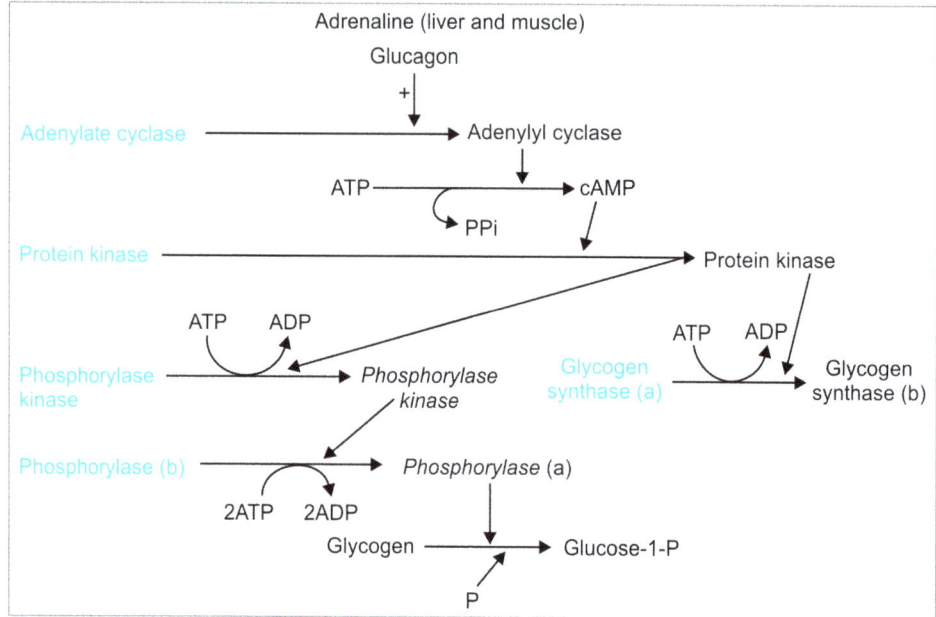

**Fig. 9.6:** Regulation of glycogen metabolism during fasting condition.
(ATP: adenosine triphosphate; cAMP: cyclic adenosine monophosphate; ADP: adenosine diphosphate)

- Activity of aminotransferase (to convert pyruvate to alanine).

### Anterior Pituitary Hormones
- Growth hormone and adrenocorticotropic hormone (ACTH) antagonize the action of insulin by elevating the blood glucose level.
- Growth hormone decreases glucose uptake in the muscle and ACTH decreases glucose utilization by the tissue.

### Thyroxine
Accelerates liver glycogenolysis and increase the rate of absorption of hexoses from the intestine.

## Hormonal Regulation of Fat Metabolism

Starvation associated with decreased insulin and increased glucagon; therefore, the hyperglycemic hormones antagonizes the action of insulin.

Norepinephrine, glucagon, ACTH, growth hormone (GH) and vasopressin accelerate the release of free FAs from adipose tissue, and raise the plasma-free FA concentration by increasing the lipolysis of the TG **(Figs. 9.7 and 9.8).**

Cyclic AMP, by stimulating cAMP-dependent protein kinase, activates hormone sensitive lipase, glucagon, epinephrine and norepinephrine, and inactivate the enzyme by cAMP-dependent phosphorylation and inhibit the FA synthesis.

## Hormonal Regulation of Cholesterol Metabolism

The $\beta$-hydroxy-$\beta$-methylglutaryl-CoA (HMG-CoA) reductase is the regulatory enzyme of cholesterol synthesis. Insulin and thyroid hormones increase HMG-CoA reductase activity through dephosphorylation of the enzyme (active).

Glucagon and glucocorticoids decrease HMG-CoA reductase activity through cAMP-dependent phosphorylation (inactive).

# CHAPTER 9: Integration of Metabolism and Homeostasis

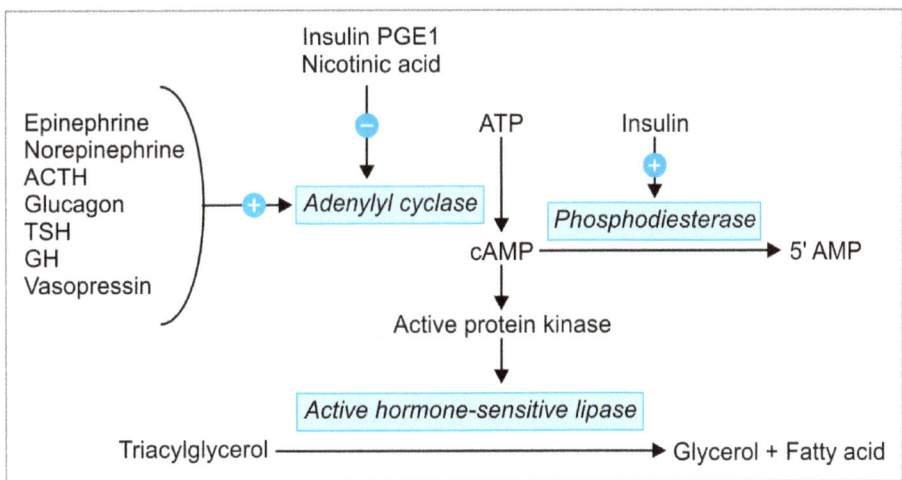

**Fig. 9.7:** Hormonal regulation of fat metabolism during fasting condition.
(ACTH: adrenocorticotropic hormone; TSH: thyroid-stimulating hormone; GH: growth hormone; PGE1: prostaglandin E1: ATP: adenosine triphosphate; AMP: adenosine monophosphate; cAMP: cyclic adenosine monophosphate)

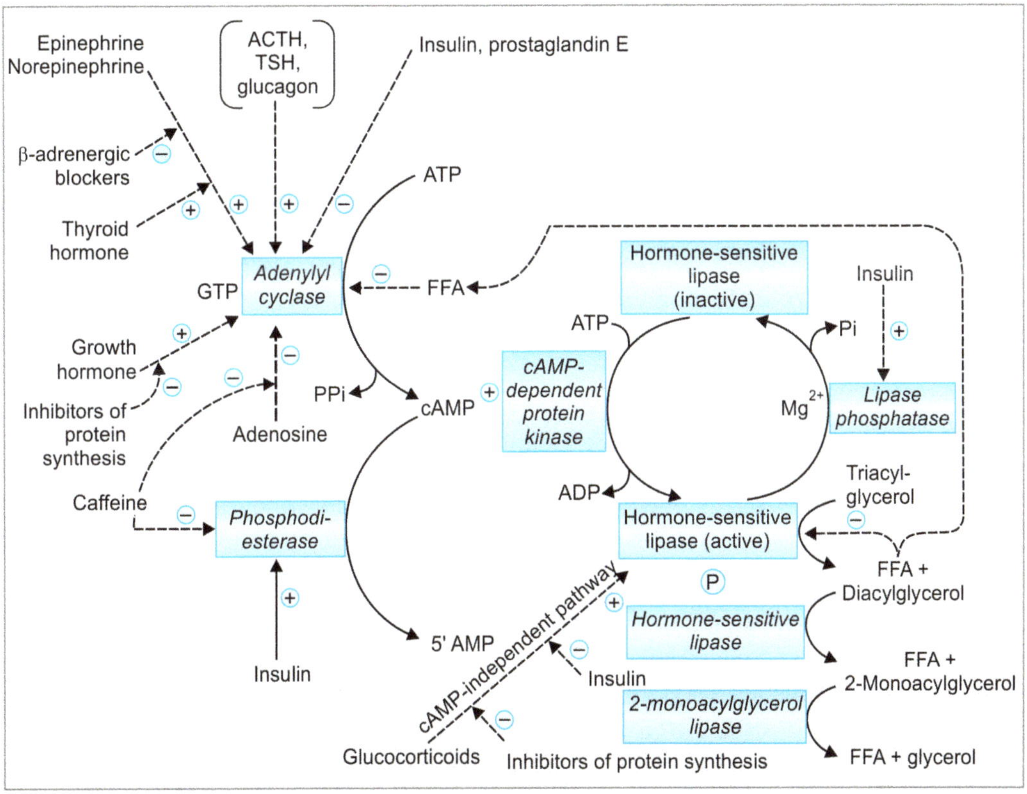

**Fig. 9.8:** Hormonal regulation of metabolism during fasting state.
(ACTH: adrenocorticotropic hormone; TSH: thyroid-stimulating hormone; ATP: adenosine triphosphate; GTP: guanosine triphosphate; FFA: free fatty acid; AMP: adenosine monophosphate; cAMP: cyclic adenosine monophosphate; ADP: adenosine diphosphate)

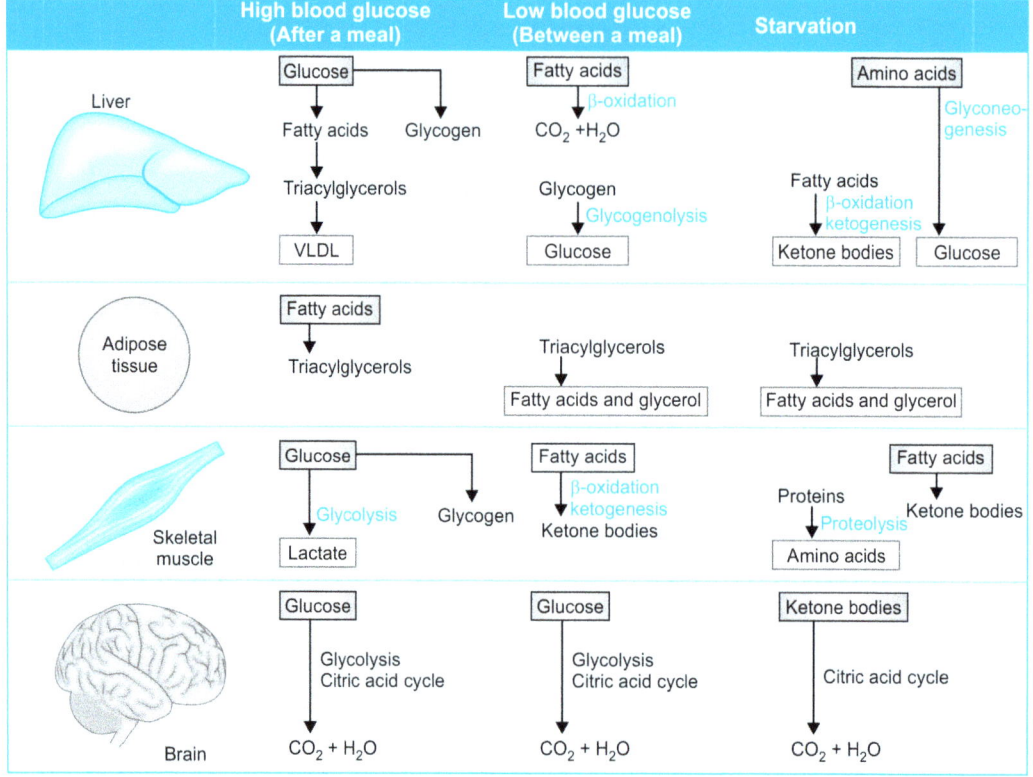

Fig. 9.9: Integration of metabolism after meal, between meals, and starvation.

Metabolism after a meal, between a meal, and during startvation are shown in **Figure 9.9. Briefly explain the role of adiponectin and leptin in hunger and satiety**

### Adipose Tissue Hormones

**Obesity:** Obesity, can be defined as: A chronic condition with excess amount of body fat, or more specifically, a body mass index (BMI) of 30 and above.

Obesity is also shown to be inversely related to *adiponectin and leptin*.

Adipose tissue plays an important role in the effect that different environmental temperatures have on appetite.

Adipokines are secreted by adipose tissue and are involved in homeostatic and appetite-regulating signaling in the body.

Leptin and adiponectin are adipokines that play a major role in energy homeostasis and appetite regulation.

Leptin signals the hypothalamus that energy requirements are being met and that no more food intake is required.

Adiponectin also acts at the hypothalamus but works to stimulate food intake.

### Adiponectin

*Adiponectin* is a 244 amino acid protein hormone. Synthesized exclusively in adipose tissue. It is a major adipokines secreted by fat cells

### Functions

- Glucose flux—decreases gluconeogenesis, increases glucose uptake
- Lipid catabolism—increases β-oxidation
- Protection from endothelial dysfunction
- Improves insulin secretion
- Biomarker for insulin sensitivity
- Weight loss
- Anti-inflammatory in action

# CHAPTER 9: Integration of Metabolism and Homeostasis

## Leptin

Leptin is a hormone predominantly made by adipose cells and enterocytes in the small intestine that helps to regulate energy balance by inhibiting hunger, which in turn diminishes fat storage in adipocytes. Leptin acts on cell receptors in the arcuate nucleus of the hypothalamus

**Leptin** is a **hormone** that is produced by our body's fat cells. It is often referred to as the "**satiety hormone**" or the "**starvation hormone**".

### Functions

- Helps to regulate the synthesis of thyroid hormones
- Decreases glucose stimulated insulin secretion
- Increases heart rate
- Regulate bone mass
- Regulating the menstrual cycle
- Regulate appetite, control metabolism and energy expenditure
- Helps in the activation of immune cells
- Increases blood pressure

Studies have shown that an absence of leptin in the body or leptin resistance can lead to uncontrolled feeding and weight gain.

## Artificial Sweeteners

Artificial sweeteners or intense sweeteners are sugar substitutes that are used as an alternative to table sugar. They are many times sweeter than natural sugar and as they contain no calories, they may be used to control weight and obesity. Extensive scientific research has demonstrated the safety of the six low-calorie sweeteners currently approved for use in foods in the US and Europe

1. Stevia
2. Acesulfame-K
3. Aspartame
4. Neotame
5. Saccharin
6. Sucralose

Table sugar has been an essential component of human diet. Its excess can lead to unhealthy effect on the body, most notably diabetes mellitus. Therefore, sugar substitutes were introduced as safer alternatives.

### Uses

Used in diabetes
- In controlling or reducing weight
- In dental caries
- In reactive hypoglycemia
- Flavor enhancement

Potential risks: Malignancy (used at very high dose), hypertriglyceridemia (fructose), weight gain and gastrointestinal symptoms.

Various natural sweeteners, which are safer, can be used instead of artificial sweeteners. Many of these include added benefits of being rich in minerals and vitamins. These include honey, coconut nectar, fruits, coconut sugar, maple syrup, molasses, sugar alcohols, stevia, dates, agave nectar, apple sauce and others.

They are safe for people with diabetes, and they can be used to reduce both your calorie and carbohydrate intake. Sugar substitutes also can help curb those cravings you have for something sweet.

## Laboratory Tests in Myocardial Infarction

A diagnosis of myocardial infarction (MI) is created by integrating the history of the presenting illness and physical examination with electrocardiogram findings and cardiac markers.

Cardiac markers or cardiac enzymes are proteins that leak out of injured myocardial cells through their damaged cell membranes into the bloodstream.

The markers most widely used in detection of MI are CK-MB subtype of the enzyme creatine kinase and cardiac troponins T and I as they are more specific for myocardial injury. The cardiac troponins T and I which are released within 4-6 hours of an attack of MI and remain elevated for up to 2 weeks, have nearly complete tissue specificity and are now the preferred markers for assessing myocardial damage.

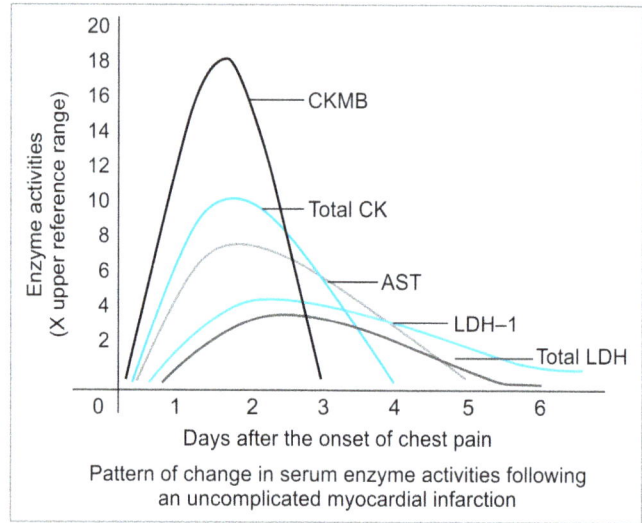

**Fig. 9.10:** Serum enzyme levels after myocardial infarction.
(CK: creatine kinase; AST: aspartate aminotransferase; LDH: lactate dehydrogenase)

Cardiac enzymes like **creatine kinase (CK), CKMB, lactate dehydrogenase (LDH), LDH1 and AST** are included in the cardiac enzyme panel **(Fig. 9.10).**

Following myocardial infarction, the 1st set of enzymes to increase is CK and CKMB. Immediately after the heart attack CKMB starts increasing reaches a maximum level by the end of 1st day. After reaching the peak level Ck and CKMB decreases and reaches normal level by 3rd day. In MI, CKMB may go up to 10-30 percent of total CK.

AST levels in plasma increase after 6-8 hours of chest pain and it reaches the peak value by 2nd day, but comes to normal by 4th or 5th day.

Total LDH and LDH1 begin to increase 8 to 12 hrs. after the chest pain. It goes on increasing and reaches the maximum value by 3rd day and slowly comes to normal by about 7th day.

The level of these enzymes in serum is related to the severe damage to heart muscle.

CKMB and LD1 are the most sensitive and specific markers for the diagnosis of MI.

## Troponin I and T

Troponin is a protein complex consisting of three subunits with different structure and function, namely:

1. Troponin T (TnT): Tropomyosin binding element. It is the myofibrilla protein of the striated muscle which is the building block of the contractile apparatus.
2. Troponin I (TnI): Actinomyosin ATPase inhibitory element.
3. Troponin C (TnC): Calcium binding.
   - Troponins have been investigated as markers of acute cardiac ischemia.
   - *Troponin-T is normally measured* because a small pool of it is not compartmentalized in the contractile apparatus and may be a precursor for synthesis of the troponin complex.
   - It is released into the blood within about 4 hours after the onset of symptoms, peaks at 12-16 hours and remains, elevated for 5-9 days' post-infarction.
   - Therefore, cardiac troponin (CTT) is very useful as a marker at any time interval after the heart attack which is its great advantage.
   - A level >1.2 µg/L is indicative of myocardial damage.
   - Troponin-T is the specific and sensitive test for the diagnosis of myocardial infarction as compared to CPK and LDH enzymes.

Its estimation indicates:
- Acute myocardial infarction
- Subacute myocardial infarction
- Micro-infarction
- Size of infarction
- Monitoring the outcome of thrombolysis therapy.

## SUMMARY

The human beings have variable demands of energy and therefore the supply is also equally variable. The absorbed metabolic fuel may be oxidized to $CO_2$ and $H_2O$ or stored to meet the energy requirement as and when the body needs. In a well-fed state, the metabolism and organs integrate themselves to meet the energy demands and to metabolize or to store the consumed dietary components. The insulin becomes active to burn the carbohydrates as well as to store the excess. Well-fed state makes hormone-sensitive lipase inhibition through insulin to reduce the release of free FAs. During starvation, the metabolism gets reorganized to meet the energy demands. Starvation is a metabolic stress, which imposes certain metabolic compulsions on the organism. The glucagon activity increases to make an effort to build up the blood glucose level. The TG of adipose tissue is the predominant energy reserve of the body. The hormone-sensitive lipase becomes active to hydrolyze the TG. The prolonged starvation results in the production of ketone bodies to provide energy to the brain. Any deficiency or reduced action of insulin causes diabetes. Obesity is one of the major causes for developing type 2 diabetes. Obesity is the deposition of excess fat and a BMI of 30 and above is considered obese. Obesity is inversely proportional to adipose tissue hormones such as adiponectin and leptin. There are several artificial sweeteners available and used by diabetic and obese people mainly to control their weight. It is better to monitor cholesterol status of our body by performing lipid profile testing. High level of cholesterol as well as LDL cholesterol results in atherosclerosis and later MI. MI can be diagnosed by analyzing blood levels of TnT and cardiac enzymes.

## SELF-ASSESSMENT QUESTIONS

1. Describe the pathway for the storage of glucose in the liver in the fed state. How is this pathway regulated?
2. What pathway provides for the production of pyruvate to be used for FA synthesis in the fed state? How is this pathway regulated?
3. During the conversion of glucose to FA, how is pyruvate, produced from glycolysis, converted to citrate in the cytosol? In which compartment does each reaction take place?
4. What are the sources of the reducing agent used for the reductive biosynthesis of FAs?
5. Which enzyme controls the pathway for the synthesis of FAs from acetyl-CoA in the cytosol? How is this pathway regulated?
6. What keeps newly formed free FA from entering the mitochondria in the fed state?
7. What happens to the product of the FA synthase complex before it is found in the blood?
8. Compare the $K_m$ for lipoprotein lipase in heart and adipose tissue. What implications does this have for the usage of blood TG in the fed and fasting state?
9. How does insulin affect the delivery of free FA into adipose cells in the fed state?
10. What are the pathways for the synthesis of TG in adipose from glucose and free FAs? How is the production of glycerol phosphate regulated?
11. What happens to the glycerol released in the lipoprotein lipase reaction in the fed state?
12. What pathways provide blood glucose during fasting? Why are these pathways active?
13. Why glycogen is not made in the liver during fasting?

14. Glycolysis does not function when gluconeogenesis is functioning. What factors turn on gluconeogenesis and turn off glycolysis?
15. What is the control enzyme for the release of free FAs during a fast and how is this enzyme regulated?
16. Why are ketone bodies produced during a fast?
17. Besides providing ATP, how does increased β-oxidation enable gluconeogenesis?
18. Explain how increased FA oxidation and decreased insulin spare blood glucose by muscle in the fasting and resting state?
19. What is the effect of exercise upon the use of blood glucose by muscle in the fasting state? What is the mechanism?

## MULTIPLE CHOICE QUESTIONS

1. An 8-year-old male patient with type 1 diabetes mellitus feels nauseated and drowsy, and has been vomiting for a few hours. Clinical examination shows mild signs of dehydration and low blood pressure. You request for laboratory tests and the results show the following:
    - Blood glucose: 380 mg/dL (above the reference range)
    - Hemoglobin A: 11.8 g/dL (reference range: 13.5–17.0 g/dL)
    - Hemoglobin A1c: 12% of total hemoglobulin (reference range: <6%)
    - Urine ketones: Positive
    - Urine glucose: Positive
    - Blood pH: 7.29
    - Partial pressure of carbon dioxide in arterial blood (PaCO$_2$): Below reference range
    - Serum bicarbonate: Below reference range
   
   Which of the following best indicates that this patient has had hyperglycemia over a period of weeks?
   (a) Ketonemia
   (b) Hemoglobin A1c
   (c) Glucosuria
   (d) Blood pH

2. Insulin facilitates energy storage in the liver. Which enzymes of carbohydrate metabolism are coordinately regulated in the liver in response to insulin signaling?
   (a) Glycogen synthase
   (b) Phosphofructokinase-2
   (c) Pyruvate kinase
   (d) All the above

3. Which one of the following enzymes of carbohydrate metabolism is not dephosphorylated in the liver in response to insulin signaling?
   (a) Glycogen synthase
   (b) Glycogen phosphorylase
   (c) Phosphofructokinase-1
   (d) Pyruvate kinase

4. Enzymes such as glycogen synthase, glycogen phosphorylase, the phosphofructokinase-2 (PFK-2)/fructose biphosphatase-2 (FBPase-2), and pyruvate kinase are phosphorylated by glucagon and/or epinephrine action. Which kinase is responsible for these phosphorylation events?
   (a) Protein kinase A
   (b) Calmodulin-dependent protein kinase
   (c) Protein kinase C
   (d) Receptor tyrosine kinase

5. The receptor to which epinephrine binds in order to stimulate phosphorylation of glycogen synthase and glycogen phosphorylase is:
   (a) α-1
   (b) α-2
   (c) β
   (d) γ

6. Insulin regulates all of the following enzymes in the liver. Which of these enzymes are also regulated by insulin in muscle?
   (a) Glycogen synthase
   (b) Glucokinase
   (c) Glycogen phosphorylase
   (d) Both a and c

# CHAPTER 9: Integration of Metabolism and Homeostasis

7. **The hormone that increases the rate of absorption of hexoses from the intestine is:**
   - (a) Glucocorticoids
   - (b) Thyroxine
   - (c) Anterior pituitary hormones
   - (d) Epinephrine
8. **In a fasting state, glucocorticoids:**
   - (a) Decrease protein catabolism
   - (b) Decrease hepatic uptake of amino acids
   - (c) Stimulate the utilization of glucose in extrahepatic tissues
   - (d) Increase the activity of aminotransferase
9. **Concerning insulin action, one of the following statements is incorrect, it:**
   - (a) Activates pyruvate kinase
   - (b) Stimulates glycerol phosphate acyltransferase
   - (c) Increases HMG-CoA reductase activity
   - (d) Activates hormone-sensitive lipase
10. **Starvation associated with:**
    - (a) Increased insulin and decreased glucagon
    - (b) Decreased epinephrine and increased insulin
    - (c) Decreased insulin and increased glucagon
    - (d) Decreased insulin and decreased glucocorticoids
11. **Lipase phosphatase is stimulated by:**
    - (a) Insulin
    - (b) Epinephrine
    - (c) Prostaglandin
    - (d) ACTH
12. **During starvation:**
    - (a) Acetyl-CoA carboxylase remains active
    - (b) Hormone-sensitive lipase becomes active
    - (c) Fructose-1,6-bisphosphatase becomes inactive
    - (d) Glycogen phosphorylase becomes inactive through cAMP-dependent phosphorylation
13. **Prolonged starvation is associated with:**
    - (a) The formation of fructose from carbohydrates
    - (b) Reduced breakdown of muscle glycogen
    - (c) Formation of fatty acids using acetyl-CoA
    - (d) Increased breakdown of triacylglycerol

## ANSWERS

| 1. b | 2. d | 3. c | 4. a | 5. c | 6. d | 7. b | 8. d |
| 9. d | 10. c | 11. a | 12. b | 13. d | | | |

# Chapter 10: Hemoglobin Metabolism

## LEARNING OBJECTIVES

*At the end of this chapter students should be able to:*
- Understand the structure of hemoglobin and its major function
- Know the difference between hemoglobin and myoglobin
- Explain the basis for different types of abnormal hemoglobin
- Explain the synthesis of hemoglobin
- Know about different types of porphyrias including their causes and symptoms

## Introduction

- Hemoglobin (Hb) is a conjugated protein.
- It is the red pigment present in red blood cell (RBC).
- It transports oxygen ($O_2$) from lungs to tissues.
- It transports carbon dioxide (CO) and $H^+$ from tissues to lungs and kidney.
- It acts as an intracellular buffer hence involved in acid–base balance.
- It is a globular, oligomeric protein made up of two parts, heme, a pigment and a protein part called globin.
- Hb synthesis takes place in the bone marrow. Its blood level is 12–16 g/dL. The synthesis of Hb depends on three important factors such as iron, folic acid, and vitamin $B_{12}$ along with amino acids. Deficiency of any of these factors decreases the ability of the bone marrow to synthesize RBC, thus causing anemia.

**Briefly describe the structure of hemoglobin.**

## Structure of Hemoglobin

Heme consists of a porphyrin ring with one iron (Ferrous $Fe^{2+}$) at the center **(Fig. 10.1)**.
- Hb is a conjugated metalloprotein of molecular weight 68,000.
- It consists of four heme molecules linked to the protein portion called "globin." Globin part consists of four polypeptide chains.

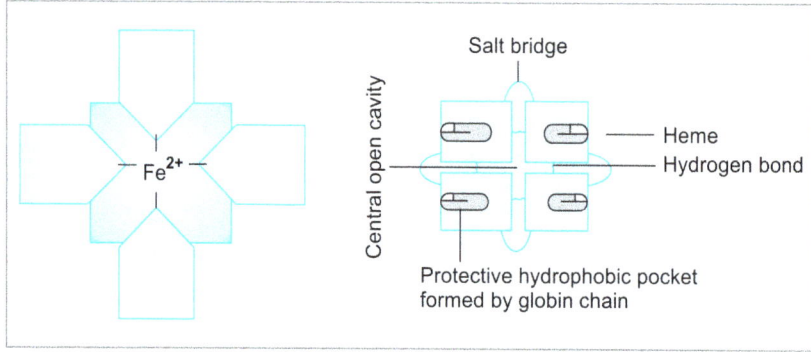

**Fig. 10.1:** Structure of hemoglobin.

# CHAPTER 10: Hemoglobin Metabolism

- Each heme molecule is located in a pocket formed by the folding of polypeptide chain.
- The quaternary structure of Hb is stabilized by hydrogen bonds, salt bridges, and van der Waals forces.
- The iron ($Fe^{2+}$) is held in the center of the protoporphyrin molecule by coordination bonds with the four nitrogen of the protoporphyrin ring.
- The iron has six coordination bonds:
    - Four bonds are formed between the iron and nitrogen atoms of the porphyrin ring system.
    - Fifth bond is formed between nitrogen atoms of histidine residue of the globin polypeptide chain, it is the proximal histidine.
    - The sixth bond is formed with oxygen.
- The oxygenated form of Hb is stabilized by H-bond between oxygen and side chain of another histidine residue of the globin chain, it is distal histidine. This distal histidine is not directly involved with the heme group but helps to stabilize the binding of oxygen to the heme molecule.
- Normal adult blood consists of two types of Hb, they are $HbA_1$ and $HbA_2$.
- $HbA_1$ comprises 97% of the total Hb and $HbA_2$ is about 3% of the total Hb.
- The blood of the newborn baby contains another type of Hb called fetal Hb (HbF). The amount of HbF is up to 90% in the neonatal stage and falls gradually by about 4–5 months.
- In normal adults, HbF concentration is about 1%.

The polypeptide chain composition of various Hb s is as follows:

| $HbA_1$ | $\alpha_2\beta_2$ | Chains |
| $HbA_2$ | $\alpha_2\delta_2$ | Chains |
| HbF | $\alpha_2\gamma_2$ | Chains |

The numbers of amino acids in the polypeptide chains are as follows:

α chain 141
β chain 146
δ chain 146
γ chain 146

## Binding Sites for Oxygen, Hydrogen, and Carbon Dioxide

Oxygen is bound to the ferrous ($Fe^{2+}$) atoms of the heme to form oxyhemoglobin. Carbon dioxide to α amino group of N-terminal end of the polypeptide chains of Hb to form carbaminohemoglobin (**Fig. 10.2**).

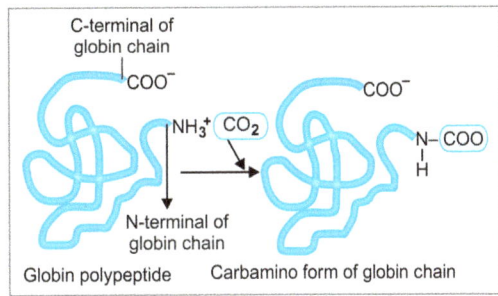

**Fig. 10.2:** Binding of carbon dioxide to hemoglobin.

## Compare Myoglobin and Hemoglobin

### Comparison of Myoglobin with Hemoglobin

The heme proteins myoglobin and Hb maintain a supply of oxygen, which is essential for oxidative metabolism.

Myoglobin is a monomeric protein of red muscle, which stores oxygen as a reserve against oxygen deprivation. It releases oxygen during severe exercise for use in muscle mitochondria for aerobic synthesis of ATP.

The tertiary structure of myoglobin is that of a typical water-soluble globular protein. Its secondary structure is unusual in that it contains a very high proportion (75%) of α-helical secondary structure. Each myoglobin molecule contains one heme prosthetic group inserted into a hydrophobic cleft in the protein. Each heme residue contains one central coordinately bound iron atom that is normally in the $Fe^{2+}$, or ferrous, oxidation state. The heme of myoglobin lies in a crevice between helices E and F oriented with its polar propionate groups facing the surface of the globin. The histidine, F8 linked iron and E7 on the sides of the heme ring are playing important roles in oxygen binding.

Hb, tetrameric protein of erythrocytes, transports oxygen to the tissues and returns $CO_2$ and protons to the lungs. The secondary structure of the polypeptide subunits of Hb resembles myoglobin. The heme and ferrous iron are responsible for storage and transport of oxygen.

**Explain the oxygen dissociation curves of myoglobin and hemoglobin.**

## Oxygen Dissociation Curves of Myoglobin and Hemoglobin

The oxygen binding curve for myoglobin is hyperbolic. Myoglobin, therefore, loads $O_2$ readily at the $PO_2$ of the lung capillary bed (100 mm Hg). However, strenuous exercise lowers the $PO_2$ of muscle tissue to about 5 mm Hg, myoglobin releases $O_2$ for mitochondrial synthesis of ATP, to keep continuing the muscular activity **(Fig. 10.3)**.

The myoglobin and β-subunit of HbA have almost identical secondary and tertiary structures except the number of amino acids. The cooperative binding nature of Hb (tetrameric) permits Hb to maximize both the quantity of $O_2$ loaded at the $PO_2$ of the lungs and the quantity of oxygen released at the $PO_2$ of the peripheral tissues.

**Discuss the cooperative binding of oxygen by hemoglobin including its importance.**

## Cooperative Oxygen Binding of Hemoglobin

The cooperative interaction between different binding sites makes Hb an unusually good oxygen-transport protein because it enables the molecule to pick up as much oxygen as possible once the partial pressure of this gas reaches a particular threshold level and then gives off as much oxygen as possible when the partial pressure of $O_2$ drops significantly below this threshold level. The hemes are too much far apart to interact directly. But, changes that occur in the structure of the globin that surrounds a heme when it picks up an $O_2$ molecule are mechanically transmitted to the other globins in this protein **(Fig. 10.4)**. These changes carry the signal that facilitates the gain or loss of an $O_2$ molecule by the other hemes.

The cooperative binding of $O_2$ by Hb enhances oxygen transport. The shape of $O_2$ binding curve of Hb is sigmoidal (S-shaped) because oxygen binding is cooperative. This shape indicates that the affinity of Hb for binding the first molecule of oxygen is relatively very low, but subsequent oxygen molecules are bound with a very much higher affinity accounting for the steeply rising portion of the S-shaped curve.

The Hb also transports $CO_2$ (by-product of respiration) and protons from peripheral tissues to the lungs. Hb carries $CO_2$ as carbamates (15%) formed with the amino terminal nitrogen of the polypeptide chains.

This favors the salt bond formation between α and β chains of Hb. The remaining $CO_2$ is carried as bicarbonate, which is formed in erythrocyte by the hydration of $CO_2$ to $H_2CO_3$ (carbonic acid), catalyzed by carbonic anhydrase. The venous blood pH dissociates $H_2CO_3$ into $HCO_3^-$ (bicarbonate) and a proton.

Deoxyhemoglobin binds one proton for every two oxygen molecules released, contributing significantly to the buffering capacity of

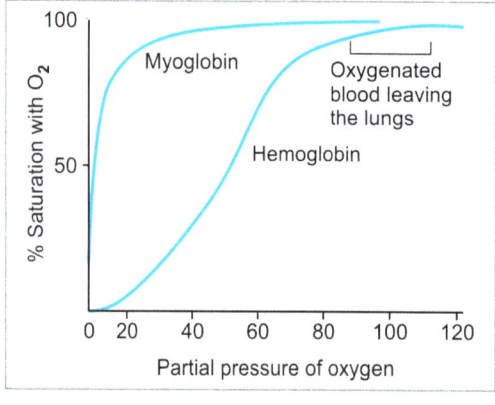

**Fig. 10.3:** Oxygen dissociation curve of hemoglobin and myoglobin.

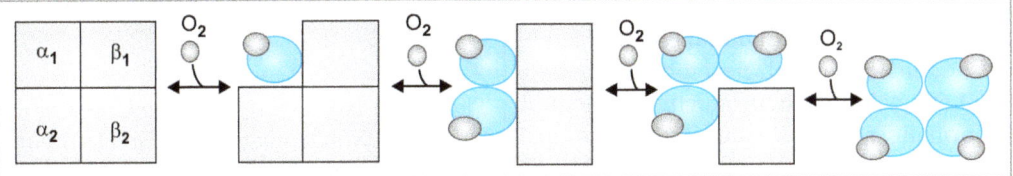

**Fig. 10.4:** Cooperative binding of oxygen to hemoglobin.

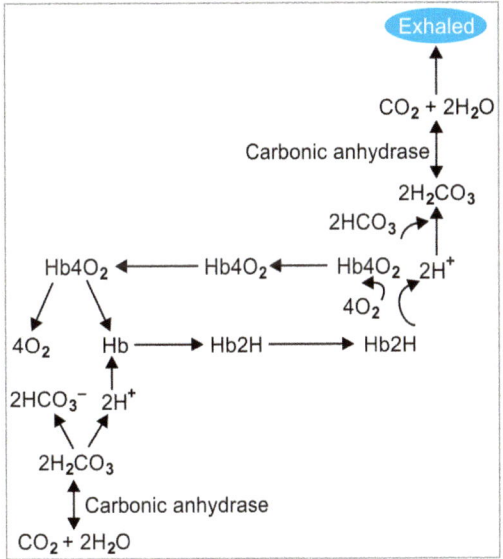

**Fig. 10.5:** Bohr effect.

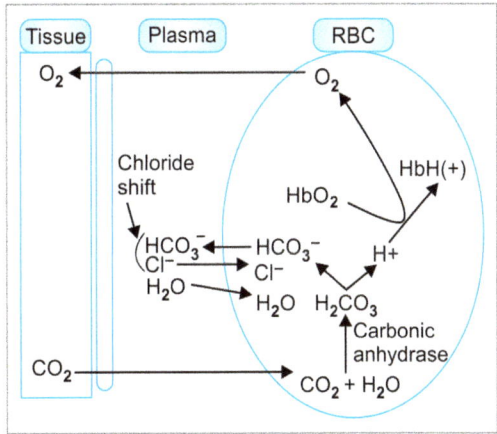

**Fig. 10.6:** Chloride shift.

blood. In the lungs, the process reverses. As oxygen binds to deoxyhemoglobin, protons are released (due to rupture of salt bridges) and combine with bicarbonate to form carbonic acid. Dehydration of $H_2CO_3$ catalyzed by carbonic anhydrase forms $CO_2$, which is exhaled. This reciprocal coupling of protons and oxygen binding is termed "Bohr effect" (**Fig. 10.5**). This effect mainly depends on cooperative interactions between the hemes of the Hb tetramer. Therefore, myoglobin (monomer) does not exhibit the Bohr effect.

Bohr effect increases hydrogen ion concentration and decreases the amount of oxygen bound by Hb at any oxygen concentration (partial pressure). Coupled to the diffusion of bicarbonate out of RBCs in the tissues there must be ion movement into the RBCs to maintain electrical neutrality. This is the role of Cl⁻ and is referred to as the chloride shift. In this way, Cl⁻ plays an important role in bicarbonate production and diffusion and thus also negatively influences $O_2$ binding to Hb (**Fig. 10.6**).

## Factors Affecting Oxygen Binding

The binding of oxygen to Hb can be dramatically altered by a small group of substances called allosteric effectors. Hydrogen ions (protons), carbon dioxide, and 2,3-bisphosphoglycerate (2,3-BPG) are effectors that can promote the release of oxygen by favoring the deoxygenated form of Hb.

## Role of 2,3-Bisphosphoglycerate

Low $PO_2$ in peripheral tissues promotes the synthesis of 2,3-BPG in erythrocytes from 1,3-BPG. This 2,3-BPG binds to deoxygenated Hb (T) and stabilizes it. The BPG binds more weakly to HbF than to HbA. Therefore, the HbF has higher affinity for $O_2$ than HbA.

## Abnormal Hemoglobin

The abnormal Hb of sickle cell anemia was first demonstrated by Linus Pauling in 1949.

Structurally each globin chain has its own genetic locus. The individual chain of Hb is under genetic control. Based on the genetics of the globin chain production, structural abnormalities can be divided into four groups:
1. Amino acid substitutions: HbS, HbC, HbD, and HbE.
2. Amino acid deletion (deletion of three nucleotides in DNA): Hb Gun Hill.
3. Elongated globin chains (resulted from chain termination, shift mutation, or other mutations).
4. Fused or hybrid chains (resulted from non-homologous crossing-over): Hb Lepore.

Most of the Hb variants arise by a single amino acid substitution, which is called "point mutations."

Deletion of one or two nucleotide bases can shift the reading frame of all code words that follow. Such an event observed in microorganisms was called "frameshift mutation."

Abnormal Hbs are inherited as autosomal codominants. Thus subjects who inherit one normal and one abnormal gene are heterozygous and those who have two identical abnormal genes are homozygous.

## Hemoglobinopathy

When biological functions of Hb are altered due to a mutation in Hb, the condition is known as hemoglobinopathy, which may be grouped into two types:
1. **Quantitative hemoglobinopathies**, characterized by a decreased synthesis of either $\alpha$ or $\beta$ globin chain, leading to altered combination of normal $\alpha$, $\beta$, $\gamma$, or $\delta$ chains, e.g. thalassemia.
2. **Qualitative hemoglobinopathies**, characterized by an altered sequence of amino acids, usually in one of the constituent chains, e.g. sickle cell disease, HbC disease, HbD disease, and HbM disease.

In normal adults, amount of HbF is about 1%. The presence of HbF in more than 1% in adults and children above the age of 1 year is abnormal and the condition is known as hemoglobinopathy.

**What causes thalassemia? Explain briefly.**

## Thalassemia

The name is derived from the Greek word, "thalassa," which means "sea." Greeks inherited this disease present around Mediterranean Sea. The absence or diminished synthesis of one of the polypeptide chains of human Hb is characterized as "thalassemias." The reduction in the chain synthesis is called $\alpha$-thalassemia and decreased synthesis of chain synthesis is called $\beta$-thalassemia. The $\beta$-thalassemia is more common.

*α-Thalassemia:* $\alpha$ globin chain is structurally normal but its production impaired, resulting in the production excess $\beta$ and $\gamma$ globin chains, which leads to:

The formation of $\beta$-globin tetramer, called HbH and tetramer of $\gamma$ globin Hb Bart. These two forms cannot deliver oxygen to the tissues, leading to fetal death.

Depressed production of Hbs but contains $\alpha$ chains, i.e., $HbA_1$, $HbA_2$, and HbF.

*β-Thalassemia:* In this type, $\beta$ globin chain is structurally normal but its production is decreased. This decreased production of $\beta$ globin chain leads to:

A large excess of $\alpha$ chains form $\alpha$-globin tetramer that precipitates immediately within the RBCs as Heinz bodies and responsible for damage of the cell membrane and premature breakdown of RBCs.

There are two types of $\beta$-thalassemias:
1. $\beta$-Thalassemia major: This is the homozygous state for the thalassemia gene. It is a severe disease. Splenomegaly and skin pigmentation are the clinical pictures. Blood picture shows anemia; erythrocyte shows marked anisocytosis. The mean corpuscular volume (MCV) and mean corpuscular hemoglobin (MCH) decreases and mean corpuscular hemoglobin concentration (MCHC) increases. Both HbA and HbF are present (HbF 10–98%).
2. $\beta$-Thalassemia minor: This is the heterozygous state for the thalassemia gene. Both HbA and HbF are present. It has less symptoms.

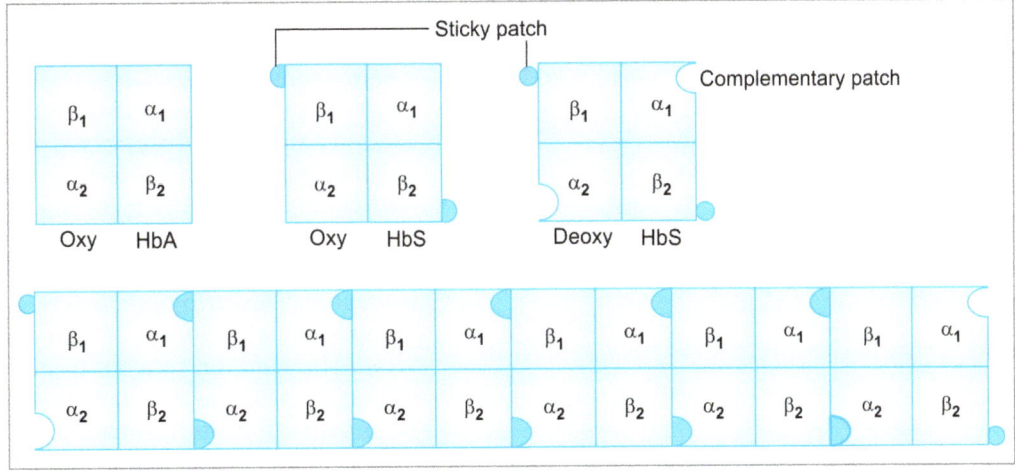

Fig. 10.7: Polymerization of deoxyhemoglobin.

**Discuss the sickle cell hemoglobin including the cause, symptoms, and the biochemical tests available to identify this.**

### Sickle Cell Hemoglobin

The sickle cell hemoglobinopathies are hereditary disorders in which the red cells contain HbS. They include the heterozygous (sickle cell trait, HbA and HbS present) and homozygous (sickle cell anemia, only HbS is present with the complete absence of HbA) for HbS. HbS causes a condition called sickle cell anemia. HbS differs from HbA in the substitution of valine for glutamic acid in the sixth position from the N-terminal end of the β chain.

HbA-Val-His-Leu-Thr-Pro-Glu-Glu-Lys
HbS-Val-His-Leu-Thr-Pro-Val-Glu-Lys

The side chain of valine is distinctly nonpolar, whereas that of glutamate is highly polar. This generates hydrophobic contact point called sticky patch, at position six of the β chain.

This sticky patch is present on the outer surface of the oxygenated and deoxygenated HbS. This is not found in normal HbA.

A complementary sticky patch is also present on the surface of the deoxygenated HbS. It is masked in oxygenated HbS.

This alteration in polarity markedly reduces the solubility of deoxygenated HbS.

When this HbS is deoxygenated, the sticky patch can bind to the complementary patch on another deoxygenated HbS molecule. This binding causes polymerization of deoxy-HbS forming insoluble long tubular fibrous precipitates **(Fig. 10.7)**.

The insoluble fibers of deoxygenated HbS distort the red cells into sickle-shaped (crescent-shaped) cells **(Fig. 10.8)**. Hence, this condition is known as sickle cell anemia. The change in the shape of the cell causes hemolysis leading to anemia.

### Clinical Symptoms

Clinical symptoms of sickle cell hemoglobin are as follows:
- Chronic hemolytic anemia.
- Hypoxia (breathlessness) due to less blood supply to the tissues and decreased oxygen.
- Pain and swelling in the joints.
- Persons with sickle cell trait show an increased resistance to malaria specifically for *Plasmodium falciparum*. This parasite

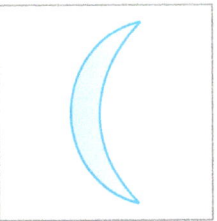

Fig. 10.8: Sickle cell red blood cell.

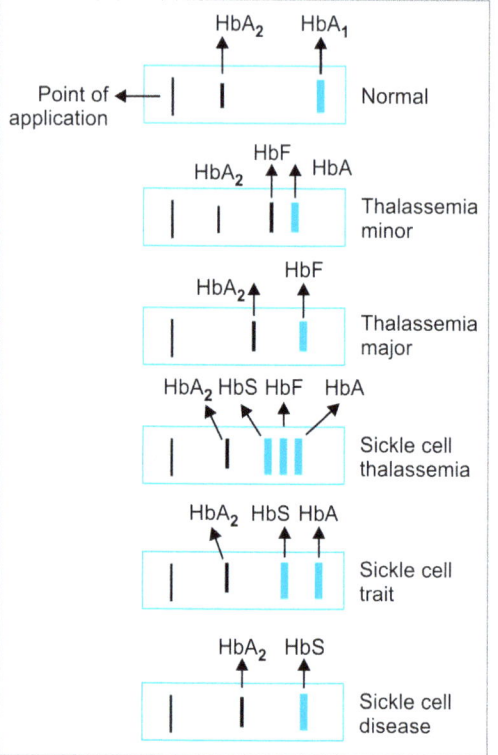

**Fig. 10.9:** Normal and abnormal hemoglobin patterns on cellulose acetate electrophoresis.

spends an obligatory part of its life cycle in the RBC.

## Detection of Abnormal Hb

### Electrophoresis of Hbs

Different types of Hbs can be separated from each other by electrophoresis. The Hb variants move with different speed in an electrical field and appear as separate bands. These differences in the migration are the result of different electrical charges of each Hb variant brought about by various amino acids in the polypeptide chains of Hb molecules. Support medium used for Hb electrophoresis is cellulose acetate strip **(Fig. 10.9)**.

1. *Detection of HbS*
   - *Sickling test*: Red cells containing HbS when mixed with a freshly prepared solution of sodium metabisulfite (reducing agent). This can be detected under microscope. This test is simple and will detect both homozygous and heterozygous sickle gene. False results may be obtained if the patient has had a recent transfusion of normal red cells or if the blood sample is infected.
   - *Solubility test*: HbS is less soluble in concentrated buffer solution at a pH of 6.5%, whereas normal Hb is soluble. This principle is used in differentiating HbS from normal Hb. When Hb is added to a solution of sodium hydrosulfite, a reducing agent in phosphate buffer, the solubility decreases and the solution becomes turbid if HbS is present.
2. Reference range
   *Percent solubility*
   Normal—90–95
   
   Hb AS—25–35
   
   Hb SS—3–10
   *Reference range*
   HbF% (alkali denaturation test)
   Normal—0.5–2
   Thalassemia major—10–100
   Thalassemia minor—0.5–8.0
   Sickle cell B-thalassemia—5–20
   Sickle cell anemia—5–30
   Normal newborn—60–90

## Derived Hb Compounds

Hb derivatives are formed by the joining of different groups with the heme part or change in the oxidation state of iron.

- *Oxyhemoglobin (Hb-O)*: It is the form of Hb present in the RBC, in the body. $O_2$ is combined to Hb through $Fe^{2+}$ (ferrous). It is dark red in color and the $\gamma$ max is 577 nm.
- *Reduced Hb or deoxyhemoglobin (Hb)*: This Hb is without oxygen. This is purple red in color.
- *Carboxy Hb (Hb-CO)*: Carboxy Hb is formed by binding of CO with Hb. CO binds with the iron atom in the same way as oxygen binds. CO has more affinity toward Hb than $O_2$; hence, even small quantity of CO present will bind to the Hb.

λ max of Hb-CO is 572 mm.
Exposure to CO occurs in the following conditions:
- In the mines (also deep wells)
- Heavy cigarette smoking
- Incomplete burning of petrol.

❖ *Methemoglobin (MetHb):* A substitution of tyrosine for the histidine at either the proximal or distal histidine residues of either the α or β chains locks the heme iron into a trivalent state ($Fe^{3+}$) or the action of oxidizing agents on ferrous form of Hb converts $Fe^{2+}$ into $Fe^{3+}$ state. $Fe^{3+}$ cannot bind oxygen; hence, oxygen transport is not possible. Increased MetHb in the blood is known as methemoglobinemia.

*Causes of methemoglobinemia*
- Congenital MetHb reductase deficiency.
- Ingestion of nitrites, nitrates sulfa drugs, or certain dyes (aniline dyes).
- Household substances such as shoe polish (nitrobenzene) and furniture.
- When MetHb in the blood increases up to 15% of the total pigment cyanosis occurs (bluish color of the skin). Normally small amount of MetHb is produced in the blood. The enzyme MetHb reductase present in the RBC converts the $Fe^{3+}$ to $Fe^{2+}$ form thus converting the MetHb to normal Hb.
- Thus under normal conditions, MetHb concentration is less than 1% of the total Hb γ max of MetHb=630 nm.
- There are again two types of methemoglobinemia:
  1. Hereditary methemoglobinemia associated with NADH-MetHb reductase deficiency. This is an autosomal recessive trait and affected subjects are persistently cyanotic.
  2. Hereditary methemoglobinemia associated with HbM: This is associated with cyanosis. This disorder is transmitted as an autosomal dominant trait.

❖ *Sulfhemoglobin (HbS):* This is an abnormal sulfur-containing Hb (attached to the porphyrin ring). It does not act as an oxygen carrier and it is not present in the normal RBCs. It is formed by the toxic action of drugs and chemical agents that contains sulfur. It results in cyanosis.

❖ *Cyanomethemoglobin:* Hb is converted to cyan-MetHb by Drabkin's reagent (potassium ferricyanide+Pot cyanide). It is a complex formed by MetHb with cyanide and it is a stable compound having max at 540 nm. This provides an accurate method for the estimation of Hb in the blood.

❖ *Carbonyl Hb (Hb-$CO_2$):* This is the form of Hb transporting $CO_2$ from tissues to the lungs.

**Briefly explain the process of heme synthesis including the regulation.**

## Heme Synthesis

Heme is synthesized in a complex series of steps involving enzymes in the mitochondrion and in the cytosol of the cell. The first step in heme synthesis takes place in the mitochondrion, with the condensation of succinyl CoA and glycine by aminolevulinic acid (ALA) synthase to form Δ-ALA. This molecule is transported to the cytosol where a series of reactions produce a ring structure called coproporphyrinogen III. This molecule returns to the mitochondrion where an addition reaction produces protoporphyrin IX **(Fig. 10.10)**.

The enzyme ferrochelatase inserts iron into the ring structure of protoporphyrin IX to produce heme. Deranged production of heme produces a variety of anemias. Iron deficiency, world's most common cause of anemia, impairs heme synthesis thereby producing anemia. A number of drugs and toxins directly inhibit heme production by interfering with enzymes involved in heme biosynthesis. Lead commonly produces substantial anemia by inhibiting heme synthesis, particularly in children.

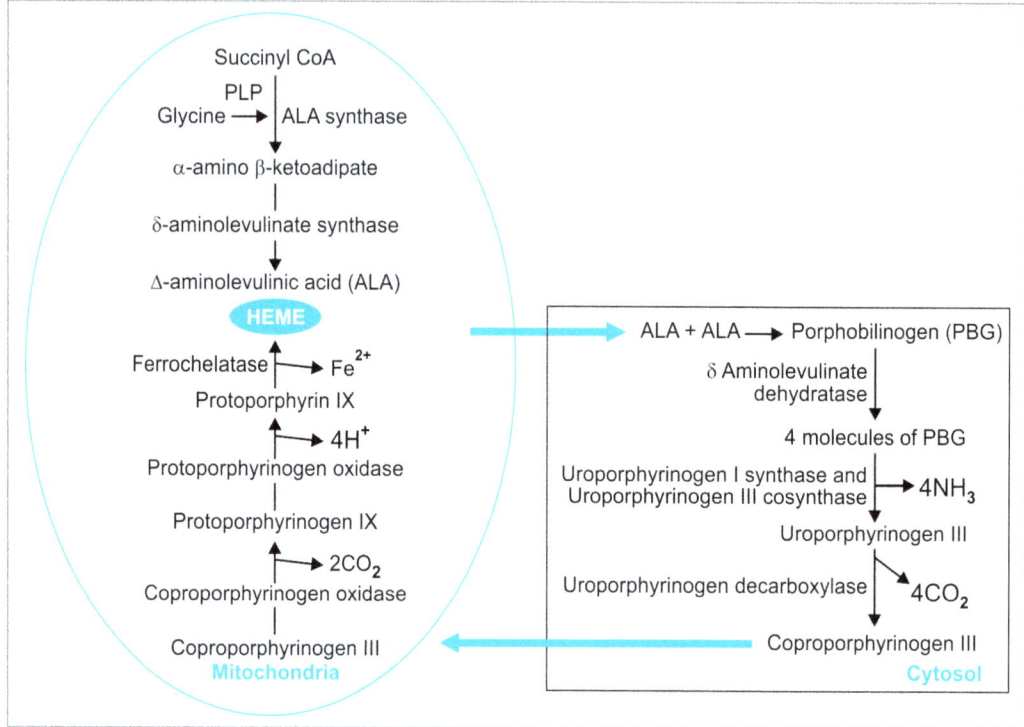

**Fig. 10.10:** Heme synthesis.

## Globin Synthesis

Two distinct globin chains (each with its individual heme molecule) combine to form Hb. One of the chains is designated α. The second chain is called "non-α." With the exception of the very first weeks of embryogenesis, one of the globin chains is always α. A number of variables influence the nature of the non-α chain in the Hb molecule. The fetus has a distinct non-α chain called gamma. After birth, a different non-α globin chain, called β, pairs with the α chain. The combination of two α chains and two non-α chains produces a complete Hb molecule (a total of four chains per molecule).

## Regulation of Heme Biosynthesis

Although heme is synthesized in virtually all tissues, the principal sites of synthesis are erythroid cells (~85%) and hepatocytes. The differences in these two tissues and their needs for heme result in quite different mechanisms for the regulation of heme biosynthesis. In hepatocytes, heme is required for incorporation into the cytochromes, in particular, the $P_{450}$ class of cytochromes that are important for detoxification. In addition, numerous cytochromes of the oxidative-phosphorylation pathway contain heme.

The rate-limiting step in hepatic heme biosynthesis occurs at the ALA synthase catalyzed step, which is the committed step in heme synthesis. The $Fe^{3+}$ oxidation product of heme is termed "hemin." Hemin acts as a feedback inhibitor on ALA synthase. Hemin also inhibits transport of ALA synthase from the cytosol (its site of synthesis) into the mitochondria (its site of action) as well as represses synthesis of the enzyme.

In erythroid cells, all of the heme is synthesized for incorporation into Hb and occurs only upon differentiation when the synthesis of Hb proceeds. When red cells mature, both heme and Hb synthesis ceases. The heme (and Hb) must, therefore, survive for the life of the erythrocyte (normally this is 120 days). In reticulocytes (immature erythrocytes), heme stimulates protein synthesis. Additionally, control of heme biosynthesis in erythrocytes occurs at numerous sites other than at the level of ALA synthase. Control has been shown to be exerted on ferrochelatase, the enzyme responsible for iron insertion into protoporphyrin IX, and on porphobilinogen deaminase.

## Heme Catabolism

Breakdown of RBC releases heme and globin. The globin goes to globin pool and heme converted hemin. The hemin loses its iron and converts to biliverdin. The biliverdin reductase reduces biliverdin to bilirubin, a yellow pigment (**Fig. 10.11**).

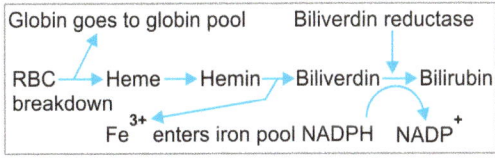

**Fig. 10.11:** Heme catabolism.

## Clinical Aspect of Heme Metabolism

Clinical problems associated with heme metabolism are of two types. Disorders that arise from defects in the enzymes of heme biosynthesis are termed the "porphyrias" and cause elevations in the serum and urine content of intermediates in heme synthesis (**Table 10.1**). An inherited disorder in bilirubin metabolism leads to hyperbilirubinemia. Bilirubin is potentially toxic waste product of heme catabolism. The body eliminates bilirubin by transporting it to the liver bound to albumin in the serum. In the liver, it is conjugated with glucuronate, which renders it water-soluble. The glucuronide conjugate is then excreted in the bile. Persons with extreme elevation in unconjugated bilirubin are susceptible to bilirubin encephalopathy, also referred to as kernicterus. Accumulation of bilirubin in the plasma and tissues results in jaundice. Gilbert syndrome and Crigler–Najjar syndrome result from predominantly unconjugated hyperbilirubinemia. Dubin–Johnson syndrome and Rotor syndrome result from conjugated hyperbilirubinemia. The porphyrias are both inherited and acquired disorders in heme synthesis. These disorders are classified as either erythroid or hepatic, depending upon the principal site of expression of the enzyme defect. Eight different porphyrias have been classified (**Table 10.1**).

**List the different types of porphyria and state the causes and features of it.**

## Role of Hemoglobin in Disease

- ❖ Decreased levels of Hb, with or without an absolute decrease of RBCs, lead to symptoms of anemia.
- ❖ Anemia has many different causes.
- ❖ Absence of iron decreases heme synthesis, RBCs in iron deficiency anemia are hypochromic (lacking the red Hb pigment) and microcytic (smaller than normal). Other anemias are rarer.
- ❖ In hemolysis (accelerated breakdown of RBCs), associated jaundice is caused by the Hb metabolite bilirubin, and the circulating Hb can cause renal failure.
- ❖ Mutations in the globin chain are associated with the hemoglobinopathies, such as sickle cell disease and thalassemia.

## Fate of Bilirubin

- ❖ Once the bilirubin is formed, it binds to albumin and is transported to the liver.
- ❖ In the liver, it is separated from the albumin and the bilirubin is taken up by the liver parenchymal cells.

**Table 10.1:** Causes and features of porphyrias.

| Porphyrias | Enzyme defect | Primary symptoms |
|---|---|---|
| Erythropoietic class | | |
| CEP | Uroporphyrinogen III cosynthase | Photosensitivity (itching and burning of skin when exposed to light). Excrete more uro- and coproporphyrinogen I, which then oxidized to uro- and coproporphyrin (red pigments) |
| EPP | Ferrochelatase | Photosensitivity, protoporphyrin IX excreted into urine and feces |
| Hepatic class | | |
| ADP | ALA dehydratase | Neurovisceral |
| AIP | PBG deaminase or uroporphyrinogen I synthase | Neurovisceral. Increased excretion of porphobilinogen and ALA and urine gets darkened |
| HCP | Coproporphyrinogen oxidase | Neurovisceral. Some photosensitivity coproporphyrinogen, ALA PBG are excreted in urine and feces |
| VP | Protoporphyrinogen oxidase | Neurovisceral, some photosensitivity. All the intermediates of heme synthesis accumulate and excreted in urine and feces |
| PCT | Uroporphyrinogen decarboxylase | Photosensitivity. Increased excretion of uroporphyrins |
| HEP | Uroporphyrinogen decarboxylase | Photosensitivity, some neurovisceral |

(ADP: ALA dehydratase deficiency porphyria; AIP: acute intermittent porphyria; PBG: porphobilinogen; ALA: aminolevulinic acid; CEP: congenital erythropoietic porphyria; EPP: erythropoietic protoporphyria; HCP: hereditary coproporphyria; HEP: hepatoerythropoietic porphyria; PCT: porphyria cutanea tarda; VP: variegate porphyria)

- In the liver, the uridine diphosphate (UDP) glucuronyl transferase enzyme conjugates the bilirubin with two molecules of UDP glucuronic acid to form a conjugated bilirubin called bilirubin diglucuronide.
- The conjugated bilirubin is secreted into the bile through bile duct and reaches the intestine.
- The intestinal bacterial enzymes β-glucuronidase hydrolyzes the conjugated bilirubin and deconjugates it.
- The portion of this free bilirubin then gets reduced by fecal flora to a colorless tetrapyrrole urobilinogen.
- Then a small percent of this urobilinogen is reabsorbed from the intestine and returned to the liver by portal blood and reexcreted through the liver known as enterohepatic urobilinogen cycle.
- More than 90% of the recirculated urobilinogen is taken up by the liver and reexcreted into the bile, the remainder is filtered by the kidneys and excreted in the urine.
- The urobilinogen is also excreted through blood, but it is negligible.
- The urobilinogen is further reduced to stercobilinogen and excreted through feces (around 200–300 mg/day).
- The urobilinogen and stercobilinogen are colorless compounds; but when they are exposed to atmospheric oxidation, they are converted to a colored urobilin and stercobilin, respectively.
- The conjugated water-soluble bilirubin when treated with diazo reagent ($NaNO^+$ sulphanilic acid) gives a red color immediately. This is called direct van den Bergh's test. The conjugated bilirubin reacts directly without adding methanol so it is also called direct bilirubin (direct positive).

- The water-insoluble unconjugated bilirubin gives a positive van den Bergh's test only if methanol is added to the serum. This is indirect van den Bergh's test. This also called indirect bilirubin (Indirect positive).
- The water-soluble free conjugated bilirubin can be filtered through the glomerular membrane and excreted in the urine when there is increase in the blood levels of conjugated bilirubin.
- The water-insoluble unconjugated bilirubin is not filtered by the glomerular membrane as it is bound to albumin; hence, it does not appear in the urine, whenever a blood level of unconjugated bilirubin is increased.

## Disorders of Hb Catabolism

Normal concentration of serum bilirubin is:
- Total bilirubin: 0.1–1.0 mg/dL
- Conjugated bilirubin: 0.1–0.2 mg/dL
- Unconjugated bilirubin: 0.2–0.8 mg/dL

The bilirubin metabolism is altered when there is:
- Increased load of bilirubin to the liver.
- Reduced hepatic uptake.
- Reduced intracellular transport.
- Reduced conjugation and excretion of bilirubin.
- Obstruction to the flow of bile.
- One or more of the above problems leads to elevated bilirubin and causing jaundice.

**What is jaundice? Explain.**

## ▪ Jaundice

- Normal serum bilirubin concentration is around 1.2 mg/100 mL.
- When the bilirubin level exceeds more than 1.2 mg/dL, it diffuses into the tissues. The skin and sclera of the eye turn yellow. This condition is called jaundice (icterus).
- The yellowish coloration is caused by an excess amount of bilirubin in the skin.
- Bilirubin is a yellowish-red pigment.
- Normally, small amounts of bilirubin are found in everyone's blood.
- When too much bilirubin is made, the excess is dumped into the bloodstream and is deposited in tissues for temporary storage.
- Jaundice in the infant appears first in the face and upper body and progresses downward toward the toes.

Hyperbilirubinemia may be acquired or inherited.

## Acquired Hyperbilirubinemia

- Prehepatic or hemolytic jaundice
- Hepatic jaundice
- Obstructive jaundice
- Neonatal or physiologic jaundice.

## Prehepatic or Hemolytic Jaundice

- This type of jaundice mainly arises due to excessive breakdown of RBC **(Table 10.2)** This excess hemolysis may be due to:
- Sickle cell Hb
- Deficiency of glucose-6-phosphate dehydrogenase
- Incompatible blood transfusions.

## Hepatic Jaundice

This type of jaundice mainly arises due to the damage of the parenchymal liver cells **(Table 10.2)**.

## Obstructive or Posthepatic Jaundice

Obstruction to the flow of bile causes the conjugated bilirubin to return to the blood. Therefore, the serum contains increased amount of direct bilirubin **(Table 10.2)**.

## Neonatal or Physiologic Jaundice

This type of jaundice mainly arises due to excessive breakdown of RBC.

This type of jaundice is common in newborn babies where there is increase bilirubin formed and released into the bloodstream

**Table 10.2:** Causes and laboratory findings of different types of jaundice.

| Specimen | Prehepatic or hemolytic | Hepatic | Posthepatic or obstructive |
|---|---|---|---|
| Causes | Abnormal red cells; antibodies; abnormal hemoglobin | Viral hepatitis; toxic hepatitis; intrahepatic cholestasis; drugs, and toxins | Extrahepatic cholestasis; gallstones; tumor of bile duct; carcinoma of pancreas |
| Unconjugated bilirubin | Present (++) | Present (++) | Normal |
| Conjugated bilirubin | Normal | Increases in early phase and later decreases | Present (++) |
| Serum enzymes | | | |
| ALP | Normal | Moderately increased | Increased markedly |
| ALT | Normal | Increased markedly | Moderately increased |
| AST | Normal | Increased markedly | Moderately increased |
| GGT | Normal | Moderately increased | Increased |

(ALP: alkaline phosphatase; ALT: alanine transferase; AST: aspertate transferase; GGT: gamma-glutamyl transferase).

when RBCs are broken down. Infants have too many RBCs. It is natural processes for the baby's body to break down these excess RBCs, forming a large amount of bilirubin. It is this bilirubin that causes the skin to take on a yellowish color. A newborn's liver is immature and deficient in UDP glucuronyl transferase, a conjugating enzyme, and cannot process bilirubin as quickly as it will be able to when it gets older.

Occasionally, there are other factors that cause jaundice in an infant. Two of the conditions known are ABO incompatibility and Rh incompatibility. Both of these conditions result in a very fast breakdown of RBCs. Also, jaundice may appear in infants with physical defects in the organs that work to eliminate the bilirubin from the body and decreased conjugating enzyme.

**List the different types of jaundice and state the causes and biochemical tests available to identify them.**

**What is Crigler–Najjar syndrome? Explain.**

## Inherited Unconjugated Hyperbilirubinemia

### Crigler–Najjar Syndrome

This is a rare autosomal recessive disorder due to deficiency of hepatic glucuronyl transferase enzyme.

There are two types of this condition:
1. *Type I*: It is characterized by the complete absence of the conjugating enzyme glucuronyl transferase. Therefore, no conjugated bilirubin is formed in this condition. It leads to severe jaundice with kernicterus.
2. *Type II*: It is a less severe form due to partial deficiency of the conjugating enzyme. The patient survives without any neurologic impairment.

### Gilbert's Syndrome

It is an inherited disease characterized by mild benign unconjugated hyperbilirubinemia due to:
* Impaired hepatic uptake from the circulation.
* Partial conjugation defect due to reduced activity of the conjugating enzyme.

**What causes the Dubin–Johnson syndrome?**

## Inherited Conjugated Hyperbilirubinemia

### Dubin–Johnson Syndrome

It is a benign autosomal recessive disorder, which causes an increase of conjugated bilirubin without elevation of liver enzymes. This condition is associated with a defect in the ability of hepatocytes to secrete conjugated bilirubin into the bile. It is usually diagnosed in early infancy.

It is also characterized by abnormal black pigment in the hepatocytes, giving a dark brown to black color to the liver.

*Rotor Syndrome*

It has many things in common with Dubin–Johnson syndrome except that in Rotor syndrome, the liver cells are not pigmented. The main symptom is a nonitching jaundice. There is a rise in bilirubin in the patient's serum, mainly of the conjugated type.

## SUMMARY

Hemoglobin is a conjugated iron containing a metalloprotein with four heme molecules linked to the protein portion called "globin." Globin part consists of four polypeptide chains. Normal hemoglobin consists of $2\alpha$ and $2\beta$ chains. Oxygen is bound to the ferrous ($Fe^{2+}$) atoms of the heme to form oxyhemoglobin. Myoglobin is a monomeric protein of red muscle, which stores oxygen as a reserve against oxygen deprivation. It releases oxygen during severe exercise for use in muscle mitochondria for aerobic synthesis of ATP. The oxygen binding curve for hemoglobin is sigmoidal in shape, whereas myoglobin is hyperbolic. Defect in the synthesis of hemoglobin results in the formation abnormal hemoglobin (sickle cell hemoglobin). The reduction in the globin chain synthesis results in thalassemia. Different types of hemoglobin can be differentiated through electrophoresis. Heme synthesis takes place in mitochondrion and cytosol, which depends on succinyl CoA, glycine, ALA synthase, and iron. Catabolism of heme results in bilirubin.

## SELF-ASSESSMENT QUESTIONS

1. Briefly explain the structure of normal hemoglobin.
2. What is sickle cell hemoglobin?
3. What is thalassemia and what are its types?
4. Name the tests used to detect abnormal hemoglobin.
5. Write the significance of alkali denaturation test.
6. What are the different types of hemoglobin derivatives?
7. Write short note on methemoglobin.

## MULTIPLE CHOICE QUESTIONS

1. **The polypeptide chains of $HbA_1$ are:**
   (a) $\alpha_2 \beta_2$
   (b) $\alpha_2 \delta_2$
   (c) $\alpha_2 \gamma_2$
   (d) $\delta_2 \gamma_2$
2. **The rate-limiting step of hemoglobin synthesis is catalyzed by:**
   (a) Ferrochelatase
   (b) Porphobilinogen deaminase
   (c) ALA synthase
   (d) Protoporphyrinogen oxidase
3. **Concerning fetal hemoglobin, all are true, *except*:**
   (a) Compared to adult hemoglobin, it is less sensitive to 2,3-bisphosphoglycerate
   (b) Its binding curve is to the right of myoglobin
   (c) It consists of $2\alpha$ and $2\gamma$ chains
   (d) Compared to adult hemoglobin, the critical substitution involves replacement of histidines with tryptophans

4. Concerning heme catabolism, one of the following statements is incorrect:
   (a) Heme converted hemin once it loses globin
   (b) Hemin loses iron and converted to biliverdin
   (c) Biliverdin reductase converts biliverdin to bilirubin
   (d) Biliverdin gains $H^+$ and changes to yellow pigment
5. Unconjugated hyperbilirubinemia results in:
   (a) Dubin–Johnson syndrome
   (b) Crigler–Najjar syndrome
   (c) Rotor syndrome
   (d) Metabolic syndrome
6. The porphyria that does not show photosensitivity is:
   (a) Acute intermittent porphyria
   (b) Variegate porphyria
   (c) Porphyria cutanea tarda
   (d) Erythropoietic protoporphyria
7. The erythropoietic protoporphyria results from the deficiency of:
   (a) Coproporphyrinogen oxidase
   (b) Protoporphyrinogen oxidase
   (c) Ferrochelatase
   (d) ALA dehydratase
8. Concerning sickle cell hemoglobin, one of the following statements is incorrect:
   (a) It results from the substitution of valine for glycine
   (b) It is determined by solubility test
   (c) It moves just behind $HbA_1$ during electrophoresis
   (d) The substitution takes place at the sixth position of β chain
9. All the following are the causes for methemoglobinemia, *except*:
   (a) Congenital MetHb reductase deficiency
   (b) Ingestion of nitrites
   (c) Continuous exposure to nitrobenzene
   (d) Exposure to lead
10. λ Max of MetHb is:
    (a) 630 nm
    (b) 540 nm
    (c) 380 nm
    (d) 700 nm
11. Which of the following trace elements may produce anemia in children by inhibiting hemoglobin synthesis?
    (a) Selenium
    (b) Lead
    (c) Iodine
    (d) Fluorine
12. Hepatic glucuronyl transferase deficiency results in:
    (a) Gilbert's syndrome
    (b) Dubin–Johnson syndrome
    (c) Lesch–Nyhan syndrome
    (d) Crigler–Najjar syndrome

## ANSWERS

| 1. a | 2. c | 3. d | 4. d | 5. b | 6. a | 7. c | 8. a |
| 9. d | 10. a | 11. b | 12. d | | | | |

# Chapter 11

# Acid–Base Balance

## LEARNING OBJECTIVES

*At the end of this chapter students should be able to:*
- List various buffer systems of our body playing their role in maintaining the acid–base status
- Understand the role of bicarbonate buffer system in maintaining the acid–base homeostasis
- Explain the renal and respiratory mechanism in regulating acid–base balance
- Understand the acid–base status in metabolic acidosis, metabolic alkalosis, respiratory acidosis and respiratory alkalosis

## Introduction

The human body can be described as a complex system, which consists of several levels and subsystems. At the chemical level, acids and bases are among those essential compounds upon which all biochemical processes depend. The biochemical reactions, which are taking place in our body, are extremely sensitive to even small changes in the acidity or alkalinity of the environment. The acid–base homeostasis should be maintained for cellular viability, enzymatic reactions, protein conformation, central nervous system (CNS) functions, etc. These functions are modified when there is change in the cellular and extracellular acid–base status. For these reactions, the acids and bases that are formed constantly should be kept in balance.

To understand acid-base homeostasis, definitions of some of the terms needed are explained below.

**Acids:** Bronsted is defined an acid as a chemical entity that donates protons in solution.

$$HCl \leftrightarrow H^+ + Cl^-$$
$$H_2CO_3 \leftrightarrow H^+ + HCO_3^-$$
$$NH_4 \leftrightarrow H^+ + NH_3$$
$$H_2PO_4 \leftrightarrow H^+ + HPO_4$$

**Bases:** Bases are those that accept protons.

**pH:** Sorenson expressed pH as the negative log of $H^+$ concentration ($-\log[H^+]$).

## Buffers

Buffer is a solution that resists changes in pH when small amount of acid or base is added. The effectiveness depends on its p$K$ or (p$K$a). p$K$ is the pH at which the buffer is 50% ionized, which means that the acid concentration is exactly equal to that of the base conjugate. The buffer is very efficient at a pH of ±1 around its p$K$.

Example—Phosphate buffer p$K$=6.8

This buffer will have the maximum buffer capacity between pH 5.8 and 7.8.

A buffer solution is a mixture of a weak acid and its Na or K salt (base).

## Henderson–Hasselbalch Equation

$$pH = pKa + \log_{10} \frac{[Base]}{[Acid]}$$

This indicates the relationship between the pH, p$K$, of the buffer and the ratio of conjugate base to the undissociated acid. It enables to relate quantitatively the changes in pH, [Acid] and [Base].

## H⁺ Balance

In a healthy individual, the normal pH of arterial blood is 7.4±0.05 and that of venous blood is 7.4±0.02. When the arterial pH raises above 7.45, then the individual is considered to have alkalosis; if the pH is below 7.35, then the individual is considered to have acidosis. In a healthy subject, the pH of blood is always between 7.35 and 7.45. The change in pH leads to serious effects; therefore, the control of pH is necessary.

There are two types of metabolic acids:
1. Fixed acids
2. Volatile acids.

$CO_2$ is the volatile acid.

Lactic acid, acetoacetic acid, β-hydroxybutyric acid, $H_2SO_4$, and $H_3PO_4$ are nonvolatile or fixed acids.

$CO_2$ is the major end product in the oxidation of carbohydrates, fats, and amino acids. It has the ability to react with $H_2O$ to form $H_2CO_3$, and again they dissociate to $H^+$ and $HCO_3^-$. The $CO_2$ can be regarded as an acid by virtue of its ability to react with $H_2O$ to form $H_2CO_3$, which in turn can dissociate to form $H^+ + HCO_3^-$. In vivo, it is the carbonic anhydrase in tissues of liver and kidney, which catalyzes the following reaction either way depending on the blood pH.

$$CO_2 + H_2O \xleftarrow{\text{Carbonic anhydrase}} HCO_3$$
$$H_2CO_3 \xleftarrow{\text{Carbonic anhydrase}} H^+ + HCO_3^-$$

The fixed acids $H_2SO_4$ and $H_3PO_4$ are the end products of the sulfur-containing amino acids, phospholipids, nucleic acids, phosphoproteins, and phosphoglycerides.

Organic acids such as lactic acid and β-hydroxybutyric acids are formed during the metabolism of carbohydrates and lipids.

Accumulation of lactic acid is called lactic acidosis. Normally lactic acid produced by the anaerobic glycolysis is taken up by the liver and converted to glucose through a Cori's cycle.

Pyruvate and lactate accumulate in conditions such as arsenic or mercury poisoning and also in thiamine deficiency. Inherited enzyme pyruvate dehydrogenase deficiency also leads to lactic acidosis.

## Regulation of Acid–Base Balance

The pH of the plasma is 7.4 and is normally maintained within a narrow range of 7.35–7.45.

Blood buffer system regulates small changes in acids or bases.

Next one is the respiratory system that by increasing the expulsion of the $CO_2$ (hyperventilation) or by conservation of $CO_2$ (hypoventilation) regulates the blood pH. These two compensatory mechanisms cannot go longer. It is only temporary balance.

The renal system maintains acid–base balance of blood by adjusting the rate of reabsorption and excretion of $H^+$ or $HCO_3^-$ or $HPO_3^-$ in addition to formation and excretion of $NH_3$ and $NH^+$.

**List the blood buffer system and explain the role of bicarbonate–carbonate buffer system in the regulation of acid–base balance.**

## Blood Buffer System

### Extracellular Fluid Buffer
* Carbonate–bicarbonate—$HCO/HCO_3^-$ (20:1)
* Phosphate buffer—$HPO_4/H_2PO_4^-$ (4:1)
* Protein buffer system.

## Bicarbonate Buffer System

The most important buffer system in the plasma is the bicarbonate–carbonate system. It accounts for 60% of buffering action in plasma and 40% in the whole body. The bicarbonate ($HCO_3^-$) level is regulated by the kidney; the acid part carbonic acid ($H_2CO_3$) is under respiratory control. The buffer is most active when the ratio of salt and acid is equal according to the Henderson–Hasselbalch equation. The normal plasma bicarbonate level is 24 mmol/L. The normal $pCO_2$ of arterial blood is 40 mm Hg. The normal carbonic acid is 1.2 mmol/L. The p$K$a of carbonic acid is 6.1. Substituting these values in Henderson–Hasselbalch equation,

$$pH = pKa + \log_{10} \frac{[Base]}{[Acid]}$$

pH of blood = $7.4 = 6.1 + \log \frac{[HCO_3^-]}{[H_2CO_3]}$

$7.4 = 6.1 + \log$

$6.1 + \log 20$ (antilog of $20 = 1.3$)

$6.1 + 1.3 = 7.4$

So the ratio between $(HCO_3^-)$ and $(H_2CO_3)$ = 20:1

$(HCO_3^-):(H_2CO_3) = 20:1$

So the ratio of $HCO_3^-$ to $H_2CO_3$ at pH 7.4 is 20 in normal conditions. The bicarbonate represents the alkali reserve, and it is sufficient to meet the acid load. During compensation, if $(HCO_3^-)$ is 24, then $(H_2CO_3)$ is adjusted to 1.2. This is how compensatory mechanism operates to bring the ratio back to 20:1.

Whenever metabolic acid is added to the blood, it reacts with the basic component of the buffer system, producing salt and water, and helps to prevent the fall in blood pH.

Reversal of this mechanism takes place in the event of addition of base by metabolic processes.

## Mechanism

When a strong acid such as HCl is added to the bicarbonate buffer solution, the increased hydrogen ions are buffered by $HCO^-$. This results in more $H_2CO_3^-$ formation and this in turn leads to more production of $CO_2 + H_2O$.

$HCl \rightarrow H^+ + Cl^-$
$HCO_3^- + H^+ \rightarrow H_2CO_3$
$H_2CO_3 \rightarrow CO_2 + H_2O$

The net result is the stimulation of respiration by $CO_2$, and this respiration tries to eliminate this $CO_2$ from the extracellular fluid.

The opposite reaction takes place when a strong base such as NaOH is added to the bicarbonate buffer system. In this case, the hydroxyl ions (OH) released combine with $H_2CO_3$ to form additional $HCO_3^-$. The $NaHCO_3$ replaces the strong base NaOH. At the same time, concentration of $H_2CO_3$ decreases, because it reacts with NaOH, causing more $CO_2$ to combine with $H_2O$ to replace $H_2CO_3$.

$NaOH \rightarrow Na + OH^- \rightarrow H_2CO_3 \rightarrow NaHCO_3 + H_2O$
Carbonic anhydrase

$CO_2 + H_2O \xleftrightarrow{\text{Carbonic anhydrase}} H_2CO_3$

The decreased $CO_2$ concentration in the blood inhibits respiration and decreases the rate of $CO_2$ removal through respiration. The rise in blood $HCO_3^-$ is compensated by bicarbonate, which is considered as the alkali reserve because any stronger acid than carbonic acids is buffered by bicarbonate as long as any bicarbonate is present in the blood.

## Phosphate Buffer System

It is the main intracellular buffer. The pKa value, 6.8, is nearer to the physiological pH 7.4. When equation is applied

$pH = pKa + \log \frac{[Base]}{[Acid]}$

$7.4 = 6.8 + \log \frac{[Base]}{[Acid]}$

$0.6 = \log \frac{[Base]}{[Acid]}$

Antilog of 0.6 is 4.

Therefore, the ratio is 4.

The phosphate buffer system is effective at wide range of pH; because of the more ionizable groups, it has different pKa values.

$H_3PO_4 \xrightarrow{\text{Pka=1.96}} H^+ + H_2PO_4^-$

$H_2PO_4^- \xrightarrow{\text{Pka=6.8}} H^+ + HPO_4^-$

$HPO_4^- \xrightarrow{\text{Pka=12.4}} H^+ + PO_4^{2-}$

The $Na_2HPO_4/NaH_2PO_4^-$ is an effective buffer system in the human body because of its pKa value nearer to the physiological pH.

## Protein Buffer System

The buffering action of protein mainly depends on the pKa value of its ionizable side chains. The effective group is histidine with a pKa value of 6.1. Therefore the albumin and hemoglobin with more histidine residues play an important role in buffering action in the body.

**Explain briefly the role of hemoglobin buffer system in the maintenance of acid–base balance.**

## Action of Hemoglobin Buffer in the Regulation of Blood pH

Hemoglobin releases $H^+$ in the lungs when it gets oxygenated because the oxygenated form of hemoglobin is a stronger acid than deoxygenated hemoglobin. This decreases the bicarbonate level and increases the carbonic acid and its anhydride $CO_2$, thus increasing $pCO_2$ of the blood **(Fig. 11.1)**.

The lungs eliminate this increased $pCO_2$ through the elimination of $CO_2$ from the blood and bring back the ratio of $HCO_3^-:H_2CO_3$ to 20:1.

Deoxyhemoglobin neutralizes carbonic acid to raise the pH and causes an increase in the bicarbonate level and a decrease in $pCO_2$. Some of the $H^+$ ions are bound by the deoxygenated Hb, and the rest are bound by the proteins and phosphate buffer in the plasma. Because all the $H^+$ formed is buffered, there is no change in the pH. This type buffering action is called isohydric shift.

The $HCO_3^-$ formed in erythrocyte as a result of $H^+$ uptake diffuses out of the cells into the plasma in exchange for $Cl^-$, which diffuses into the red blood cell (RBC) from the plasma. This increase in $Cl^-$ is termed "chloride shift." This chloride will come out of the RBC when $CO_2$ comes out of lungs.

## Respiratory Regulation of Acid–Base Balance

The second line of defense against acid–base disturbance is the control of $CO_2$ by the lungs by increasing or decreasing the rate of respiration.

The rate of respiration is known to be controlled by the receptors in the respiratory center, which are sensitive to changes in pH and $pCO_2$ of blood. When there is a fall in pH of plasma, the respiratory center is stimulated, resulting in hyperventilation, which eliminates more $CO_2$ thus lowering $H_2CO_3$ concentration in blood. If the blood pH increases, the respiratory center is inhibited so that elimination of $CO_2$ is decreased by hypoventilation till the blood pH comes to normal.

The hemoglobin transports $CO_2$ formed in the tissues and also it serves to generate bicarbonate or alkali reserve by the activity of carbonic anhydrase system.

**Discuss the role of kidney in the regulation of acid–base balance.**

## Renal Regulation of pH

An important function of kidney is to regulate the function by excreting either acidic or basic urine. The pH of urine ranges from to 9.5 because the renal system plays a significant role in long-term pH maintenance of the blood at 7.4 ± 0.05. This is possible by its capacity of reabsorption, secretion, and excretion of the nonvolatile acids such as lactic acid; lungs cannot excrete pyruvic acid and inorganic acid, HCl, phosphoric acid, and $H_2SO_4$, which are produced in the body. The first mechanism for removal of acids from the body is by renal excretion. The major mechanisms by which the kidney regulates the level of $HCO_3^-$ in plasma are reabsorption of filtered $HCO_3^-$, generation of new $HCO_3^-$, and by secreting $HCO^-$ under condition of chronic alkalosis **(Fig. 11.2)**.

The filtered $HCO_3$ combined with $H^+$ forming $H_2CO_3$, carbonic anhydrase presents in the

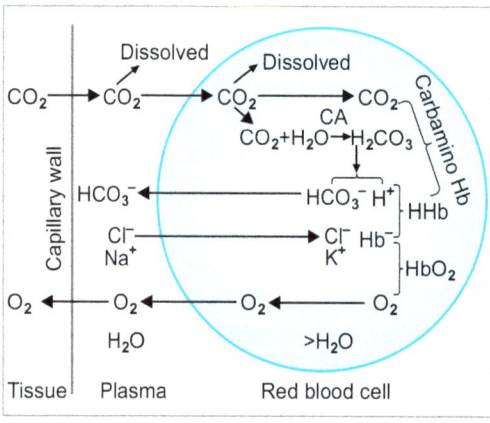

**Fig. 11.1:** Hemoglobin buffer system.

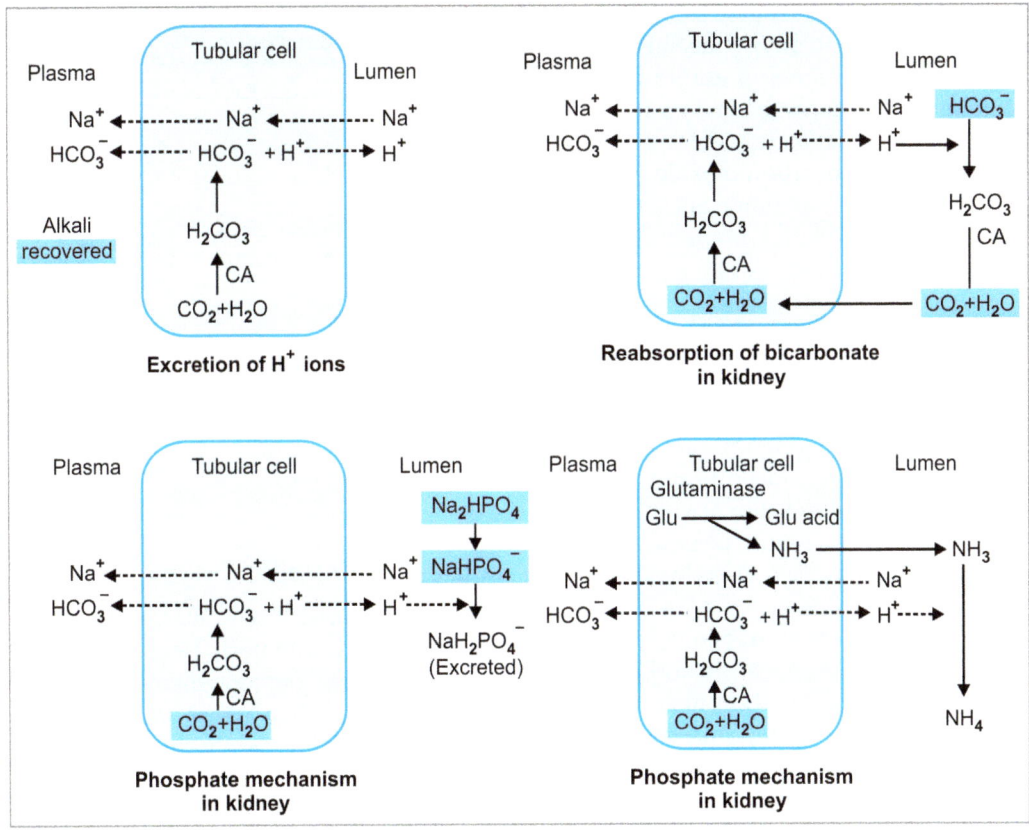

Fig. 11.2: Role of kidney in the regulation of acid–base balance.

brush border of the cell wall dissociate $H_2CO_3$ into $H_2O$ and $CO_2$. The $CO_2$ diffuses into the cell; in the cell carbonic anhydrase again ionizes $H_2CO_3$ into $HCO_3^-$ and $H^+$. It is secreted into the lumen in exchange for $Na^+$ and $HCO_3^-$ and is reabsorbed into plasma along with $Na^+$. There is no net excretion of $H^+$ or generation of new $HCO_3^-$ so that this mechanism helps to maintain a steady state of acid–base balance.

Another function of the kidney is to buffer acids and thus to conserve fixed base, through the production of $NH_3$ from amino acids with the help of an enzyme, glutaminase. Whenever there is excess acid generated, the $NH_3$ production is also increased, which combines with $H^+$ to form $NH^+$, which is excreted as $NH_4Cl$. This occurs in the event of acidosis. When alkali is in excess, $H^+$ is reabsorbed into the cell in exchange to $Na^+/K^+$.

## Acid–Base Disorders

- Acid–base disorders result from a variety of pathological conditions. If the pH is more than the normal range, it is termed "alkalemia" and if pH is lesser than the normal range, it is called acidemia and the conditions are called alkalosis and acidosis, respectively.
- There are two reasons for the pH abnormalities in blood, which are metabolic or respiratory causes. Metabolic causes are responsible for metabolic acidosis and metabolic alkalosis. The respiratory causes are responsible for respiratory acidosis and respiratory alkalosis.

## Compensation

The body's acid–base balance is tightly regulated. Several buffering agents exist, which reversibly bind hydrogen ions and slow down any change in pH. Extracellular buffers include bicarbonate and ammonia, while proteins and phosphate act as intracellular buffers. The bicarbonate buffering system is especially key, as carbon dioxide ($CO_2$) can be shifted through carbonic acid ($H_2CO_3$) to hydrogen ions and bicarbonate ($HCO_3^-$) as shown below.

$$HCO_3^- + H^+ \leftrightarrow H_2CO_3 \leftrightarrow CO_2 + H_2O$$

Acid–base imbalances that overcome the buffer system can be compensated in the short term by changing the rate of ventilation. This alters the concentration of carbon dioxide in the blood. For instance, if the blood pH drops too low (*acidemia*), the body will compensate by increasing breathing and expelling $CO_2$.

The kidneys are slower to compensate, but renal physiology has several powerful mechanisms to control pH by the excretion of excess acid or base. In responses to acidosis, tubular cells reabsorb more bicarbonate from the tubular fluid, collecting duct cells secrete more hydrogen and generate more bicarbonate, and ammoniagenesis leads to increased formation of the $NH_3$ buffer. In responses to alkalosis, the kidney may excrete more bicarbonate by decreasing hydrogen ion secretion from the tubular epithelial cells and lowering rates of glutamine metabolism and ammonia excretion.

**Explain the causes and biochemical findings of metabolic acidosis.**

## Metabolic Acidosis ($HCO_3^-$ Deficit or Fall in pH)

* It is the most common acid–base disturbance **(Fig. 11.3)**.
* In this condition, the $HCO_3^-$ concentration is reduced. This is due to the increased production of acids. These acids dissociate to give $H^+$ ions, which are buffered by $HCO_3^-$.

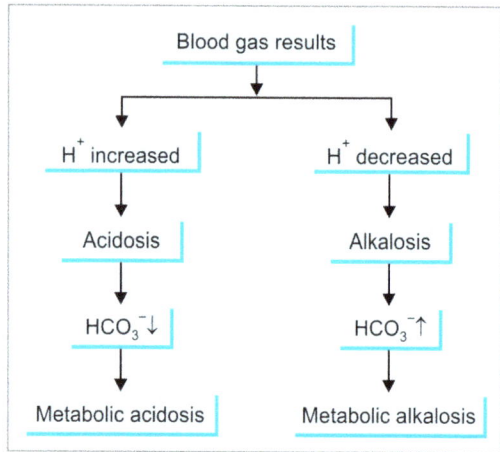

**Fig. 11.3:** Metabolic acid–base disorders.

### Causes: Uncontrolled Diabetes Mellitus

* Lactic acidosis: This results from a number of causes, particularly tissue anoxia. In acute hypoxia condition such as respiratory failure or cardiac arrest, lactic acidosis develops immediately. Lactic acidosis may also be caused by liver disease. The presence of lactic acidosis can be determined by plasma lactate.
* Diabetic ketoacidosis: **Ketoacidosis** is a metabolic state associated with high concentrations of ketone bodies, formed by the breakdown of fatty acids and the deamination of amino acids due to lack of insulin. The two common ketones produced in humans are acetoacetic acid and β-hydroxybutyrate.
  Ketoacidosis is most common in untreated type 1 diabetes mellitus, when the liver breaks down fat and proteins in response to a perceived need for respiratory substrate.
* Chronic renal failure (accumulation of sulfates, phosphates, and urea).
* Intoxication:
  - Organic acids (salicylates, ethanol, methanol, formaldehyde, ethylene glycol, paraldehyde, and INH).
  - Sulfates, metformin (glucophage).

- Metabolic acidosis is also due to ingestion of acids such as ammonium chloride. The ammonia part after detoxification leaves behind the $H^+$.
- It also occurs in diarrhea, which leads to loss of $HCO_3^-$ from the intestinal fluid.
- The primary compensatory mechanism in metabolic acidosis is through hyperventilation that removes $CO_2$. The deep, rapid, and gasping respiratory pattern is known as kussmaul breathing.
- There is also elimination of acids in the urine and the urinary ammonia is also increased.

e.g., = $[HCO_3^-]$ = 15 mEq/L, $pCO_3$ = 1.2 mEq/L
pH = pKa + log $[HCO_3^-]/pCO_2$
6.1 + log15/1.2
6.1 + 12.5
6.1 + 1.2 = 7.3 (antilog of 12.5 is 1.2)

**List the causes and biochemical findings of metabolic alkalosis.**

## Metabolic Alkalosis ($HCO_3^-$ Excess or Rise in pH)

- This condition occurs due to the gain of more $HCO_3^-$ **(Fig. 11.3)**.
- This occurs in (a) vomiting (loss of gastric HCl) and (b) ingestion of bicarbonate in the treatment of peptic ulcer. (c) Potassium depletion: Hypokalemic alkalosis is caused by the kidneys' response to an extreme lack or loss of potassium, which can occur when people take certain diuretic medications.
- The compensatory mechanism is through hypoventilation to prevent $CO_2$ loss. $CO_2$ is then consumed toward the formation of the carbonic acid intermediate, thus decreasing pH.
- The secondary compensatory mechanism is by increasing the excretion of $HCO_3^-$ by kidney.

e.g., = $[HCO_3^-]$ = 36 mEq/L, $pCO_2$ = 1.2 mEq/L
pH = pKa + log $[HCO_3^-]/pCO_2$
6.1 + log 36/1.2 = 6.1 + 30 = 6.1 + 1.45 = 7.55

**Explain the causes and biochemical findings of respiratory acidosis and alkalosis.**

## Respiratory Acidosis (Excess $CO_2$)

- The retention of $CO_2$ leads to change in $HCO_3^-$ **(Fig. 11.4)**.
- The ratio of $[HCO_3^-]:[CO_2]$ decreases.
- This is caused by hypoventilation, which occurs due to an obstruction of respiration that is in pneumonia, emphysema, asthma, and depression of the respiratory centers in morphine bicarbonate poisoning and alcohol ingestion.
- The primary compensatory mechanism is reabsorption of $HCO_3^-$ from the kidney, for example, $[HCO_3^-]$ = 27 mEq/L, $pCO_2$ = 1.8 mEq/L pH = pKa + log $[HCO_3^-]/pCO_2$ 6.1 + log 27/1.8 = 6.1 + 15 = 6.1 + 1.17 = 7.27.

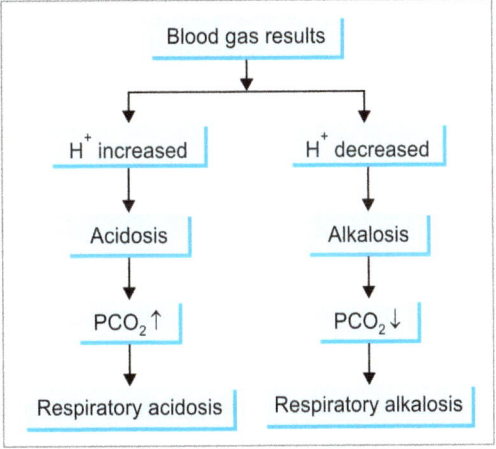

**Fig. 11.4:** Respiratory acid–base disorders.

## Respiratory Alkalosis ($CO_2$ Deficit)

- This is caused by hyperventilation that leads to reduced concentration of $CO_2$ **(Fig. 11.4)**.
- The $HCO_3^-$ level also slightly varies.
- This occurs when respiration is stimulated as in fever, hot bath, lack of oxygen at high altitude, and increased environmental temperature.

Table 11.1: Laboratory findings in acid–base disturbances.

| | pH | pCO$_2$ | HCO$_3^-$ | HCO$_3^-$/H$_2$CO$_3$ |
|---|---|---|---|---|
| Normal | 7.4 ± 0.05 | 40 mm Hg | 20 mm Hg | 20 |
| Metabolic acidosis | <7.3 | <22 mmol/L or normal | Decreased | Decreased |
| Metabolic alkalosis | >7.4 | >33 mmol/L or normal | Increased | Increased |
| Respiratory acidosis | <7.3 | >45 mm Hg | Varied or normal | Decreased |
| Respiratory alkalosis | >7.4 | <35 mm Hg | Varied or decreased | Increased |

* Compensatory mechanism is by increasing the excretion of HCO$_3^-$ by kidney.
  e.g., [HCO$_3^-$] = 27 mEq/L, pCO$_2$ = 0.68 mEq/L
  pH = p$K$a + log [HCO$_3^-$]/pCO$_2$
  6.1 + log 27/0.68 = 6.1 + 39.7 = 6.1+1.6 = 7.7.
  **Summary of laboratory findings in acid–base disturbances are shown in Table 11.1.**

### Mixed Acid–Base Disorders

Mixed acid–base disorders occur when there is more than one primary acid–base disturbance present simultaneously. They are frequently seen in hospitalized patients, particularly in the critically ill.

Mixed acid–base disorder occurs when:
* The expected compensatory response does not occur.
* Compensatory response occurs, but level of compensation is inadequate or too extreme.
* Whenever the PCO$_2$ and [HCO$_3^-$] become abnormal in the opposite direction (i.e. one is elevated while the other is reduced). In simple acid–base disorders, the direction of the compensatory response is always the same as the direction of the initial abnormal change.
* pH is normal, but PCO$_2$ or HCO$_3^-$ is abnormal.
* In anion gap metabolic acidosis, if the change in bicarbonate level is not proportional to the change of the anion gap. More specifically, if the delta ratio is greater than 2 or less than 1.
* In simple acid–base disorders, the compensatory response should never return the pH to normal. If that happens, suspect a mixed disorder.

Mixed acid–base disorders usually produce arterial blood gas results that could potentially be explained by other mixed disorders.

### Anion Gap

* The sum of cations and anions in extracellular fluid is always equal so as to maintain the electrical neutrality.
* 95% of the cations were maintained by Na$^+$ and K$^+$.
* Chloride and HCO$_3^-$ account for 86% of anions.
* These are the commonly measured electrolytes; hence, there is a difference between cations and anions.
* The difference between cations and anions or the unmeasured anions constitutes the anion gap, which is due to the presence of phosphorous, SO$_4^-$, PO$_{43}^-$, and organic acid salts.
* The difference between Na$^+$+K$^+$ and Cl$^-$+HCO$_3^-$ is normally about 12 ± 5 mEq/L (mmol/L).
* Measurement of anion gap is extremely useful in the clinical assessment with acid–base disorders.

### Assessment of Acid–Base Analysis

The blood gas analyzer that measures pH, pCO$_2$, and pO$_2$ by means of electrodes is usually used to measure acid–base parameters of arterial blood. Heparinized blood is collected and directly introduced into the analyzer. The blood should be analyzed within 20 minutes of collection. There should not be any contact of collected blood with the external air during either during collection or analysis.

## Procedure

Usually, blood is taken from an artery. The blood may be collected from the radial artery in the wrist, the femoral artery in the groin, or the brachial artery in the arm.

The healthcare provider will insert a small needle through the skin into the artery. You can choose to have numbing medicine (anesthesia) applied to the site before the test begins.

After the blood is taken, pressure is applied to the site for a few minutes to stop the bleeding. The healthcare provider will watch the site for signs of bleeding or circulation problems.

The sample must be quickly sent to a laboratory for analysis to ensure accurate results.

There is no special preparation. If you are on oxygen therapy, the oxygen concentration must remain constant for 20 minutes before the test.

## SUMMARY

The human body is a complex system, which consists of several levels and subsystems. At the chemical level, acids and bases are among those essential compounds upon which all biochemical process depends. The acid–base homeostasis should be maintained for cellular viability, enzymatic reactions, protein conformation, CNS functions, etc. These functions are modified when there is change in the cellular and extracellular acid–base status. Carbonate-bicarbonate buffer, phosphate buffer, and protein buffer (hemoglobin) are the major buffer systems of our body, which help to maintain the balance. The respiratory system also participates in the regulation of acid–base balance whenever there is a change in the acid–base concentration either by eliminating or retaining $CO_2$. Kidney plays an important role in the regulation of acid–base concentration by excreting either acidic or basic urine. Metabolic acidosis and alkalosis are the two acid–base disorders whenever there is a disturbance in the metabolism. Hypo- or hyperventilation causes respiratory acidosis and alkalosis.

## SELF-ASSESSMENT QUESTIONS

1. Name the blood buffer systems.
2. Briefly discuss the bicarbonate buffer system to show how it helps to regulate the blood pH.
3. Explain the regulation of blood pH through renal mechanism.
4. Discuss the various acid– base disorders. Mention the causes and findings of each disorder.
5. Mention the laboratory findings of metabolic acidosis and respiratory alkalosis.
6. What is metabolic alkalosis and respiratory acidosis?

## Case Studies

1. A 30-year-old drug addict is found unconscious in a valley with an empty syringe beside him.
   The test is used to evaluate respiratory diseases and conditions that affect the lungs. It helps determine the effectiveness of oxygen therapy. The test also provides information about the body's acid–base balance, which can reveal important clues about lung and kidney function and the body's general metabolic state.
   In the absence of blood gas analyzer, venous blood may be collected under paraffin. Bicarbonate is estimated by titration to pH 7.5. If acid–base disturbance is suspected, the electrolytes should also be estimated. From the values of electrolytes and bicarbonate, the anion gap is calculated.

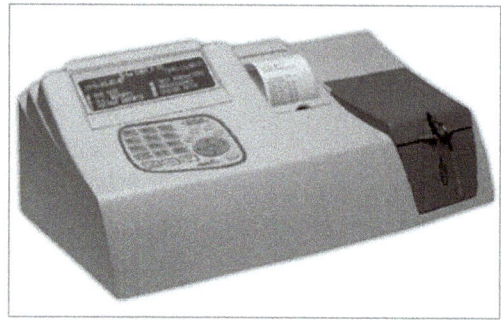

When his blood gases are checked, which of the following would be expected?
(a) Metabolic acidosis
(b) Metabolic alkalosis
(c) Respiratory acidosis
(d) Respiratory alkalosis

**Answer is c.** Opioids, such as heroin, depress respiration centrally by reducing the responsiveness of brainstem respiratory centers to $CO_2$. The resulting hypoventilation leads to $CO_2$ retention because of the inability of the patient to "blow off" the $CO_2$. This increases the production of carbonic acid ($H_2CO_3$) by carbonic anhydrase present in red blood cells (which converts $CO_2$ to carbonic acid). Dissociation of carbonic acid to bicarbonate and protons produces a respiratory acidosis.

2. Arterial blood gases (ABG) were obtained twice on the day of birth and 2 days later with the following results:

Day of birth: Serum bicarbonate 24 mEq/L
Day 1, 63% $O_2$ by hood; Day 3, 25% $O_2$

| | | | |
|---|---|---|---|
| $pO_2$ | 107 | 63 | 57 |
| $pCO_2$ | 48 | 45 | 36 |
| pH 7.35 | 7.37 | 7.44 | |

1. What is the infant's initial acid–base status?
2. What does a comparison of the second day 1 measurement with the day 3 measurement suggest?
3. What clinical conditions could this pattern produce?

## Initially it is Respiratory Acidosis

The pH is acidotic and the $PCO_2$ is greater than 40 mm Hg, indicating that the lung has retained acid in the body and is at least a partial cause for the acidosis. The serum bicarbonate is 24, indicating that the kidney has not had time to compensate for the respiratory problem.

## A Pulmonary Shunt may be Present

The important thing to notice here is that the oxygen level in inspired air was dropped by more than half between the second specimen on days 1 and 3, with essentially no change in the blood $PO_2$. If the $PO_2$ of 63 was due to a selective block in oxygen transfer (VQ mismatch or pulmonary fibrosis), decreasing the oxygen content of the inspired air should have dramatically affected $PO_2$.

Remember that shunts normally do not affect $PCO_2$ unless they are very large, because the lung has a lot of excess capacity to remove $CO_2$. Thus in this case where $CO_2$ retention is occurring, we would be postulating a very big shunt.

Shunts might be produced in this setting by:
1. Large cardiac defects
2. Pulmonary vascular defects
3. Lung tissue that is perused but not ventilated

3. A 40-year-old woman was admitted to the hospital for evaluation. Her evaluation at admission, including arterial blood gases obtained before, during, and after an exercise stress test, showed the following results:
Serum bicarbonate 27 mEq/L
Arterial blood gases

|  | At rest | During exercise | Rest/oxygen |
|---|---|---|---|
| $pO_2$ | 91 | 67 | 541 |
| $pCO_2$ | 32 | 37 | 29 |
| pH 7.46 | 7.41 | 7.49 | |

## Respiratory Alkalosis

The pH is alkalotic and the $PCO_2$ is below 40, indicating that the lung is producing the alkalosis by removing acid ($CO_2$) from the body. Interestingly, the bicarbonate concentration of 27 mEq/L is slightly higher than the normal of 24. This indicates that there is no renal response to the respiratory alkalosis. Perhaps the current alkalosis is partly triggered by stress or nervousness in the patient and her usual resting pH is nearer to normal. Also note that the patient's $PO_2$ is adequate, indicating that the lungs can keep up with the body's oxygen demand, but it is probably lower than it should be for the patient's level of respiration.

Exercise uncovers her basic defect in oxygen transfer by increasing the body's demand for oxygen. Under these conditions, the lungs cannot keep up with the oxygen demand and the $pO_2$ drops to 67. These results suggest VQ mismatch or pulmonary fibrosis. Other causes for hypoxemia don't really fit her pattern.

The patient's hypoxia corrects with oxygen, which would not occur if a shunt was present. Note that the patient's $PCO_2$ is still quite low (29), indicating that she is still breathing rapidly. She probably had not been on oxygen long when this sample was drawn.

## MULTIPLE CHOICE QUESTIONS

1. **Concerning acid–base balance, one of the following statements is incorrect:**
   (a) Blood buffer system helps in maintaining the acid–base balance
   (b) Respiratory system is regulating the blood pH through expulsion of $CO_2$
   (c) Renal mechanism regulates the pH through the absorption or excretion of $H^+$
   (d) Carbon dioxide and bicarbonate buffer system is first mechanism which regulates blood pH

2. **The buffering action of protein mainly depends on the:**
   (a) pKa value of its ionizable side chains of histidine  (b) pKa value of tyrosine
   (c) Basic amino acid content  (d) Neutral amino acid content

3. **Concerning renal regulation of acid–base balance, one of the following statements is incorrect:**
   (a) Reabsorption of filtered $HCO_3^-$  (b) Generation of new $HCO_3^-$
   (c) Generation of $H^+$  (d) Excretion of $H^+$

4. **Metabolic acidosis occurs in all the following conditions, *except*:**
   (a) Vomiting  (b) Uncontrolled diabetes mellitus
   (c) Starvation  (d) Severe exercises

5. **Deficit of $HCO_3^-$ results in:**
   (a) Metabolic alkalosis  (b) Metabolic acidosis
   (c) Respiratory acidosis  (d) Respiratory alkalosis

6. Respiratory acidosis results from:
   (a) Excess $CO_2$
   (b) Excess $HCO_3^-$
   (c) Excess $H^+$
   (d) Excess $H_2CO_3$
7. All of the following are the laboratory findings of metabolic alkalosis, *except*:
   (a) pH increased
   (b) $pCO_2$ decreased
   (c) $HCO_3^-$ increased
   (d) $HCO_3/H_2CO_3$ decreased
8. In uncompensated metabolic alkalosis:
   (a) The plasma pH, the plasma $HCO_3^-$ concentration, and the arterial $PCO_2$ are all low
   (b) The plasma pH is high and the plasma $HCO_3^-$ concentration and arterial $PCO_2$ are low
   (c) The plasma pH and the plasma $HCO_3^-$ concentration is low and the arterial $PCO_2$ is normal
   (d) The plasma pH and the plasma $HCO_3^-$ concentration is high and the arterial $PCO_2$ is normal
9. Concerning angiotensin II, one of the following statements is false:
   (a) It is produced from angiotensin I in the lungs
   (b) It is a vasoconstrictor
   (c) It stimulates aldosterone secretion
   (d) It is a decapeptide
10. One of the following is a recognized cause of metabolic acidosis with increased anion gap:
    (a) Diabetic ketoacidosis
    (b) High-fat diet
    (c) Hyperparathyroidism
    (d) Diarrhea
11. Concerning metabolic acidosis, which of the following statement is false?
    (a) Caused by severe diarrhea is associated with a normal anion gap
    (b) Caused by renal tubular acidosis is associated with a normal anion gap
    (c) Caused by lactic acidosis is associated with an increase in the anion gap
    (d) Caused by diabetic ketoacidosis is associated with a decrease in the anion gap
12. The metabolism of the following amino acids results in the production of acids:
    (a) Histidine
    (b) Aspartate
    (c) Glutamate
    (d) Alanine
13. Respiratory alkalosis:
    (a) Occurs in hyperventilation
    (b) Occurs in normal pregnancy
    (c) Does not occur in type I respiratory failure
    (d) May occur in type II respiratory failure
14. A 19-year-old man has the following arterial blood results: pH = 7.50, $PCO_2$ = 48 mm Hg, $[HCO_3^-]$ = 37 mM, oxygen saturation = 98% on air. His plasma potassium concentration is 2.5 mM:
    (a) There is a respiratory alkalosis
    (b) There is a metabolic alkalosis
    (c) His urine is likely to be alkaline
    (d) Pulmonary embolism is a likely diagnosis
15. Concerning renal regulation of acid–base balance, one of the following statement is false:
    (a) Ammonium ions are mainly produced in the loop of Henle
    (b) Glutamine metabolism by the kidneys results in bicarbonate production
    (c) Ammonia production by the kidneys is increased in acidosis
    (d) Secreted hydrogen ions are buffered by the phosphate buffer system in tubular fluid
16. Arterial blood gas analysis from a 20-year-old woman shows: pH = 7.36, $PCO_2$ = 32 mm Hg, $[HCO_3^-]$ = 17 mM, oxygen saturation = 99% on air:
    (a) Pulmonary embolism is a likely diagnosis
    (b) She is acidotic
    (c) Aspirin overdose is a possible diagnosis
    (d) The anion gap is likely to be decreased
17. Which of the following statements is false with respect to the bicarbonate buffer system:
    (a) Within extracellular fluid is made up of carbonic acid and sodium bicarbonate
    (b) Within intracellular fluid is made up of carbonic acid and potassium bicarbonate
    (c) The majority of carbonic acid exists as dissolved carbon dioxide
    (d) The pH is proportional to the log of the bicarbonate ion concentration

# CHAPTER 11: Acid–Base Balance

18. **With respect to acid–base status, the:**
    (a) pH is calculated from log of hydrogen ion concentration
    (b) pH of arterial blood is 7.35
    (c) pH of venous blood is 7.4
    (d) pH of interstitial fluid is 7.35
19. **Respiratory acidosis:**
    (a) Occurs in type I respiratory failure
    (b) If chronic, it is associated with a fall in plasma bicarbonate concentration
    (c) Occurs in chronic bronchitis
    (d) Is associated with a high arterial $PO_2$
20. **The following are recognized causes of metabolic acidosis with a normal anion gap:**
    (a) Salicylate poisoning
    (b) Starvation
    (c) Diarrhea
    (d) Pancreatic secretion
21. **A 36-year-old woman has the following arterial blood gas results: pH = 7.33 [$HCO_3^-$] = 16 mM, $PCO_2$ = 30 mm Hg:**
    (a) Pulmonary embolism is a likely diagnosis
    (b) She has a respiratory acidosis
    (c) She has a metabolic acidosis
    (d) There is a respiratory compensation to a metabolic acidosis
22. **Concerning acid–base balance:**
    (a) The plasma proteins represent the major extracellular buffer
    (b) The normal range for the plasma pH is 7.36–7.44
    (c) The normal range for the plasma bicarbonate is 30–34 mmol/L
    (d) Most of the hydrogen that is excreted in the urine is in the form of free H⁺ ions

## ANSWERS

| | | | | | | | |
|---|---|---|---|---|---|---|---|
| 1. d | 2. a | 3. c | 4. a | 5. b | 6. a | 7. d | 8. d |
| 9. d | 10. a | 11. d | 12. a | 13. a | 14. b | 15. a | 16. c |
| 17. d | 18. d | 19. c | 20. c | 21. c | 22. b | | |

# Chapter 12

# Biological Oxidation

## LEARNING OBJECTIVES

*At the end of this chapter students should be able to:*
- Understand transport of reducing equivalents across mitochondria
- Know about the electron transport chain organization and its components
- Explain the oxidative phosphorylation and chemiosmotic theory
- List the inhibitors of electron transport chain and oxidative phosphorylation
- Know about the uncouplers and their significance

## Introduction

- Oxidation-reduction reactions are coupled chemical reactions in which one atom or molecule loses one or more electrons (oxidation), while another atom or molecule gains those electrons (reduction).
- The compound that loses electrons becomes oxidized.
- The compound that gains those electrons becomes reduced.
- In covalent compounds, however, it is usually easier to lose a whole hydrogen (H) atom—a proton and an electron—rather than just an electron.
- An oxidation reaction during which both a proton and an electron are lost is called dehydrogenation.
- A reduction reaction during which both a proton and an electron are gained is called hydrogenation.
- The large quantity of NADH resulting from tricarboxylic acid (TCA) cycle activity can be used for reductive biosynthesis.
- The reducing potential of mitochondrial NADH is most often used to supply the energy for ATP synthesis via oxidative phosphorylation.
- The oxidation of NADH with phosphorylation of ADP to form ATP is processes supported by the mitochondrial electron transport assembly and ATP synthase, which are integral protein complexes of the inner mitochondrial membrane.
- The electron transport assembly comprises a series of protein complexes that catalyze sequential oxidation-reduction reactions; some of these reactions are thermodynamically competent to support ATP production via ATP synthase provided a coupling mechanism, such as a common intermediate, is available. Proton translocation and the development of a transmembrane proton gradient provide the required coupling mechanism.

## Principles of Reduction–Oxidation Reactions

- Redox reactions involve the transfer of electrons from one chemical species to another.
- An example of a coupled redox reaction is the oxidation of NADH by the electron transport chain (ETC):
  $NADH + (1/2)O + H^+ \rightarrow NAD^+ + H O$
- The description of ATP synthesis through oxidation of reduced electron carriers indicated 3 mol of ATP could be generated for every mole of NADH and 2 mol for

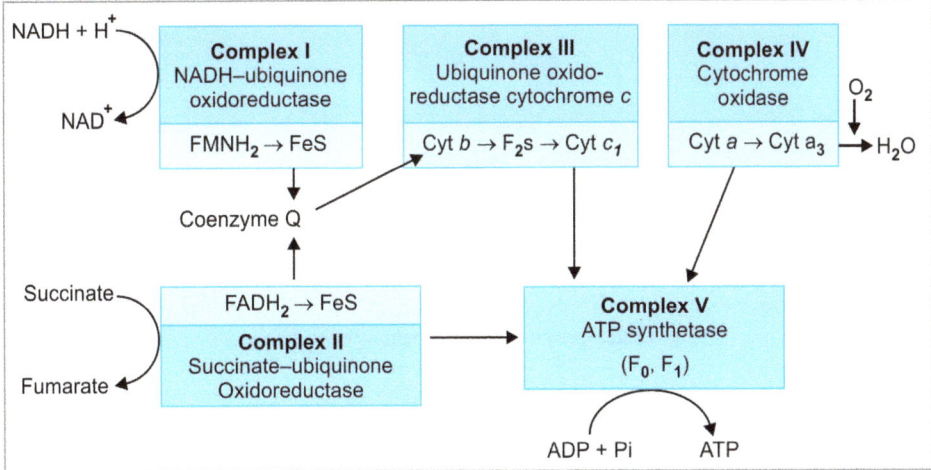

Fig. 12.1: Complexes in electron transport chain.

every mole of $FADH_2$. However, direct chemical analysis has shown that for every 2 electrons transferred from NADH to oxygen, 2.5 equiv of ATP are synthesized and 1.5 for $FADH_2$.

# Structural Organization of Respiratory Chain and Electron Transport Structure of the Mitochondria

The mitochondrion consists of outer membrane, the inner membrane, the intermediate space, the cristae, and the matrix.

The components of the ETC are located in the inner mitochondrial membrane. The inner mitochondrial membrane is a specialized structure that is impermeable to ions ($H^+$, $Na^+$, and $K^+$) and small molecules such as ATP, ADP, pyruvate, and other metabolites. Therefore, the specialized carriers or transport systems are required to move ions or molecules across membrane. The inner membrane is rich in protein. The inner membrane is highly folded to form **cristae** and serve to increase greatly the surface area of the membrane.

The inner membrane particles attached to the inner surface of the inner mitochondrial membrane are called ATP synthetase complexes.

The gel-like solution in the interior of the mitochondria is mitochondrial matrix. This is rich in enzymes responsible for oxidation of fatty acid, pyruvate, amino acids, and TCA cycle.

# Organization of the Chain

The inner mitochondrial membrane can be disrupted into five separate enzyme complexes, called complex I, II, III, IV, and V. Complexes I–IV are carriers of electrons, whereas complex V catalyzes ATP synthesis. There are certain mobile electron carriers in the respiratory chain. Each carriers of the ETC can receive electrons from an electron donor and donate subsequently to next carrier. The greater portion of the oxygen supplied to the body is utilized by the mitochondria for the operation of ETC (Fig. 12.1).

# Reactions of the Electron Transport Chain Formation of NADH

NADH is more actively involved in the ETC. $NAD^+$ is reduced to NADH + $H^+$ by removal of two hydrogen atoms from the substrate glyceraldehyde-3-phosphate, pyruvate, malate, etc. The NADPH is not substrate for ETC (Figs. 12.2 and 12.3).

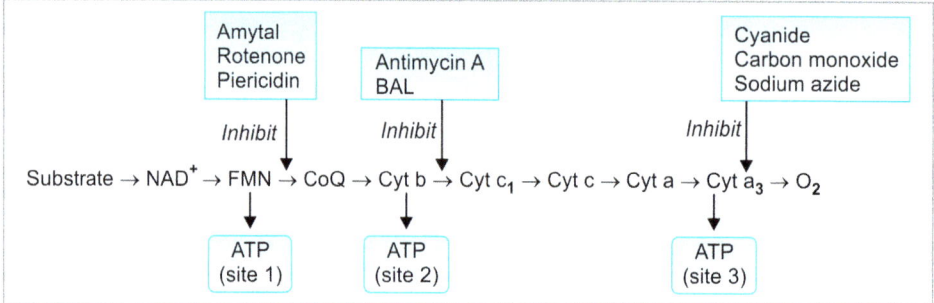

Fig. 12.2: Electron transport chain with inhibitors.

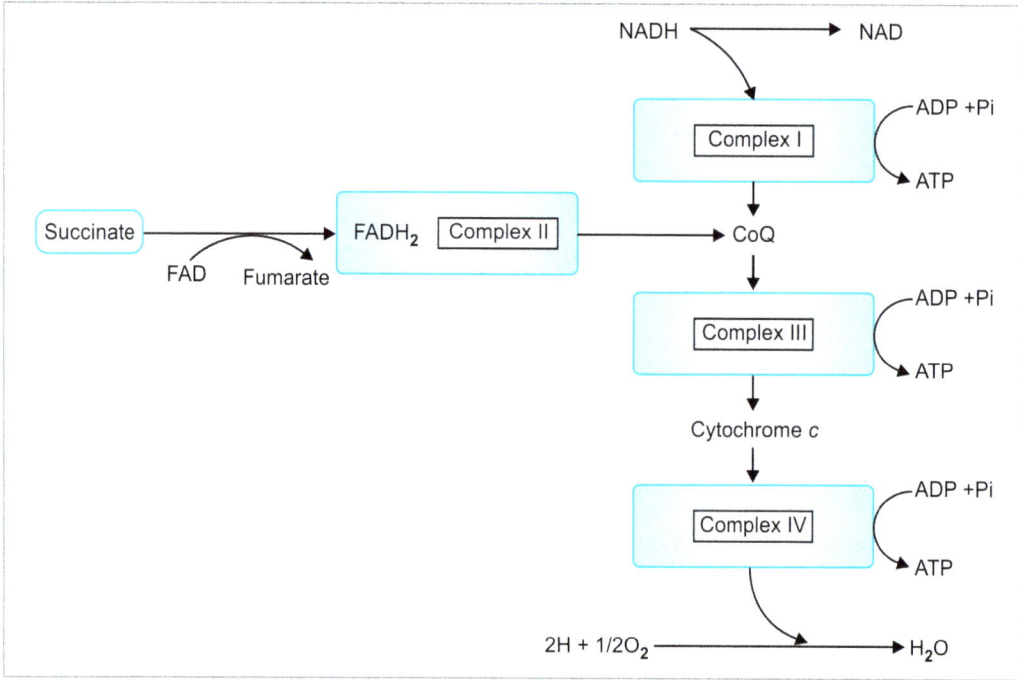

Fig. 12.3: Electron transport chain with sites of ATP synthesis.

## Flavoproteins

The NADH dehydrogenase (NADH-CoQ reductase) is a flavoprotein with FMN, which accepts two electrons and a proton to form $FMNH_2$. NADH dehydrogenase is a complex enzyme, which contains several iron atoms paired with sulfur.

Succinate dehydrogenase (succinate-coenzyme Q reductase) is an enzyme found in the inner mitochondrial membrane. It is a flavoprotein with FAD as the coenzyme which accepts two hydrogen atoms from succinate.

## Iron–Sulfur Protein

It exists in the oxidized ($Fe^{3+}$) or reduced ($Fe^{2+}$) state. One FeS is involved in the transfer of electron.

## Coenzyme Q

It is a quinine derivative with a long isoprenoid tail. It is also called ubiquinone because it is ubiquitous in biologic systems. It can accept hydrogen atoms both from $FMNH_2$, produced by NADH dehydrogenase, and from FADH, which is produced by succinate dehydrogenase.

## Cytochromes

These are conjugated proteins containing heme group made of a porphyrin ring containing an atom of iron. Unlike the heme groups of hemoglobin and myoglobin, the cytochrome iron atom is reversibly converted from its ferric ($Fe^{3+}$) to its ferrous ($Fe^{2+}$), which is essential for the transport of electrons in the ETC. Electrons are transported from CoQ to cytochromes $b$, $c_1$, $c$, $a$, and $a_3$.

## Cytochromes $a$ and $a_3$

The term "cytochrome oxidase" is used to represent cytochromes $a$ and $a_3$, which is the terminal component of ETC. This cytochrome is the only electron carrier, the heme iron of which can directly react with molecular oxygen. This also contains copper atoms that are required for this complex reaction to occur.

Electrons from FMN CoQ and the other associated with cytochromes $b$ and $c_1$.

## Oxidative Phosphorylation

The transfer of electrons through the ETC is linked with the release of free energy.

The process of synthesizing ATP from ADP and Pi coupled with the ETC is called oxidative phosphorylation. The complex V is the site of oxidative phosphorylation.

There are three sites of oxidative phosphorylation in ETC, which result in the synthesis of three ATP molecules:
1. Oxidation of $FMNH_2$ by CoQ
2. Oxidation of cytochrome by cytochrome $c_1$
3. Cytochrome oxidase reaction

Each one of the above reactions represents a coupling site for ATP production.

The first reaction is bypassed for the oxidation of $FADH_2$ (two ATP molecules synthesized).

### Mechanism

Important hypothesis to explain the process of oxidative phosphorylation are:
- Chemical coupling: According to chemical coupling hypothesis, during the course of electron transfer in respiratory chain, a series of phosphorylated high-energy intermediates is first produced and is utilized for the synthesis of ATP. However, this hypothesis does not have the experimental evidence.
- Conformational coupling hypothesis: According to this hypothesis, induced conformational change in the membrane protein may be responsible for the synthesis of ATP.
- Chemiosmotic hypothesis: This hypothesis explains how the free energy generated by the transport of electrons by the ETC is used to produce ATP (**Figs. 12.4 and 12.5**).
  - Proton gradient: Electron transport is coupled to transport of protons ($H^+$) across the inner mitochondrial membrane from the matrix to the intermembrane space. This process creates across the inner mitochondrial membrane, an electrical gradient (with more positive charges on the outside of the membrane than on the inside of the membrane) and a pH gradient (lower pH outside). The energy generated through this proton gradient is more than sufficient to drive ATP synthesis.
  - ATP synthetase: This enzyme complex (complex V) synthesizes ATP, utilizing the energy of the proton gradient generated by the ETC. The chemiosmotic hypothesis proposes that after protons have been transferred to the cytosolic side of the inner mitochondrial membrane, they can reenter the mitochondrial matrix by passing through a channel in the ATP synthetase molecule, resulting in the

synthesis of ATP from ADP + Pi and at the same time dissipating the pH and electrical gradients **(Figs. 12.4 and 12.5)**.

## Uncouplers

The oxidation and phosphorylation proceed simultaneously. There are certain compounds, which can uncouple (delink) the electron transport from oxidative phosphorylation. Such compounds increase the permeability of the inner mitochondrial membrane to protons. An example is 2.4 dinitrophenol, a small lipophilic proton carrier molecule readily diffuse through the mitochondrial membrane. This uncoupler causes electron transport to proceed at a rapid rate without creating a proton gradient.

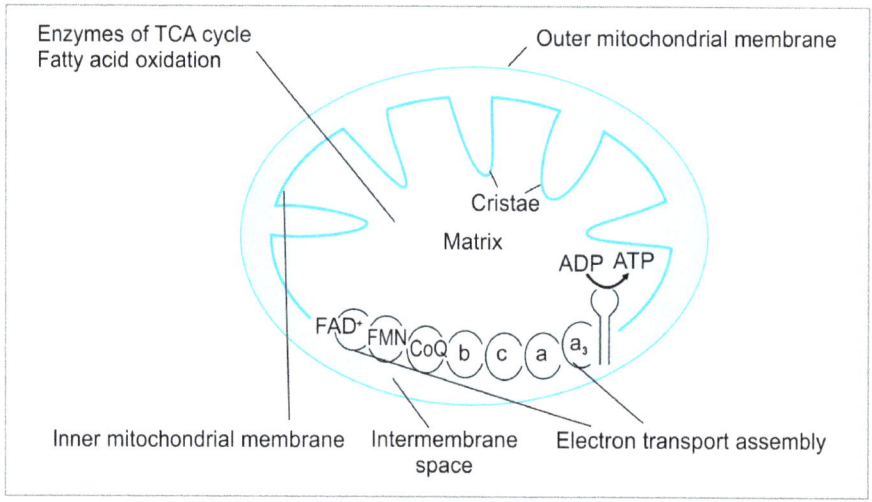

**Fig. 12.4:** Mitochondrion showing chemiosmotic hypothesis.

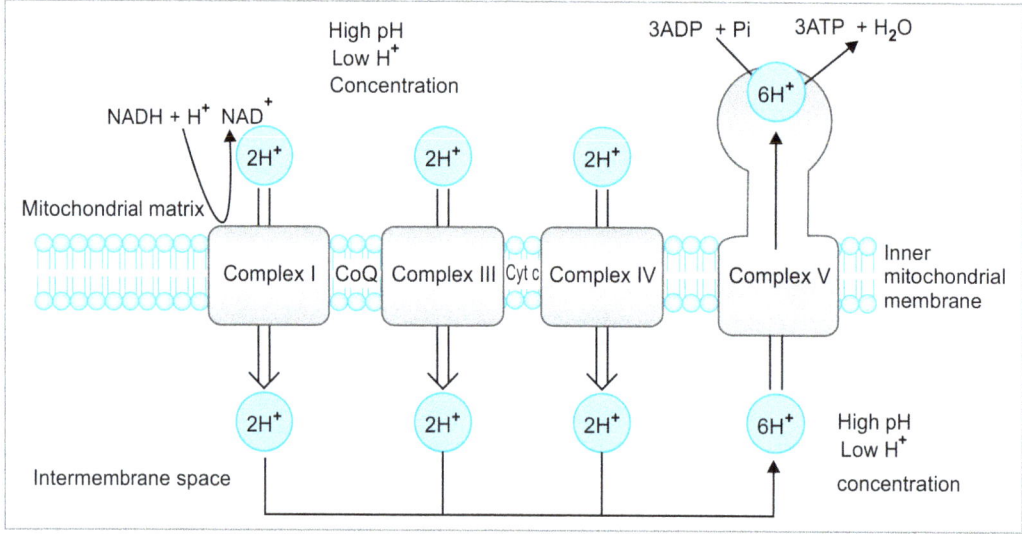

**Fig. 12.5:** Chemiosmotic hypothesis for oxidative phosphorylation.

The energy produced by the transport of electrons is released as heat rather than being used to synthesize ATP. As a result, ATP synthesis does not occur. The uncouplers allow oxidation substrates (via NADH or FADH) without ATP formation.

Other uncouplers are dinitrocresol, pentachlorophenol, trifluoro carbonyl cyanide phenylhydrazone, and high-dose aspirin. The thyroxine and long-chain fatty acids act as uncoupler at high concentration.

## Significance of Uncoupling

Uncoupling agents also occur naturally. Newborn and hibernating animals contain brown fat. Brown fat mitochondria contain the protein thermogenin, which provides a channel through the inner mitochondrial membrane. The heat energy released as the protons rush down their concentration gradient through this channel keeps the animal warm.

## Oligomycin

This antibiotic binds to the stalk of the ATP synthetase, closes the H⁺ channel, and prevents reentry of protons into the mitochondrial matrix. Due to this, protons get accumulated at higher concentration in the intermediate space. Electron transport ultimately stops because of the difficulty of pumping any more protons against the steep gradients. This indicates that the electron transport and phosphorylation are tightly coupled processes.

## SUMMARY

Oxidation–reduction reactions are coupled chemical reactions in which one atom or molecule loses one or more electrons (oxidation), while another atom or molecule gains those electrons (reduction). NADH and FADH resulting from metabolic pathway can be used for reductive biosynthesis. Reducing potential of mitochondrial NADH is most often used to supply the energy for ATP synthesis by electron transport chain and then via oxidative phosphorylation.

## SELF-ASSESSMENT QUESTIONS

1. Briefly discuss how the reactions of the electrons transport chain.
2. Write the flowchart to show the flow of electrons.
3. List the sites where ATP is synthesized.
4. What is oxidative phosphorylation?
5. Describe the chemiosmotic hypothesis.
6. List the inhibitors of electron transport chain and write the site of inhibition.
7. Explain the term "uncouplers" and give any two examples.
8. What is the P:O ratio? Write its significance.
9. What is the significance of uncouplers in animals?
10. Describe the action of oligomycin on electron transport chain and oxidative phosphorylation.

## MULTIPLE CHOICE QUESTIONS

1. **The site of oxidative phosphorylation is:**
   (a) Complex I
   (b) Complex II
   (c) Complex IV
   (d) Complex V

2. Concerning chemiosmotic hypothesis, all of the following statements are true, *except*:
   (a) Electron transport is coupled to transport of $H^+$ across the inner mitochondrial membrane
   (b) Energy generated through proton gradient is not sufficient to drive ATP synthesis
   (c) ATP synthetase complex synthesizes ATP, utilizing the energy of the proton gradient
   (d) Proton gradient creates low pH outside the mitochondrial membrane
3. The components of electron transport chain are located in the:
   (a) Intermediate space of the mitochondrial membrane
   (b) Inner mitochondrial membrane
   (c) Outer mitochondrial membrane
   (d) Cytosolic portion of the cell
4. The inner mitochondrial membrane is not permeable to:
   (a) Hydrogen ions
   (b) Sodium
   (c) Potassium
   (d) Selenium
5. All the following are the sites of ATP synthesis in a respiratory chain, *except*:
   (a) Complex I
   (b) Complex II
   (c) Complex III
   (d) Complex IV
6. 2,4 Dinitrophenol is:
   (a) Uncoupler causes electrons to stop flowing from one complex to other
   (b) Inhibitor causes electrons transport at slower speed without creating a proton gradient
   (c) Uncoupler causes electron transport to proceed at a rapid rate without creating a proton gradient
   (d) Inhibits the complex IV
7. All of the following are the uncouplers of oxidative phosphorylation, *except*:
   (a) Dinitrocresol
   (b) Carbon tetrachloride
   (c) Pentachlorophenol
   (d) Trifluorocarbonylcyanide phenylhydrazone
8. Which of the following applies to the statement "heat energy released as the protons rush down their concentration gradient through this channel keeps the animal warm"?
   (a) It is a significance inhibition mechanism
   (b) It is a significance oxidative phosphorylation
   (c) It is a significance of uncoupling mechanism
   (d) None of the above
9. All of the following inhibit the complex II, *except*:
   (a) Amytal
   (b) Rotenone
   (c) Piericidin
   (d) Antimycin

### ANSWERS
1. d    2. b    3. b    4. d    5. b    6. c    7. b    8. c
9. d

# Chapter 13

# Hormones

## LEARNING OBJECTIVES

*At the end of this chapter students should be able to:*
- Classify the hormones understand the mechanism of hormonal action
- Discuss the functions of pituitary hormones including the pathophysiology
- Explain the actions and pathophysiology of various hormones like thyroid, parathyroid, adrenal, pancreatic, ovarian and testicular hormones

## Introduction

Hormones are the substances secreted by highly specialized cells and carried by the extracellular fluid (mainly blood) and act through the receptor on the target organ to alter the activity of the cells quantitatively to influence:
- Metabolism
- Growth
- Reproduction
- Adaptation to the environment.
  - Hormones carry messages from glands to cells to maintain chemical levels in the bloodstream that achieve homeostasis (glands manufacture hormones).
  - Hormones circulate freely in the bloodstream, waiting to be recognized by a target cell, their intended destination.
  - The target cell has a receptor that can only be activated by a specific type of hormone. Once activated, the cell knows to start a certain function within its walls.
  - There are two types of hormones known—steroids and peptides.
  - In general, steroids are sex hormones related to sexual maturation and fertility. Steroids are made from cholesterol. Cortisol, testosterone, and estrogen are examples of steroid hormone.
  - Peptides regulate other functions such as sleep and sugar level. They are made from long strings of amino acids, so sometimes they are referred to as "protein" hormones.
  - Growth hormone (GH) helps us to burn fat and build up muscles.
  - Insulin starts the process to convert sugar into cellular energy.
  - As special categories, autocrine hormones act on the cells of the secreting gland, while paracrine hormones act on nearby, but unrelated, cells.

## Chemical Classes of Hormones

Vertebrate hormones fall into three chemical classes:
1. Amine-derived hormones are derivatives of the amino acids, tyrosine and tryptophan. Examples are catecholamines and thyroxine.
2. Peptide hormones consist of chains of amino acids. Examples of small peptide hormones are thyrotropin-releasing hormone (TRH) and vasopressin. Peptides composed of scores or hundreds of amino acids are referred to as proteins. Examples of protein hormones include insulin and

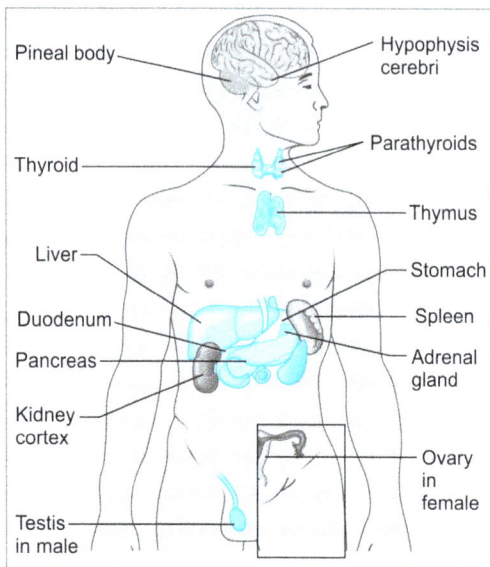

Fig. 13.1: Endocrine glands location in humans.

GH. More complex protein hormones bear carbohydrate side chains and are called glycoprotein hormones. Luteinizing hormone (LH), follicle-stimulating hormone (FSH), and thyroid-stimulating hormone (TSH) are glycoprotein hormones.

3. Lipid- and phospholipid-derived hormones are derived from lipids such as linoleic acid and arachidonic acid and phospholipids. The main classes are the steroid hormones that derive from cholesterol and the eicosanoids. Examples of steroid hormones are testosterone and cortisol. Sterol hormones such as calcitriol are a homologous system. The adrenal cortex and the gonads are primary sources of steroid hormones. Examples of eicosanoids are the widely studied prostaglandins.

In classical endocrinology, the hormones are (Fig. 13.1):
- Pituitary hormones
- Thyroid hormones
- Parathyroid hormones (PTHs)
- Pancreatic hormones
- Suprarenal cortical hormones
- Suprarenal medullary hormones
- Ovarian hormones
- Testicular hormones
- Hypophyseal hormones.

**Briefly explain the mechanism of hormonal action.**

## Mechanism of Hormonal Action

- The hormone binds to a site on the extracellular portion of the receptor (Fig. 13.2).

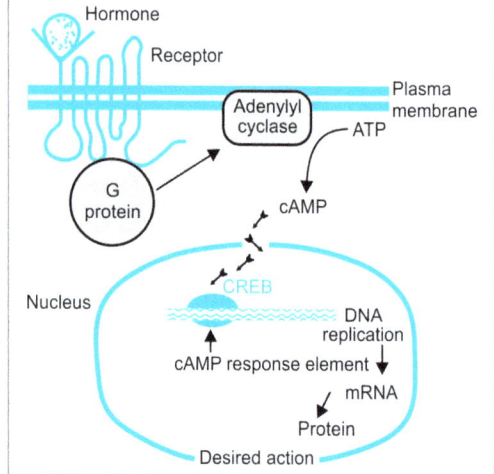

Fig. 13.2: Mechanism of hormonal action.
(ATP: adenosine triphosphate; cAMP: cyclic adenosine monophosphate; CREB: cAMP response element binding protein; DNA: deoxyribonucleic acid; mRNA: messenger ribonucleic acid)

- The receptors are transmembrane proteins that pass through the plasma membrane seven times, with their N-terminal exposed at the exterior of the cell and their C-terminal projecting into the cytoplasm.
- Binding of the hormone to the receptor activates a G protein.
- This initiates the production of a second messenger such as cyclic AMP (cAMP), which is produced by adenylyl cyclase from ATP, inositol-1,4,5-trisphosphate.
- The second messenger, in turn, initiates a series of intracellular events such as phosphorylation and activation of enzymes; release of $Ca^{2+}$ into the cytosol from stores within the endoplasmic reticulum.

- In the case of cAMP, these enzymatic changes activate the transcription factor CREB (cAMP response element binding protein).
- Bound to its response element in the promoters of genes that are able to respond to the hormone, activated CREB turns on gene transcription.
- This results in translation to produce the desired protein.
- The cell begins to produce the appropriate gene products in response to the hormonal signal it had received at its surface.

## Pituitary Hormones

The endocrine is a gland, which secretes hormone also called ductless glands, as the hormone is carried not by the duct, but by blood.

Pituitary gland comprises:
- Anterior pituitary
- Posterior pituitary
- Intermediate lobe.

**List the anterior pituitary hormones.**

## Anterior Pituitary Hormones

- Growth hormone
- Thyroid stimulating hormone
- Follicle stimulating hormone
- Luteinizing hormone
- Adrenocorticotropic hormone (ACTH)
- Prolactin (PRL)
- Alpha-melanocyte-stimulating hormone.

**Discuss the growth hormone including its major functions.**

### Growth Hormone

Human GH (also called somatotropin) is a protein of 191 amino acids.

The GH-secreting cells are stimulated to synthesize and release GH by the intermittent arrival of GH-releasing hormone (GHRH) from the hypothalamus.
- Direct effects are the result of GH binding its receptor on target cells. Fat cells (adipocytes), for example, have GH receptors, and GH stimulates them to break down triglyceride and suppresses

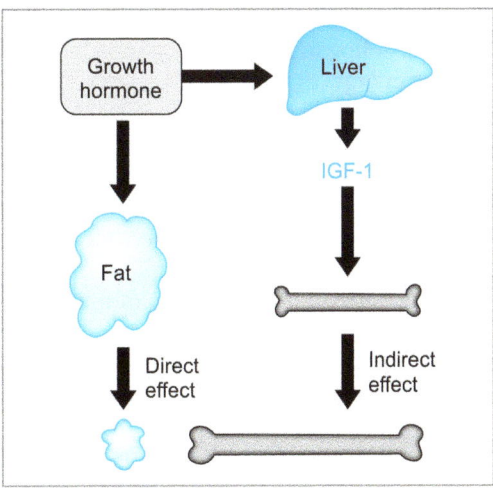

**Fig. 13.3:** Role of growth hormone.

their ability to take up and accumulate circulating lipids.
- Indirect effects are mediated primarily by an insulin-like growth factor-I (IGF-I), a hormone that is secreted from the liver and other tissues in response to GH. A majority of the growth-promoting effects of GH are actually due to IGF-I acting on its target cells (e.g., on long bones) **(Fig. 13.3)**.

**State the signs and symptoms of growth hormone deficiency in children and adults.**

### Pathophysiology

- In childhood, hyposecretion of GH produces the stunted growth of a dwarf.
- Dwarfism can also result from an inability to respond to GH.
- This can result from inheriting two mutant genes encoding the receptors for:
  - Growth hormone releasing hormone
  - Growth hormone.

*GH deficiency symptoms:* Symptoms of GH deficiency in children include the following:
- Short stature
- Low growth velocity (speed) for age and pubertal stage.
- Increased amount of fat around the waist.
- The child may look younger than other children of his or her age.
- Delayed tooth development
- Delayed onset of puberty

Symptoms of GH deficiency in adults include the following:
* Low energy
* Decreased strength and exercise tolerance
* Decreased muscle mass
* Weight gain, especially around the waist
* Feelings of anxiety, depression, or sadness causing a change in social behavior.

The effect of excessive secretion of GH is also very dependent on the age of onset and is seen as two distinctive disorders:
1. Hypersecretion leads to gigantism.
2. Gigantism is the result of excessive GH secretion that begins in young children or adolescents. It is a very rare disorder, usually resulting from a tumor of somatotropes.

In adults, hypersecretion of GH leads to acromegaly.

**Mention the important role of thyroid-stimulating hormone.**

## Thyroid-stimulating Hormone

TSH (also known as thyrotropin) is a glycoprotein. The secretion of TSH is:
* Stimulated by the arrival of TRH from the hypothalamus
* Inhibited by the arrival of somatostatin from the hypothalamus.

As its name suggests, TSH stimulates the thyroid gland to secrete its hormone thyroxine ($T_4$) (**Fig. 13.4**).

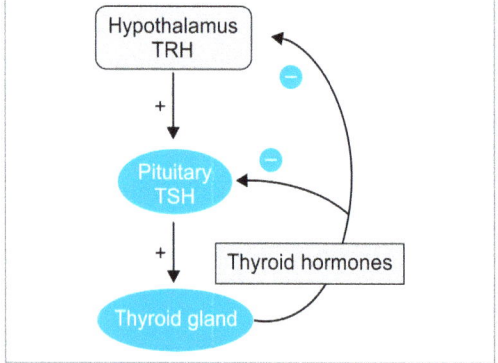

**Fig. 13.4:** TSH role.
(THS: thyroid-stimulating hormone; TRH: thyrotropin-releasing hormone)

## Follicle-stimulating Hormone
* *In females*: FSH acts on the ovary to stimulate the development of ovarian follicle.
* *In males*: It acts on the testes for the maturation of sperm.

## Luteinizing Hormone
* *In females*: LH stimulates the ovarian follicle to mature and also to secrete the estrogen.
* *In males*: It stimulates the secretion of testosterone.

## Adrenocorticotrophic Hormone
* ACTH is a peptide of 39 amino acids.
* It is cut from a larger precursor proopiomelanocortin.
* It acts on the cells of the adrenal cortex stimulating them to produce their hormone.

*Pathophysiology*
* If ACTH secretion is increased by the pituitary or by ectopic production from a tumor, it results in Cushing's syndrome.
* The decreased ACTH production leads to Addison's disease.

## Prolactin (Somatomammotropin)
* PRL is a protein of 198 amino acids.
* During pregnancy, it helps in the preparation of the breasts for future milk production. After birth, PRL promotes the synthesis of milk.
* PRL secretion is stimulated by TRH and repressed by estrogens and dopamine.

*Pathophysiology*
* Hyperprolactinemia is a cause of infertility in females.
* Secretion of PRL is stimulated by TRH and inhibited by prolactin inhibiting factor (PIF).

- *Normal range*: Females: 5.4–22.5 ng/mL (mid-cycle) 4.5–15 ng/mL (menopausal women).
- *Males*: 4.2–15 ng/mL

**List the posterior pituitary hormones and state their functions.**

## Posterior Pituitary Hormones
### Vasopressin
- It was originally named because of its ability to control blood pressure when administered in pharmacological amounts.
- But more appropriately it is called antidiuretic hormone (ADH), because of its important function to promote reabsorption of water from the distal convoluted tubules.
- If there is defect in the ADH secretion or the decreased action, it may lead to diabetes insipidus.
- Diabetes insipidus is characterized by excretion of large volumes of diluted urine.
    - Primary *diabetes insipidus*: An insufficient secretion of hormone, which is due to the destruction of the hypothalamic–hypophyseal tract.
    - Arises due to basal skull fractures.
    - Tumor or infection
    - It may be hereditary as well.

### Biochemical Findings
- Decreased specific gravity
- Decreased ADH
- Diluted urine
- Polyuria

### Oxytocin
- Produced in hypothalamus and transported to posterior pituitary gland.
- Appropriate stimulation releases the hormones into the blood.
- The neural impulses that result from stimulation of the nipples are the primary stimuli for oxytocin release.
- Vaginal and uterine distension is the secondary stimuli.
- Estrogen also stimulates the production of oxytocin.
- Oxytocin causes contraction of uterine smooth muscles and thus is used in pharmacological amount to induce labor in humans.
- The most likely physiologic function of oxytocin is stimulation for the contraction of cells surrounding mammary alveoli. This promotes the movement of milk into the system and allows milk ejection.

**State the functions of thyroid hormones.**

## Thyroid Hormones
- The thyroid gland synthesizes and secretes: $T_4$ and $T_3$.
- Thyroxine ($T_4$) is a derivative of the amino acid tyrosine with four atoms of iodine.
- In the liver, one atom of iodine is removed from $T_4$ converting it into triiodothyronine ($T_3$).
- $T_3$ is the active hormone
- Thyroid hormones have many effects on the body. Among the most prominent of these are:
    - Increase metabolic rate (seen by a rise in the uptake of oxygen)
    - Increase the rate and strength of the heartbeat.
- The thyroid cells are responsible for the synthesis of $T_4$, take up circulating iodine from the blood.

**What are the different types of hypothyroid diseases? State the biochemical findings, signs, and symptoms of them.**

## Pathophysiology
*Hypothyroid diseases*: Caused by inadequate production of $T_3$.

*Cretinism:* Hypothyroidism in infancy and childhood leads to stunted growth and intelligence. It can be corrected by giving thyroxine if started early enough.

*Myxedema:* Hypothyroidism in adult's leads to lowered metabolic rate and vigor.

It can be reversed by giving thyroxine.

*Goiter:* enlargement of the thyroid gland. Can be caused by:
- Inadequate iodine in the diet with resulting low levels of $T_4$ and $T_3$.
- An autoimmune attack against components of the thyroid gland (called Hashimoto's thyroiditis).
- The region for hypothyroid disease produces an enlarged gland.
- The activity of the thyroid is under negative feedback control.
- The synthesis and release of TRH and TSH are normally inhibited as the levels of $T_4$ and $T_3$ rise in the blood.
- When the iodine supply is inadequate, $T_4$ and $T_3$ levels fall. This stimulates the hypothalamus and pituitary to increase TRH and TSH activity, respectively, which prompts the thyroid gland to enlarge (fruitlessly).

## Symptoms
- Decrease basal metabolic rate (BMR)
- Slow heart rate
- Diastolic hypertension
- Sluggish behavior
- Sleepiness
- Constipation
- Sensitivity to cold
- Dry skin and hair

## Biochemical Findings
- Decreased $T_3$, $T_4$, and increased TSH especially in primary hypothyroidism.
- Decreased $T_3$, $T_4$, and decreased TSH in secondary hypothyroidism.

**What happens to the level of TSH and thyroid hormones in hyperthyroidism and which symptoms help the clinician to diagnose it?**

## Hyperthyroid Diseases
Caused by excessive secretion of thyroid hormones
- Graves's disease
- *Osteoporosis*: High levels of thyroid hormones suppress the production of TSH through the negative feedback mechanism mentioned above. The resulting low level of TSH causes an increase in the numbers of bone-reabsorbing osteoclasts resulting in osteoporosis.

## Symptoms
- Rapid heart rate
- Nervousness
- Inability to sleep
- Weight loss in spite of hyperthyroidism
- Weakness
- Excessive sweating
- Sensitivity to heat

## Biochemical Findings
Increased $T_3$ and $T_4$ and TSH decreased.

## Normal Levels
- $T_3$ = 0.8–2.0 mg/mL
- $T_4$ = 4.5–12.0 mg/dL.

**Show with the help of diagram the role of parathyroid hormone in maintaining the calcium homeostasis.**

## Parathyroid Hormones

### Functions

*Calcium Homeostasis (Regulation)*

Parathyroid hormone restores normal calcium concentration by acting directly on bone and kidney and acting indirectly on intestinal mucosa **(Fig. 13.5)**.

*Bone:* It increases the resorption in both organic and inorganic phases, which lose $Ca^{2+}$ into extracellular fluid (ECF).

*Kidney:* It reduces renal clearance or excretion of calcium and hence increases ECF concentration of calcium.

*Gastrointestinal tract (GIT):* It increases efficiency of calcium absorption from the intestine by promoting the synthesis of

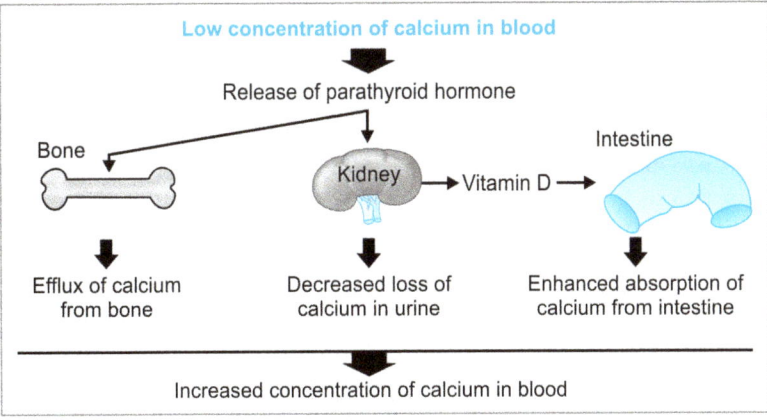

**Fig. 13.5:** Regulation of calcium by parathyroid hormone.

calcitriol. It acts upon the intestine to increase $Ca^{2+}$ absorption and plays a permissive role of PTH on bone and kidney.

Parathyroid hormone also increases renal phosphate clearance. Thus the net effect of PTH on bone and kidney is to increase ECF calcium concentration and decrease ECF $PO_4$ concentration.

Excessive secretion of PTH is seen in two forms:
1. Primary hyperparathyroidism is the result of parathyroid gland disease, most commonly due to a parathyroid tumor (adenoma), which secretes the hormone without proper regulation. Common manifestations of this disorder are chronic elevations of blood calcium concentration (hypercalcemia), kidney stones, and decalcification of bone.
2. Secondary hyperparathyroidism is the situation where disease outside of the parathyroid gland leads to excessive secretion of PTH. A common cause of this disorder is kidney disease—if the kidneys are unable to reabsorb calcium, blood calcium levels will fall, stimulating continual secretion of PTH to maintain normal calcium levels in blood. Secondary hyperparathyroidism can also result from inadequate nutrition, e.g., diets that are deficient in calcium or vitamin D, or which contain excessive phosphorus. A prominent effect of secondary hyperparathyroidism is decalcification of bone.

Inadequate production of PTH—hypoparathyroidism—results in decreased concentrations of calcium and increased concentrations of phosphorus in blood. Common causes of this disorder include surgical removal of the parathyroid glands and disease processes that lead to destruction of parathyroid glands. The resulting hypocalcemia often leads to tetany and convulsions and can be acutely life threatening.

**List the hormones secreted by adrenal gland.**

### Adrenal Gland

The adrenal gland comprises cortex and medulla.

Cortex has three zones:
1. Zona glomerulosa: Produces mineralocorticoids
2. Zona fasciculata: Produces glucocorticoids
3. Zona reticularis: Secretes sex steroids such as androgens and estrogens.

**Explain the functions of glucocorticoid hormones.**

### Glucocorticoids

It is a steroid hormone; it is mainly derived from cholesterol.

The functions of glucocorticoid in the human body are as follows:
* The glucocorticoids get their name from their effect of raising the level of blood sugar. They do this by stimulating gluconeogenesis in the liver.
* The conversion of fat and protein into intermediate metabolites that are ultimately converted into glucose.
* The most abundant glucocorticoid is cortisol (also called hydrocortisone).
* Cortisol and the other glucocorticoid also have a potent anti-inflammatory effect on the body.
* They depress the immune response, especially cell-mediated immune response.
* They are widely used in therapy:
   - To reduce the inflammatory destruction of rheumatoid arthritis and other autoimmune diseases.
   - To prevent the rejection of transplanted organs.
   - To control asthma

**Explain the regulation of cortisol secretion and its mode of action.**

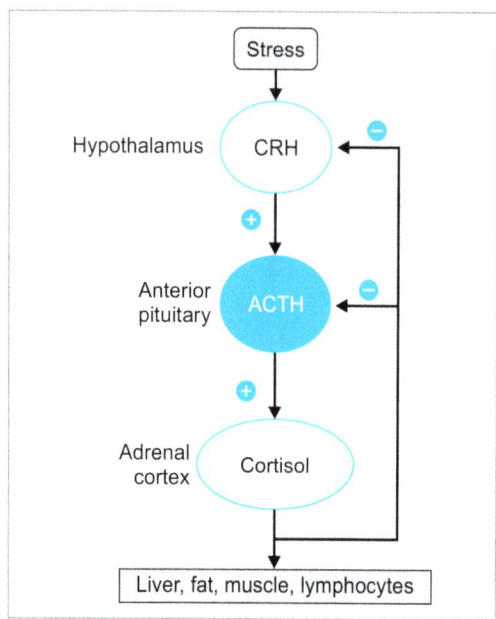

**Fig. 13.6:** Cortisol secretion.
(CRH: corticotropin-reseasing hormone; ACTH: adrenocorticotropic hormone)

## Control of Cortisol Secretion

* Cortisol and other glucocorticoids are secreted in response to a single stimulator: ACTH from the anterior pituitary. ACTH is itself secreted under control of the hypothalamic peptide corticotropin-releasing hormone (CRH). The central nervous system is thus the commander and chief of glucocorticoid responses, providing an excellent example of close integration between the nervous and endocrine systems **(Fig. 13.6)**.
* Virtually any type of physical or mental stress results in elevation of cortisol concentrations in blood due to enhanced secretion of CRH in the hypothalamus.
* Cortisol secretion is suppressed by classical negative feedback loops. When blood concentrations rise above a certain threshold, cortisol inhibits CRH secretion from the hypothalamus, which turns off ACTH secretion and leads to a turning off of cortisol secretion from the adrenal. The combination of positive and negative control on CRH secretion results in pulsatile secretion of cortisol. Typically pulse amplitude and frequency are highest in the morning and lowest at night.
* ACTH binds to receptors in the plasma membrane of cells in the zona fasciculata and reticularis of the adrenal. Hormone receptor engagement activates adenyl cyclase, leading to elevated intracellular levels of cAMP, which leads ultimately to activation of the enzyme systems involved in the biosynthesis of cortisol from cholesterol.

## Mode of Action

Glucocorticoids bind to the cytosolic glucocorticoid receptor. This type of receptor is activated by ligand binding. After a hormone binds to the corresponding receptor, the newly formed receptor–ligand complex translocates itself into the cell nucleus, where it binds to many glucocorticoid response elements in the promoter region of the target genes.

**Discuss the Addison's disease and Cushin syndrome including causes and symptoms.**

## Pathophysiology

### Addison's Disease (Adrenal Insufficiency)

- Addison's disease is a rare endocrine or hormonal disorder that occurs in all age-groups.
- In this condition, the adrenal gland releases insufficient amounts of steroid hormones (glucocorticoids and often mineralocorticoids).
- The disease is also called adrenal insufficiency or hypocortisolism.

### Causes

- Failure to produce adequate levels of cortisol can occur for different reasons. The problem may be due to a disorder of the adrenal glands themselves (primary adrenal insufficiency):
  - Destruction of the adrenal glands by infection or by autoimmune attack.
- Inadequate secretion of ACTH by the pituitary gland (secondary adrenal insufficiency).
  - An inherited mutation in the ACTH receptor on adrenal cells.

Another cause of secondary adrenal insufficiency is the surgical removal of benign, or noncancerous, ACTH-producing tumors of the pituitary gland (Cushing's disease).

### Other Causes

Less common causes of primary adrenal insufficiency are:
- Cancer cells spreading from other parts of the body to the adrenal glands.
- Amyloidosis
- Surgical removal of the adrenal glands.

### Symptoms
- Hypoglycemia
- Extreme sensitivity of insulin
- Intolerance to stress
- Weight loss
- Nausea
- Severe weakness
- Patients have low blood pressure.

The essential role of the adrenal hormones means that a deficiency can be life threatening. Fortunately, replacement therapy with glucocorticoid and mineralocorticoids can permit a normal life.

A diagnosis of Addison's disease is made by laboratory tests. The aim of these tests is to determine whether levels of cortisol are insufficient and then to establish the cause.

### ACTH Stimulation Test

This is the most specific test for diagnosing Addison's disease. In this test, blood cortisol, urine cortisol, or both are measured before and after a synthetic form of ACTH is given by injection. In the so-called short, or rapid, ACTH test, measurement of cortisol in blood is repeated 30–60 minutes after an intravenous ACTH injection. The normal response after an injection of ACTH is a rise in blood and urine cortisol levels. Patients with either form of adrenal insufficiency respond poorly or do not respond at all.

Routine investigation may show:
- Hypoglycemia
- Hyponatremia
- Hypokalemia
- Eosinophilia and lymphocytosis

### Cushing's Syndrome

Cushing's syndrome is a hormonal disorder caused by prolonged exposure of the body's tissues to high levels of the hormone cortisol **(Fig. 13.7)**.

In Cushing's syndrome, the level of adrenal hormones, especially of the glucocorticoids (cortisol) is too high.

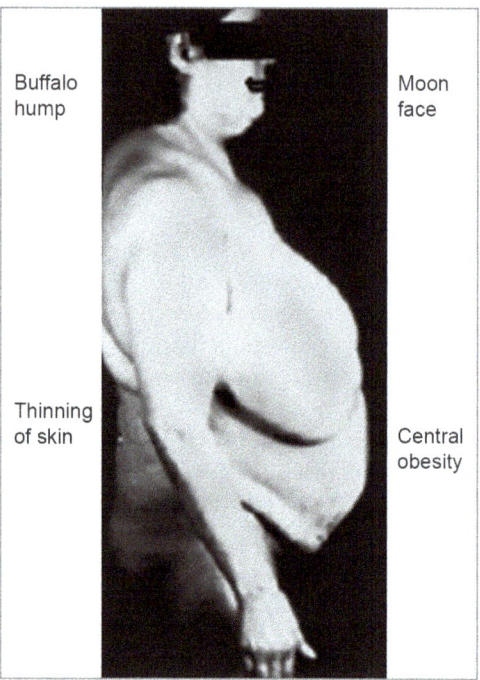

**Fig. 13.7:** Features of Cushing's syndrome.

## Causes

- Excessive production of ACTH by the anterior lobe of the pituitary.
- Excessive production of adrenal hormones themselves (e.g., because of a tumor).
- Ectopic ACTH syndrome: Some benign or malignant (cancerous) tumors that arise outside the pituitary can produce ACTH. This condition is known as ectopic ACTH syndrome. Lung tumors cause over 50% of these cases.
- As a result of glucocorticoid therapy for some other disorder such as rheumatoid arthritis or decreased glucocorticoid hormone synthesis.

## Symptoms

- Hyperglycemia
- High blood pressure
- Severe protein catabolism results in thinning of skin, muscle wasting, osteoporosis, and negative nitrogen balance.
- There is a peculiar redistribution of fat in trunks.
- Moon face
- Central obesity and typical buffalo hump.
- Impaired resistant to infection and inflammatory response.
- Facial hair growth

Diagnosis is based on a review of the patient's medical history, physical examination, and laboratory tests.

## Twenty-four Hour Urinary-free Cortisol Level

This is the most specific diagnostic test. The patient's urine is collected over a 24-hour period and tested for the amount of cortisol. If the cortisol level is higher than 50–100 µg a day for an adult suggests Cushing's syndrome. The normal range may vary from laboratory to laboratory depending on the techniques they use.

**Write the procedure and the importance of dexamethasone suppression test.**

## Dexamethasone Suppression Test

This test is used to distinguish patients with excess production of ACTH due to pituitary adenomas from those with ectopic ACTH-producing tumors. Patients are given dexamethasone, a synthetic glucocorticoid, by mouth every 6 hours for 4 days. For the first 2 days, low doses of dexamethasone are given, while for the last 2 days, higher doses are given. Twenty-four-hour urine sample collections are made before dexamethasone is administered and on each day of the test. Since cortisol and other glucocorticoids signal the pituitary to lower secretion of ACTH, the normal response after taking dexamethasone is a drop in blood and urine cortisol levels. Different responses of cortisol to dexamethasone are obtained depending on whether the cause of Cushing's syndrome is a pituitary adenoma or an ectopic ACTH-producing tumor.

The dexamethasone suppression test can produce false-positive results in patients with depression, alcohol abuse, high estrogen levels, acute illness, and stress. Conversely, drugs such as phenytoin and phenobarbital may cause false-negative results in response to dexamethasone suppression. For this reason, patients are usually advised by their physicians to stop taking these drugs at least 1 week before the test.

## Mineralocorticoids

- It is a steroid hormone and mainly derived from the cholesterol.
- The mineralocorticoids get their name from their effect on mineral metabolism. The most important of them is the steroid aldosterone.
- Aldosterone acts on the kidney promoting the reabsorption of sodium ions ($Na^+$) into the blood.
- Water follows the salt and this helps maintain normal blood pressure.
- Aldosterone also acts on sweat glands to reduce the loss of sodium in perspiration.
- It acts on taste cells to increase the sensitivity of the taste buds to sources of sodium.
- The secretion of aldosterone is stimulated by:
  - A drop in the level of sodium ions in the blood.
  - A rise in the level of potassium ions in the blood.
  - Angiotensin II
  - Adrenocorticotropic hormone

## Primary Aldosteronism or Cohn's Syndrome

- Results from an aldosterone-secreting tumor, which leads to elevated levels of plasma aldosterone.
- The plasma pH in this condition increases because of hypokalemic alkalosis and the plasma osmolality also increases.

## Adrenal Medulla

It secretes:
- Dopamine
- Adrenaline (epinephrine)
- Noradrenaline (norepinephrine)

## Functions

- The adrenal medulla consists of masses of neurons that are part of the sympathetic branch of the autonomic nervous system.
- Instead of releasing their neurotransmitters at a synapse, these neurons release them into the blood. Thus although part of the nervous system, the adrenal medulla functions as an endocrine gland.
- The adrenal medulla releases:
  - Adrenaline (also called epinephrine).
  - Noradrenaline (also called norepinephrine). Both are derived from the amino acid tyrosine.
- Release of adrenaline and noradrenaline is triggered by nervous stimulation in response to physical or mental stress.

Some of the effects are:
- Increase in the rate and strength of the heartbeat, resulting in increased blood pressure.
- Blood shunted from the skin and viscera to the skeletal muscles, coronary arteries, liver, and brain.
- Rise in blood sugar
- Increased metabolic rate
- Bronchi dilate
- Pupils dilate
- Hair stands on end
- Reduced clotting time
- Increased ACTH secretion from the anterior lobe of the pituitary.

## Pathophysiology

The tumor of the adrenal medulla results in oversecretion of its hormones and leads to a condition called pheochromocytoma.

## Pancreas

Alpha cells of pancreas secrete glucagon and beta cells of islets of Langerhans of pancreas secrete insulin.

**State the functions of insulin.**

## Insulin

- Insulin is a polypeptide hormone synthesized from the beta cells of islets of Langerhans of pancreas.
- It is synthesized as a larger precursor called preproinsulin. Preproinsulin has 109 amino acids. It is immediately converted into proinsulin in the endoplasmic reticulum by the removal of 23 amino acids. So the proinsulin formed contains 86 amino acids. The proinsulin is transported to Golgi apparatus and is cleaved to from insulin and C-peptide
- The C-peptide contains 33 amino acids. Insulin formed from proinsulin contains 53 amino acids from which 2 amino acids are cleaved to from insulin with 51 amino acids.

Insulin mainly controls blood glucose by the following mechanisms:
- Increases the uptake of glucose by the peripheral cells.
- Increases the utilization of glucose by stimulating the glycolysis.
- Stimulates glycogenesis and inhibits glycogenolysis.
- Inhibits lipolysis
- Inhibits gluconeogenesis

## Glucagon

It is a polypeptide secreted by alpha cells of islets of Langerhans of pancreas. It is called anti-insulin hormone since its actions are entirely opposite to that of insulin. Glucagon stimulates the production of glucose in the liver by promoting glycogenolysis and gluconeogenesis (refer to blood sugar regulation).

**Discuss in detail the secretion and role of female sex hormones at different stages including the infancy and puberty.**

## Female Sex Hormones

It is very important to know how hormones can affect the female body, mind, and emotions. Then we will be able to minimize their negative effects and enhance their positive ones.

## Infancy

Newborn babies (boys and girls) may have slightly enlarged breasts, sometimes accompanied by a little milk production, due to the female hormone, estrogen, in the mother's body passing through the placenta during pregnancy and stimulating breast development in the baby, which finally, disappears during childhood.

## Puberty

- At puberty, hormones will begin to make major, lasting changes to a girl's body.
- Breasts will get bigger and take on the shape of an adult woman's breasts.
- She will develop underarm and pubic hair and will get noticeably taller as a significant growth spurt occurs.
- Her periods will start, usually as the growth spurt is beginning to slow down.
- From beginning to end, the process of puberty usually takes at least 4 years.
- The hypothalamus starts to release hormone, which stimulates the pituitary gland to produce LH and FSH, which in turn causes a girl's ovaries to start producing other hormones.

## Female Sex Hormones at Different Stages

The most important hormones made by the ovaries are known as female sex hormones such as estrogen and progesterone. The ovaries also produce some of the male hormone, testosterone. During puberty, estrogen stimulates breast development and causes the vagina, uterus, and fallopian tubes to mature. It also plays a role in the growth spurt and alters the distribution of fat on a girl's body, typically resulting in more being deposited around the hips, buttocks, and thighs. Testosterone helps to promote muscle and bone growth.

From puberty onward, LH, FSH, estrogen, and progesterone all play a vital part in regulating a woman's menstrual cycle, which results in her periods. Each individual hormone follows its own pattern, rising and falling at different points in the cycle but together they produce a predictable chain of events. One egg (out of several hundred thousand in each ovary) becomes mature and is released from the ovary to and run toward fallopian tube and into the womb. If that egg is not fertilized, the levels of estrogen and progesterone produced by the ovary begin to fall. Without the supporting action of these hormones, the lining of the womb, which is full of blood, is shed, resulting in a period.

## Pregnancy

If the egg released from the ovary is fertilized and a pregnancy results, a woman's hormones change dramatically. The usual fall in estrogen and progesterone at the end of the menstrual cycle does not occur, so no period is seen. A new hormone, human chorionic gonadotropin produced by the developing placenta, stimulates the ovaries to produce the higher levels of estrogen and progesterone that are needed to sustain a pregnancy. By the fourth month of pregnancy, the placenta takes over from the ovaries as the main producer of estrogen and progesterone. These hormones cause the lining of the womb to thicken, increase the volume of blood circulating, and relax the muscles of the womb sufficiently to make room for the growing baby. Around the time of childbirth, other hormones such as oxytocin come into play that help the womb to contract during and after labor as well as stimulate the production and release of breast milk.

## After Childbirth

The levels of estrogen, progesterone, and other hormones fall sharply, causing a number of physical changes. The womb shrinks back to its nonpregnant size, pelvic floor muscle tone improves, and the volume of blood circulating round the body returns to normal.

## The Menopause

The next significant hormonal change for most women occurs around the time of the last period—the menopause. Over 3–5 years leading up to a woman's last period, the normal functioning of her ovaries begins to deteriorate. This can cause her menstrual cycle to become shorter or longer, and sometimes it becomes quite erratic. Eventually, the ovaries produce so little estrogen and finally periods stop altogether.

## Ovary

The ovarian follicles secrete the following hormones:
- Estrogen is secreted from the follicular tissue.
- Progesterone is secreted from the corpus luteum.
- Androgens

## Estrogen

- Are primarily responsible for the conversion of girls into sexually mature women
  - Development of breasts
  - Further development of the uterus and vagina
  - Broadening of the pelvis
  - Growth of pubic and axillary hair
  - Increase in adipose (fat) tissue

- Participates in the monthly preparation of the body for a possible pregnancy.
- Participates in pregnancy, if it occurs.

## Progesterone

- It is steroid hormone synthesized from parent compound cholesterol:
  - It causes the development of endometrium and prepares it for the implantation of fertilized ovum for conception.
  - It stimulates the mammary glands.
- Normal range:
  - 0.175–0.7 ng/mL—follicular and mid cycle
  - 4.7–20 ng/mL—luteal cycle.

## Testes

- It secretes testosterone
- It promotes the growth and function of epididymis, vas deference, prostate, and seminal vesicles.
- It enhances and maintains the mobility and fertilizing power of the sperms.
- It promotes protein synthesis in the body.

## SUMMARY

Hormones are the substances secreted by highly specialized cells and carried by the extracellular fluid and act through the receptor on the target organ to alter the activity of the cells quantitatively to influence metabolism, growth, reproduction, and adaptation to the environment. Steroids and peptides are the two types of hormones. Steroids are sex hormones related to sexual maturation and fertility. Peptides regulate sleep and sugar level. The pituitary hormones are of two types—anterior and posterior. Growth hormone, TSH, ACTH, FSH, LH, and prolactin are the anterior pituitary hormones. Oxytocin and ADH are the posterior pituitary hormones. Thyroid gland secretes $T_3$ and $T_4$. Parathyroid secretes PTH. Mineralocorticoids, glucocorticoids, and sex steroids are secreted from adrenal gland. Insulin and glucagon are secreted from pancreas. Testes secrete testosterone and progesterone and estrogen are secreted from ovary.

## SELF-ASSESSMENT QUESTIONS

1. What are hormones?
2. Name the hormones secreted from anterior and posterior pituitary gland.
3. Describe the mechanism of hormonal action.
4. Explain the pathophysiology of growth hormone.
5. Mention the hormones secreted from thyroid gland and which hormones stimulate the thyroid hormone release?
6. Add a note on the following:
   (a) Cretinism             (b) Goiter
   (c) Myxedema
7. How the parathyroid hormones act to maintain the calcium homeostasis?
8. Mention the hormones secreted from three zones of adrenal cortex.
9. List the functions of glucocorticoid and mineralocorticoid hormones.
10. Write the causes, signs, and symptoms of:
    (a) Addison's disease     (b) Cushing's syndrome
11. List the adrenal medullary hormones and their functions.
12. Mention few functions of female sex hormones and mention on what influence they enter into the circulation to act finally.
13. What are the hormones secreted from pancreas?

# CHAPTER 13: Hormones

## Case Studies

1. A patient presents with a blood pressure of 175/90 mm Hg, and complaints of tiredness and muscle weakness. The laboratory result reveals that plasma sodium is slightly increased and plasma potassium is significantly decreased compared to normal. Hematocrit is also low. Plasma renin activity is markedly decreased, and serum aldosterone is increased. Which of the following is the most likely diagnosis?
   (a) Addison's disease
   (b) Conn's syndrome
   (c) Cushing's syndrome
   (d) Pheochromocytoma

   **Answer is b.** Conn's syndrome, or primary hyperaldosteronism, results from an adrenal tumor that secretes excessive aldosterone. The increased mineralocorticoid effects of aldosterone lead to renal sodium and water retention and increased renal potassium excretion (hypokalemia). The volume expansion also explains the decrease in hematocrit. The increased blood volume, increased blood pressure, and hypernatremia will all tend to suppress renin secretion in an attempt to compensate for the increased aldosterone.

2. A 65-year-old woman presents to her physician prior to beginning chemotherapy for newly diagnosed small cell lung carcinoma. Her examination is notable for obesity, blood pressure of 170/100, facial hair, abdominal striae, and an acneiform rash on her chest and back. Laboratory values are normal except for serum glucose of 300 mg/dL. Her chest X-ray shows a right perihilar mass and severe diffuse osteoporosis. Which of the following accounts for her physical exam, lab, and X-ray findings?
   (a) Adrenal gland destruction by metastases
   (b) Anterior pituitary gland disruption by metastases
   (c) Ectopic production of PTH
   (d) Ectopic production of ACTH

   **The correct answer is d.** This woman has all the classic findings of Cushing's syndrome—obesity, hypertension, hirsutism, acne, striae, glucose intolerance, and osteoporosis. Cushing's syndrome may be caused by an excess production of cortisol by bilateral adrenal hyperplasia or an adrenal neoplasm; by excess production of ACTH by a pituitary adenoma; or by ectopic production of ACTH by a tumor, most commonly a small cell lung carcinoma.

3. A 35-year-old woman with disseminated histoplasmosis complains of profound weakness, easy fatigability, anorexia, weight loss, and diarrhea. Laboratory investigation reveals serum sodium of 131 mEq/L, serum potassium of 5.8 mEq/L, and pH of 7.58. Skin hyperpigmentation is seen on physical examination. Which of the following is the most likely diagnosis?
   (a) Primary adrenocortical insufficiency
   (b) Conn's syndrome
   (c) Cushing's syndrome
   (d) Secondary adrenocortical insufficiency

   **Answer is c.** The evidences shown indicate that this patient has adrenal insufficiency due to diminished aldosterone production. The primary form of adrenocortical insufficiency results from any condition that destroys the adrenal cortex. Clinical manifestations of hypoaldosteronemia appear when 90% of the adrenal cortex is destroyed. The most frequent form is due to an autoimmune process. The remaining cases are secondary to infections (such as tuberculosis or fungal infections) or metastatic disease involving both adrenals. Secondary adrenocortical insufficiency differs from the primary form, (1) it is caused by disorders affecting the pituitary gland or hypothalamus and leading to reduced ACTH production, and (2) it is not associated with skin hyperpigmentation. Skin hyperpigmentation results from increased production of ACTH precursor (which stimulates melanocytes), presenting Addison's disease, but obviously lacking in secondary adrenocortical insufficiency.

4. A 50-year-old man is evaluated for congestive heart failure. In addition to a dilated cardiomyopathy, she displays multiple signs and symptoms, including intellectual function, fatigue, lethargy, cold intolerance, listlessness, thickened facial features, periorbital edema, dry and coarse skin, and peripheral edema. Serum studies demonstrate a $T_4$ of 1.4 µg/dL and a TSH of 22 µU/mL. Which of the following diagnoses is supported by these data?
   (a) Cretinism
   (b) Graves' disease
   (c) Hashimoto's thyroiditis
   (d) Myxedema

**Answer is d.** The diagnosis of myxedema, due to long-standing hypothyroidism in adults, is warranted. The clinical manifestations are those listed in above with the question. Myxedema can result from the many causes of hypothyroidism: Hashimoto's thyroiditis, idiopathic primary hypothyroidism, iodine deficiency, drugs, pituitary lesions, hypothalamic lesions, and damage to the thyroid by surgery or radiation.

5. A 50-year-old woman develops swelling in her neck and diarrhea. X-ray shows dense calcification in her thyroid. Physician asked her to have a nuclear scan and it showed a cold nodule that does not concentrate radioiodine. Her doctor does serum assays for several hormones. After the hormone is assayed, he tells her general practitioner that the patient probably has medullary carcinoma of the thyroid since one of the hormones is markedly raised. What hormone did the physician order?
   (a) Calcitonin
   (b) Thyroid-stimulating hormone
   (c) Thyroid hormone
   (d) Parathyroid hormone

   **Answer is a.** Medullary thyroid cancer is a malignancy of the thyroid parafollicular cells. Thyroid parafollicular cells normally produce the hormone calcitonin. A malignancy of these cells, therefore, can also produce calcitonin. Assay of calcitonin is a very good diagnostic test for medullary carcinoma of the thyroid. Thyroid-stimulating hormone is an anterior pituitary hormone and is not produced by the thyroid gland at all.

6. A patient with small-cell carcinoma of the lung complains of muscle weakness, fatigue, confusion, and weight gain. Serum sodium is found to be 115 mEq/L. Which of the following abnormal laboratory results would also be expected in this patient?
   (a) Decreased plasma atrial natriuretic peptide concentration
   (b) Decreased serum osmolarity
   (c) Decreased urinary sodium concentration
   (d) Increased plasma aldosterone concentration

   **Answer is b.** Bronchogenic carcinomas can secrete ectopic vasopressin (ADH), leading to the syndrome of inappropriate ADH (SIADH). As long as water intake is not decreased, the increased plasma vasopressin causes excessive water reabsorption by the renal distal tubule and collecting duct. The increased total body water can explain the weight gain. Edema is usually absent because the extra free water is distributed to both intracellular and extracellular volumes. The extra plasma water produces a dilutional hyponatremia, which can explain the weakness, fatigue, and confusion. There will also be a dilutional decrease in serum osmolarity. With SIADH, the urine sodium is usually increased compared to normal. This leads to an inappropriately concentrated urine. The volume expansion resulting from the excessive water retention may be responsible for the increased urinary sodium. Volume expansion would increase plasma ANP and increase renal sodium excretion. The volume expansion would also inhibit renin secretion from the kidney with subsequent decrease in plasma aldosterone. Decreased plasma aldosterone would then allow for increased renal excretion of sodium.

7. A 48-year-old woman presents with complaints of moderate weight loss over the past 4 months, heat intolerance, palpitations, and fine tremors in the hands. Physical examination reveals the presence of a diffuse goiter and exophthalmos. Which of the following laboratory findings would be expected in this individual?
   (a) Decreased serum $T_4$
   (b) Decreased resin $T_3$ uptake
   (c) Increased plasma concentration of thyroid-stimulating hormone
   (d) Increased plasma concentration of thyroglobulin

   **Answer is d.** The above case is of an individual with Graves' disease. Hypersecretion of thyroid hormone because of stimulation of the TSH receptor by thyroid-stimulating immunoglobulins results in excessive movement of thyroglobulin from the colloid to the plasma. The presence of exophthalmos is thought to be part of the autoimmune disorder in Graves' disease. It is postulated that the thyroid and orbital muscles may share a common antigen. Lymphocytic infiltration and inflammation of orbital muscle then produces the ophthalmopathy.

8. A 45-year-old man presents with complaints of recurrent headaches. He also admits to impotence and loss of libido that has gradually worsened during the past year. Visual field examination reveals a bitemporal hemianopsia. Laboratory examination reveals an increase in serum prolactin, while serum luteinizing hormone (LH) and testosterone are decreased. Which of the following is the most likely diagnosis?
    (a) Idiopathic panhypopituitarism
    (b) Pituitary infarction
    (c) Prolactinoma
    (d) LH deficiency

    **Answer is d.** Hyperprolactinemia is the most common hypothalamic pituitary disorder. A tumor in the pituitary (prolactinoma) that secretes excessive prolactin is the most common functional pituitary tumor. The increase in serum prolactin suppresses the normal GnRH-gonadotropin-gonadal steroid axis. Hypogonadism, manifested as amenorrhea in females or loss of libido and/or impotence in males, is a prominent symptom. Blood levels of sex steroids are usually decreased. Although not present in this patient, galactorrhea may occur due to the action of prolactin on the mammary gland. Since the anterior pituitary is located just below the optic chiasm, space-filling tumors that compress this structure may produce visual field defects.

9. At 26 weeks of pregnancy, an unidentified infection greatly compromises the viability of a developing fetus. The level of which of the following hormones in the mother's blood is most likely to be affected?
    (a) Human chorionic gonadotropin
    (b) Human chorionic somatomammotropin
    (c) Progesterone
    (d) Estriol

    **Answer is d.** Plasma levels of maternal estrogens during pregnancy are dependent on a functioning fetus. The fetal adrenal cortex and liver produce the weak androgens, DHEA-S and 16-OH DHEA-S, which are carried to the placenta by the fetal circulation. The placenta then desulfates the androgens and aromatizes them to estrogens (16-OH DHEA-S, estriol) prior to delivery to the maternal circulation. Estradiol and estrone increase approximately 50-fold during pregnancy, but estriol increases about 1000-fold. When estriol is assayed daily, a significant drop may be a sensitive early indicator of fetal jeopardy.

10. A patient with signs and symptoms consistent with hypothyroidism exhibits a decrease in both serum TSH and serum $T_4$. Injection of TRH fails to produce the expected increase in TSH. Which of the following is the most likely cause of the patient's hypothyroidism?
    (a) Secondary hypothyroidism
    (b) Hashimoto's thyroiditis
    (c) Iodine deficiency
    (d) Tertiary hypothyroidism

    **Answer is a.** A decrease in both serum $T_4$ and TSH could result from either a pituitary defect or a hypothalamic defect. In the case of the hypothalamic defect, decreased secretion of TRH leads to decreased TSH secretion and, hence, decreased $T_4$ secretion. In the secondary hypothyroidism, a decrease in TSH secretion due to a pituitary defect is responsible for the decreased $T_4$. The TRH stimulation test can be used to distinguish between these two possibilities. Failure of TSH to increase after injection of TRH indicates a pituitary defect.

## MULTIPLE CHOICE QUESTIONS

1. **Binding of hormones to receptor activates:**
    (a) Glycoprotein
    (b) G protein
    (c) M protein
    (d) Lipoproteins

2. **The hormonal action on the target organs depends on all the following factors, *except*:**
    (a) Cyclic AMP
    (b) Adenylate cyclase
    (c) Receptor
    (d) ADP

3. **Which of the following is NOT an anterior pituitary hormone:**
    (a) Prolactin
    (b) Follicle-stimulating hormone
    (c) Antidiuretic hormone
    (d) Alpha-melanocyte-stimulating hormone

4. **Human growth hormone is also called:**
   - (a) Cortisol
   - (b) Somatomammotropin
   - (c) Alpha-melanocyte-stimulating hormone
   - (d) Somatotropin
5. **Concerning prolactin, all of the following statements are true, *except*:**
   - (a) Hypoprolactinemia is a cause of infertility in females
   - (b) It is a protein of 198 amino acids
   - (c) Its secretion is stimulated by TRH
   - (d) Its secretion is repressed by dopamine
6. **Vasopressin:**
   - (a) Is secreted from anterior pituitary gland
   - (b) Deficiency results in diabetes mellitus
   - (c) Deficiency occurs due to basal skull fractures
   - (d) Deficiency leads to oliguria
7. **Which one of the following is not a hypothyroid disease?**
   - (a) Cretinism
   - (b) Myxedema
   - (c) Graves' disease
   - (d) Goiter
8. **Concerning the hypothyroidism, one of the following is incorrect:**
   - (a) Sensitivity to heat
   - (b) Rapid heart rate
   - (c) Increased BMR
   - (d) Reduced TSH
9. **Concerning calcium homeostasis by PTH, all of the following statements are true, *except*:**
   - (a) It increases the resorption bone
   - (b) It reduces renal clearance or excretion of calcium during hypocalcemia
   - (c) It acts upon the intestine to increase $Ca^{2+}$ absorption
   - (d) It increases renal phosphate clearance
10. **Concerning the glucocorticoids, all of the following statements are true, *except*:**
    - (a) It stimulates glycolysis
    - (b) It has antiinflammatory effect
    - (c) It prevents the rejection of transplanted organs
    - (d) It is used to control asthma
11. **Cushing's syndrome:**
    - (a) Results from deficiency of glucocorticoids
    - (b) Presents with low blood glucose
    - (c) Is sensitive to infection
    - (d) Means that patients have obesity
12. **Cohn's syndrome results from the deficiency of:**
    - (a) Elevated aldosterone
    - (b) Elevated cortisol
    - (c) Reduced mineralocorticoids
    - (d) Reduced dopamine
13. **Concerning the adrenal gland hormones, one of the following statements is incorrect:**
    - (a) They are derived from tyrosine
    - (b) They rise the blood pressure
    - (c) Elevated BMR
    - (d) Reduced ACTH secretion from the anterior pituitary
14. **Insulin:**
    - (a) Stimulates gluconeogenesis
    - (b) Is synthesized directly
    - (c) Inhibits lipolysis
    - (d) Increases the uptake of glucose from the peripheral cells
15. **Concerning the estrogen, all of the following are true, *except*:**
    - (a) Stimulates the mammary gland
    - (b) Increases the adipose tissue fat
    - (c) Participates in pregnancy if it occurs
    - (d) Broadens the pelvis

16. **All of the following are the adrenal gland hormones, *except*:**
    (a) Epinephrine
    (b) ADH
    (c) Mineralocorticoids
    (d) Glucocorticoids
17. **Which one of the following does not secret steroid hormones?**
    (a) Ovary
    (b) Testes
    (c) Adrenal medulla
    (d) Placenta
18. **Receptors within cell cytoplasm are specific to:**
    (a) Peptide hormones
    (b) Protein hormones
    (c) Catecholamine
    (d) Cortisol
19. **The maximum number of hormone-secreting cells of anterior pituitary are:**
    (a) Thyrotropes
    (b) Corticotropes
    (c) Lactotropes
    (d) Somatotropes
20. **Which of the following is rapid acting?**
    (a) $T_4$
    (b) TBG
    (c) $T_3$
    (d) Thyroglobulin
21. **In myxedema, serum findings are all except:**
    (a) Low $T_3$, $T_4$
    (b) High TSH
    (c) Low cholesterol
    (d) Normal creatinine
22. **Conversion of vitamin $D_3$ to 1–25 dihydroxycholecalciferol occurs in:**
    (a) Kidney
    (b) Adrenal cortex
    (c) Bone
    (d) Intestine
23. **Thyroid hormone:**
    (a) Decreases the absorption of carbohydrate from the intestine
    (b) Exerts a positive feedback action on TSH production
    (c) Indirectly increases the nitrogen excretion
    (d) Does not have any action on the cardiac muscle
24. **Concerning aldosterone, one of the following statements is incorrect:**
    (a) Deficiency results in hypotension
    (b) Increases sodium reabsorption from urine
    (c) Release is stimulated by an increase in angiotensin II
    (d) Is secreted by the zona fasciculata
25. **Concerning Insulin, all the following are true, *except*:**
    (a) Stimulates glycolysis in liver
    (b) Stimulates lipogenesis in liver and fat tissues
    (c) Is synthesized in the endoplasmic reticulum of the beta cells
    (d) Receptors are increased in the presence of uremia
26. **Calcitonin:**
    (a) Is produced by the parafollicular cells outside the thyroid glands
    (b) Is a steroid hormone
    (c) Is decreased in the presence of hypercalcemia
    (d) Increases incorporation of calcium into bone matrix
27. **Parathyroid hormone:**
    (a) Is not a peptide hormone
    (b) Is released in response to hypocalcemia
    (c) Increases phosphate reabsorption in the kidneys
    (d) Increases calcium excretion in the kidneys

28. **Amyloidosis:**
    (a) The protein stained with eosin
    (b) The deposition is intracellular
    (c) Has a polymorphous structure
    (d) All types are seen in 15% of patients with multiple myeloma

| ANSWERS | | | | | | | | | |
|---|---|---|---|---|---|---|---|---|---|
| 1. b | 2. d | 3. c | 4. d | 5. a | 6. c | 7. c | 8. b |
| 9. d | 10. a | 11. d | 12. a | 13. d | 14. c | 15. a | 16. b |
| 17. c | 18. d | 19. d | 20. c | 21. c | 22. a | 23. c | 24. d |
| 25. d | 26. d | 27. b | 28. d | | | | |

# Chapter 14

# Immunochemistry

## LEARNING OBJECTIVES

*At the end of this chapter students should be able to:*

- Know about humoral and cellular immunity, antigen and vaccine development, types of vaccines, and the role of recombinant DNA technology in the development of vaccine
- Explain the structure, types, and functions of immunoglobulin
- Describe the process of antibody production
- Explain multiple myeloma and human leukocyte antigen (HLA).

## Introduction

Immunology is the study of the immune system and is a very important branch of the medical and biological sciences. The immune system protects us from infection through various lines of defense. If the immune system does not function as it should, it can result in disease, such as autoimmunity, allergy, and cancer. It is also now becoming clear that immune responses contribute to the development of many common disorders not traditionally viewed as immunologic, including metabolic, cardiovascular, and neurodegenerative conditions.

From Edward Jenner's pioneering work in the 18th century that would ultimately lead to vaccination in its modern form to the many scientific breakthroughs in the 19th and 20th centuries that would lead to safe organ transplantation, the identification of blood groups, and the now ubiquitous use of monoclonal antibodies throughout science and health care, immunology has changed the face of modern medicine. Immunological research continues to extend horizons in our understanding of how to treat significant health issues, with ongoing research efforts in immunotherapy, autoimmune diseases, and vaccines for emerging pathogens, such as Ebola.

## Humoral and Cellular Immunity

There are two main mechanisms of immunity within the adaptive immune system—humoral and cellular.

**Humoral immunity** is also called antibody-mediated immunity. With assistance from helper T cells, B cells will differentiate into plasma B cells that can produce antibodies against a specific antigen. The humoral immune system deals with antigens from pathogens that are freely circulating, or outside the infected cells. Antibodies produced by the B cells will bind to antigens, neutralizing them, or causing lysis (dissolution or destruction of cells by a lysin) or phagocytosis.

**Cellular immunity** occurs inside infected cells and is mediated by T lymphocytes (the name refers to the organ from which they are produced—the thymus). The antigens are expressed on the cell surface or on an antigen-presenting cell. Helper T cells release cytokines that help activated T cells bind to the infected cells' major histocompatibility complex (MHC)-antigen complex and differentiate the T cell into a cytotoxic T cell. The infected cell then undergoes lysis.

# Vaccine Development

The process of taking a new **antigen** or immunogen identified in the research process and **developing** this substance into a final **vaccine** that can be evaluated through preclinical and clinical studies to determine the safety and efficacy of the final **vaccine**.

## Vaccination

It is the administration of a **vaccine** to help the immune system develop protection from a disease. **Vaccines** contain a microorganism or virus in a weakened or killed state, or proteins or toxins from the organism.

**There are four main types of vaccines:**
1. Live-attenuated vaccines
2. Inactivated vaccines
3. Subunit, recombinant, polysaccharide, and conjugate vaccines
4. Toxoid vaccines

A **recombinant vaccine** is a **vaccine** produced through **recombinant DNA technology**. This involves inserting the **DNA** encoding an antigen (such as a bacterial surface protein) that stimulates an immune response into bacterial or mammalian cells, expressing the antigen in these cells and then purifying it from them.

**What are immunoglobulins? Explain the structure of it.**

# Immunoglobulin

The defense strategies of the body are collectively known as immunity.

Two types of immunity identified as explained above:
1. Cellular immunity: This is mediated by T lymphocytes or T cells (thymic origin).
2. Humoral immunity: This is mediated by a specialized group of proteins known as immunoglobulins or antibodies.
   - The B lymphocytes or B cells (mature in bone) are responsible for the production of immunoglobulins.

The immunoglobulins are also known as gamma-globulins.
- Protective in function
- Function as antibodies
- Synthesized in response to a foreign substance called antigen
- Provide immunity
  - Five different types of immunoglobulins.
  - They are IgA, IgG, IgM, IgD, and IgE [remember it as Government (IgG) MADE] **(Table 14.1)**.

**Table 14.1:** Different types of immunoglobulin and their properties.

| Type | Heavy chains | Light chains | Serum conc. mg% | Placental transfer |
|---|---|---|---|---|
| IgG | γ | κ or λ | 800–1500 | + |
| IgM | μ | κ or λ | 50–200 | – |
| IgA | α | κ or λ | 150–400 | – |
| IgD | δ | κ or λ | 1–10 | – |
| IgE | ε | κ or λ | 0.02–0.05 | – |

## Structure of Immunoglobulin

- All the immunoglobulin molecules consist of two identical heavy (H) chains MW = 53,000–75,000 and two identical light (L) chains MW = 23,000.
- They are held together by disulfide bridges **(Fig. 14.1)**.

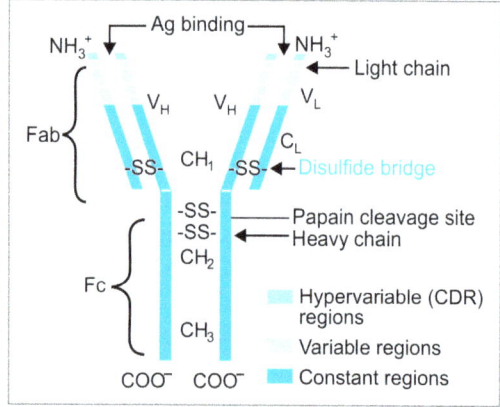

**Fig. 14.1:** Structure of immunoglobulin.

- Heavy chains of immunoglobulins are linked to carbohydrates; hence, immunoglobulins are glycoproteins.
- Each chain (L or H) of Ig has two regions (domains), namely the constant and the variable.
- The amino-terminal half of the light chain is the variable region ($V_L$).
- The carboxy-terminal half is the constant region ($C_L$).
- There are five types of heavy chains: $\alpha$, $\delta$, $\varepsilon$, $\gamma$, and $\mu$.
- Light chains are of two types: kappa ($\kappa$) and lambda ($\lambda$).
- One quarter of the amino-terminal region of heavy chain is variable ($V_H$). The remaining three quarters are constant ($CH_1$, $CH_2$, and $CH_3$).
- The amino acid sequence of variable regions of light and heavy chains is responsible for the specific binding of immunoglobulin (antibody) with antigen.
- There are certain hypervariable regions within the variable regions of $V_L$ and $V_H$.
- Light chains have three hypervariable regions.
- Heavy chains have four hypervariable regions.
- The hypervariable regions more specifically determine the antigen-binding site.

## Functions of Immunoglobulin

The main function of immunoglobulin (antibodies) is to protect body against infectious agents.

The immunoglobulins are able to provide resistance because they can neutralize viruses, opsonize microbes (the process by which antibodies make microorganisms more easily ingested by phagocytic cells) and activate complement, and prevent the attachment of microbes to mucosal surfaces.

Immunoglobulins act in direct and indirect way to protect the body against infections.

### Direct Effect

Binding of antigen via antigen-binding fragment of antibody (Fab) results in any one of the methods mentioned below:
- Precipitation of soluble antigens
- Agglutination by the cross-linking of particulate antigens (viruses or bacteria).
- Neutralization: By blocking of the attachment of viruses or bacterial toxins to membrane receptors, in which the antibodies cover the toxic sites of the antigenic substance.
- Lysis of the cell membrane of the organisms to destroy them.

### Indirect Effect

It is through the activation of the complement system, which is mediated through complement-binding site (Fc).

Indirect action is stronger compared to direct effect.

The binding of one of the complement molecules to Fc portion results in any one of the following:
- Opsonization and phagocytosis: Activation of neutrophils and macrophages to engulf bacteria.
- Chemotaxis (movement of large number of phagocytes to the site of antigenic agent).
- Agglutination of foreign bodies
- Neutralization
- Activation of mast cells and basophils liberates histamine. This histamine dilates the blood vessels and increases capillary permeability. This results in the entry of plasma proteins from the blood to tissues to inactivate the antigenic products.

**What are the different types of immunoglobulins? Explain with their functions.**

## IgG

It comprises the following:
* Composed of a single unit (monomer).
* Major immunoglobulin of plasma (75–80%).
* Produced in response to various infections and protects the body against infections.

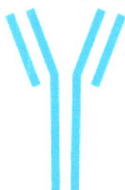

* IgG can cross the placenta from the mother's blood to the fetus and provide immunity to the fetus.
* It triggers foreign cell destruction mediated by complement system.

## IgA

It comprises the following:

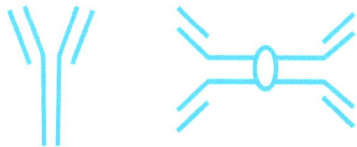

* It occurs as a single (monomer) or double unit (dimer) held together by J chain.
* It is produced by the secretary cells of the respiratory tract, digestive tract, urinary tract, etc., and is present in the mucous secretions of these cells.
* It prevents the entry of bacteria into the body through these cells.

## IgM

It comprises the following:
* Largest immunoglobulin composed of 5 Y-shaped units held together by a J polypeptide chain.
* It cannot traverse blood vessels; hence, it is restricted to bloodstream.
* It is the first antibody to be produced whenever bacteria or virus attack the body.
* It is also produced in the fetal stage itself.

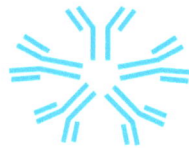

## IgD

It comprises the following:
* It is composed of single Y-shaped unit.
* It is present in very small amount.
* IgD molecules are present on the surface of B cells.
* The synthesis and function of this are still unknown.

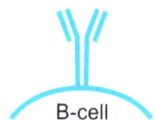

## IgE

It comprises the following:
* It is composed of single Y-shaped monomer.
* IgE molecules tightly bind with mast cells which release histamine and cause allergy.
* It is produced by the plasma cells of the respiratory tract.
* It increases in allergic diseases.

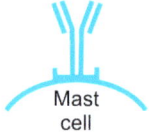

## ■ Mechanism of Antibody Production

The following animal model experiment explains the mechanism of antibody production (**Fig. 14.2**).

A mouse is immunized by injection of an antigen X to stimulate the production of antibodies targeted against X. The antibody-forming cells are isolated from the mouse's spleen.

Monoclonal antibodies are produced by fusing single antibody–forming cells to tumor

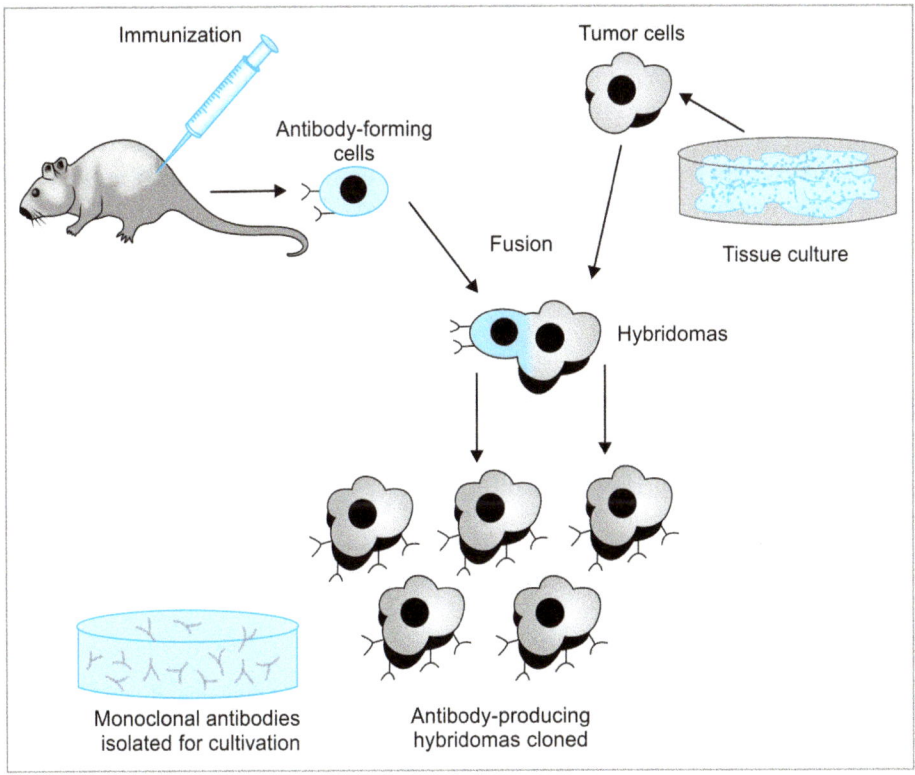

**Fig. 14.2:** Mechanism of antibody production.

cells grown in culture. The resulting cell is called a hybridoma.

Each hybridoma produces relatively large quantities of identical antibody molecules. By allowing the hybridoma to multiply in culture, it is possible to produce a population of cells, each of which produces identical antibody molecules. These antibodies are called "monoclonal antibodies" because they are produced by the identical offspring of a single, cloned antibody-producing cell.

Once a monoclonal antibody is made, it can be used as a specific probe to track down and purify the specific protein that induced its formation.

## Immunoglobulins: Blood Test

This test measures the amount of immunoglobulins, also known as antibodies, in the blood. Antibodies are proteins made by the immune system to fight disease-causing substances, such as viruses and bacteria. Our body makes different types of immunoglobulins to fight different types of these substances.

An immunoglobulins test usually measures three specific types of immunoglobulins. They are called IgG, IgM, and IgA. If these immunoglobulins are too low or too high, it may be a sign of a serious health problem.

## Quantitative Determination of Serum Immunoglobulins in Antibody-Agar Plates Radial Immunodiffusion Method

The antibody in agar plate test has proved valuable for the quantitative measurement of individual serum immunoglobulins. With this technique, specific antiserum is mixed uniformly in an agar gel plate. Antigen-containing solutions are placed in small antigen wells cut in the agar. A concentric ring of antigen-antibody precipitate forms around the antigen well. By graphically comparing the ring diameters with those of appropriate standards, the protein concentration of the test sera can be determined. This procedure has been used to quantify protein concentrations as low as 0.003 mg/mL. Multiple samples can be easily tested.

## A Sensitive Tube Method Developed by Eva and Peter

A sensitive and simple method for the quantitative determination of antibodies is reported. Tubes coated with antigen are incubated with antiserum followed by an enzyme-labeled preparation of anti-immunoglobulin. The enzyme remaining in the tubes after washing provides a measure of the amount of specific antibodies in the serum. Coating of polystyrene tubes with antigen is described, as well as the preparation of specifically purified antibodies against rabbit IgG, and their conjugation to alkaline phosphatase.

When rabbit antisera against human serum albumin or against the dinitrophenyl group were incubated in tubes coated with antigen, less than 1 ng/mL of specific antibody could be detected in both systems.

Antibodies in unknown sera could be quantitated by comparison with a standard antiserum.

## Quantitative Determination of Serum Immunoglobulin by Enzyme-linked Immunosorbent Assay

In enzyme-linked immunosorbent assay (ELISA) technique, enzymes are used to label the antigens in place of radioactive isotopes in RIA.

The presence of antigen-specific antibodies can be detected in an antigen-specific ELISA in which the plate is coated with the antigen. The total amount of immunoglobulin (e.g., IgG) can be quantified in a sandwich ELISA using immunoglobulin-specific antibodies (e.g., anti-IgG) for capture and detection. Antibodies directly conjugated to an enzyme can be used for detection of total IgG, IgA, and IgM, whereas the use of biotinylated detection antibody together with streptavidin-conjugated enzyme is the optimum method for detection of total IgE.

There are two types of methods in ELISA.

1. **Single antibody method (competitive binding method)**

    Principle

    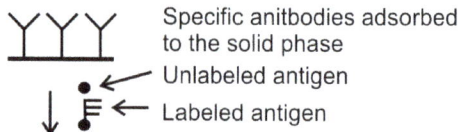
    Specific anitbodies adsorbed to the solid phase
    Unlabeled antigen
    Labeled antigen

    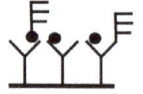
    Labeled and unlabeled antigen bound to the antibody

    ↓ Substrate for enzyme added and plates incubated

    **Enzyme activity measured**

2. **Double antibody method**

    Principle

    Specific antibodies to the solid phase

    ↓ Putative antigen solution added; incubated and then washed

    Specific antigen bound

    ↓ Enzyme labeled specific antibody added, incubated and washed

    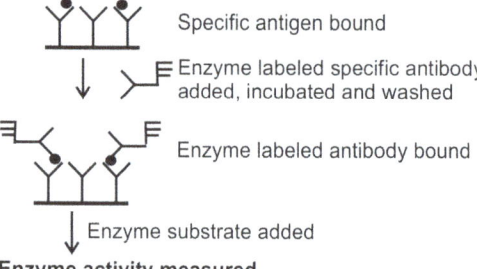
    Enzyme labeled antibody bound

    ↓ Enzyme substrate added

    **Enzyme activity measured**

# Quantitative Determination of Serum Immunoglobulin by Immunoelectrophoresis

Immunoelectrophoresis is a technique used to detect the presence of monoclonal immunoglobulin proteins and to evaluate for immune system disorders.

Immunoelectrophoresis consists of a combination of an electrophoretic step with the subsequent precipitation of antigen–antibody complexes (immunoprecipitates). The most common procedures in the analysis rely upon the migration of antigenic proteins through or into an antibody-containing gel. Buffers and pH values are usually chosen so that only the antigens migrate, and the antibodies either do not move at all or, at most, migrate only very slowly and thus remain evenly distributed throughout the gel during the whole electrophoresis. The most popular techniques are as follows:

## Grabar/Williams Method

It is the classical method of immunoelectrophoresis. Proteins are separated by electrophoresis, then antibodies are applied in a trough next to the separated proteins and immunoprecipitates are formed after a period of diffusion of the separated proteins and antibodies against each other.

## Crossed Immunoelectrophoresis

It is also called two-dimensional quantitative immunoelectrophoresis *ad modum* Clarke and Freeman or *ad modum* Laurell. In this method, the proteins are first separated during the first dimension electrophoresis, then instead of the diffusion toward the antibodies, the proteins are electrophoresed into an antibody-containing gel in the second dimension. Immunoprecipitation will take place during the second dimension electrophoresis and the immunoprecipitates have a characteristic bell shape, each precipitate representing one antigen, the position of the precipitate being dependent on the amount of protein as well as the amount of specific antibody in the gel, so relative quantification can be performed.

## Laurell Rocket Technique

In this antigen, proteins are transported electrophoretically through a gel slab containing antibodies at a pH value at which the antibodies remain essentially immobile, resulting in the formation of "rocket"-shaped precipitate peaks, the height and area of which are linearly related to the antigen concentration. These techniques allow quantitative analysis of antigens but are not applicable to complex mixtures.

## Fused Rocket Immunoelectrophoresis

It is a modification of one-dimensional quantitative immunoelectrophorsis used for the detailed measurement of proteins in fractions from protein separation experiments.

## Affinity Immunoelectrophoresis

This is based on changes in the electrophoretic pattern of proteins through specific interaction or complex formation with other macromolecules or ligands. Affinity immunoelectrophoresis has been used for estimation of binding constants, as for instance with lectins or for characterization of proteins with specific features such as glycan content or ligand binding. Some variants of affinity immunoelectrophoresis are similar to affinity chromatography by the use of immobilized ligands.

**An immunoglobulins blood test may be used to help diagnose a variety of conditions, including:**

- Bacterial or viral infections.
- Immunodeficiency, a condition that reduces the body's ability to fight infections and other diseases.
- An autoimmune disorder, such as rheumatoid arthritis or lupus. An autoimmune

disorder causes system to attack healthy cells, tissues, and/or organs by mistake.
* Certain types of cancer, such as multiple myeloma.
* Infections in newborns.

## Hypogammaglobulinemia

Serum immunoglobulin tests are used for the evaluation of antibody (humoral) immunodeficiency. A low level of immunoglobulin is termed "hypogammaglobulinemia."

**Causes of secondary or acquired hypogammaglobulinemia:**

Conditions that cause an abnormal loss or increased catabolism of immunoglobulin:
* Nephrotic syndrome and other severe renal diseases
* Severe burns
* Sepsis
* Protein-losing enteropathy
* Intestinal lymphangiectasia.

Conditions/factors affecting immunoglobulin production:
* Nutritional due to malnutrition or alcoholism.
* Drugs such as phenytoin, carbamazepine, immunosuppressive drugs, or chemotherapy agents.
* Malignancies, especially hematological malignancies (chronic lymphocytic leukemia, lymphoma, and multiple myeloma).
* Rheumatological disease, including rheumatoid arthritis or systemic lupus erythematosus (SLE).
* Viruses, including HIV, Epstein–Barr virus, rubella, cytomegalovirus.

## Hypergammaglobulinemia

**Causes of increased immunoglobulin levels:**

Polyclonal increase in any or all of the three classes (IgG, IgA, and/or IgM):
* Infections, acute and chronic (including HIV, Epstein–Barr virus, and cytomegalovirus).
* Connective tissue diseases (rheumatoid arthritis, SLE, and scleroderma).
* Chronic active autoimmune hepatitis (IgG)
* Primary biliary cirrhosis (IgM)
* Hematologic disorders

Monoclonal increase in one class with or without decrease in other two classes:

Monoclonal (discrete) hypergammaglobulinemia is a group of disorders characterized by an abnormal benign or malignant proliferation of a single clone of B lymphocytes and or plasma cells that produce homogeneous monoclonal immunoglobulins.

The discrete dense immunoglobulin bands seen with serum electrophoresis are known as paraprotein or monoclonal components.

This is due to the production of a single immunoglobulin fragment (light or heavy chain) by a single clone B cell.
* Multiple myeloma (IgG, IgA, and rarely IgM).
* Monoclonal gammopathy of uncertain significance.
* Chronic lymphocytic leukemia
* Non-Hodgkin lymphoma
* Waldenström's macroglobulinemia (IgM)
* Primary systemic amyloidosis
* Monoclonal cryoglobulinemia
* Benign paraproteinemia

## Multiple Myeloma

This is a malignant disease of the plasma cell.

In this case, one type of plasma cell multiplies abnormally and produces one type of immunoglobulin (IgG or IgA) in excess quantities.

The electrophoresis of such a serum shows a thick deeply stained protein band in the $\gamma$-globulin region. This band is called "M" band.

### The Biochemical Findings

The biochemical findings of multiple myeloma are increased total proteins, decreased albumin, and increased globulins and $Ca^{2+}$ levels in plasma. Some cases of multiple myeloma patients excrete light chains of immunoglobulins in the urine which are known as Bence-Jones proteins.

*Bence-Jones Proteins*
It comprises the following:
* Bence-Jones proteins are light chain fragments of immunoglobulins, which are excreted in urine, in some cases of multiple myeloma.
* It was discovered in the urine by its characteristic behavior on heating.
* Bence-Jones proteins precipitate between 40 and 60°C. But as the temperature increases above 60°C the protein redissolves. Again on cooling the protein gets precipitated.

## Waldenström's Macroglobulinemia

It is a malignant disease of the lymphoid elements, characterized by high serum level of IgM.

## Amyloidosis

It is characterized by the deposition of insoluble fibrillar protein complexes in various tissues.

The deposition may contain fragments of light chains. This also occurs in multiple myeloma.

## Cryoglobulinemia

Cryoglobulin is a serum IgM protein that precipitates at temperature lower than body temperature.

The patients with this disorder may develop thrombosis in cold environment.

Therefore, the cryoglobulin examination maintenance of 37°C is very important during blood collection.

## Benign Paraproteinemia

In this condition, paraproteins are found in patients, where there is no association of pathological features.

It may be transient occurs during acute infection and in autoimmune diseases due to antigen stimulation.

Or it may be persistent due to a benign tumor of B cells.

## Human Leukocyte Antigen

The HLA region, located on the short arm of chromosome 6, is a highly polymorphic region containing about 200 genes. The HLA system is the name of the MHC in humans **(Fig. 14.3)**.

The super locus contains a large number of genes related to immune system function in humans. This group of genes resides on chromosome 6 and encodes cell-surface antigen-presenting proteins and many other genes. The proteins encoded by certain genes are also known as antigens.

The major HLA antigens are essential elements in immune function.

Different classes have different functions. The Class I proteins, classically involved in presenting endogenous antigens to CD8+ T cells, are expressed by genes located in the HLA-A, -B, and -C loci. In contrast, the Class

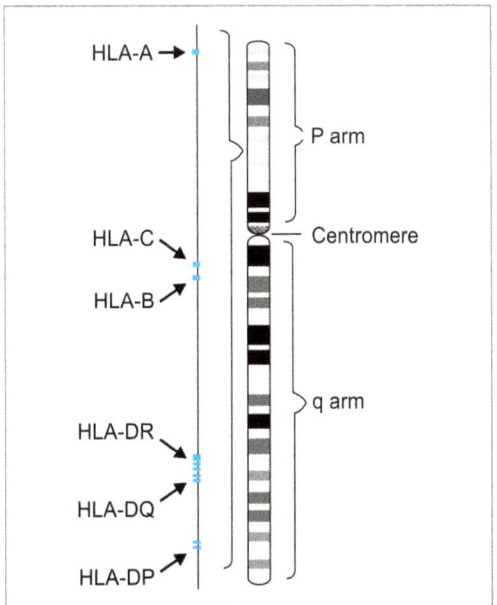

**Fig. 14.3:** HLA region of chromosome 6. (HLA: human leukocyte antigen)

II proteins, which associate with and present exogenous antigens to CD4+ T cells, are expressed by the HLA-DR, -DQ, and -DP loci.

HLAs have other roles. They are sometimes involved in mate selection. They may protect against or allow cancer. They may mediate autoimmune disease.

HLA in human population is one aspect of disease defense, and, as a result, the chance of two unrelated individuals having identical HLA molecules on all loci is very low. Historically, HLA genes were identified as a result of the ability to successfully transplant organs between HLA similar individuals.

## Human Leukocyte Antigen Typing

HLA typing refers to the tissue type matching for transplant purposes.

HLA antigens are detected on the surface of white cells (leukocytes), from blood specimen, but they reside on the surface of all body cells.

These antigens regulate how the body can recognize and reject foreign tissues.

The phasing out of serological tissue typing and its replacement with DNA-based tissue typing has increased the accuracy and specificity of HLA typing, which allows for more precise HLA matching between donors and transplant patients.

Several large-scale studies have demonstrated that more precise HLA matching between donor and patient significantly:
- Improves overall transplant survival.
- Reduces the incidence and severity of both acute and chronic graft-versus-host disease
- Improves rates of engraftment.
- Studies on HLA and transplant outcome have also demonstrated HLA loci which are critical to match in order to maximize the success of hematopoietic cell transplantation. Although matching at the three HLA loci traditionally associated with hematopoietic cell transplantation (HLA-A, -B, and -DR) can lead to successful transplantation outcomes, recent research has shown matching at HLA-C can also improve outcome.

## Examining Human Leukocyte Antigen Types Serotyping

In order to create a typing reagent, blood from animals or humans would be taken, the blood cells allowed to separate from the serum, and the serum diluted to its optimal sensitivity and used to type cells from other individuals or animals. Thus serotyping became a way of crudely identifying HLA receptors and receptor isoforms.

## Gene Sequencing

Minor reactions to subregions that show similarity to other types can be observed to the gene products of alleles of a serotype group. The sequence of the antigens determines the antibody reactivates and so having a good sequencing capability (or sequence-based typing) obviates then need for serological reactions. Therefore, different serotype reactions may indicate the need to sequence persons HLA to determine a new gene sequence.

## Phenotyping

Gene typing is different from gene sequencing and serotyping. With this strategy, PCR primers specific to a variant region of DNA are used (called SSP-PCR), if a product of the right size is found, the assumption is that the HLA allele has been identified.

## Haplotypes

An HLA haplotype is a series of HLA "genes" (loci-alleles) by chromosome, one passed from the mother and father.

These haplotypes can be used to trace migrations in the human population because they are often much like a fingerprint of an event that has occurred in evolution.

## Antibodies

HLA antibodies are typically not naturally occurring, with few exceptions are formed as a result of an immunologic challenge of a foreign material containing non-self HLAs via blood transfusion, pregnancy (paternally inherited antigens), or organ or tissue transplant.

Antibodies against disease associated HLA haplotypes have been proposed as a treatment for severe autoimmune diseases.

Donor-specific HLA antibodies have been found to be associated with graft failure in kidney, heart, lung, and liver transplantation.

## SUMMARY

Immunology is the study of the immune system and is a very important branch of the medical and biological sciences. There are two main mechanisms of immunity within the adaptive immune system—humoral and cellular. Vaccination is the administration of a vaccine to help the immune system develop protection from a disease. Vaccines contain a microorganism or virus in a weakened or killed state, or proteins or toxins from the organism. There are four main types of vaccines: live-attenuated vaccines; inactivated vaccines; subunit, recombinant, polysaccharide, and conjugate vaccines; and toxoid vaccines. Immunoglobulins provide immunity; hence, they are considered as antibodies. There are five types of immunoglobulins such as IgG, IgM, IgA, IgD, and IgE. They are classified on the basis of heavy chains. Hypergammaglobulinemia means elevated gamma globulins in the blood and this will be seen in inflammation and diseases such as multiple myeloma, a plasma cell cancer. Reduced level of immunoglobulins is hypogammaglobulinemia. Human leukocyte antigen (HLA) typing refers to the tissue type matching for transplant purposes. The HLA region, located on the short arm of chromosome 6, is a highly polymorphic region containing about 200 genes. HLA antigens are detected on the surface of white cells (leukocytes), from blood specimen, but they reside on the surface of all body cells.

## SELF-ASSESSMENT QUESTIONS

1. How do you differentiate humoral and cellular immunity?
2. Discuss the structure of immunoglobulin.
3. List the functions of immunoglobulin.
4. What is vaccination?
5. Briefly explain, how the antibody can be developed using mouse model.
6. List the different immunoelectrophoresis methods for the quantitative determination of immunoglobulin.

## MULTIPLE CHOICE QUESTIONS

1. Which of the following immunoglobulin will be elevated in blood during allergies?
   a. IgA
   b. IgD
   c. IgE
   d. IgM
2. In which of the following procedure enzyme will be tagged to antigen for the determination of immunoglobulin?
   a. RIA
   b. FIA
   c. MEIA
   d. ELISA

3. The first immunoglobulin formed when bacteria or virus enters the body is:
   a. IgA
   b. IgM
   c. IgD
   d. IgE
4. All of the following will be seen with the blood sample of multiple myeloma patients, *except*:
   a. Elevated level of calcium
   b. High gamma globulin
   c. Presence of Bence jones protein in urine
   d. High albumin

### ANSWERS

1. c    2. d    3. b    4. d

# Chapter 15: Free Radicals and Antioxidants

## LEARNING OBJECTIVES

*At the end of this chapter students should be able to:*
- Understand about the free radicals and their effects
- Know about different types of antioxidants available in the body to scavenge the free radicals and preventing the cellular damage

## Introduction

Free radicals are chemical species possessing an unpaired electron that can be considered as fragments of molecules and which are generally very reactive **(Fig. 15.1)**.

The free radicals are produced continuously in cells either as accidental by-products of metabolism or deliberately during phagocytosis.

The main danger from free radicals comes from the damage they can do when they react with important cellular components such as DNA or the cell membrane.

Reactive radicals formed within cells can oxidize biomolecules and lead to cell death and tissue injury.

To prevent free-radical damage, the body has a defense system of **antioxidants**. These include enzymes to decompose peroxides, proteins to sequester transition metals and a range of compounds to "scavenge" free radicals.

**How free radicals are formed?**
- Normally, bonds do not split in a way that leaves a molecule with an odd, unpaired electron. But, when weak bonds split, free radicals are formed.

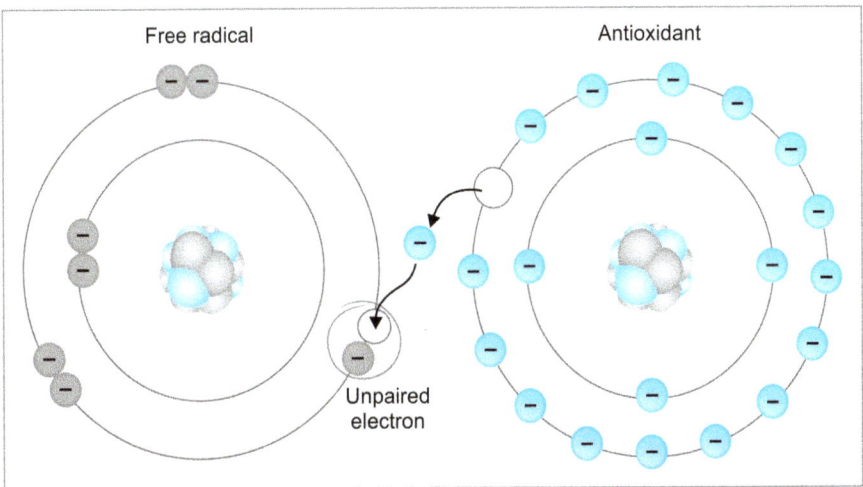

**Fig. 15.1:** Free radical and antioxidant.

- Free radicals are very unstable and react quickly with other compounds, trying to capture the needed electron to gain stability. Generally, free radicals attack the nearest stable molecule, taking its electron. When the "attacked" molecule loses its electron, it becomes a free radical itself, beginning a chain reaction. Once the process is started, it can cascade, finally resulting in the disruption of a living cell.
- Some free radicals arise normally during metabolism and sometimes the cells of the immune system purposefully create them to neutralize viruses and bacteria. However, environmental factors such as pollution, radiation, cigarette smoke, and herbicides can also spawn free radicals.

**Describe the reactive oxygen species.**

## Reactive Oxygen Species

There are many types of radicals, but those of most concern in biological systems are derived from oxygen and known collectively as *reactive oxygen species* (ROS). Oxygen has two unpaired electrons in separate orbitals in its outer shell. This electronic structure makes oxygen especially susceptible to radical formation.

Sequential reduction of molecular oxygen leads to formation of a group of ROS:
- **Superoxide anion**
- **Peroxide** (hydrogen peroxide)
- **Hydroxyl radical**

The structure of these radicals is shown in the figure below. One can observe the difference between hydroxyl radical and hydroxyl ion (not a radical) **(Fig. 15.2)**.

Another radical derived from oxygen is **singlet oxygen**, designated as $^1O_2$. This is an exciting form of oxygen in which one of the electrons jumps to a superior orbital following absorption of energy.

## Formation of Reactive Oxygen Species

Oxygen-derived radicals are generated constantly as part of normal aerobic life. They are formed in mitochondria as oxygen is reduced along the electron transport chain. ROS are also formed as necessary intermediates in a variety of enzyme reactions. Examples of situations in which oxygen radicals are overproduced in cells include:
- **White blood cells** such as neutrophils specialize in producing oxygen radicals, which are used in host defense to kill invading pathogens.
- **Cells exposed to abnormal environments** such as hypoxia or hyperoxia generate abundant and often damaging ROS. There are many drugs that have oxidizing effects on cells and lead to production of oxygen radicals.
- **Ionizing radiation** is well known to generate oxygen radicals within biological systems. Interestingly, the damaging effects of radiation are higher in well-oxygenated tissues than in tissues deficient in oxygen.

## Biological Effects of Reactive Oxygen

Free radicals are generated in a number of reactions essential to life and, as mentioned above, phagocytic cells generate radicals to kill invading pathogens.

Despite their beneficial activities, ROS clearly can be toxic to cells. By definition, radicals possess an unpaired electron, which

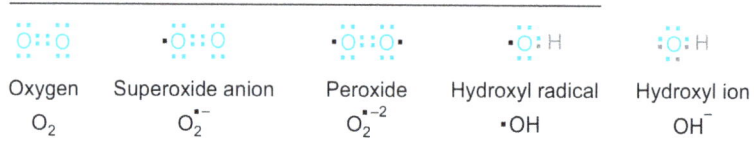

**Fig. 15.2:** Reactive oxygen species.

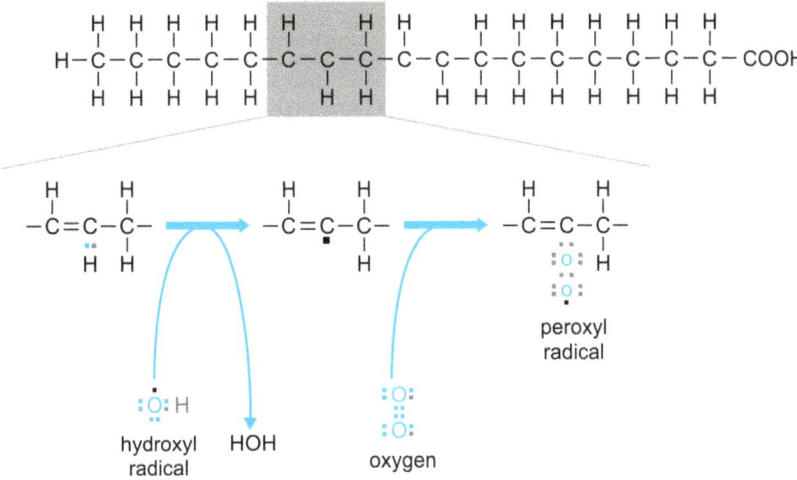

**Fig. 15.3:** Peroxidation reaction involving a fatty acid.

makes them highly reactive and thereby able to damage all macromolecules, including lipids, proteins, and nucleic acids.

One of the known toxic effects of oxygen radicals is damage to cellular membranes (plasma, mitochondrial, and endomembrane systems), which is initiated by a process known as *lipid peroxidation*. A common target for peroxidation is unsaturated fatty acids present in membrane phospholipids. A peroxidation reaction involving a fatty acid is depicted in **Figure 15.3**.

Reactions involving radicals occur in chain reactions. In **Figure 15.3**, the hydrogen is abstracted from the fatty acid by hydroxyl radical, leaving a carbon-centered radical as part of the fatty acid. The same radical then reacts with oxygen to yield the peroxy radical, which can then react with other fatty acids or proteins. Peroxidation of membrane lipids can:

* Increase membrane rigidity
* Decrease activity of membrane-bound enzymes (e.g. sodium pumps).
* Alter activity of membrane receptors
* Alter permeability

In addition to effects on phospholipids, radicals can also directly attack membrane proteins and induce lipid–lipid, lipid–protein, and protein–protein crosslinking, all of which obviously have effects on membrane function.

## Mechanisms for Protection against Radicals

Life on Earth evolved in the presence of oxygen and necessarily adapted by the evolution of a large battery of antioxidant systems. Some of these antioxidant molecules are present in all life forms examined, from bacteria to mammals, indicating their appearance early in the history of life.

Many antioxidants work by transiently becoming radicals themselves. These molecules are usually part of a larger network of cooperating antioxidants that end up regenerating the original antioxidant. For example, vitamin E becomes a radical but is regenerated through the activity of the antioxidants vitamin C and glutathione.

### ■ Antioxidants

* Antioxidants are involved in the prevention of cellular damage—the common pathway for cancer, aging, and a variety of diseases.
* An antioxidant is a molecule capable of slowing or preventing the oxidation of other molecules. Oxidation is a chemical reaction that transfers electrons from a substance to an oxidizing agent.
* Oxidation reactions can produce free radicals, which start chain reactions that

damage cells. Antioxidants terminate these chain reactions by removing free-radical intermediates and inhibit other oxidation reactions by being oxidized themselves.

- Plants and animals maintain complex systems of multiple types of antioxidants (e.g., glutathione, vitamin C, and vitamin E) as well as enzymes [e.g., catalase, superoxide dismutase (SOD)], and various peroxidases. Additionally, selenium is required for proper functioning of one of the body's antioxidant enzyme systems.
- The body cannot manufacture these micronutrients, so they must be supplied in the diet. Low levels of antioxidants, or inhibition of the antioxidant enzymes, cause oxidative stress and may damage or kill cells.
- Antioxidants are also widely used as ingredients in dietary supplements in maintaining health and preventing diseases (cancer and coronary heart disease). In addition to the uses of medicine, antioxidants have many industrial uses, such as preservatives in food and cosmetics.

## Enzymatic Antioxidants

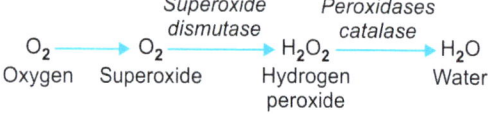

## Enzyme Systems

The released superoxide is first converted to hydrogen peroxide and then further reduced to water. This detoxification pathway is the result of multiple enzymes, with SODs catalyzing the first step and then catalases and various peroxidases removing hydrogen peroxide.

## Superoxide Dismutase

SODs are a class of closely related enzymes that catalyze the breakdown of the superoxide anion into oxygen and hydrogen peroxide. They are present in almost all aerobic cells and in extracellular fluids. SOD enzymes contain metal ion cofactors such as copper, zinc, manganese or iron that depending on the isoenzyme. In humans, the copper or zinc-dependent SOD is present in the cytosol, while manganese dependent SOD is present in the mitochondrion. There is a third form of SOD in extracellular fluids, which has copper and zinc in its active sites.

## Catalase

Catalases are enzymes that catalyze the conversion of hydrogen peroxide to water and oxygen, using either an iron or manganese cofactor. This protein is localized to peroxisomes in eukaryotic cells. It is an unusual enzyme; since hydrogen peroxide is its only substrate, it follows a ping-pong mechanism.

## Peroxiredoxins

Peroxiredoxins are peroxidases that catalyze the reduction of hydrogen peroxide, organic hydroperoxides, as well as peroxynitrite. They are divided into three classes—typical 2-cysteine peroxiredoxin, atypical 2-cysteine peroxiredoxins, and 1-cysteine peroxiredoxins. These enzymes share the same basic catalytic mechanism in which a redox-active cysteine (the peroxidatic cysteine) in the active site is oxidized to a sulfonic acid by the peroxide substrate.

## Thioredoxin and Glutathione Systems

The thioredoxin system contains the 12-kDa protein thioredoxin and its companion thioredoxin reductase. Proteins related to thioredoxin are present in all sequenced organisms, with plants such as *Arabidopsis thaliana* having a particularly great diversity of isoforms. In its active state, thioredoxin acts as an efficient reducing agent, scavenging ROS and maintaining other proteins in their reduced state. After being oxidized, the active thioredoxin is regenerated by the action of thioredoxin reductase, using NADPH as an electron donor.

## Glutathione

The glutathione system includes glutathione, glutathione reductase, glutathione peroxidases, and glutathione S-transferases. This system is found in animals, plants, and microorganisms. Glutathione peroxidase is an enzyme containing four selenium cofactors that catalyze the breakdown of hydrogen peroxide and organic hydroperoxides. There are at least four different glutathione peroxidase isozymes in animals. Glutathione peroxidase 1 is the most abundant and is a very efficient scavenger of hydrogen peroxide, while glutathione peroxidase 4 is most active with lipid hydroperoxides.

## Nonenzymatic Antioxidants

### Melatonin

Melatonin is a powerful antioxidant that can easily cross cell membranes and the blood–brain barrier. Unlike other antioxidants, melatonin does not undergo redox cycling, which is the ability of a molecule to undergo repeated reduction and oxidation.

### Vitamin E

- Vitamin E is the collective name for a set of eight related tocopherols and tocotrienols, with antioxidant properties.
- It is the abundant and efficient chain-breaking antioxidant available in the body (Fig. 15.4).
- Primary defender against oxidation and lipid peroxidation.

### Vitamin C

- Vitamin C is the most abundant water-soluble chain-breaking antioxidant in the body.
- It acts primarily in cellular fluid and combating free-radical formation caused by pollution and cigarette smoke.
- It also helps in returning the vitamin E to its active form.

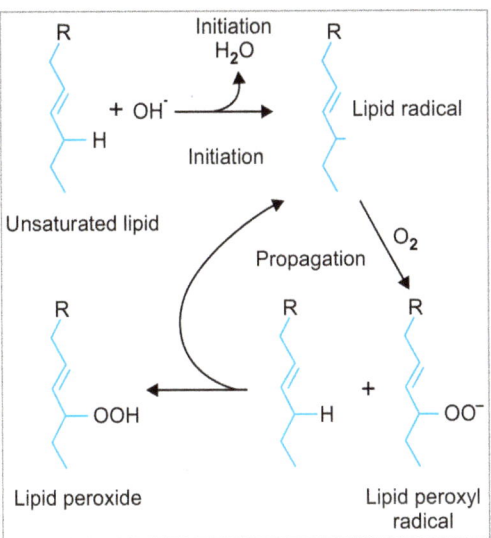

Fig. 15.4: Chain-breaking antioxidation.

### β-Carotene (Carotenoids)

β-Carotene acts as a chain-breaking antioxidant by trapping peroxy radicals in tissues at low pressure of oxygen.

### Selenium

Selenium is a trace element and is an important constituent of various enzymes, such as glutathione peroxidase, which is an important scavenger for inorganic–organic peroxides. Deiodinase is an example.

Selenium deficiency results in the downregulation of glutathione peroxidase enzyme synthesis. Selenium and vitamin E reinforce each other in their action against lipid peroxides.

### Transferrin and Ferritin

Transferrin and ferritin bind free $Fe^{2+}$ and prevent it from initiating the formation of free radicals.

### Ceruloplasmin

Ceruloplasmin binds $CU^{2+}$ and prevents it from initiating any oxidative damage.

## Uric Acid

Uric acid has the capacity of scavenging free electron (e–) and thus prevents the progression of free-radical damage in the blood. It is also having the sparing action on vitamin C. It prevents the initiation of free-radical formation by transition elements ions by forming complex with them.

## Ubiquitone

Ubiquitone is a lipid-soluble, radical-trapping antioxidant in membrane and plasma lipoproteins.

## Bilirubin

Bilirubin also works as an antioxidant in plasma. A molecule of unconjugated bilirubin scavenges two hydroperoxy radicals and itself gets oxidized to bilirubin.

# Oxidative Stress in Disease

Oxidative stress can damage the cells, leading to a range of diseases and causes symptoms of aging, such as wrinkles.

Oxidative stress is thought to contribute to the development of a wide range of diseases including Alzheimer's disease, Parkinson disease, diabetes, rheumatoid arthritis, and neurodegenerative diseases. Low-density lipoprotein (LDL) oxidation appears to trigger the process of atherogenesis, which results in atherosclerosis and finally cardiovascular disease.

## Impairment of Cognitive Function

Memory capabilities decline with age, evident in human degenerative diseases such as Alzheimer's disease, which is accompanied by an accumulation of oxidative damage.

## Cause of Aging

Oxidative damage initiated by ROS is a major contributor to the functional decline that is characteristic of aging.

## Male Infertility

Exposure of spermatozoa to oxidative stress is a major causative agent of male infertility. Sperm DNA fragmentation, caused by oxidative stress, appears to be an important factor in the etiology of male infertility.

## Cancer

ROS are constantly generated and eliminated in the biological system and are required to drive regulatory pathways. Under normal physiological conditions, cells control ROS levels by balancing the generation of ROS with their elimination by scavenging system. But under oxidative stress conditions, excessive ROS can damage cellular proteins, lipids, and DNA, leading to fatal lesions in cell that contribute to carcinogenesis.

Cancer cells exhibit greater ROS stress than normal cells do, partly due to oncogenic stimulation, increased metabolic activity and mitochondrial malfunction.

ROS, at low levels, facilitates cancer cell survival since cell-cycle progression driven by growth factors and receptor tyrosine kinases requires ROS for activation and chronic inflammation, a major mediator of cancer, is regulated by ROS. ROS at a high level can suppress tumor growth through the sustained activation of cell-cycle inhibitor and induction of cell death as well as senescence by damaging macromolecules. In fact, most of the chemotherapeutic and radio-therapeutic agents kill cancer cells by augmenting ROS stress.

## Carcinogenesis

ROS-related oxidation of DNA is one of the main causes of mutations, which can produce several types of DNA damage.

## Cell Proliferation

Both exogenous and endogenous ROS have been shown to enhance proliferation of cancer cells.

## Cell Death

A cancer cell can die in three ways: apoptosis, necrosis, and autophagy. Excessive ROS can induce apoptosis through both the extrinsic and intrinsic pathways.

## Chronic Inflammation and Cancer

ROS induces chronic inflammation by the induction of COX-2, inflammatory cytokines [TNFα, interleukin 1 (IL-1), IL-6], chemokines (IL-8, CXCR4), and proinflammatory transcription factors (NF-κB).

## Disease Treatment

Antioxidants are commonly used as medications to treat various forms of brain injury. SOD memetic, sodium thiopental, and propofol are used to treat reperfusion injury and traumatic brain injury. These compounds appear to prevent oxidative stress in neurons and prevent apoptosis and neurological damage. Antioxidants are also being investigated as possible treatments for neurodegenerative diseases such as Alzheimer's disease and Parkinson disease.

## Antioxidants and Disease Prevention

### Heart Disease

Vitamin E may protect against cardiovascular disease by defending against LDL oxidation and artery-clogging plaque formation.

### Cancer

Many studies have shown intake of high-vitamin C reduces the rate of cancer, particularly cancers of the mouth and larynx.

## SUMMARY

Free radicals are chemical species, possessing an unpaired electron, which can be considered as fragments of molecules. These are produced continuously in cells either accidental by products of metabolism or during the processes of phagocytosis. Oxidation reactions can produce free radicals, which start chain reactions that damage cells. Antioxidants terminate these chain reactions by removing free-radical intermediates and inhibit other oxidation reactions by being oxidized themselves. Antioxidants are also widely used as ingredients in dietary supplements in the hope of maintaining health and preventing diseases such as cancer and coronary heart disease. The important antioxidants are SOD, catalase, and glutathione.

## SELF-ASSESSMENT QUESTIONS

1. What are free radicals, explain?
2. Why do they have a damaging effect to human body?
3. How do vitamin E and the other antioxidant nutrients help to protect the body against free-radical damage?
4. Explain the role of antioxidants in disease treatment and prevention.

# Chapter 16: Specialized Proteins

## LEARNING OBJECTIVES

*At the end of this chapter students should be able to:*
- Explain the different types of collagen including their functions
- Describe the elastin and keartin
- Explain the structure and function of actin and myosin

## Introduction

Extracellular matrix (ECM) is a complex structural entity surrounding and supporting cells that are found within mammalian tissues. It is often referred to as the connective tissue. The ECM is composed of three major classes of biomolecules:
1. Structural proteins: Collagen and elastin.
2. Specialized proteins: Fibrillin, fibronectin, and laminin.
3. Proteoglycans: Protein core attached with long chains of repeating disaccharide units termed glycosaminoglycans.

## Collagen

- It is the main protein of connective tissue in animals and the most abundant protein in mammals, making up about 25% of the total protein.
- It is the major protein comprising the ECM.
- It is one of the long, fibrous structural proteins.
- Its functions are quite different from those of globular proteins such as enzymes.
- It is tough and inextensible, with great tensile strength.
- It is the main component of cartilage, ligaments, and tendons.
- Main protein component of bone and teeth.
- Along with soft keratin, it is responsible for skin strength and elasticity, and its degradation leads to wrinkles that accompany aging.
- It strengthens blood vessels and plays a role in tissue development.
- It is present in the cornea and lens of the eye in crystalline form.
- It is also used in cosmetic surgery, for example, lip enhancement.

## Types of Collagen

Collagen occurs in many places throughout the body and occurs in different types, which include:

*Type I collagen:* This is the most abundant collagen of the human body. It has a triple helical structure. The mature collagen type I contains approximately 1,000 amino acids. Each alpha-chain is twisted into a left-handed helix of three residues per turn. Three alpha-chains are wound into a right-handed super-helix, forming a rod-like molecule 1.4 nm in diameter and about 300 nm long. It is present in scar tissue (the end product when tissue heals by repair). Found in tendons and the organic part of bone.

*Type II collagen:* Articular cartilage.

*Type III collagen:* This is the collagen of granulation tissue and is produced quickly by young fibroblasts before the tougher type I collagen is synthesized.

*Type IV collagen:* The well-characterized example of collagen discontinuous triple helices is an important component of basement membrane. It occurs in basal lamina and eye lens.

*Type V collagen:* Most interstitial tissue, associated with type I.

*Type VI collagen:* Most interstitial tissue, associated with type I.

*Type VII collagen:* Epithelia.

*Type VIII collagen:* Some endothelial cells.

*Type IX collagen:* Cartilage, associated with type II.

*Type XI collagen:* Cartilage.

*Type XII collagen:* Interacts with types I and III.

*Type XIII collagen:* Interacts with types I and II.

There are 27 types of collagen in total.

Collagens are predominantly synthesized by fibroblasts, but epithelial cells also synthesize these proteins.

Lateral interactions of triple helices of collagens result in the formation of fibrils roughly 50 nm diameter. This staggered array produces a striated effect that can be seen in the electron microscope **(Fig. 16.1)**.

Collagen is synthesized on ribosomes in a precursor form, preprocollagen.

As it enters the endoplasmic reticulum, it becomes procollagen (removal leader sequence).

Type I procollagen contains an additional 150 amino acids at the N-terminus and 250 at the C-terminus.

Specific proline residues are hydroxylated by prolyl 4-hydroxylase and prolyl 3-hydroxylase. Specific lysine residues also are hydroxylated by lysyl hydroxylase. Both hydroxylases depend upon vitamin C as a cofactor.

The processed procollagens are secreted into the extracellular space where extracellular enzymes remove the prodomains.

The collagen molecules then polymerize to form collagen fibrils.

The oxidation of certain lysine residues by the extracellular enzyme lysyl oxidase forming reactive aldehydes.

These reactive aldehydes form specific cross-links between two chains, thereby stabilizing the staggered array of the collagens in the fibril. Methyl violet, trichrome, and van Gieson are the stains used to stain the collagen in tissue samples.

## Elastin

- It is a connective tissue protein that is responsible for extensibility and elastic recoil in tissues.
- It is present in large amounts in lungs, large arterial blood vessels, and some elastic ligaments.
- It is also present in skin, ear cartilage, and other tissues in smaller amounts.
- It is synthesized as a soluble monomer called tropoelastin.
- Some of the proline residues of tropoelastin are hydroxylated to hydroxyproline by prolyl hydroxylase. After secretion from the cell, certain lysyl residues of tropoelastin are oxidatively deaminated to aldehydes by lysyl oxidase. The cross-links formed in elastin are the desmosines, which result from the condensation of three of these lysine-derived aldehydes with an unmodified lysine to form a tetrafunctional cross-link. The cross-linked extracellular

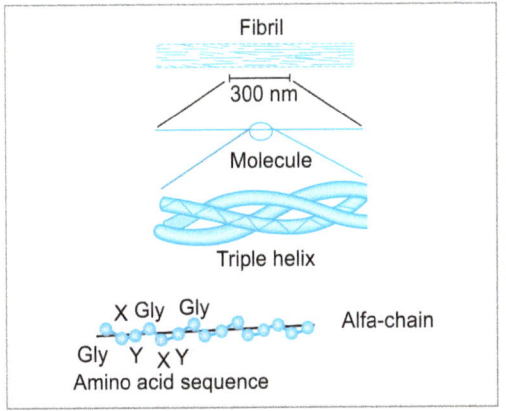

**Fig. 16.1:** Structure of collagen.

elastin is highly insoluble and stable with a low turnover rate.
- Elastin exhibits a variety of random coil conformations that permit the elastin to stretch and recoil during its physiological functions.
- It does not contain hydroxylysine.
- It is not synthesized in pro-form like collagen.
- Elastin does not contain repeat Gly-X-Y sequences, triple helical structure.
- The deletions of elastin gene have been found in majority of the subjects with William's syndrome. It is a disorder affecting connective tissue and central nervous system.

## Keratin

- Keratin is a strong protein, which is a major component in skin, hair, nails, hooves, horns, and teeth.
- The amino acids that combine to form keratin have several unique properties, and depending on the levels of the various amino acids, keratin can be inflexible and hard.
- Most of the keratin that people interact with is actually dead; hair, skin, and nails are all formed from dead cells, which the body sheds as new cells push up from underneath. If the dead cells are kept in good condition, they will serve as an insulating layer to protect the delicate new keratin below them.

There are two main forms of keratin—alpha-keratin and beta-keratin. Alpha-keratin is seen in humans and other mammals, beta-keratin is present in birds and reptiles. Beta-keratin is harder than alpha-keratin. Structurally alpha-keratin has alpha-helical-coiled coil structure while beta-keratin has twisted beta-sheet structure.

Keratin is difficult to dissolve, because it contains cysteine disulfide, which means that it is able to form disulfide bridges. These disulfide bridges create a helix shape that is extremely strong. Depending on how much cysteine disulfide keratin contains, the bond can be extremely strong to make hard cells like those found in hooves, or it can be softer to make flexible keratin like hair and skin.

Keratin is formed by keratinocytes, living cells that make up a large part of skin, hair, nails, and other keratin containing parts of the body. The cells slowly push their way upwards, eventually dying and forming a protective layer of cells.

## Actin

- Actin is the thin filament of sarcomere.
- Actin exists as a polymer of repeating globular proteins called G-actin.
- Two actin filaments are twisted into a single-stranded filament. These strands are anchored at one end to the Z-disk.
- An ADP molecule on each G-actin molecule is thought to be the active or binding site on the actin filament.
- Lying in the groove formed by the actin filaments are a series of rod-shaped protein molecules called tropomyosin. Each tropomyosin molecule is six to seven G-actin molecules in length.
- Bound to the end of each tropomyosin is a third protein called troponin (**Fig. 16.2**).
- Troponin consists of three small bound proteins molecules. One molecule is bound to the actin filament, one to the tropomyosin, and the third is available to bind with $Ca^{2+}$.

## Myosin

Myosins are a large superfamily of motor proteins that move along actin filaments while hydrolyzing ATP. About 20 classes of myosin have been distinguished on the basis of the sequence of amino acids in their ATP-hydrolyzing motor domains. The different classes of myosin also differ in structure of their tail domains.

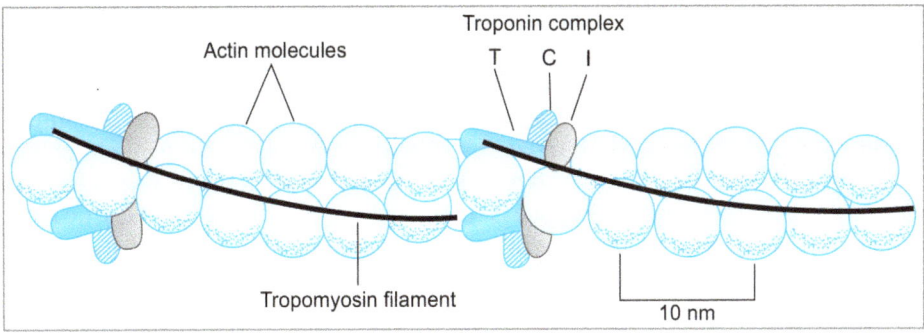

**Fig. 16.2:** Structure of actin.

Myosin II was first studied for its role in muscle contraction, but it functions also in nonmuscle cells.

* Each myosin filament is composed of two twisted strands called heavy chains and two other, but each different, pairs of twisted strands, called light chains. These light chains are found in the myosin heads **(Fig. 16.3)**. Two light chains designated essential and regulatory, wrap around the neck region of each myosin II heavy chain. In addition to regulatory roles, light chains may help to stiffen the neck regions.
* Myosin filament is flexible at the point of the myosin head, and the stacking of the myosin molecules leaves the myosin heads protruding from the filament at ~60°. This spacing maximizes the chances of interaction with actin-binding sites.
* Myosin II light chains are similar in structure to calmodulin, but in many organisms have lost the ability to bind $Ca^{2+}$. However, the calmodulin-like light chains of some myosins do bind $Ca^{2+}$.

Myosin I has only one heavy chain with a single globular motor domain. Its relatively

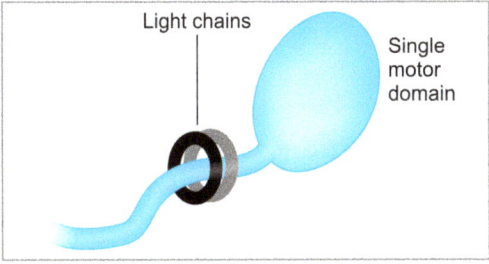

**Fig. 16.4:** Structure of myosin I.

short tail lacks the heptad repeats that would be involved in dimerization via formation of a coiled coil **(Fig. 16.4)**.

Myosin VI tail domain includes a short segment of heptad repeats. Myosin VI is found to be either monomeric or dimeric under different conditions.

Myosin V has two heavy chains like myosin II. But myosin V has a longer neck region that has six binding sites for calmodulin light chains. Its shorter coiled coil region is followed by a globular domain at the end of each heavy chain tail.

## Lens Protein

Protein found in the lens is a transparent body at the front of the vertebrate eye. The lens, which is behind the iris, refracts light entering the eye through the pupil, thus focusing it on the retina. The perfect physiochemical balance of the lens proteins gives it transparency. Any alteration in the optical homogeneity of the lens or decrease in its transparency is known as a cataract.

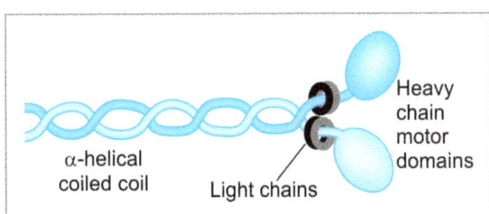

**Fig. 16.3:** Structure of myosin II.

## SUMMARY

Collagen, elastin, keratin, actin, myosin, and lens proteins are the specialized proteins responsible for various functions of our body. Collagen main is the protein of connective tissue in animals and the most abundant protein in mammals, making up about 25% of the total protein. There are about 27 types of collagen present in the extracellular matrix. Elastin is a connective tissue protein that is responsible for extensibility and elastic recoil in tissues. Keratin is a strong protein, which is a major component in skin, hair, nails, hooves, horns, and teeth. Actin is the thin filament of sarcomere. Myosins are a large superfamily of motor proteins that move along actin filaments while hydrolyzing ATP. About 20 classes of myosin have been distinguished on the basis of the sequence of amino acids in their ATP-hydrolyzing motor domains. Lens protein found in the lens is a transparent body at the front of the vertebrate eye.

## SELF-ASSESSMENT QUESTIONS

### Essay Questions

1. Explain, why collagen is the important tissue of human body?
2. What is the main biochemical composition of collagen and list the various types of collagen found in the human body?

### MULTIPLE CHOICE QUESTIONS

1. **Collagen is the:**
    (a) Major protein of the extracellular fluid (ECF)
    (b) Main protein of connective tissue in animals
    (c) Minor protein comprising the ECM
    (d) Non-fibrous protein

2. **Concerning collagen:**
    (a) It is the minor glycoprotein found in bone
    (b) Its degradation leads to wrinkles that accompany aging
    (c) It gives strength to ligaments
    (d) It is used in the treatment of ulcers

3. **Collagen synthesis depends on:**
    (a) Hydroxylysine and vitamin K
    (b) Glycine and fluoride
    (c) Epinephrine and vitamin C
    (d) Hydroxyproline and vitamin C

4. **The cofactor essential for hydroxylation of proline is:**
    (a) Pantothenic acid
    (b) Vitamin $B_{12}$
    (c) Vitamin C
    (d) Folic acid

### ANSWERS

1. b    2. b    3. d    4. c

# Chapter 17: Vitamins

## LEARNING OBJECTIVES

At the end of this chapter students should be able to:
- Understand the sources, daily requirement, functions, metabolism and deficiency manifestation of vitamins A, D E and K
- Discuss the sources, functions and disorders associated with vitamin C
- Explain the sources, requirement, coenzyme forms, functions and disorders associated with vitamins thiamine, riboflavin, pyridoxine, niacin, biotin, pantothenic acid, folic acid and $B_{12}$

## Introduction

- Vitamins are naturally occurring organic substances.
- Their coenzyme forms are essential in metabolic processes.
- They serve nearly the same roles in all forms of life.
- The daily requirement of any vitamin depends on a number of factors and may increase during growth, pregnancy, and lactation.
- They are essential nutrients and have various roles in the human body.

The vitamins are divided into two groups:
1. Fat-soluble vitamins (A, D, E, and K). Foods that contain these vitamins will not lose them when cooked.
2. Water-soluble vitamins (B complex).

## Fat-soluble Vitamins

Vitamins A, D, E, and K are called *fat-soluble* vitamins as they dissolve in fat. They are absorbed from the small intestines, along with dietary fat. Fat-soluble vitamins are primarily stored in the liver and adipose tissues. With the exception of vitamin K, fat-soluble vitamins are generally excreted more slowly than water-soluble vitamins and vitamins A and D can accumulate and cause toxic effects in the body (**Table 17.1**).

## Vitamin A

- Vitamin A comprises the preformed retinoid and the precursor forms, the provitamin A carotenoids.
- Preformed retinoid is a collective term for retinol, retinal, and retinoic acid, all of which are biologically active.
- The provitamin A carotenoids include β-carotene and others, which are converted to retinoids. Retinoids are sensitive to heat, light, and oxidation by air. β-carotene is relatively more stable.
- Retinoids are converted to retinol in the intestines and transported with dietary fat to the liver, where it is stored. A special transport protein, retinol-binding protein, transports vitamin A from the liver to other tissues. Carotenoids are absorbed intact at a much lower absorption rate than retinol. Of all the carotenoids, β-carotene has the highest potential vitamin A activity. The active forms of vitamin A have three basic functions: vision, growth and development of tissues, and immunity.

Retinol

Retinoic acid

Retinal

## Sources

Cod liver oils, fish liver oils, animal liver, milk and milk products, and eggs.

The carotenoid pigments present in carrots, sweet potato, and green leafy vegetables such as spinach and amaranth.

The yellow pigment, β-carotene present in vegetables is a precursor of vitamin A.

It has two ionone rings connected by a polyprenoid chain.

One molecule of β-carotene can theoretically give rise to two molecules of vitamin A, but it may produce only one in biological systems.

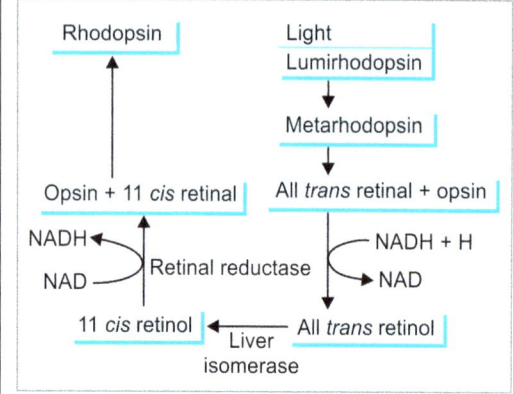

Fig. 17.1: Wald's visual cycle.

## Recommended Dietary Allowance

- *Adult*: 800–1,000 µg/day (5,000 IU/day).
- *Pregnancy and lactation*: 1,000–1,200 µg/day (4,000 IU/day).
- *Infants and children*: 400–600 µg/day (3,000 IU/day).

## Physiological Role

- *Role of vitamin A in vision*: Retina of the eye contains two types of cells.
  1. Rod cells (vision in dim light)
  2. Cone cells (vision in bright light colored vision)
- Rod cells have a photosensitive pigment called rhodopsin, which is a conjugated protein made up of opsin and 11-*cis* retinal (**Fig. 17.1**).
- When rhodopsin exposed to light, it dissociates into all-*trans* retinal and opsin. All-*trans* retinal is reduced to all-*trans* retinol in the retina and transported to liver where it is isomerized to 11-*cis* retinol. This is transported back to retina then oxidized to 11-*cis* retinal, which combines with opsin to form rhodopsin.
- Retinoic acid form of vitamin A maintains structural and functional integrity of epithelium.
- Retinol form of vitamin A is required for growth and reproductive function.
- Retinol is also known to require for the formation of bone and teeth.

## Deficiency

- Night blindness
- Keratinization of lacrimal glands
- *Keratomalacia*: Dryness of the cornea, corneal epithelium becomes keratinized and opaque and may become softened and ulcerated (**Fig. 17.2**).
- *Follicular hyperkeratosis*: Deficiency will affect hair follicles and causes scaly skin (**Fig. 17.3**).
- Xerophthalmia
- Bitot's spot

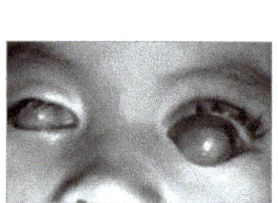

Fig. 17.2: Keratomalacia.

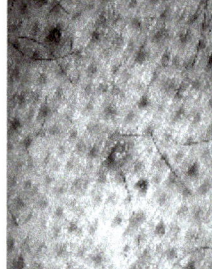

Fig. 17.3: Follicular hyperkeratosis.

## Vitamin D

**Ergocalciferol [D₂]**

**Cholecalciferol [D₃]**

## Vitamin D (Cholecalciferol)

### Sources
- $D_2$ in plants
- $D_3$ in fish, egg, and liver
  - Ergosterol $\xrightarrow[\text{Dehydrogenation}]{\text{UV light}}$ Vitamin D (ergocalciferol)
  - Cholesterol→7-dehydrocholesterol $\xrightarrow{\text{Sunlight}}$ Vitamin D (cholecalciferol)
  - The 7-dehydrocholesterol, an intermediate of a minor pathway of cholesterol synthesis, is available in the epidermis. The skin on exposure to sunlight the 7-dehydrocholesterol converted to cholecalciferol.

### Recommended Dietary Allowance
- *Children*: 10 µg/day (400 IU/day).
- *Adults*: 5–10 µg/day (400 IU/day).
- *Pregnancy and lactation*: 10 µg/day (400 IU/day).

Vitamin $D_2$ or $D_3$ is not active biologically but converted to active form by hydroxylation.

### Regulation of Formation of 1,25(OH)₂ Vitamin D₃
- Low plasma calcium level stimulates parathyroid hormone (PTH) secretion, this in turn acts on kidney to secrete 1-α-hydroxylase **(Fig. 17.4)**.
- High level of $1,25(OH)_2D_3$ inhibits the secretion of 1-α-hydroxylase.

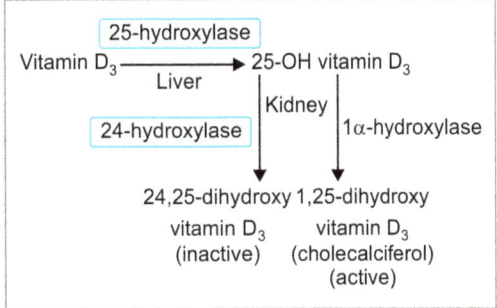

Fig. 17.4: Formation of active vitamin $D_3$.

- High plasma calcium level inhibits the activity of 1-α-hydroxylase.
- Low plasma phosphate level also activates the 1-α-hydroxylase but independent of PTH.
- High plasma phosphate inhibits the activity of 1-α-hydroxylase.
- When calcium level is normal, the production of $1,25(OH)_2$ vitamin $D_3$ suppressed resulting in the stimulation of 24-hydroxylase, which converts 25-hydroxy vitamin $D_3$ to $24,25(OH)_2$ vitamin $D_3$.

### Functions
It maintains an adequate calcium level by the following mechanisms:
- Increases the absorption of calcium from the intestine on vitamin $D_3$ enters the

intestinal cell then binds to cytoplasmic receptor. This complex interacts with DNA in the nucleus results in the synthesis of mRNA. This in turn forms a calcium-binding protein (CBP) known as calbindins and osteocalcin. This CBP increases the absorption of calcium.
- Reabsorption of calcium and phosphate from the kidney, 1,25-dihydroxycholecalciferol causes the increased reabsorption of calcium and phosphate in the distal convoluted tubule from glomerular filtrate.
- Mobilization of calcium and phosphate from bone. Vitamin D has both anabolic and catabolic role on bone causing removal of calcium from bone (resorption of bone calcium).

## Deficiency

- The deficiency of vitamin D leads to rickets in children.
- Signs and symptoms are bowlegs, knock knee, pigeon chest, hypocalcemia, and hypophosphatemia (**Fig. 17.5**).
- Osteomalacia in adults
- Soft and pliable bones

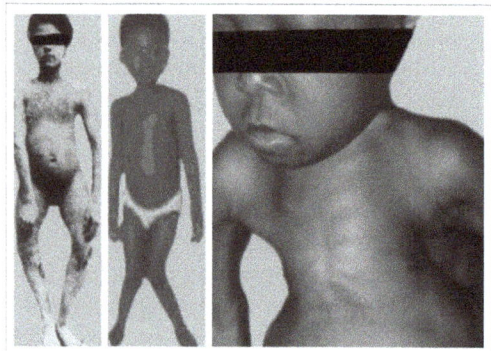

**Fig. 17.5:** Features of vitamin $D_3$ deficiency.

## Vitamin E (Tocopherol)

### Sources
- Vegetable oils such as wheat germ oil, corn oil, cottonseed oil, and safflower oil.
- Vitamin E is absorbed from intestine together with dietary lipid. It is delivered to the tissues via chylomicrons. The major site of vitamin E storage is in the adipose tissue.

### Recommended Dietary Allowance
- *Adult male*: 15 mg/day (22 IU/day).
- *Female*: 15 mg/day (22 IU/day).
- *Children*: 10 mg/day (16 IU/day).

### Functions
- Potent physiological antioxidant: Protects membranes with lipids from oxidative damage.
- Vitamin E, which is present in cell membranes, prevents the destructive nonenzymatic oxidation of polyunsaturated fatty acids by molecular oxygen, and it maintains the membrane integrity.
- Protects erythrocytes from hemolysis by oxidizing agents ($H_2O_2$).
- Required for normal reproduction in animals.
- Prevents liver necrosis and muscular dystrophy.
- Protects cellular and subcellular membranes.

### Deficiency
- Reproductive failure in animals.
- Hemolysis of erythrocytes which may lead to anemia.
- Muscular weakness, fragile RBCs.

## Vitamin K

### Sources
- Green leafy vegetables (spinach, alfalfa grass, cauliflower, and cabbage), tomato, and putrid fish meal.

- It is also synthesized by microorganisms in the intestinal tract.

## Functions

- Required for the maintenance of normal concentration of following blood clotting factors.
  - Prothrombin
  - Stable factor
  - Plasma thromboplastin component
  - Stuart–Prower factor
- Each of these is synthesized in the liver in an inactive form.
- Conversion of inactive to active form involves gamma carboxylation of glutamic acid residues from the N-terminal end. This process creates negative charges (**Fig. 17.6**). This process depends on vitamin K.
- The $Ca^{++}$ and phospholipids bind with negative charges and activate prothrombin to thrombin.

  Fibrinogen $\xrightarrow{\text{Thrombin}}$ Fibrin

- In the absence of gamma carboxylation, chelation with $Ca^{++}$ is impaired.
- The vitamin-dependent gamma carboxylation is also necessary for the functional activity of C-reactive protein

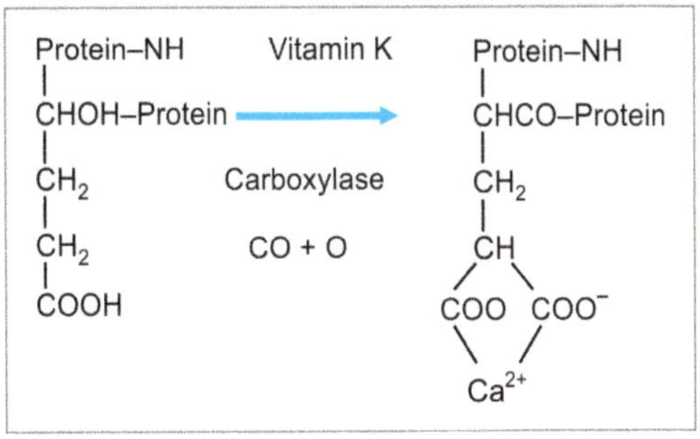

**Fig. 17.6:** Gamma carboxylation of inactive clotting factors.

and osteocalcin. The osteocalcin binds to hydroxyapatite crystals of bone; this binding is mainly dependent on the level of gamma carboxylation. The vitamin K helps to retain calcium by this mechanism.

- The vitamin K-dependent carboxylase enzyme requires oxygen, $CO_2$, nicotinamide adenine dinucleotide phosphate (NADPH), and reduced vitamin K. In this process, the vitamin passes through a cycle. For reconversion of vitamin K, reduced lipoamide is necessary. This process is inhibited by a vitamin K antagonist, warfarin, and dicoumarol (**Fig. 17.7**).

Phylloquinone ($K_1$)

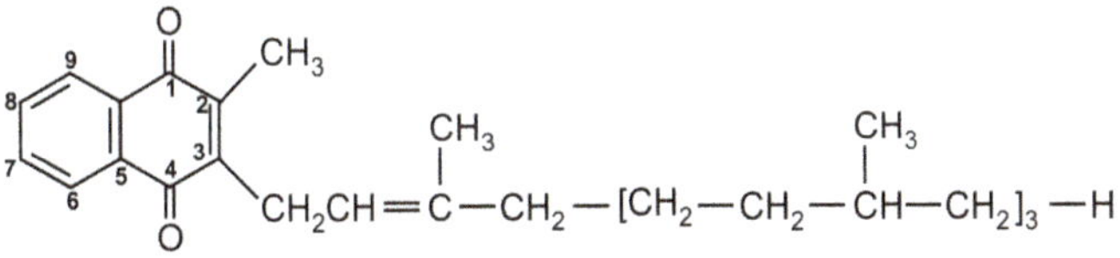

Menaquinone ($K_2$)

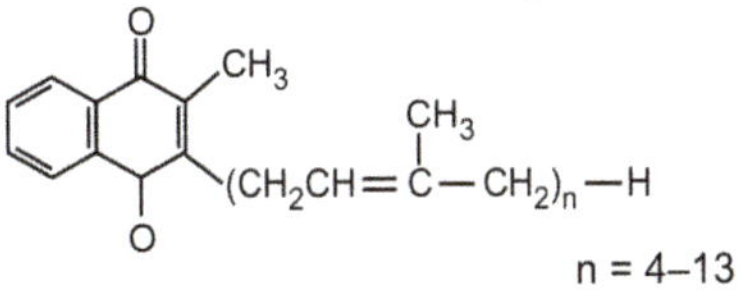

n = 4–13

Menadione ($K_3$)

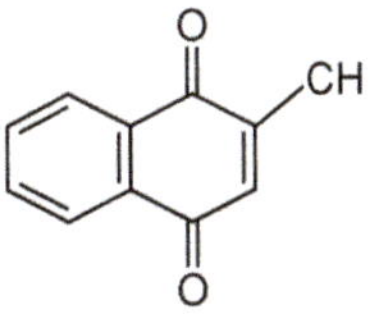

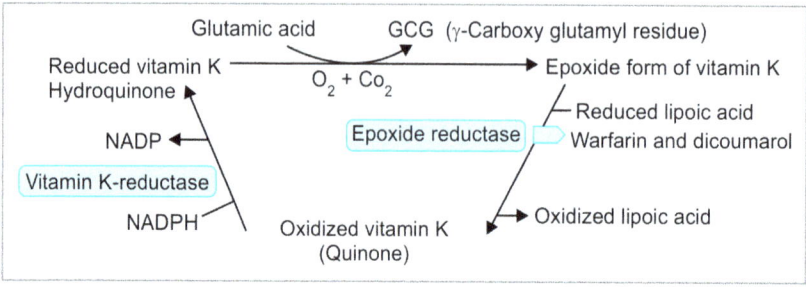

**Fig. 17.7:** Vitamin K cycle.

## Recommended Dietary Allowance

Intestinal bacteria synthesize vitamin K.
* *Newborn and infancy:* 2.0 µg/day
* *Children:* 60 µg/day
* *Adults:* 60–140 µg
* *Pregnancy and lactation:* 90 µg/day.

## Deficiency

* Normally does not occur.
* The drug therapy (sulfa drugs) inhibits the bacteria that help in vitamin K synthesis.
* Steatorrhea and pancreatic failure with decreased fat absorption result in vitamin K deficiency.

* *If deficiency arises:* Profuse bleeding and prolonged clotting time are the main symptoms.

## Antagonists

Dicoumarol

Warfarin

Summary of fat-soluble vitamins are shown in **Table 17.1**.

**Table 17.1:** Summary of fat-soluble vitamins.

| Vitamins | Sources | Functions | Deficiency | Overconsumption |
|---|---|---|---|---|
| Vitamin A (retinol, retinoic acid, and retinal) | Liver, fortified milk, and dairy products. Provitamin A: Carrots, green leafy vegetables, sweet potatoes, apricots | Skin and mucous membrane formation; night vision bones and teeth development, and β-carotene is an antioxidant and may protect against cancer | Night blindness, intestinal infections, impaired vision, inflammation of eyes, keratinization of skin and eyes, and blindness in children | Nausea, irritability, growth retardation, enlargement of liver and spleen, loss of hair, bone pain |
| Vitamin D | Vitamin D: Fortified dairy products, fortified margarine, fish oils, egg yolk and synthesized by sunlight action on skin | Promotes hardening of bones and teeth, increases the absorption of calcium | Rickets in children; osteomalacia in adults | Nausea, weight loss, movement of calcium from bones into soft tissues |
| Vitamin E | Vegetable oil, margarine, butter, green leafy vegetables, wheat germ | Spares the action of vitamins A and prevents damage to cell membranes and antioxidant | Possible anemia in low birth weight infants | Nontoxic under normal conditions |
| Vitamin K | Dark green leafy vegetables, liver; also made by bacteria in the intestine | Helps blood to clot | Excessive bleeding | None reported |

# Water-soluble Vitamins

## Vitamin C (Ascorbic Acid)

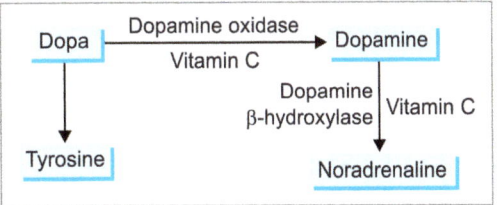

- B-complex vitamins and vitamin C are water-soluble vitamins that are not stored in the body and must be replaced each day.
- These vitamins are easily destroyed or washed out during food storage and preparation.
- The B-complex group is found in a variety of foods: cereal grains, meat, poultry, eggs, fish, milk, legumes, and fresh vegetables.
- Citrus fruits are good sources of vitamin C.
- Use of heavy doses of vitamins is not recommended **(Table 17.2)**.

### Sources

The rich sources are citrus fruits (orange, lemon) and also tomatoes, strawberries, green vegetables, guava fruit, and green pepper.

### Recommended Dietary Allowance

- *Adults*: 60 mg/day
- *Children*: 40 mg/day.

### Functions

- *Collagen synthesis*: Vitamin C is very important for the hydroxylation of proline and lysine residues (via prolyl hydroxylase and lysyl hydroxylase), which are the collagen precursors.
- It helps in the absorption of iron by reducing $Fe^{3+}$ to $Fe^{2+}$ in the stomach.
- Vitamin C acts as an electron donor for eight different enzymes.
- Reaction between amino groups of protein and nitrites formed in the intestine produces nitrosamines that may cause cancer. So, vitamin C acts as an antioxidant, scavenging the free radicals and reduces the nitrosamine formation.
- The conversion of dopa to dopamine and dopamine to noradrenaline requires vitamin C as an activator **(Fig. 17.8)**.
- The vitamin C in high dose (1 g/day) decreases the severity of cold.

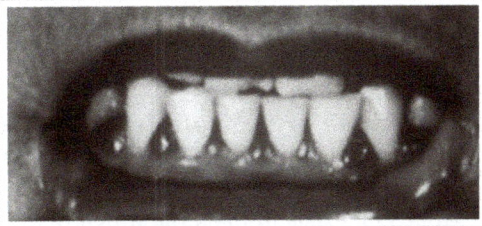

**Fig. 17.8:** Role of vitamin c in the formation of dopa and dopamine.

### Deficiency

- The vitamin C deficiency results in **scurvy** **(Fig. 17.9)**.
- Signs and symptoms are as follows:
  - Spongy gums
  - Loose teeth
  - Fragile blood vessels
  - Aching swollen joints
  - Anemia
  - Delay in wound healing.

**Fig. 17.9:** Symptoms of scurvy.

## B-complex Vitamins

### Thiamine ($B_1$)

Thiamine ($B_1$)

It is a sulfur-containing vitamin with thiazole and pyrimidine rings.

### Sources

The major sources are whole grains (unpolished rice, wheat), legumes (beans, peas), meat, bananas, and soybeans.

### Recommended Dietary Allowance

- *Children*: 1.2 mg/day
- *Adults*: 1.5 mg/day
- *Pregnancy and lactation*: 2.0 mg/day.

### Functions

- The coenzyme form of thiamine is thiamine pyrophosphate (TPP).
- TPP is required as coenzyme for several reactions, which are taking place in the human body.

  Pyruvate dehydrogenase complex

  Pyruvate $\xrightarrow{TPP}$ Acetyl CoA

  α-KG dehydrogenase complex

  α-ketoglutarate $\xrightarrow{TPP-FAD}$ Succinyl CoA

  Fructose-6-P+Glyceraldehyde-3-P $\xrightarrow{Transketolase\ TPP}$ Xylulose-5-P+Erythrose-4-P

- Thiamine monophosphate and thiamine triphosphate are the other two derivatives of thiamine.
- Thiamine triphosphate was long considered a specific neuroactive form of thiamine. However, recently it was shown that TPP exists in bacteria, fungi, plants, and animals suggesting a much more general cellular role.

### Deficiency

- Caused by alcoholism and malnutrition.
- Thiamine deficiency leads to failure of carbohydrate metabolism, where the TPP is required in for many enzymes to catalyze the reactions. This results in the decreased production of ATP and thus impaired cellular functions of central nervous system, heart, and gastrointestinal tract. The overall picture of this vitamin deficiency, including neurological, cardiovascular, and gastrointestinal disorders, is referred to as beriberi.

Beriberi is of four types:
1. Dry beriberi (peripheral neuritis)
2. Wet beriberi (cardiac manifestation)
3. Cerebral beriberi (Wernicke–Korsakoff syndrome)
4. Infantile beriberi

*Dry beriberi*

Symptoms

It comprises the following symptoms:
- Loss of appetite
- Weight loss
- Muscle wasting
- Peripheral neuritis with numbness (**Fig. 17.10**)

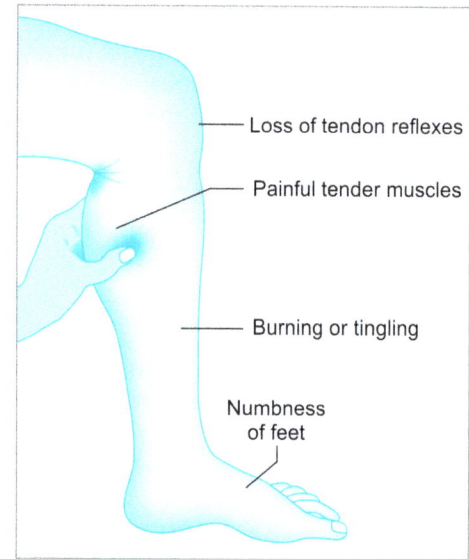

**Fig. 17.10:** Symptoms of dry beriberi.

- Tingling sensations in the lower legs and feet.
- Ataxic gait

*Wet Beriberi*
- Symptoms of dry beriberi
- Edema
- Foot drop and wrist drop
- Enlargement of heart

*Cerebral Beriberi (Wernicke-Korsakoff Syndrome)*
It occurs in alcoholics who consume less food and characterized by intelligence disturbance:
- Ataxia
- Double vision
- Nystagmus (rapid involuntary movement of the eyes)
- If this condition untreated progresses to Korsakoff's psychosis, which is irreversible.

*Infantile Beriberi*
It is due to the low thiamine content of breast milk from a deficient mother and it is characterized by:
- Anorexia
- Tachycardia
- Vomiting
- Convulsions
- Edema

Thiaminase present in raw fish and sea food may destroy the thiamine.

# Riboflavin (B$_2$)

*Chemistry:* Riboflavin has a dimethyl isoalloxazine ring attached to ribitol (the reduced form or ribose) B$_2$ is stable to heat but is sensitive to light.

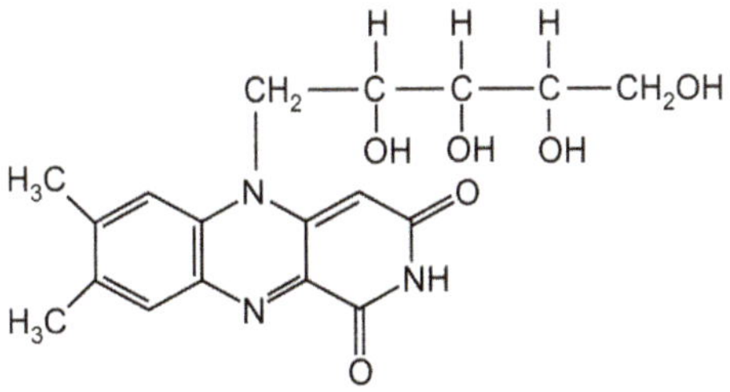

*Sources*
The major sources are animal liver, yeast, green leafy vegetables, milk, and eggs.

*Recommended Dietary Allowance*
- Adults: 2.0 mg/day
- Children: 1.2 mg/day
- Pregnancy and lactation: 2.0 mg/day.

*Active Form of Riboflavin*
- The riboflavin has two coenzyme forms they are flavin mononucleotide (FMN) and flavin adenine dinucleotide (FAD); both are nucleotides.
- Some enzymes have FMN and FAD as their integral part. Such enzymes are called flavoproteins.

*Functions of Flavin Mononucleotide and Flavin Adenine Dinucleotide*

They take part in oxidation reactions.
FMN is required for:
- L-Amino acid oxidase
- Cytochrome *c* reductase

FAD is required as coenzyme for:
- Succinate dehydrogenase
- Pyruvate dehydrogenase complex
- α-Ketoglutarate dehydrogenase complex
- Xanthine oxidase

*Deficiency Manifestations*

*Causes*
- Malabsorption
- Malnutrition
- Anorexia
- Chronic alcoholism

*Ariboflavinosis*
It is the medical condition caused by deficiency of riboflavin. It is often associated with protein energy malnutrition and alcoholism.

Ariboflavinosis is characterized by:
* Glossitis (magenta-colored tongue).
* Cheilosis (fissuring of the lips).
* Fissuring at the corners of mouth (**Fig. 17.11**).
* Seborrheic dermatitis and corneal vascularization are the symptoms of riboflavin deficiency.

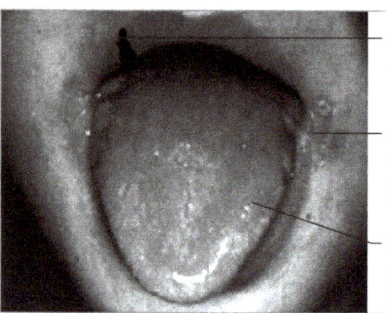

**Fig. 17.11:** Signs and symptoms of ariboflavinosis.

## Niacin (Nicotinic Acid) (B$_3$)

Niacin is also known as nicotinic acid. The amide form of niacin is nicotinamide. Both of these have equal biological activities. The compounds have pyridine ring. The niacin is stable in nature.

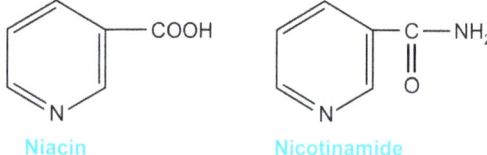

### Sources

The major sources are lean meats (liver), legumes, peanuts (ground nuts), green vegetables, and whole grains.
* Amino acid tryptophan can be converted to the coenzyme nicotinamide adenine dinucleotide (NAD).
* About 60 mg of tryptophan yields 1 mg of niacin.
* Milk and eggs are low in niacin but are rich in tryptophan.

### Recommended Dietary Allowance

* *Adults*: 16–20 mg/day
* *Children*: 9–16 mg/day
* *Infants*: 5–8 mg/day

### Coenzyme Forms

The active form of niacin is:
* NAD.
* NAD phosphate (NADP)
* They take part mainly in oxidation–reduction reactions of our body.
* NAD is required as a coenzyme for pyruvate dehydrogenase complex, α-ketoglutarate dehydrogenase complex to mediate the reactions.
* NADP is required for glucose-6-phosphate dehydrogenase and 6-phosphate gluconate dehydrogenase mediated reactions.

### Deficiency

* The deficiency of niacin leads to a condition called pellagra.
* It involves skin, gastrointestinal tract, and central nervous system (**Figs. 17.12A and B**).
* Its symptoms are called 3D symptoms, ***diarrhea, dermatitis, and dementia*** [disturbances of central nervous system (CNS)] and if untreated is followed by death.
* Fate of these vitamins when given in large doses: Nicotinic acid and nicotinamide are converted to their corresponding *N*-methyl derivatives before they are excreted in urine. This is an example of detoxication by transmethylation.

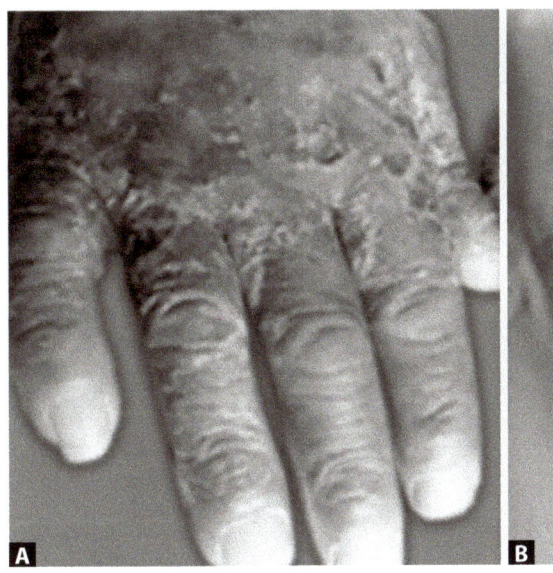 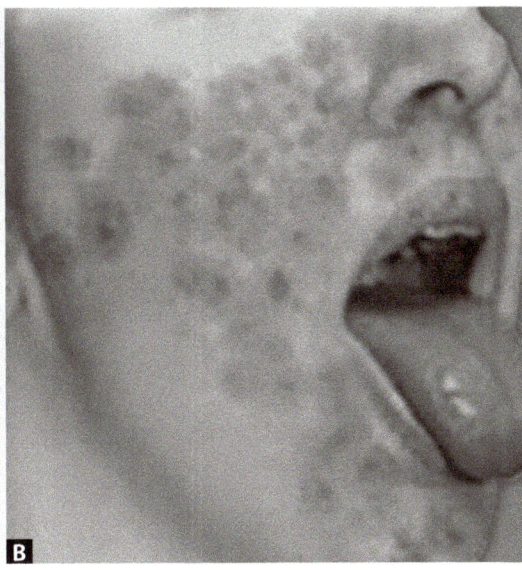

**Figs. 17.12A and B:** Signs of pellagra.

## Pyridoxine (B₆)

### Chemistry
- Pyridoxine, pyridoxal, and pyridoxamine as a group are designated vitamin B₆.
- All are equally active
- They have a pyridine ring
- Pyridoxine is heat stable but decomposes in the light or in alkaline solutions.

### Sources
The sources are whole grains, poultry fish, potatoes, organ meats, eggs, and legumes.

### Recommended Dietary Allowance
- *Adults*: 2.2 mg/day
- *Children*: 1.2 mg/day
- *Infants*: 3.0 mg/day

### Active Form of Pyridoxine
The coenzyme form of pyridoxine is pyridoxal phosphate (PLP), which is active.

PLP is required as coenzyme in the reactions involved amino acid metabolism for the enzymes such as:
- Transaminases
- Decarboxylases
- Kynureninase
- Cystathionine α-synthase
- Cystathionine gamma-lyase and aminolevulinic acid (ALA) synthase.

Enzymes such as serine hydroxymethyltransferase and phosphorylase contain PLP, but the role of PLP in their action is not known.

### Deficiency Manifestations
The deficiency leads to:
- Cheilosis **(Fig. 17.13A)**
- Hypochromic microcytic anemia
- Glossitis **(Fig. 17.13B)**
- Pigmented scaly dermatitis similar to pellagra.
- Numbness and tingling sensations in the extremities.
- Irritability, depression, and convulsive seizures.

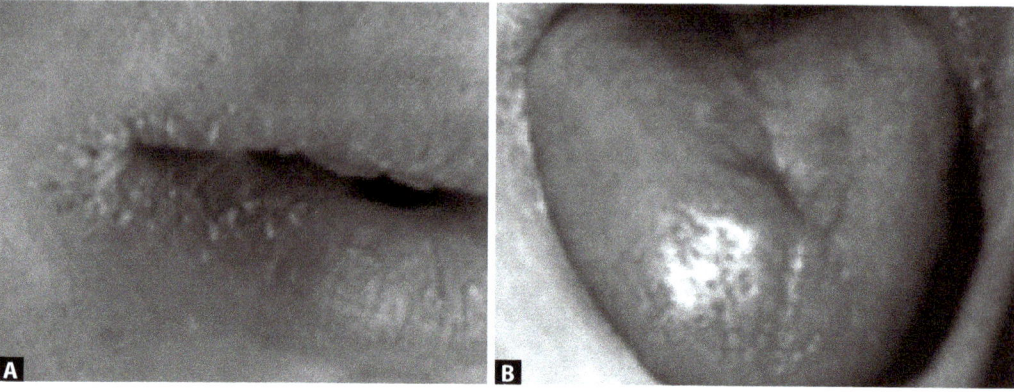

**Figs. 17.13A and B:** Signs of pyridoxine deficiency: (A) Cheilosis; (B) Gliossitis.

Tuberculous patients who are on long-term therapy with antituberculosis drug iso-nicotinic acid hydrazide (INH) suffer from B6 deficiency. This drug has a structure similar to B6 and antagonizes the action of B6. Hence, along with INH, they have to be given large doses of B6. The deficiency occurs also in women taking oral contraceptives.

- Pyridoxine is used in the treatment of seizures, Down syndrome, autism (psychiatric disorder of childhood), and premenstrual syndrome.

### Antagonists

Deoxypyridoxine

Methoxypyridoxine

### Biotin (B$_7$)

Sulfur-containing vitamin consists of two fused rings, one is imidazole and the other is thiophane and an attached valeric acid side chain.

Oxybiotin

### Sources

The sources are egg yolk, organ meats (liver, kidney), milk, legumes, and nuts.

### Recommended Dietary Allowance

- *Adults*: 0.3 mg/day
- The intestinal bacteria also synthesize biotin to some extent.
- *The coenzyme form*: Biotin itself acts as coenzyme.
- It functions as a coenzyme in the reactions involving fixation of $CO_2$.

$$Pyruvate \xrightarrow[H_2O + CO_2\,biotin]{Pyruvate\ carboxylase} Oxaloacetate$$

$$Propionyl\ CoA \xrightarrow[CO_2\,biotin]{Propionyl\ CoA\ carboxylase} \text{D-methyl malonyl CoA}$$

Acetyl CoA + $CO_2$ + ATP $\xrightarrow[\text{Biotin}]{\text{Acetyl CoA carboxylase}}$ Malonyl CoA + ADP + Pi

## Antivitamin

Avidin, a glycoprotein, presents in raw egg white when fed to animals can produce biotin deficiency. Since avidin causes egg white injury, biotin is called anti-egg white injury factor. Avidin being protein on heating will be denatured and loses its biotin-binding activity.

## Deficiency and Symptoms

It is rare; experimental animals show the symptoms such as anorexia, depression, insomnia, muscle pain, and dermatitis.

## Antagonists

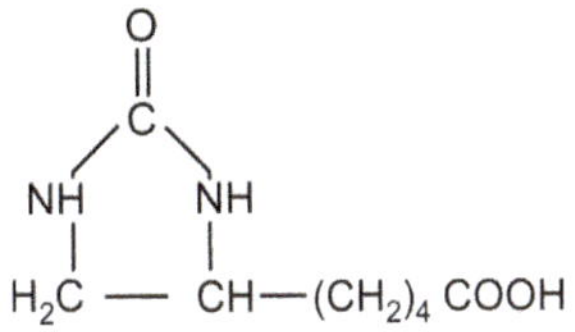

**Desthiobiotin**

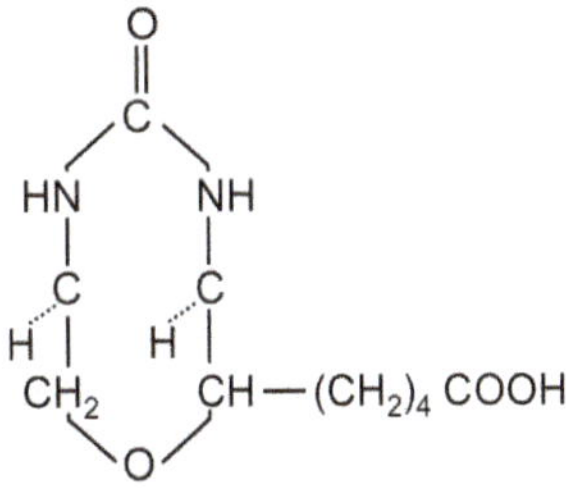

**Oxybiotin**

## Pantothenic Acid ($B_5$)

Consists of a dihydroxy dimethyl butyric acid joined to an α-alanine by a peptide bond.

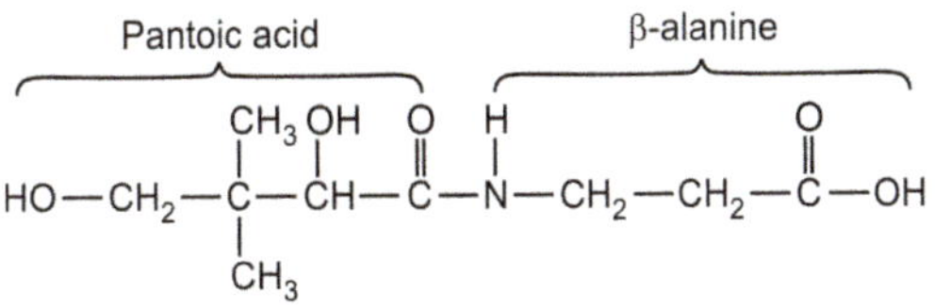

## Sources

The good sources are eggs, animal liver, meat, milk, vegetables, and grains.

## Required Dietary Allowance

* Adults: 5–10 mg/day
* Children: 4–5 mg/day
* Infants: 1–2 mg/day

**Active form:**

* The coenzyme form: Coenzyme A (CoASH).
* Its reactive group is sulfhydryl group (–SH).

CoASH is required for:
Pyruvate dehydrogenase that converts acetyl CoA to pyruvate
α-ketoglutarate dehydrogenase that converts α-ketoglutarate to succinyl CoA
Thiokinase that activates fatty acid to acyl CoA
Thiolase that converts α-ketoacyl CoA to acyl CoA and acetyl CoA
Detoxication of benzoic acid
Synthesis of bile salts

## Deficiency

It is rare. When it is produced experimentally have the symptoms, fatigue, sleep disorders, weakness, abdominal cramp, and a burning sensation of the feet.

## Folic Acid

Composed pteridine ring attached to *para* amino benzoic acid and conjugated with glutamic acid residues.

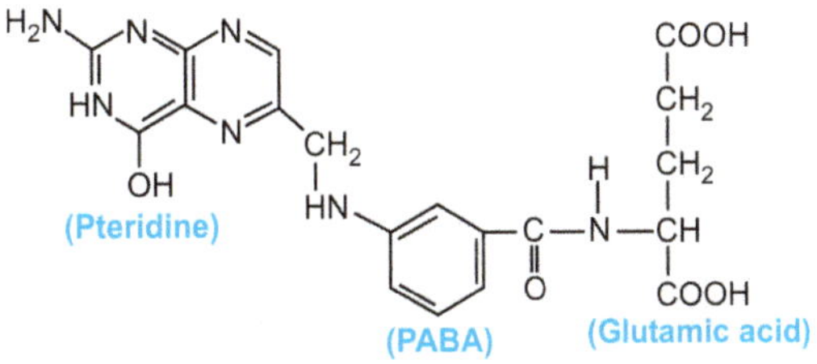

## Sources

Fresh green, vegetables, liver, whole grains, meat, and legumes.

## Recommended Dietary Allowance

- Children: 300 µg/day
- Adults: 400 µg/day
- Pregnancy and lactation: 800 µg/day.

## Active Form of Folic Acid

- The coenzyme form of folic acid is tetrahydro folic acid [THF] ($FH_4$) is the active form.
- It is formed from folic acid **(Fig. 17.14)**.
- The THF is a carrier of single carbon and it is involved in single carbon transfer reactions.
- The single carbon may be in the form of:
  - Formyl (-CHO)
    Tryptophan
    ↓ THF
    Formate → $N_{10}$ formyl THF → C-2 of purine ring
  - Methenyl (=CH)
  - Methylene

## Combined Roles of Vitamin $B_{12}$ and Folate in the Synthesis of Methionine

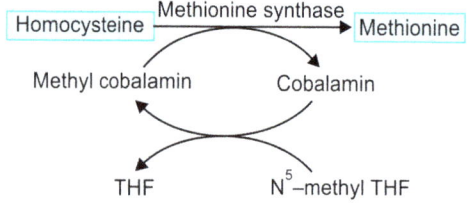

## Deficiency

- Megaloblastic anemia
- Growth failure

The deficiency of folate leads to impairment of the methionine synthase reaction due to which purine ring synthesis is impaired. The impaired synthesis of DNA prevents cell division and formation of the nucleus of new red blood cells. Megaloblasts are formed instead

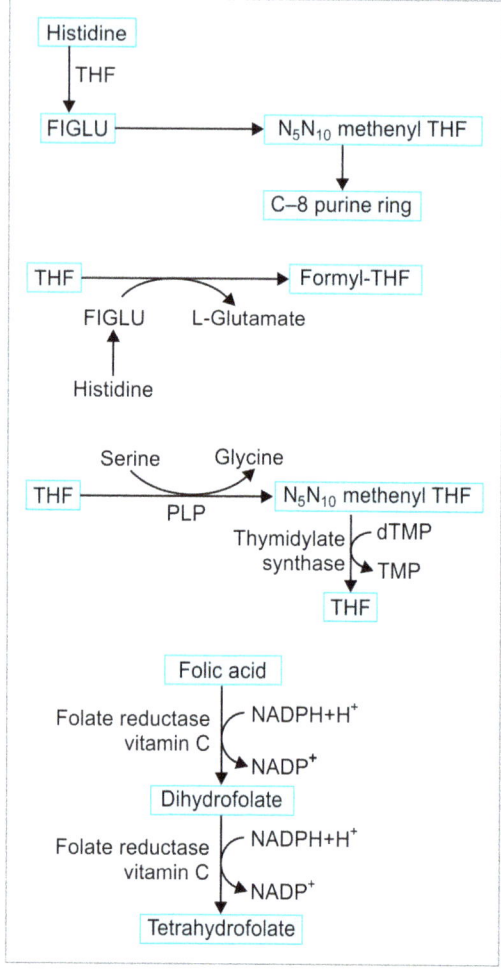

**Fig. 17.14:** Formation of tetrahydrofolate.

of normoblast. These megaloblasts are accumulated in the bone marrow and leads to megaloblastic anemia.

*Causes:* Low dietary intake, malabsorption syndrome, and during pregnancy.

*Formiminoglutamic (FIGLU) excretion test:* In the deficiency of folic acid, the availability of $FH_4$ is less or totally absent. So, the intermediate of histidine metabolism, formiminoglutamate accumulates in the blood and excreted in the urine. This is one of the tests to detect the megaloblastic anemia to check whether it is due to folic acid or vitamin $B_{12}$ deficiency.

## Vitamin B$_{12}$ (Cobalamin)

It has a corrin ring linked to cobalt atom held in the center of the corrin ring, by four coordination bonds with the nitrogen of the pyrrole groups. The remaining coordination bonds of the cobalt are linked with the nitrogen of dimethylbenzimidazole nucleotide and sixth bond is linked either methyl or 5'-deoxyadenosyl or hydroxyl group to form methylcobalamin, adenosylcobalamin, or hydroxycobalamin, respectively.

### Sources

The sources are liver, meat, fish, eggs, milk.
Human beings get small amount of vitamin B$_{12}$ from their intestinal flora.

### Recommended Dietary Allowance

* Children: 2 µg/day
* Adults: 3 µg/day
* Pregnancy and lactation: 4 µg/day.

### Active Form of Vitamin B$_{12}$

Methylcobalamin and deoxyadenosylcobalamin are the two active forms of vitamin B$_{12}$.

### Absorption

* A glycoprotein is the castle's intrinsic factor.
* Vitamin B$_{12}$ is called extrinsic factor.
* Vitamin B$_{12}$ of food binds to intrinsic factor in the stomach, this complex moves to ileum there it bind to specific receptors. Then the B$_{12}$ is transported to mucosal cell and then to blood and carried by B$_{12}$-binding proteins. The coenzyme form of vitamin B$_{12}$ is 5'-deoxyadenosylcobalamin.
* Vitamin B$_{12}$ along with folic acid is required for the development of red blood cells beyond megaloblastic stage.
* It acts as coenzyme for the mutase enzyme which converts methyl malonyl CoA into succinyl CoA.
* Methylcobalamin is required in the conversion of homocysteine to methionine.
* It is involved in the conversion of ribonucleotides to deoxyribonucleotide.

### Deficiency

The common cause of deficiency is malabsorption. Pernicious anemia is caused by the deficiency of an intrinsic factor, which leads to impaired absorption of cobalamin.

* Megaloblastic anemia
* Glossitis and inflammation of mouth
* Methyl malonic aciduria

*Folate trap:* Deficiency of this vitamin produces megaloblastic anemia due to its role in folate metabolism. During the many transformations of folate from one form to another, a proportion gets accidentally converted to $N^5$-methyl-THF, an inactive metabolite. This is called the "folate trap," since there is no way for active $N^5,N^{10}$-THF to be regenerated except through a reaction for which a form of vitamin B$_{12}$, methyl-B$_{12}$, is a cofactor. Deficiency of B$_{12}$ then produces a situation where more and more folate is trapped in an inactive form with no biochemical means of escape. The end result is failure to synthesize adequate DNA.

Summary of water-soluble vitamins are shown in **Table 17.2**.

**Table 17.2:** Summary of water-soluble vitamins.

| Sources | Functions | Deficiency symptoms | Overconsumption symptoms | Characteristics |
|---|---|---|---|---|
| **Vitamin C (ascorbic acid)** | | | | |
| Citrus fruits, broccoli, Strawberries, melon, green pepper, tomatoes, dark green vegetables, potatoes | Formation of collagen, wound healing; maintaining blood vessels, bones, teeth; absorption of iron, production of brain epinephrine and norepinephrine, antioxidant | Bleeding gums; poor wound healing, bruise easily; dry, rough skin; scurvy; sore joints and bones | Nontoxic under normal conditions | Most unstable under heat, drying, storage; very soluble in water |
| **Vitamin $B_1$ (thiamine)** | | | | |
| Liver, whole grains, enriched grain products, peas, meat, legumes | Helps release energy from foods; promotes normal appetite; important in function of nervous system | Mental confusion; muscle weakness, wasting; edema; impaired growth; beriberi | Not known | Losses depend on cooking method |
| **Vitamin $B_2$ (riboflavin)** | | | | |
| Liver, milk, dark green vegetables, whole and enriched grain products, eggs | Helps release energy from foods; promotes good vision, healthy skin | Cracks at corners of mouth; dermatitis around nose and lips; eyes sensitive to light | Not known | Sensitive to light |
| **Vitamin $B_3$ [niacin (nicotinamide, nicotinic acid)]** | | | | |
| Liver, fish, poultry, meat, peanuts, whole and enriched grain products | Energy production from foods; aids digestion, promotes normal appetite; promotes healthy skin, nerves | Skin disorders; diarrhea; weakness; mental confusion; irritability | Abnormal liver function; cramps; nausea; irritability | |
| **Vitamin $B_6$ (pyridoxine, pyridoxal, and pyridoxamine)** | | | | |
| Pork, meats, whole grains and cereals, legumes, green, leafy vegetables | Helps in protein metabolism, absorption; aids in red blood cell formation; helps body use fats | Skin disorders, dermatitis, cracks at corners of mouth; anemia | Not known | Considerable losses during cooking |
| **Folacin (folic acid)** | | | | |
| Liver, kidney, dark green leafy vegetables, meats, fish, whole grains, fortified grains and cereals, legumes, citrus fruits | Aids in protein metabolism; promotes red blood cell formation; prevents birth defects of spine, brain; lowers homocysteine levels and thus coronary heart disease risk | Anemia; diarrhea | May mask pernicious anemia | Easily destroyed by storing and cooking |

*Contd...*

Contd...

| | | Vitamin B$_{12}$ | | |
|---|---|---|---|---|
| Animal foods such as meats, liver, kidney, fish, eggs, milk and milk products, oysters, shellfish | Aids in building of genetic material; development of normal red blood cells; maintenance of nervous system | Pernicious anemia, anemia; neurological disorders; degeneration of peripheral nerves that may cause numbness, tingling in fingers and toes | Not known | |
| | | Vitamin B$_5$ (pantothenic acid) | | |
| Liver, kidney, meats, egg yolk, whole grains, legumes; also made by intestinal bacteria | Involved in energy production; aids in formation of hormones | Fatigue; nausea, abdominal cramps | Not known | About half of pantothenic acid is lost in the milling of grains |
| | | Vitamin B$_7$ (biotin) | | |
| Liver, kidney, egg yolk, milk, most fresh vegetables, also made by intestinal bacteria | Helps release energy from carbohydrates; aids in fat synthesis | Fatigue; loss of appetite, nausea, vomiting, depression | Not known | |

## SUMMARY

Vitamins are naturally occurring organic substances. Most of the metabolic reactions require coenzyme forms of these vitamins to catalyze the metabolic reactions. They serve nearly the same roles in all forms of life. The daily requirement of any vitamin depends on a number of factors and may increase during growth, pregnancy, and lactation. The vitamins are divided into fat-soluble vitamins (A, D, E, and K) and water-soluble vitamins (B complex) and vitamin C. Dietary deficiency of vitamins results in many symptoms. For example, vitamin A deficiency leads to night blindness, D deficiency results in rickets in children, K deficiency leads to clotting disorder, C deficiency to scurvy, B-complex deficiency results in dermatitis (niacin), magenta-colored tongue (riboflavin), and anemia (folic acid).

## SELF-ASSESSMENT QUESTIONS

### Long Answer Questions

1. Write a note on the sources and requirement of vitamin A.
2. Discuss the functions and deficiency manifestations of vitamin A.
3. What are the functions of vitamin D?
4. What are the deficiency symptoms of vitamin D?
5. Describe the sources and functions of vitamins E and K.
6. Add a note on the requirement, sources, functions, and deficiency manifestations of vitamin C.
7. Name the B-complex vitamins.

8. Mention is the coenzyme form of thiamine.
9. Discuss the sources and functions of thiamine.
10. What is beriberi? Explain briefly.
11. Name the enzymes that are dependent on PLP as coenzyme.
12. Mention the symptoms of pyridoxine deficiency.
13. Briefly describe the sources, requirement, functions, and deficiency manifestations of niacin.
14. What are the functions of biotin in the body?
15. Mention the coenzyme form for pantothenic acid.
16. Mention the enzymes that need FMN and FAD as coenzymes.
17. Write the deficiency symptoms of riboflavin.
18. Discuss the sources, functions, and deficiency manifestations of vitamin $B_{12}$.
19. Write a note on the requirement and deficiency diseases of folic acid.
20. What is FIGLU excretion test?

## Short Answer Questions

1. Which form of vitamin A has a role in vision?
2. Cod liver oil is a rich source for which vitamin?
3. Which vitamin deficiency leads to night blindness?
4. Name the two forms of vitamin.
5. In adults and children, deficiency of vitamin D leads to what?
6. The antioxidant property is observed in which vitamin?
7. Name the naturally occurring form of vitamin K.
8. Which vitamin involved in gamma carboxylation of the glutamic acid residues of the inactive clotting factor?
9. Name the important source for vitamin.
10. Which vitamin is responsible for the hydroxylation of prolyl residues?
11. The vitamin C deficiency leads to what?
12. Name the coenzyme form of thiamine.
13. Which vitamin deficiency leads to beriberi?
14. Which vitamin deficiency leads to pellagra?
15. Mention the coenzyme form of pyridoxine.
16. Name the two coenzyme forms of niacin.
17. Which vitamin deficiency leads magenta-colored tongue?
18. Write the requirement of niacin for adults and children.
19. Name the coenzyme forms of riboflavin.
20. Which vitamin is called anti-egg white injury factor?
21. CoASH is the coenzyme form of which vitamin?
22. Give the requirement of folic acid for pregnant and lactating women.
23. What is the other name for vitamin $B_{12}$?
24. The folic acid deficiency leads to what?
25. Mention the importance of FIGLU excretion test.

## Fill in the Blanks

1. _____ form of vitamin A has a role in vision.
2. Cod liver oil is a rich source for vitamin _____.
3. Night blindness is due to the deficiency of _____.
4. The two forms of vitamin D are _____ and _____.
5. The deficiency of vitamin D leads to _____ in adults and _____ in children.
6. The antioxidant property is observed in vitamin _____.

7. Phylloquinone is the naturally occurring form of vitamin _____.
8. The vitamin K is involved in _____ of the glutamic acid residues of the inactive clotting factor.
9. The requirement of vitamin C for children is _____.
10. The hydroxylation of prolyl residues is brought about by vitamin _____.
11. The vitamin C deficiency leads to _____.
12. The coenzyme form of thiamine is _____.
13. The beriberi is due to the deficiency of _____.
14. The pellagra is due to the deficiency of _____.
15. The coenzyme form of pyridoxine is _____.
16. The coenzyme forms of niacin are _____ and _____.
17. The magenta-colored tongue is due to the deficiency of _____.
18. The requirement of niacin for adults is _____.
19. The coenzyme forms of riboflavin are _____ and _____.
20. Anti-egg white injury factor is called for _____.
21. CoASH is the coenzyme form of _____.
22. The requirement of folic acid for pregnant and lactating women is _____.
23. The vitamin $B_{12}$ is also called _____.
24. The folic acid deficiency leads to _____.
25. The coenzyme form of vitamin $B_{12}$ is _____.

## MULTIPLE CHOICE QUESTIONS

1. **All the following are the symptoms of vitamin A deficiency, except:**
   (a) Night blindness
   (b) Fragile RBCs
   (c) Keratinization of lacrimal glands
   (d) Keratomalacia
2. **Concerning the vitamin D, one of the following statements is incorrect:**
   (a) Low calcium stimulates the 1-hydroxylase
   (b) Vitamin $D_3$ increases the absorption of calcium from the intestine
   (c) Deficiency leads to scurvy
   (d) Deficiency leads to rickets
3. **One of the following is not a form of vitamin K:**
   (a) Phylloquinone
   (b) Menaquinone
   (c) Menadione
   (d) Ubiquinone
4. **Concerning the functions of vitamin E, all of the following statements are correct, except:**
   (a) Antioxidant
   (b) Normal reproduction in animals
   (c) Helps in vision
   (d) Protects cellular membrane
5. **Scurvy is the result of:**
   (a) Deficiency of vitamin A
   (b) Deficiency of vitamin C
   (c) Deficiency of vitamin D
   (d) Deficiency of vitamin E
6. **The incorrect statement regarding vitamin $B_{12}$ is:**
   (a) It is extrinsic factor.
   (b) Vitamin $B_{12}$ of food binds to intrinsic factor in the stomach
   (c) The coenzyme form of vitamin $B_{12}$ is 5'-deoxyadenosylcobalamin
   (d) Vitamin $B_{12}$ along with vitamin C is required for the development of red blood cells beyond megaloblastic stage

7. The tetrahydro folic acid (FH$_4$) does the following, *except*:
   (a) Carrier of single carbon and it is involved in single carbon transfer reactions
   (b) Contributes to C-2 purine ring
   (c) Contributes to C-8 purine ring
   (d) Synthesis of UMP
8. One of the following enzymes does not require coenzyme A (CoASH):
   (a) Pyruvate dehydrogenase complex
   (b) α-Ketoglutarate DH complex
   (c) Hexokinase
   (d) Thiokinase
9. Deficiency of vitamin B$_6$ leads to the following, *except*:
   (a) Hypochromic microcytic anemia
   (b) Glossitis
   (c) Pigmented scaly dermatitis similar to pellagra
   (d) Megaloblastic anemia
10. All the following statements are correct regarding the riboflavin, *except*:
    (a) Has a dimethyl isoalloxazine ring attached to ribitol
    (b) RDA for adults is 2.0 mg/day
    (c) Nicotinamide dinucleotide (NAD) is its coenzyme form
    (d) Flavin adenine dinucleotide (FAD) is its coenzyme form
11. One of the following is not dependent on the coenzyme pyridoxal phosphate (PLP) for its activity:
    (a) Transaminases
    (b) Decarboxylases
    (c) Pyruvate dehydrogenase
    (d) ALA synthase
12. All the following statements are correct regarding riboflavin, *except*:
    (a) Nicotinamide adenine dinucleotide (NAD) is its coenzyme
    (b) Flavin adenine dinucleotide (FAD) is its coenzyme form
    (c) Nicotinamide adenine dinucleotide phosphate (NADP) is its coenzyme form
    (d) The deficiency of niacin leads to a condition called pellagra
13. Thiamine is essential for all the following, *except*:
    (a) Pyruvate dehydrogenase complex
    (b) α-Ketoglutarate dehydrogenase complex
    (c) Protects against night blindness
    (d) Protects against beriberi
14. Concerning warfarin, one of the statements is incorrect:
    (a) Reduces the concentration of vitamin A-dependent clotting factors
    (b) Has a half-life of about 36 hours
    (c) Crosses the placenta and should be avoided in pregnancy
    (d) Doses should be reduced in liver disease
15. Which of the following is not a dietary antioxidant?
    (a) Vitamin C
    (b) Vitamin K
    (c) Vitamin A
    (d) Vitamin E
16. Osteoporosis is associated with:
    (a) Vitamin D deficiency
    (b) Vitamin K deficiency
    (c) Prolonged bed rest
    (d) Hyperparathyroidism
17. Hemolysis is a feature of the deficiency of:
    (a) Vitamin A
    (b) Vitamin B$_1$
    (c) Vitamin K
    (d) Vitamin E
18. Reduced RBC transketolase activity is the indication of:
    (a) Vitamin B$_1$
    (b) Vitamin B$_6$
    (c) Vitamin B$_{12}$
    (d) Vitamin E

19. All of the following are vitamin K-dependent clotting factors, *except*:
    (a) Prothrombin
    (b) Factor XII
    (c) Factor VII
    (d) Factor X
20. The enzyme that requires vitamin $B_{12}$ as the coenzyme is:
    (a) Isocitrate dehydrogenase
    (b) Lactate dehydrogenase
    (c) G-6-P dehydrogenase
    (d) Homocysteine methyl transferase
21. Which of the following helps in blood coagulation?
    (a) Heparin
    (b) Ethylene diamine tetraacetic acid
    (c) Warfarin
    (d) Phylloquinone
22. Conversion of ribonucleotides to deoxyribonucleotides by ribonucleotide reductase requires:
    (a) Tetrahydrofolate
    (b) NADPH
    (c) Coenzyme A
    (d) Pyridoxal phosphate
23. If a person had glossitis and cheilosis, the physician may suspect a deficiency of:
    (a) Niacin
    (b) Thiamine
    (c) Riboflavin
    (d) Pyridoxal phosphate
24. Defective parietal cells would result in malabsorption of which vitamin?
    (a) Vitamin C
    (b) Vitamin $B_2$
    (c) Vitamin $B_{12}$
    (d) Folic acid

## ANSWERS

| | | | | | | | |
|---|---|---|---|---|---|---|---|
| 1. b | 2. c | 3. d | 4. c | 5. b | 6. d | 7. d | 8. c |
| 9. d | 10. c | 11. c | 12. b | 13. c | 14. a | 15. b | 16. c |
| 17. d | 18. a | 19. b | 20. d | 21. d | 22. a | 23. c | 24. c |

# Minerals

**Chapter 18**

## LEARNING OBJECTIVES

*At the end of this chapter students should be able to:*
- Understand the daily requirement, functions and disorders associated with calcium, iron, phosphorous, sodium, potassium and chloride
- Explain the daily requirement, important functions and the deficiency manifestations of trace elements like copper, zinc, selenium, fluoride, iodine, magnesium and molybdenum

## Introduction

Minerals are required in trace amount and are usually cofactors and enzymes. There are two types of minerals present in the human body:
1. Bulk elements (macronutrients)
2. Trace elements (micronutrients).

Bulk elements are calcium, magnesium, sodium, potassium, phosphorus, sulfur, and chloride. They constitute 60–80% of all inorganic materials in the body.

**What are the trace elements? Name them.**
Trace elements are those, which are required in very small amounts. They are iron, iodine, cobalt, manganese, molybdenum, zinc, lead, selenium, and fluoride.

**Discuss the calcium under the following headings:**
a. Sources
b. Requirement
c. Functions.

## Calcium (Ca$^{2+}$)

### Calcium Content of Body and Blood

- Calcium is the major inorganic element comprising nearly 2% of our body weight.
- Human body contains around 1,200 g. Major amount (99% of this) presents in bone and teeth as hydroxyapatite. The remaining 1% is present in blood and soft tissues.
- Calcium level of serum in adult is 9–11 mg/100 mL.
- Blood calcium present in three different forms:
  1. Ionized calcium (Ca$^{++}$) is the physiologically active form. It constitutes 50% of the total calcium (4.5–5.5 mg%).
  2. Protein (albumin) bound form. This is 45% of total level.
  3. Calcium complexes with citrate, phosphate, and bicarbonate. This fraction is only 5%.

### Sources

- *Rich sources:* Milk and its products.
- *Good sources:* Meat, fish, green leafy vegetables, cereals, and pulses.

### Recommended Dietary Allowance

- *Children:* 1.2 g/day.
- *Adults:* 0.8 g/day.
- *Pregnancy and lactation:* 1.2 g/day.

## Absorption

*Factors favoring absorption are as follows:*
1,25-Dihydroxy vitamin $D_3$, gastric acidity, lactose, amino acids and citrate, *and* calcium:phosphate ratio of the diet.

Low level of phosphate increases absorption.

*The substances, which decrease absorption, are:*
Oxalate and phytates of food, fatty acids form insoluble salts with calcium and decreases the absorption.

Chronic renal failure.

## Functions

- Calcium is a mineral
- It is a cation of the extracellular fluid (ECF).
- Calcium is required for the formation of bone and teeth.
- Gives hardness and strength to bone and teeth.
- Required for blood coagulation process.
- Required for contraction of heart and muscle.
- Controls the permeability of cell membranes.
- Activates pancreatic lipase in the digestion of fats.
- Activates phosphorylase during the break down of glycogen.
- Regulates the excitability of nerve fibers.
- Serves as a second messenger in the action of hormones such as adrenaline.
- Responses of calcium are mediated by interaction with a receptor protein called calmodulin. This cytosolic protein has calcium-binding sites. Calmodulin–calcium complex activates protein kinases, which in turn activates other enzymes and through these, it brings about metabolic effects. In this mechanism, cyclic adenosine monophosphate (cAMP) is also involved.

It is required for the formation of Ca⁻ paracaseinate (insoluble curd).

## Regulation of Serum Calcium Level

The ionic calcium level is maintained by vitamin D, parathyroid hormone (PTH), and calcitonin.

## Action of Vitamin D

- Increases the absorption of calcium (and phosphate) from the small intestine.
- Causes removal of calcium from bone (bone resorption).

The mechanism by which 1,25-dihydroxy vitamin $D_3$ increases calcium absorption from intestine is as follows:

The 1,25-dihydroxy vitamin $D_3$ enters the intestinal cell and binds to a cytoplasmic receptor. The vitamin $D_3$ receptor complex then moves to the nucleus where it interacts with DNA. This results in the synthesis of mRNA and this in turn forms a calcium-binding protein. The calcium-binding protein increases the absorption of calcium from intestine.

## Action of Parathyroid Hormone on Kidney and Bone

- PTH increases the activity of 1-α-hydroxylase in kidney, which increases the synthesis of 1,25-dihydroxy vitamin $D_3$ and this in turn enhances the absorption of calcium from intestine **(Fig. 18.1)**.
- It increases the reabsorption of calcium from glomerular filtrate in kidneys.
- It causes the resorption of bone calcium.
  These three actions correct the hypocalcemia and bring it to normal level.
- PTH also causes excretion of phosphate in urine by inhibiting phosphate reabsorption in kidney.

## Action of Calcitonin

This is a hormone from C cells of thyroid glands.

Hypercalcemia stimulates its secretion.

Calcitonin inhibits calcium reabsorption from kidneys and resorption from bone. Thus it corrects hypercalcemia.

Normal value ranges from 9 to 10.6 mg/100 mL serum or 4.5–5.4 mEq/L.

## Hypocalcemia

- Hypoparathyroidism
- Vitamin D deficiency: Decreased dietary intake, decreased sun exposure, defective

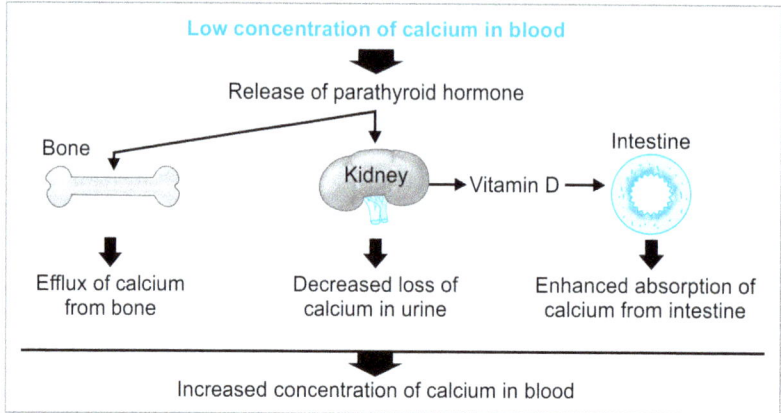

**Fig. 18.1:** Role of parathyroid hormone in restoring low plasma calcium to normal.

vitamin D metabolism, ineffective active vitamin D, and intestinal malabsorption.
* Magnesium deficiency (hypomagnesaemia).
* Eating disorders
* Chronic renal failure: The kidney loses its capacity to synthesize 1,25-dihydroxycholecalciferol. Increased PTH secretion in response to hypocalcemia may lead to bone disease if untreated.
* **Pseudohypoparathyroidism** is a condition associated primarily with resistance to the PTH. Patients have a low serum calcium and high phosphate, but the PTH level is actually appropriately high (due to the hypocalcemia).

## Symptoms

Convulsions, arrhythmias, tetany, and numbness in hands, feet, around mouth, and lips.
* Petechiae, which appear as on–off spots, then later become confluent, and appear as purpura (larger bruised areas).
* Oral, perioral, and acral paresthesias, tingling or "pins and needles" sensation in and around the mouth and lips, and in the extremities of the hands and feet. This is often the earliest symptom of hypocalcemia.
* Carpopedal and generalized tetany are seen.
* Latent tetany.
  1. Trousseau sign of latent tetany (eliciting carpal spasm by inflating the blood pressure cuff and maintaining the cuff pressure above systolic).
  2. Chvostek's sign (tapping of the inferior portion of the zygoma will produce facial spasms).
* Tendon reflexes are hyperactive.
* Life-threatening complications.
  1. Laryngospasm
  2. Cardiac arrhythmias

## Treatment

Two ampoules of intravenous calcium gluconate. Ten percent is given slowly in a period of 10 minutes, or if the hypocalcemia is severe, calcium chloride is given instead.

## Hypercalcemia

Elevated calcium level in the blood causes:
* Primary hyperparathyroidism
  1. Solitary parathyroid adenoma
  2. Primary parathyroid hyperplasia
  3. Parathyroid carcinoma
* Solid tumor with humoral mediation of hypercalcemia (e.g., nonsmall cell lung cancer or kidney cancer, pheochromocytoma).
* Hematologic malignancy (multiple myeloma, lymphoma, and leukemia).

- Hypervitaminosis D (vitamin D intoxication).
- Elevated 1,25(OH)$_2$D (see calcitriol under vitamin D) levels (e.g., sarcoidosis and other granulomatous diseases).
- Idiopathic hypercalcemia of infancy.
- Rebound hypercalcemia after rhabdomyolysis.
- Renal diseases
- Disorders related to high bone turnover rates
    1. Hyperthyroidism
    2. Prolonged immobilization
    3. Paget's disease of the bone
    4. Multiple myeloma

## Signs and Symptoms

Signs and symptoms are stones (renal or biliary), bones (bone pain), thrones (sit on throne—polyuria), fatigue, anorexia, and pancreatitis.

## Treatment

- Hydration, increasing salt intake, and forced diuresis.
- Bisphosphonates are pyrophosphate analogs with high affinity for bone, especially areas of high bone turnover.

# Phosphorus

List the sources and functions of phosphorous.

## Sources

Good sources: milk, meat, cereals.
In general, a diet supplying sufficient calcium will supply an adequate amount of phosphorus also.

## Recommended Dietary Allowance

- *Adult*: 800 mg/day.
- Extraallowance is needed for growth and pregnancy.

## Phosphorus Content of Body and Blood

Phosphorus forms 1% of the body weight.
Whole body contains 700 g of phosphorus, 80% of this is present in bones and teeth as hydroxyapatite.

## Functions

- Helps in the formation of bone and teeth. Inorganic phosphorous is a major constituent of hydroxyapatite in bone, thereby playing an important part in structural support of the body.
- Acts as a buffer in blood. Mixture of $HPO_4^-$ and $H_2PO_4^-$ constitutes the phosphate buffer, which plays a role in maintaining the pH of the body fluid.
- Helps in the formation of compounds such as nucleic acids and nucleotides such as adenosine triphosphate (ATP), guanosine triphosphate (GTP), and adenosine diphosphate (ADP) as organic phosphate esters in glycolysis and other metabolic reactions.
- It is also required in energy metabolism, synthesis of phospholipids, cAMP, phosphoproteins, and coenzymes such as thiamine pyrophosphate (TPP).

**Normal serum inorganic phosphate level:**
- *Adults*: 2.5–4.5 mg%.
- *Children*: 4–6 mg%.

**Hypophosphatemia (decreased level of phosphorous):**
- Rickets
- Hyperparathyroidism
- Condition associated with decrease in the reabsorption of phosphate from the glomerular filtrate (Fanconi syndrome).
    1. In the treatment of diabetes, the effect of insulin in causing the shift of glucose into cells also enhances the transport of phosphate into cells, which may result into hypophosphatemia.

2. Clinical symptoms are muscle pain and weakness with respiratory failure and decreased myocardial output.

## Hyperphosphatemia (Increased Phosphorous Level)

- Seen in hypoparathyroidism
- Hypervitaminosis D
- Renal failure

Elevated phosphate may cause a decrease in serum calcium concentration. Therefore, it may lead to tetany and seizures.

## ■ Magnesium (Mg$^{2+}$)

Magnesium (Mg$^{2+}$) is the major intracellular cation (15 mEq/L) next to potassium. About 70% of total magnesium is in skeletal tissues. The remainder is in muscle, brain, and other tissues.

## Sources

- Abundant in chlorophyll pigment of vegetables.
- Good sources are whole grains, nuts, milk, and meat.

## Recommended Dietary Allowance

- *Adults:* 300 mg/day.
- *Children:* 250 mg/day.

## Functions

- It is an essential activator of many enzymes especially those involving transfer of phosphate groups from ATP (hexokinase and phosphofructokinase).
- It also activates a number of enzymes such as:.
    1. Enolase
    2. Glucose-6-P dehydrogenase
    3. Pyruvate carboxylase
    4. Thiokinase.
    5. Glucose-6-phosphogluconate dehydrogenase.

- Magnesium along with sodium, potassium, and calcium controls neuromuscular irritability.
- It is important constituent of bone.

## Deficiency

Deficiency symptoms bear some resemblance to those seen in hypocalcemia, with muscle twitching, spasms, and tetany.

## ■ Sodium (Na$^+$)

- Sodium (Na$^+$) is the major cation of the ECF.
- Most of the body's sodium is located in the blood and in the fluid in the space surrounding the cells. Sodium is required by all cells in the body to maintain a normal fluid balance.

## Sources

The major sources are table salt, cereals, legumes, egg, carrot, tomato, and milk.
- Average intake from table salt is 5–10 g/day.
- Requirement: 5 g/day.
- The normal range in blood: 130–145 mEq/L (intracellular Na$^+$ is 10 mEq/L).

## Functions

- Maintains the osmotic pressure, thus to maintain the volume of blood and blood pressure (i.e., protection against fluid loss), sodium loss causes blood volume to decrease. When blood volume decreases, blood pressure also decreases, heart rate increases, and light-headedness and sometimes shock occur.

Conversely, the blood volume increases when there is too much sodium in the body. When excess sodium accumulates in the body, extra fluid accumulates in the space surrounding the cells. As a result, the tissues, especially in the feet and ankles, swell.

- Regulates the electrolyte and pH balance of the extracellular compartment.
- Controls the electronic potentials of excitable tissues such as nerve and muscle.
- Helps in the active transport of glucose, galactose, and amino acids across intestinal mucosa and for $Na^+/K^+$-ATPase.

Average serum sodium level is 142 mEq/L (intracellular sodium is 10 mEq/L).

## Osmolality

*Plasma osmolality/osmolarity measures the body's electrolyte-water balance.*

Osmolality and osmolarity are the measures that are technically different, but functionally the same for normal use.

Osmolality is a measure of the osmoles (Osm) of solute per kilogram of solvent (osmol/kg or Osm/kg); osmolarity is defined as the number of osmoles of solute per liter (L) of solution (osmol/L or Osm/L).

### Clinical Relevance

Cell membranes are freely permeable to water, the osmolality of the ECF is approximately equal to that of the intracellular fluid (ICF). Therefore, plasma osmolality is a guide to intracellular osmolality. This is important as it shows that changes in ECF osmolality have a great effect on ICF osmolality—changes that can cause problems with normal cell functioning and volume. If the ECF was to become too hypotonic, water would readily fill surrounding cells, increasing their volume and potentially lysing them (cytolysis).

Osmolality of blood increases with dehydration and decreases with overhydration. In normal people, increased osmolality in the blood will stimulate secretion of antidiuretic hormone (ADH). This will result in increased water reabsorption, more concentrated urine, and less concentrated blood plasma. A low serum osmolality will suppress the release of ADH, resulting in decreased water reabsorption and more concentrated plasma.

Osmolality of a serum or plasma sample can be measured directly or it may be calculated if the concentrations of the major solutes are already known. There are many formulae used to calculate the serum osmolality. Clinically, the simplest is:

Serum osmolality = 2 × serum (sodium)
(mmol/kg)              (mmol/L)

### Clinical use

Serum osmolality is used in two main circumstances: investigation of hyponatremia and identification of an osmolar gap. Urine osmolality is an important test of renal concentrating ability, for identifying disorders of the ADH mechanism, and identifying causes of hyper- or hyponatremia.

### Serum Osmolality

Serum osmolality is a useful preliminary investigation for identifying the cause of hyponatremia.

### Urine Osmolality

Urine osmolality is an important test for the concentrating ability of the kidney. Interpretation of urine osmolality must always be made in the light of the appropriate physiological response to the state of hydration of the patient. The test is useful in the following areas:

- For determining the differential diagnosis of hyper- or hyponatremia.
- For identifying syndrome of inappropriate ADH secretion (SIADH) (urine osmolality >200 mmol/kg, urine sodium >20 mmol/L, low serum sodium, patient not dehydrated and no renal, adrenal, thyroid, cardiac, or liver disease or interfering drugs).
- For differentiating prerenal from renal kidney failure (high urine osmolality is consistent with prerenal impairment, in renal damage the urine osmolality is similar to plasma osmolality).

* For identifying and diagnosing diabetes insipidus.

## Atrial Natriuretic Peptide

**Atrial natriuretic peptide** (ANP) is a potent vasodilator and a protein secreted by cardiac muscle cells. ANP is a circulating hormone, which regulates atrial blood pressure **(Fig. 18.2)**.

It controls the body water, Na, K, and fat. This hormone is released by muscle cells of upper chamber of heart when BP elevated.

ANP reduces water and sodium and blocks the release of several hormones. ANP is produced, piled up, and secreted by myocytes. ANP level usually increase in state of hypertension and excessive of fluids. Human heart secretes ANP and brain natriuretic peptide (BNP). Both BNP and ANP levels increase hypertension, secondary hypertensions, and chronic heart failure during heart pacing, chronic renal failure, and acute myocardial infarction is determined. These receptors are having their own functions and purposes. ANP has four receptors, namely renal, vascular, cardiac, and adipose tissues.

ANP attaches to a specific group of receptors. These receptors are designed to cause a reduction in blood volume and reduction in cardiac output and systematic blood pressure. Renal reduces aldosterone secretion by adrenal cortex. Renal inhibit rennin secretion. In vascular, it relaxes vascular smooth muscles in arterioles. Adipose tissues increase the release of fatty acids from adipose tissues.

The ANP in combination with the BNP helps in reducing the volume of blood as well as the excessive pressure on the blood, which allows keeping everything related to the heart and blood to normal levels. This ensures best control over the blood flow in your body as well as a great control over your entire body and its functions.

## Deficiency

* A nutritional deficiency is highly important.
* On a low-sodium diet, the kidney decreases the excretion of sodium in urine.
* Low blood sodium triggers the kidney to release angiotensin, which causes the adrenal cortex to secrete aldosterone, the latter induces the renal tubules to reabsorb sodium from the glomerular filtrate.

## Hyponatremia (Reduced Sodium in the Blood)

**Causes:** Imbalance of water and sodium. Most frequently it occurs when excessive water

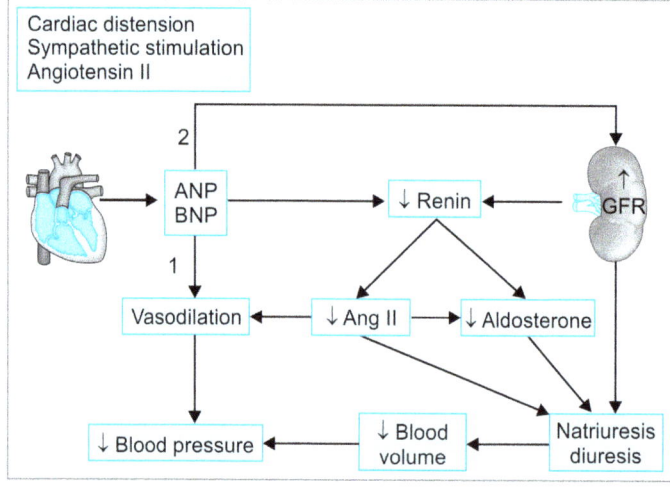

**Fig. 18.2:** Role of atrial natriuretic peptide (ANP) and brain natriuretic peptide (BNP).

dilutes the amount of sodium in the body or when not enough total sodium is present in the body. A common classification of hyponatremia is based on the amount of total body water that is present.
* Decrease in plasma sodium may be due to defect in kidneys or adrenal cortex.
* Sweating, burns, vomiting, or diarrhea, which can cause loss of sodium-containing fluids.
* In adrenocortical insufficiency (Addison's disease), decrease of serum sodium and increase in sodium excretion are seen.

## Normal Volume (Euvolemic) Hyponatremia

The amount of water in the body is normal, but an ADH is being inappropriately secreted (SIADH) from the pituitary gland. This may be seen in patients with pneumonia, small cell lung cancer, bleeding in the brain, or brain tumors.

## Excess Volume (Hypervolemic) Hyponatremia

Too much total body water dilutes the amount of sodium contained in the body. This can be seen in heart failure, kidney failure, and liver diseases such as cirrhosis. This situation is somewhat misnamed because while there is increased total body water, there may be a relative decrease of fluid within the bloodstream. Because of the underlying disease, fluid leaks into the space between tissues (called the third space) causing swelling of the extremities or ascites, fluid within the abdominal cavity.

## Inadequate Volume (Hypovolemic) Hyponatremia

The amount of water in the body is too low as can occur in dehydration. The antidiuretic hormone is stimulated, causing the kidneys to make very concentrated urine and hold onto water. This may be seen with excessive sweating and exercising in a hot environment. It can also occur in patients with excess fluid loss due to vomiting and diarrhea, pancreatitis, and burns.

**Other specific situations hyponatremia seen:**
* Hyponatremia may be a side effect of medications, especially diuretics or water pills used to help control blood pressure. This class of drugs can cause excessive loss of sodium in the urine.
* Hormonal diseases such as Addison's disease or adrenal insufficiency and hypothyroidism may be associated with low-sodium levels.
* Polydipsia, or excessive water intake, may cause "water intoxication," diluting sodium levels. This is occasionally associated with psychiatric illness.
* In some people who exercise, their concern about the potential for dehydration causes them to drink more water than they lose by perspiration. This may cause significant hyponatremia and has been known to be fatal in marathon participants who drink too much fluid without replacing lost sodium, in excess of what their thirst mechanism dictates.

## Symptoms
* Confusion
* Nausea and fatigue
* Seizures
* Some individuals do not show any symptoms.

## Diagnosis

The diagnosis of hyponatremia is made by a blood test that measures the concentration of sodium in the bloodstream. The normal sodium level is between 135 and 145 mEq/L, and levels below 110 mEq/L constitute a true emergency.

Other tests may help decide what type of hyponatremia situation exists. The amount of sodium that is being excreted in the urine may be measured, as well as the concentration of urine.

## Hypernatremia

**Hypernatremia** or **hypernatraemia** is an electrolyte disturbance with elevated sodium level in the blood.

Hypernatremia is generally not caused by an excess of sodium, but rather by a relative deficit of free water in the body. For this reason, hypernatremia is often synonymous with the less precise term, "dehydration."

Even a small rise in the serum sodium concentration above the normal range results in a strong sensation of thirst, an increase in free water intake, and correction of the abnormality.

### Causes

Decreased activity of ADH
Hyperactivity of the adrenal cortex (in Cushing's syndrome).

Common causes of hypernatremia include:
- Hypovolemic
  1. Inadequate intake of water typically in elderly or otherwise disabled patients who are unable to take in water as their thirst dictates. This is the most common cause of hypernatremia.
  2. Excessive losses of water from the urinary tract, which may be caused by glycosuria, or other osmotic diuretics.
  3. Water losses associated with extreme sweating.
  4. Severe watery diarrhea.
- Euvolemic
  1. Excessive excretion of water from the kidneys caused by diabetes insipidus, which involves either inadequate production of the hormone, vasopressin from the pituitary gland or impaired responsiveness of the kidneys to vasopressin.

### Signs and Symptoms
- Lethargy
- Restlessness
- Spasticity
- Edema
- Seizures

### Treatment

The treatment is administration of free water to correct the relative water deficit. Water can be replaced orally or intravenously. Water alone cannot be administered as intravenously rather can be given with addition to dextrose or saline infusion solutions (**Fig. 18.3**).

Rapid lowering the sodium concentration with free water may cause water to flow into brain cells and causes them to swell. This can lead to cerebral edema, potentially resulting in seizures, permanent brain damage, or death. Therefore, significant hypernatremia should be treated carefully by a physician or other medical professional with experience in treatment of electrolyte imbalances.

### Deficiency

- A nutritional deficiency is highly important.
- On a low-sodium diet, the kidney decreases the excretion of sodium in urine.
- Low blood sodium triggers the kidney to release angiotensin. Angiotensin causes the adrenal cortex to secrete aldosterone. The aldosterone induces the renal tubules to reabsorb sodium from the glomerular filtrate.

Another mechanism involves the pituitary gland, which secretes ADH. ADH causes the kidneys to conserve water. The retained sodium and water lead to decreased urine production, which eventually leads to an increase in blood volume.

## Potassium (K$^+$)

- Potassium (K$^+$) is the most important cation of ICF.

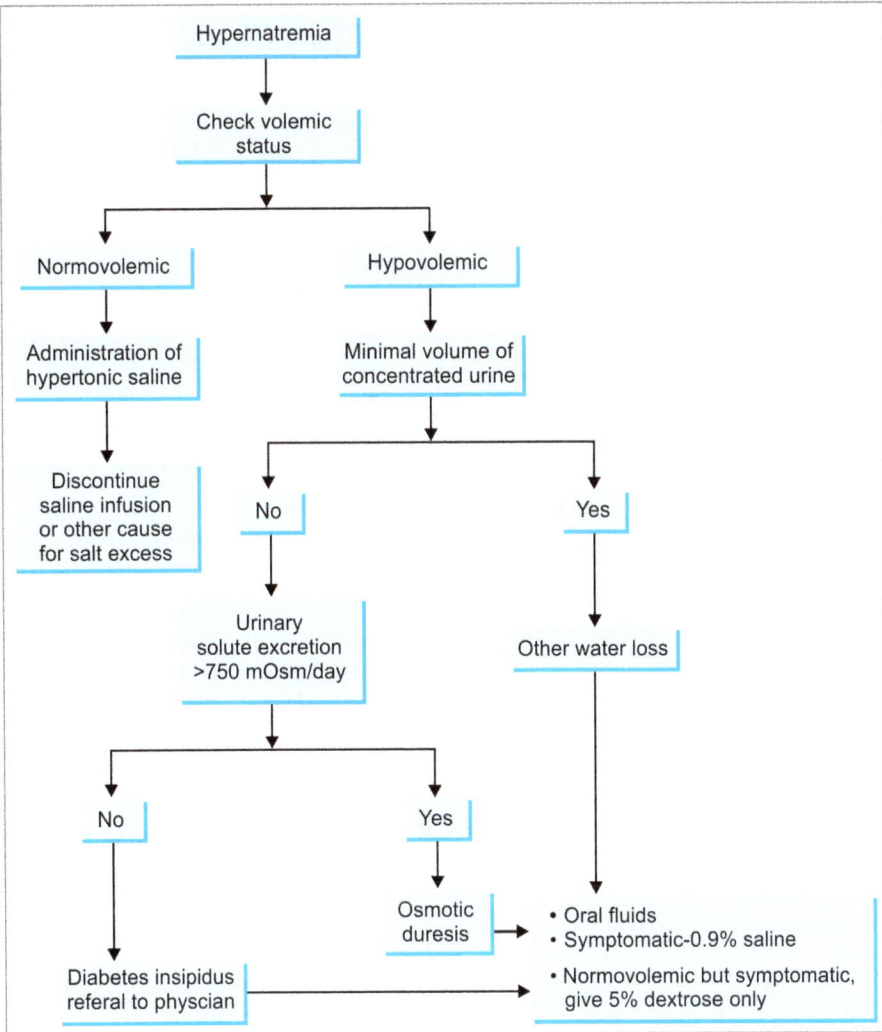

Fig. 18.3: Treatment option for hyponatremia.

- Average concentration in the ICF is 150 mEq/L.
- **Extracellular** potassium concentration is normally kept within a tight range of 3.5–5.0 mEq/L.
- **Extracellular** potassium is important for its controlling influence upon neuromuscular irritability, cardiac muscle (a proper balance between potassium and calcium is essential for the contraction of heart muscle), and the operation of $Na^+/K^+$-ATPase ($Na^+$ pump) against the concentration gradient.
- In cells, there is a significant concentration gradient of sodium and potassium across cell membranes.
- The high intracellular potassium is maintained by an energy requiring extrusion of three sodium out of the cell with replacement by two potassium **(Fig. 18.4)**.

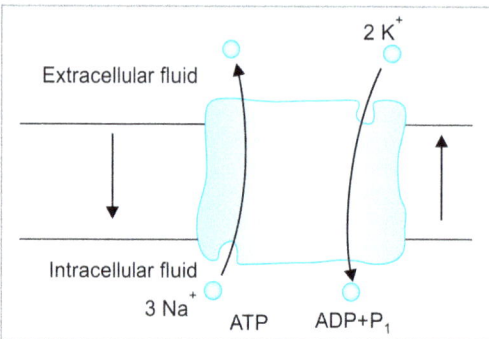

**Fig. 18.4:** Movement of potassium and sodium across the compartments.

- Intracellular potassium is essential for a number of enzyme reactions (such as pyruvate kinase, glycogen synthesis, and protein synthesis), for maintaining osmotic and acid–base balance.
- Nearly all of the total body potassium (98%) is inside cells. If, for example, there is significant tissue damage, the contents of cells, including potassium, leak out into the extracellular compartment, causing potentially dangerous increases in serum potassium.

## Sources

The sources are orange, banana, and fresh vegetables.
- An average diet provides 4 g $K^+$/day.
- Normal serum level: 3–5.0 mEq/L.

## Functions

- Potassium is the principal cation of ICF.
- It is required for the functioning of nerves, skeletal muscle, and cardiac muscles. Either decreased potassium or increased potassium levels finally cause cardiac arrest.
- It is required as a cofactor in several enzymatic reactions in the body.
- It is involved in acid–base balance.

## Hypokalemia

Hypokalemia is a metabolic disorder that occurs when the level of potassium in the blood drops too low.

This condition decreases the heartbeat and interferes with vital muscles such as those involved in respiration.

Possible causes:
- Antibiotics (penicillin, nafcillin, carbenicillin, gentamicin, amphotericin B, and foscarnet).
- Diarrhea
    - Gastrointestinal loss
- Diseases that affect the kidneys' ability to retain potassium.
- Diuretic medications, which can cause excess urination (Certain diuretics increase the excretion of potassium. It is, therefore, important to supplement enough potassium when these diuretics are used).
- Eating disorders (such as bulimia)
- Sweating
- Vomiting
- Aldosterone increases the excretion of potassium or administration of cortisone leads to hypokalemia.
- Reduced intake but it is rare.

## Pseudohypokalemia

Pseudohypokalemia is a decrease in the amount of potassium that occurs due to excessive uptake of potassium by metabolically active cells in a blood sample after it has been drawn. It is a laboratory artifact that may occur when blood samples remain in warm conditions for several hours before processing.

## Symptoms

A small drop in potassium usually does not cause symptoms. However, a big drop in the level can be life-threatening.

Symptoms of hypokalemia include:
- Abnormal heart rhythms (dysrhythmias), especially in people with heart disease.
- Constipation
- Fatigue
- Muscle damage (rhabdomyolysis)
- Muscle weakness or spasms
- Paralysis (which can include the lungs)

## Treatment

Mild hypokalemia can be treated by taking potassium supplements by mouth. Persons with more severe cases may need to get potassium through a vein (intravenously).

If diuretics used, doctor may try to keep potassium in the body (such as triamterene and amiloride).

One type of hypokalemia that causes paralysis occurs when there is too much thyroid hormone in the blood (thyrotoxic periodic paralysis). Treatment lowers the thyroid hormone level and raises the potassium level in the blood.

## Hyperkalemia

- Elevated plasma potassium concentration.
- It occurs in Addison's disease and in intravenous infusion of potassium at a rate excess of 25 mmol/h.
- Treatment using concentrated potassium solutions.

### Causes

- Renal insufficiency (renal failure)
- Medication that interferes with urinary excretion.
- Mineralocorticoid deficiency or resistance, such as:
  1. Addison's disease
  2. Aldosterone deficiency
  3. Some forms of congenital adrenal hyperplasia.
  4. Type IV renal tubular acidosis (resistance of renal tubules to aldosterone).
- Excessive release from cells
  1. Rhabdomyolysis, burns, or any cause of rapid tissue necrosis, including tumor lysis syndrome.
  2. Massive blood transfusion or massive hemolysis.
  3. Shifts/transports out of cells caused by acidosis, low insulin levels, beta-blocker therapy, digoxin overdose, or the paralyzing agent succinylcholine.
- **Excessive intake:** Excess intake with salt-substitute, potassium-containing dietary supplements, or potassium chloride (KCl) infusion.
- **Pseudohyperkalemia:** Pseudohyperkalemia is a rise in the amount of potassium that occurs due to excessive leakage of potassium from cells, during or after blood is drawn. It is typically caused by hemolysis during venipuncture.

Tissue trauma causing the cells to release potassium into the ECF includes burns, traumatic injury, and intestinal bleeding.

### Signs and Symptoms

- Fatigue
- Weakness
- Tingling
- Numbness
- Paralysis
- Palpitations and difficulty in breathing

### Treatment

Several agents are used to transiently lower $K^+$ levels. Choice depends on the degree and cause of the hyperkalemia, and other aspects of the patient's condition.

### Normal Range

- In serum—3.5–5 mEq/L
- In plasma—3.5–4.5 mEq/L

**Note:** Serum potassium level above 7 mEq/L and below 2.5 mEq/L is serious, life-threatening and requires immediate attention.

***Specimen required for test:*** Serum, heparinized plasma, sweat, urine.

Hemolyzed samples are not suitable for electrolyte analysis because of the release of potassium from the RBC, which will cause a false increase in the potassium values.

- Urine collection for electrolyte estimation should be made without any preservative.
- Serum, plasma, or urine must be stored at 2–4°C or frozen if the analysis is delayed.

## Chloride (Cl⁻)

- Chloride ($Cl^-$) is the major extracellular anion.
- Serum concentration is 105 mEq/L.

## Functions

The functions of chloride are as follows:
- It is involved in maintaining osmotic pressure, proper body hydration, and electric neutrality.
- In the central nervous system, the inhibitory action of glycine and some of the action of gamma aminobutyric acid (GABA) rely on the entry of $Cl^-$ into specific neurons.
- The chloride–bicarbonate exchanger biological transport protein relies on the chloride ion to increase the blood's capacity of carbon dioxide, in the form of the bicarbonate ion.
- Dietary chloride is almost completely absorbed by the intestinal tract. It is filtered out by the glomerulus and passively reabsorbed in conjunction with $Na^+$ by the proximal tubules. Excess chloride is excreted in urine and through sweating. Excessive sweating stimulates aldosterone secretion, which acts on the sweat glands to conserve $Na^+$ and chloride.

## Hypochloremia (A Low Serum Chloride)

- Metabolic alkalosis
- Vomiting
- Diarrhea
- Diuretics
- Gastric suction
- Respiratory losses
- Steroid medications.
  Any conditions associated with hyponatremia cause hypochloremia.
- Adrenal insufficiency (Addison's disease), salt-losing nephritis, SIADH, and renal failure.

## Hyperchloremia (High Serum Chloride)

- Metabolic acidosis
- Dehydration
- Decreased renal blood flow
- Medications containing ammonium chloride.
- Hyperparathyroidism

## Micro Minerals or Trace Elements

Trace elements are present in the body in very small amounts and are essential for certain biochemical processes. They are iron, iodine, cobalt, copper, manganese, molybdenum, zinc, lead, selenium, and fluoride.

## Iron (Fe)

- Iron (Fe) is a trace element.
- Total body iron is about 5 g.

## Sources

The sources are liver, meat, egg yolk, vegetables, whole wheat, legumes, cashew nuts, and dates.

## Functions

The functions of iron are as follows:
- Iron is necessary for the synthesis of certain proteins.

- Iron-containing proteins in the body are of two types:
  1. Heme proteins (proteins with heme group)
     *Hemoglobin*: This accounts for 70% total body iron.
     *Myoglobin*: This is the muscle $O_2$-binding protein, 5% of total Fe is in this form. Both proteins function in the transport of $O_2$.
     *Catalase and peroxidase*: Function of this is in the decomposition of $H_2O_2$, a toxic compound.
     *Cytochromes b, c1, c, a, a3*: These take part in respiratory chain.
  2. Nonheme proteins (proteins with nonheme group)
     *Ferritin and hemosiderin*: These are iron storage proteins in liver, spleen, and bone marrow. These comprise 15% of body iron.
     *Transferrin*: This is the iron transport protein in blood.
     Aconitase of Kreb's TCA cycle.
     Iron sulfur proteins. Succinate dehydrogenase is an example.

## Recommended Dietary Allowance

- *Adult males*: 12 mg/day
- *Females*: 20 mg/day
- *Pregnancy and lactation*: 40 mg/day.

## Iron Absorption

Absorption takes place mainly in the duodenum **(Table 18.1)**.

## Mechanism of Iron Absorption and Transport

Normally, about 5–10% of dietary iron is absorbed by the active transport process in the duodenum. Heme of food is absorbed directly from the intestine and nonheme iron is absorbed in the ferrous state ($Fe^{2+}$) into the mucosal cell as described here **(Fig. 18.5)**:

**Table 18.1:** Factors favoring and reducing iron absorption.

| Factors favoring absorption | Factors reducing absorption |
| --- | --- |
| • Ferrous form | • Ferric form |
| • Inorganic iron | • Organic iron |
| • Acids—HCl | • Alkalis, antacids |
| • Vitamin C | • Pancreatic secretions |
| • Iron deficiency | • Iron excess |
| • Increased erythropoiesis | • Decreased erythropoiesis |
| • Pregnancy | • Infection |

HCl of stomach liberate $Fe^{3+}$ from nonheme iron compounds of food.
Iron is absorbed as $Fe^{2+}$.

The gastric HCl and organic acids in the diet convert organic ferric compound of the diet into free ferric ($Fe^{3+}$) ions. These ferric ions are reduced with ascorbic acid and glutathione of food to more soluble ferrous form ($Fe^{2+}$), which is more readily absorbed than ferric form ($Fe^{3+}$). In the intestinal mucosa, the iron is either stored in the form of ferritin in the mucosal cells or transported across the mucosal cells to the plasma in the form of transferrin. The mucosal cell storage is dependent on body's iron status.

- After absorption of $Fe^{2+}$ into the intestinal mucosal cell, it is oxidized to $Fe^{3+}$.
- This combines with intracellular carrier protein.
- This complex either delivers a fixed amount of Fe to mitochondria or transfers some iron to another protein called apoferritin, which binds $Fe^{3+}$ to form ferritin.
- The ferritin is a storage form of iron.
- Some iron binds with plasma a1-globulin called apotransferrin, to form transferrin. Each molecule of apotransferrin binds two ferric ions. The transferrin is a transport form of iron. As mentioned above the proportions of iron transferred to apoferritin and apotransferrin depend upon the iron status of the person. Iron always transport in the ferric form.

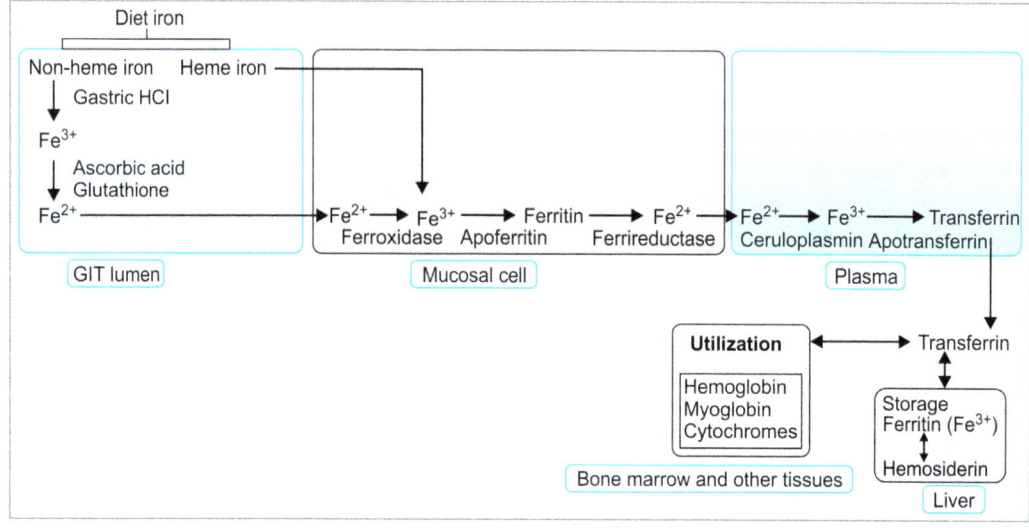

**Fig. 18.5:** Absorption and transport of dietary iron.

The transfer of storage ferritin ($Fe^{3+}$) to plasma involves reduction of $Fe^{3+}$ to $Fe^{2+}$ in the mucosal cell with the help of ferrireductase. This ferrous enters the plasma and there it is reoxidized to ferric form by a copper protein, ceruloplasmin. Or serum ferroxidase and then this ferric form incorporated into transferrin by combining with apotransferrin.

* In the iron deficient state, more iron is delivered to apotransferrin and much less to apoferritin.
* In the case of iron overload, more iron is transferred to apoferritin and much less to apotransferrin. Thus entry of iron in to the body is regulated at the intestine level.

Ferritin is the major storage form of iron and it is readily available for metabolic requirements. The storage occurs in liver, spleen, and bone.

### Hemosiderin

In addition to ferritin, iron can also be found in a form of hemosiderin. This hemosiderin is insoluble in aqueous medium and iron is released slowly from this. Normally very little hemosiderin is found in the liver, but the quantity increases during iron overload and it may represent protective role against iron overload.

### Serum Content

Transferrin of 300 mg/dL is capable of carrying 360 µg of Fe, but normally it carries an average of only 100 µg of Fe. In deficiency, this level is much less.

### Deficiency

Hypochromic microcytic anemia (microcytic RBC of reduced size).

*Causes*

* Hemorrhage
* Malabsorption
* Hookworm infestation depletes the body iron even if the diet is adequate.
* The pronounced and repeated Fe loss from menstruation, pregnancy, and lactation.
* Anemic patients are found to be pale, tired, and restless and have palpitation, lesions of oral cavity, and spoon-shaped nails **(Fig. 18.6)**.

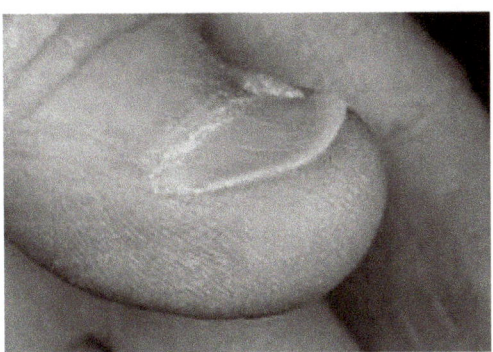

**Fig. 18.6:** Spooning of nail.

## Iron Overload

Hemosiderosis and hemochromatosis and iron poisoning are the conditions associated with iron overload.

### Hemochromatosis

- It is an excessive hemosiderin accumulation in tissues such as liver, spleen, and skin. caused by an excessive intestinal absorption of iron due to a genetic disorder.
- This results in bronze-colored skin, cirrhosis of liver, and damage to pancreas leading to diabetes. This is called bronze diabetes.
- Hemosiderosis is an excessive accumulation of iron. This may be seen in the Bantu people of Africa who consume large amount of Fe obtained from their cooking pots made of iron.

## ■ Copper (Cu$^{2+}$)

### Sources

The major sources are fish, liver, nuts, and green vegetables.
Milk and cereals are poor sources.

### Recommended Dietary Allowance

Adult: 3 mg/day.

### Functions

A need for copper is linked to its functional role in several copper-containing enzymes.

- Ceruloplasmin, a copper-containing protein catalyzes the oxidation of Fe$^{2+}$ to Fe$^{3+}$.
- Cytochrome oxidase of the respiratory chain contains Fe$^{3+}$ and Cu$^{2+}$.
- Dopamine oxidase of catecholamine synthetic pathway.
- Monoamine oxidase and diamine oxidase.
- Cytoplasmic superoxide dismutase contains Cu$^{2+}$ and Zn$^{2+}$.
- P-hydroxyphenyl pyruvate hydroxylase of tyrosine catabolism.
- Lysyl oxidase involved in cross-linking process in the conversion of tropocollagen to collagen.
- Tyrosinase of melanin synthetic pathway is a Cu-dependent enzyme.

## Absorption and Transport in Blood

About 50% of the average daily dietary copper is absorbed from the stomach and the small intestine, then transported to the liver bound to albumin and exported to peripheral tissues (90%) bound to ceruloplasmin and to a lesser extent (10%) to albumin. The route of excretion of copper is through bile.

## Deficiency

- Hypochromic microcytic anemia due to copper deficiency in milk-fed infants has been observed. It responds to copper but not to iron therapy.
- Wilson's disease or hepatolenticular degeneration.
  It is a fatal inherited disease. Blood copper level decreases.
  There is an excessive storage of copper in the liver, probably owing to defective synthesis of ceruloplasmin by the liver cells. Besides deposition in liver, copper is also deposited in kidney, brain, and cornea (brown ring called Kayser-Fleischer ring at the margin of cornea). Cirrhosis of liver, neurological disorders, tubular damage, and high urinary copper are also seen.

Penicillamine, a copper-chelating agent, is used in its treatment. Excess copper is, thus, excreted.

Menkes' syndrome or Kinky-hair disease. It is a rare X-linked recessive disorder. The genetic defect is in absorption of copper from intestine. Both serum copper and ceruloplasmin and liver copper content are reduced.

The clinical manifestations are Kinky or twisted brittle hair due to loss of copper catalyzed disulfide bond formation.

- Depigmentation of the skin and hair.
- Seizures
- Mental retardation
- Lesions of the blood vessels.

## Zinc (Zn)

### Sources

The sources are meat, egg, marine fish, unmilled cereals, legumes corn, spinach, and lettuce.

### Recommended Dietary Allowance

- *Adults*: 10–15 mg/day
- *Children*: 3–15 mg/day
- *Pregnancy and lactation*: 20–25 mg/day.

### Functions

- Carbonic anhydrase
- Alkaline phosphatase
- Liver alcohol dehydrogenase
- Carboxyl peptidase A
- DNA polymerase
- Cytosolic superoxide dismutase (both $Cu^{2+}$ and $Zn^{2+}$).

It is required for the wound healing processes and it is a necessary factor in the biosynthesis and integrity of connective tissue.

### Deficiency

- Zinc deficiency may cause dwarfism.
- Other deficiency manifestations are hypogonadism.
- Loss of taste sensation
- Impaired wound healing

*Acrodermatitis enteropathica:* It is an autosomal recessive disorder and its clinical manifestations appear to be related to zinc deficiency. The clinical manifestations of this are chronic diarrhea, alopecia, wasting, and thickened ulcerated skin around the body orifices and extremities.

## Manganese ($Mn^{2+}$)

### Sources

The sources are wheat germs seeds, nuts, leafy vegetables, and meat.

### Recommended Dietary Allowance

- *Adults*: 3.5 mg/day
- *Children*: 0.2 mg/day

### Functions

Manganese acts as a cofactor or an activator for several enzymes.

The manganese-containing enzymes are:
- Acetyl CoA carboxylase
- Mitochondrial superoxide dismutase.
- Arginase
- 6-phosphogluconate dehydrogenase
- Squalene synthetase
- Isocitrate dehydrogenase
- Glutamine synthetase
- Manganese also functions with vitamin K in the formation of prothrombin.

### Deficiency

In both birds and mammals, the manganese deficiency is characterized by defective growth, bone abnormalities, reproductive dysfunction, and central nervous system (CNS) manifestations.

The toxicity has been seen in miners as a result of absorption of manganese through respiratory tract after prolonged exposure to manganese dust.

## Molybdenum (Mo)

### Sources

The sources are legumes, whole grains, milk, leafy vegetables, and organ meat.

### Recommended Dietary Allowance

*Adults:* 0.5 mg/day.

### Metabolic Functions

It is required as a catalytic component of the metalloenzymes such as:
* Xanthine oxidase
* Aldehyde oxidase
* Sulfite oxidase.

### Deficiency

It is reported to cause xanthinuria.

## Cobalt (Co)

### Sources

The sources are liver, kidney, muscle meats, oysters, and clams.

### Functions

* This occurs in vitamin $B_{12}$ and its coenzymes.
* Cofactor for glycyl-glycine dipeptidase of intestinal juice.

### Deficiency

A cobalt deficiency is accompanied by all the signs and symptoms of a vitamin $B_{12}$ deficiency. The most important is anemia.

### Toxicity

Polycythemia.

## Selenium (Se)

### Sources

The sources are fish, whole grain, meat, liver, and kidney.

### Recommended Dietary Allowance

* *Adult:* 0.2 mg/day
* Selenium is an integral component of glutathione peroxidase. This enzyme scavenges the free radicals and protects the cells and membranes against oxidative damage.

So this mineral complements the action of vitamin E. Thus it acts as an antioxidant. Selenium also is a constituent of iodothyronine deiodinase, the enzyme that converts thyroxine to triiodothyronine.

### Absorption

The principal dietary forms of selenium, selenocysteine and selenomethionine, are absorbed from gastrointestinal tract.

### Deficiency

Selenium deficiency has been associated in some areas of China with Keshan disease, a cardiomyopathy, primarily affects children. Symptoms are loss of appetite, nausea, and congestive heart failure.

## Fluoride (F)

### Sources

The sources are fish, tea, and drinking water.

### Recommended Dietary Allowance

* Adults 1–2 mg/day
* Drinking water provides fluoride [1 part per million (1 ppm) fluoride. 2 L water consumed by an individual provides 2 mgF].

## Functions

- Fluoride is a component of a hydroxyapatite.
- It is needed for bone and teeth formation. The surface layer of enamel contains a higher content of fluoride than deeper layers of enamel or dentine. It strengthens the enamel surface of teeth and renders it resistant to dental caries (decay).

   Deficiency causes dental caries and osteoporosis.

   Excess fluoride causes fluorosis. In this condition, there is mottling of enamel. The mottled enamel is discolored, corroded, and pitted. High concentrations of fluoride inhibit magnesium-requiring enzymes, enolase.

## Chromium (Cr)

### Sources

The sources are Brewer's yeast, molasses, meat products, and cheese.

### Recommended Dietary Allowance

0.05–20 mg for adults.

### Functions

- Chromium functions in the control of glucose and lipid metabolism.
- It acts as cofactor for insulin in increasing glucose utilization and transport of amino acids into cells.
- Organochromium complex is known as the glucose tolerance factor. The researchers showed that it enhances the action of insulin.

### Deficiency

May develop the symptoms of glucose intolerance and weight loss.

### Toxicity

- Known to cause inflammation and necrosis of the skin and nasal passages.
- Oral ingestion can lead to GI tract and renal damage.

## Iodine ($I_2$)

- The adult human body contains about 50 mg of iodine.
- The blood plasma contains 4–8 µg of protein-bound iodine per 100 mL.

### Sources

The sources are seafood, drinking water, iodized table salt, onions, vegetables, etc.

### Recommended Dietary Allowance

150 µg/day.

### Functions

The most important role of iodine in the body is in the synthesis of thyroid hormones, triiodothyronine ($T_3$) and tetraiodothyronine ($T_4$), which influence a large number of metabolic functions.

### Deficiency Manifestation

A deficiency of iodine in children leads to cretinism and in adults' endemic goiter.

### Cretinism

Severe iodine deficiency in mothers leads to intrauterine or neonatal hypothyroidism, which results in cretinism in their children, a condition characterized by mental retardation, dwarfism, and slow growth.

### Goiter

It is an enlarged thyroid with decreased thyroid hormone production **(Fig. 18.7)**. The iodine deficiency in adults stimulates the proliferation of epithelial cells, resulting in enlargement of the thyroid gland. Normally thyroid gland collects iodine from the blood to synthesize thyroid hormones. In iodine-deficient state the thyroid gland undergoes compensatory enlargement in order to extract iodine from blood.

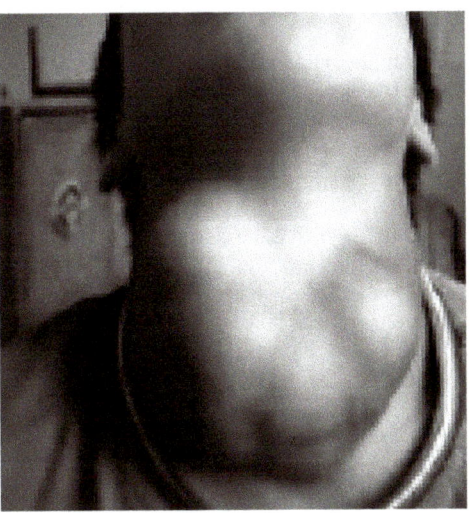

**Fig. 18.7:** Goiter.

## SUMMARY

Minerals are the essential chemical elements required by living organism and they are of bulk and trace elements. Bulk elements are seven in number such as calcium, magnesium, sodium, potassium, phosphorus, sulfur, and chloride. They constitute 60–80% of all inorganic material in the body. Trace elements are those, which are required in very small amounts. They are nine in number and they are iron, iodine, cobalt, manganese, molybdenum, zinc, lead, selenium, and fluoride. The deficiency of minerals results in various disorders. For example, hypocalcemia may lead to numbness and bone disorders, iodine deficiency results in goiter, fluoride deficiency causes dental decay, and iron deficiency results in anemia.

## SELF-ASSESSMENT QUESTIONS

### Long Answer Questions

1. Write a note on the requirement and functions of calcium.
2. What are the factors, which favor iron absorption?
3. Add a note on the absorption and transport of iron.
4. Name the heme and nonheme proteins, which contain iron.
5. Mention the functions of phosphorous.
6. Name any four enzymes, which need magnesium as an activator ion.
7. Which trace element deficiency leads to Wilson's disease?
8. Mention the important source of fluoride. What is fluorosis?
9. What are the sources of copper?
10. What are the trace elements? Name any four of them.
11. What are the importance of sodium and potassium in the human body?
12. Give the normal values of $Na^+$ and $K^+$.

## Short Answer Questions

1. State whether copper is an example of trace element or bulk element.
2. Give the normal serum value of calcium.
3. Name the nonheme protein, which contains iron.
4. Which form of iron is absorbed from GI tract?
5. The deficiency of iron leads to what?
6. Name the storage form of iron.
7. Antioxidant property is observed in which trace element?
8. Give an example for copper-containing enzyme.
9. The fluoride deficiency leads to what?
10. Name the major cation of the extracellular fluid.
11. What is hyponatremia?
12. Mention the name of the major extracellular anion.

## Fill in the Blanks

1. Copper is a/an _____ element.
2. The normal serum value of calcium is _____.
3. The example of nonheme protein, which contains iron, is _____.
4. The form of iron, which absorbed from GI tract, is _____.
5. The deficiency of iron leads to _____.
6. Storage form of iron is called _____.
7. Antioxidant property observed in the trace element is _____.
8. Cytochrome oxidase is a/an _____ containing enzyme.
9. The fluoride deficiency leads to _____.
10. The major cation of the extracellular fluid is _____.
11. Hyponatremia means _____.
12. The major extracellular anion is _____.

## MULTIPLE CHOICE QUESTIONS

1. **All of the following factors affecting calcium absorption, *except*:**
    - (a) 1,25-dihydroxy vitamin $D_3$
    - (b) Gastric acidity
    - (c) Lactose
    - (d) Calcium: magnesium ratio of the diet
2. **Oxalates may:**
    - (a) Decrease the calcium absorption
    - (b) Increase the calcium absorption
    - (c) Regulate the calcium metabolism
    - (d) Not have any effect on calcium
3. **Concerning calcium content of the body, one of the following statements is incorrect:**
    - (a) It is the major inorganic element comprising nearly 2% of the body weight
    - (b) Human body contains 1,200 g of calcium
    - (c) Major amount (99%) present in bone and teeth
    - (d) Blood calcium exists only in as ionized form
4. **Concerning the functions of calcium, all of the following statements are true, *except*:**
    - (a) It is required for the formation of bone and teeth
    - (b) It increases the absorption of iron
    - (c) It is required for blood coagulation process
    - (d) It activates phosphorylase during the break down of glycogen

5. **All of the following are the symptoms of true, *except*:**
   (a) Rickets
   (b) Hyperparathyroidism
   (c) Fanconi syndrome
   (d) Renal failure
6. **Magnesium is the second major:**
   (a) Intracellular cation
   (b) Intracellular anion
   (c) Extracellular cation
   (d) Extracellular anion
7. **All of the following are the functions of sodium, *except*:**
   (a) It maintains the osmotic pressure
   (b) It regulates the electrolyte and pH balance of the extracellular compartment
   (c) It controls the movement of ions in muscle
   (d) It helps in the active transport of glucose
8. **Cushing's disease presents with:**
   (a) Hypernatremia
   (b) Hypophosphatemia
   (c) Hyperphosphatemia
   (d) None of the above
9. **The major intracellular cation is:**
   (a) Sodium
   (b) Magnesium
   (c) Calcium
   (d) Potassium
10. **All of the following conditions result in hyperkalemia, *except*:**
    (a) Burns
    (b) Renal failure
    (c) Malnutrition
    (d) Hock
11. **Major extracellular anion is:**
    (a) Fluoride
    (b) Chloride
    (c) Bicarbonate
    (d) Selenium
12. **All of the following are the heme proteins, which contain iron, *except*:**
    (a) Ferritin
    (b) Myoglobin
    (c) Catalase
    (d) Cytochrome b
13. **Which of the following does not contain iron?**
    (a) Transferrin
    (b) Succinate dehydrogenase
    (c) Aconitase
    (d) Hexokinase
14. **All of the following favors iron absorption, *except*:**
    (a) Vitamin C
    (b) Ferric iron
    (c) Pregnancy
    (d) Increased erythropoiesis
15. **Concerning iron metabolism, one of the following statements is incorrect:**
    (a) Ferritin is the storage form of iron
    (b) Transferring is the transport from of iron
    (c) Iron oxidized to $Fe^{3+}$ after absorption
    (d) In the case of iron overload, more iron is transported as transferrin
16. **All of the following conditions result in iron deficiency, *except*:**
    (a) Shock
    (b) Malabsorption
    (c) Hookworm infestation
    (d) Hemorrhage
17. **Concerning the functions of copper, all of the following statements are true, *except*:**
    (a) Ceruloplasmin is a copper-containing protein
    (b) Glutaminase is a copper-dependent enzyme
    (c) Superoxide dismutase is a copper-dependent enzyme
    (d) Tyrosinase is a copper-dependent enzyme

18. **Acrodermatitis enteropathica results from the deficiency of:**
    (a) Zinc
    (b) Copper
    (c) Magnesium
    (d) Fluoride
19. **Which of the following vitamin has cobalt in its structure?**
    (a) Vitamin $B_6$
    (b) Vitamin C
    (c) Vitamin $B_{12}$
    (d) Vitamin $B_1$
20. **The trace element, which has antioxidant property, is:**
    (a) Fluoride
    (b) Selenium
    (c) Molybdenum
    (d) Manganese
21. **Concerning fluoride, one of the following statements is incorrect:**
    (a) 2 L water consumed by an individual provides 10 mg of fluoride
    (b) It is a component of a hydroxyapatite
    (c) Excess fluoride causes fluorosis
    (d) Its reduced levels cause to dental caries
22. **The blood level of sodium in a normal individual is:**
    (a) 3.5–5.0 mEq/L
    (b) 103 mEq/L
    (c) 8–11 mEq/L
    (d) 130–145 mEq/L
23. **The following causes hypercalcemia:**
    (a) Sarcoidosis
    (b) Primary hyperparathyroidism
    (c) Acute pancreatitis
    (d) Metastatic bronchial carcinoma
24. **With respect to iron metabolism:**
    (a) The body contains about 40 g of iron
    (b) Part of the iron in the body is contained in ferritin
    (c) Iron is transported in plasma as ferritin
    (d) Hemosiderin is the main form in which iron is stored in tissues
25. **Glucose intolerance is the feature of the deficiency of:**
    (a) Cobalt
    (b) Chromium
    (c) Selenium
    (d) Iodine

## ANSWERS

| | | | | | | | | | |
|---|---|---|---|---|---|---|---|---|---|
| 1. d | 2. a | 3. d | 4. b | 5. d | 6. a | 7. c | 8. a |
| 9. d | 10. c | 11. b | 12. a | 13. d | 14. b | 15. d | 16. a |
| 17. b | 18. a | 19. c | 20. b | 21. a | 22. d | 23. c | 24. b |
| 25. c | | | | | | | |

# Chapter 19
# Water and Electrolyte Balance

## LEARNING OBJECTIVES

*At the end of this chapter students should be able to:*
- Importance of water to human body
- Causes and symptoms of high and low body water content including the mechanism involved in the regulation
- Importance of electrolytes and their regulation
- Causes and symptoms of high and low sodium, potassium and chloride

## Water Balance

### Introduction

**Water balance** is the concept of human homeostasis that the amount of fluid lost from the body is equal to the amount of fluid taken in. Humans can survive for 4–6 weeks without food, but for only a few days without water. The amount of water varies with the individual, as it depends on the condition of the subject, the amount of physical exercise, and the environmental temperature and humidity.

- Water constitutes 60% of the total body weight.
- The body's water is distributed between two compartments.
- That is extracellular fluid (ECF) and intracellular fluid (ICF).
- Fluid found within the cells is called ICF and that found outside cells is called ECF **(Fig. 19.1)**.
- The ECF is further divided into that which is found as blood plasma within blood vessels and that which is found in the microscopic spaces between cells called interstitial fluid.
- Approximately two-thirds of body fluid are intracellular and one third is extracellular **(Table 19.1)**.
- Of the ECF, approximately 80% is interstitial fluid and 20% is blood plasma.
- Selectively permeable membranes separate body fluids into distinct compartments.
- Plasma membranes of individual cells separate ICF from ECF and blood vessel walls separate blood plasma from interstitial fluid.
- The major components of these fluids include water and solutes.
- The solute is mostly composed of electrolytes—inorganic compounds that dissociate into ions. Electrolytes include cations and anions.
- The cations are positively charged atoms. Examples are sodium, potassium, calcium, and magnesium.
- The anions are negatively charged atoms, and examples are chloride, sulfide, phosphate, bicarbonate, and carbonate.
- The exchange of interstitial and ICF is controlled mainly by the presence of the electrolytes: sodium and potassium.

Potassium is the chief intracellular cation, and sodium is the chief extracellular cation.

The body water is maintained at a constant volume by a regulation between intake and output water **(Fig. 19.2)**.

**Briefly discuss the regulation of fluid balance in the human body.**

### Regulation of Fluid Balance

The term "fluid balance" defines the state where a body's required amount of water is

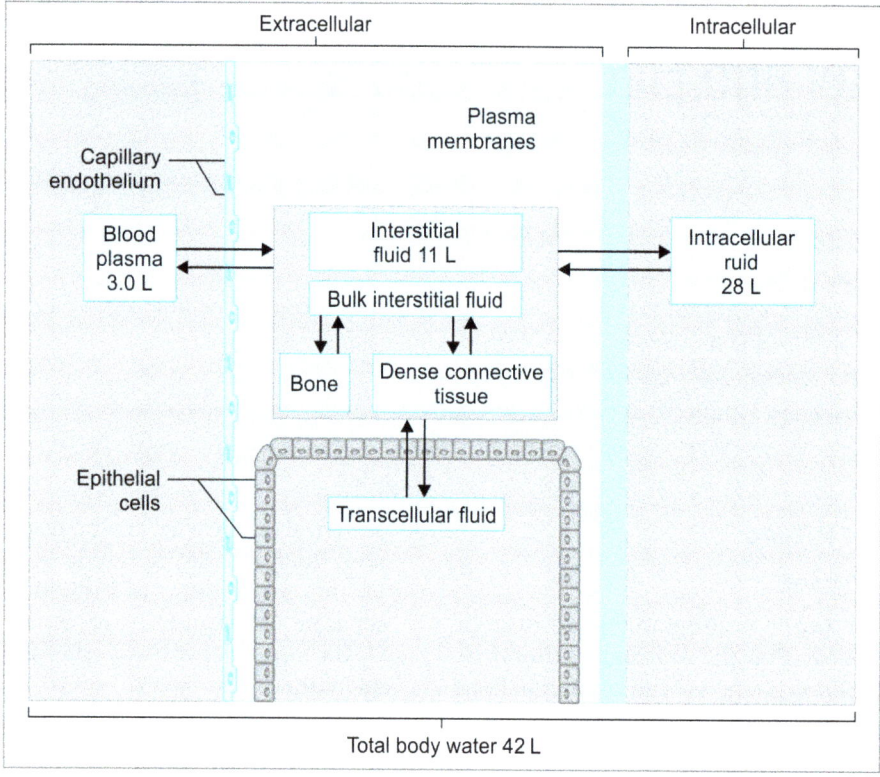

**Fig. 19.1:** Fluid distribution in different compartments.

**Table 19.1:** Fluid distribution in various compartments.

| Fluid distribution | % of total body weight (70 kg) | Volume (L) |
|---|---|---|
| Body water | 60 | 42 |
| 1. Intracellular | 40 | 28 |
| 2. Extracellular | 20 | 14 |
|    – Plasma (blood) | 5 | 3.0 |
|    – Cerebrospinal fluid (CSF) | | |
|    – Interstitial fluid | 15 | 10.5 |
|    – Lymph | | |
|    – Synovial fluid | | |
|    – Ocular fluid | | |
|    – Pleural fluid | | |
|    – Pericardial fluid | | |

CHAPTER 19: Water and Electrolyte Balance

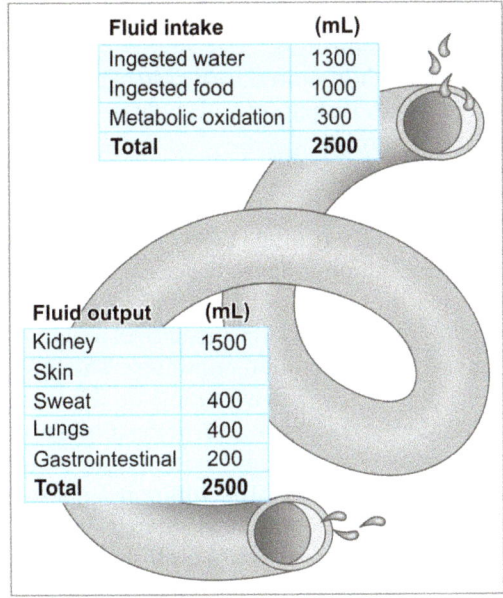

Fig. 19.2: Fluid input and output.

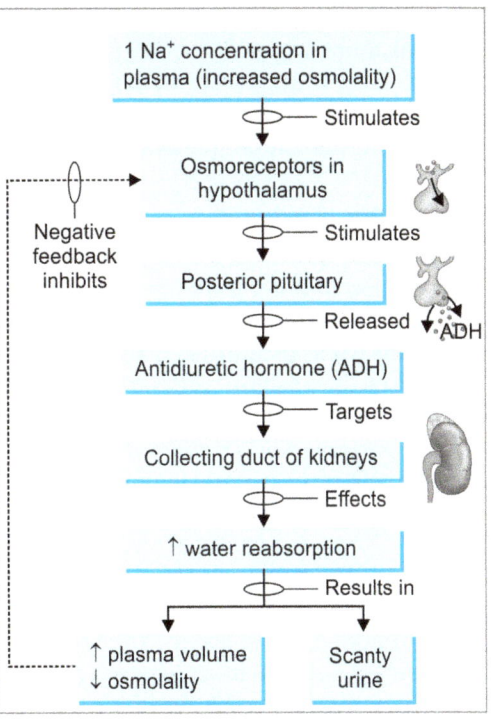

Fig. 19.3: Regulation of fluid balance.

present and proportioned normally among the various compartments **(Fig. 19.3)**.

Under normal conditions, water loss equals water gain and a body's water volume remains constant.

Water loss takes place through the kidneys, skin, lungs, feces, and menstruation.

Gain water mostly from dietary intake; this is called preformed water.

Metabolic processes such as cellular respiration and dehydration synthesis reactions generate a small component.

Water is not produced by the body to maintain homeostasis.

Metabolic water production is simply a by-product of cellular respiration.

The body regulates water intake via the thirst reflex, which stimulates us to drink. When water loss is greater than water gain, the body reaches a state of dehydration, and dehydration stimulates the thirst reflex in three ways:
- Saliva level drops resulting in a dry mucosa in the mouth and pharynx.

- Increase in blood osmotic pressure that stimulates osmoreceptors in the hypothalamus.
- There is a drop in blood volume, which leads to the renin/angiotensin II pathway stimulating the thirst center in the hypothalamus.

## Mechanism

### Thirst Center

- The intake of water is regulated by the thirst center, situated in the brain.
- When there is a decrease in the body fluid volume, it leads to increase in the salt concentration, and hence, there is increased osmolality and an increase in the osmotic pressure the ECF.
- As a result, the intracellular water comes out and cells become dehydrated.
- The dehydration of the cells stimulates the thirst center, which sends messages

to tongue and throat causing dryness and drink more water.
* Drinking inhibits the thirst center by stretching the stomach and intestines and reducing the osmotic pressure of the blood.

## Antidiuretic Hormone

Antidiuretic hormone (ADH) helps in the reabsorption of water from renal tubules and thereby loss of water from the body is regulated.

Antidiuretic hormone is the hormone secreted by the posterior pituitary.

When there is a decrease in body fluid, osmotic pressure of ECF increases which stimulates the cells of the hypothalamus, which then stimulates the posterior pituitary to secrete ADH.

Antidiuretic hormone acts on the kidney tubules and increases the reabsorption of water, thus conserving water. When the body fluid content is sufficient, the osmotic pressure of ECF is normal or low. During this condition, there is no stimulation of the hypothalamic cells or posterior pituitary, so ADH is not secreted. As a result, there is a decrease in the reabsorption of water from the renal tubules and more water is lost in the urine.

**Explain the causes and symptoms of hypovolemia and hypervolemia.**

## Dehydration (Hypovolemia)

* Loss of water from the body in excess amounts leads to dehydration.
* First, the plasma becomes concentrated followed by the ECF and then the ICF.
* When water comes out of the cells, it passes into ECF in exchange of $K^+$ and $Na^+$ passes into ICF from ECF.
* Loss of more than 20% of body water results in death.

## Causes of Dehydration

* Severe diarrhea and vomiting
* Excessive heat
* Difficulty in swallowing and state of unconsciousness.
* Loss of fluid from skin in case of burns
* Diabetes insipidus (ADH polyurea)
* Heart stroke
* Excitement
* Fever
* Excessive sweating

Dehydration induces water to move from the cells into the blood. Body tissues begin to dry out and the cells start to shrivel and malfunction if dehydration continues. The most susceptible cells to dehydration are the brain cells. Mental confusion, one of the most common signs of severe dehydration, may result and can lead to **coma**. Dehydration can occur when excessive water is lost with such diseases as **diabetes mellitus**, diabetes insipidus, and Addison's disease.

Dehydration is often accompanied by a deficiency of electrolytes, sodium, and potassium in particular. Water does not move as rapidly from the cells into the blood when electrolyte concentration is decreased. Blood pressure can decline due to a lower volume of water circulating in the bloodstream. A drop in blood pressure can cause light headedness, or a feeling of impending blackout, especially upon standing (orthostatic hypotension). Continued fluid and electrolyte imbalance may further reduce blood pressure, causing **shock** and damage to many internal organs including the brain, kidneys, and **liver**.

## Features of Dehydration

* Dryness of skin, tongue, and throat **(Table 19.2)**.
* Changes in the values of packed cell volume, Hb, plasma protein, plasma electrolytes, urea, and decreased blood pressure.

## Treatment

* Consuming plenty of plain water or water containing sugar and salt (depends upon the cause of dehydration).

## CHAPTER 19: Water and Electrolyte Balance

**Table 19.2:** Observations related to fluid balance.

| Observation | Fluid depletion | Fluid overload |
|---|---|---|
| Weight | Loss | Gain |
| Blood pressure | Lowered smaller pulse pressure | Normal or raised |
| Respirations | Rapid, shallow | Rapid, moist cough |
| Pulse | Rapid, weak | Rapid |
| Urine output | Reduced, concentrated | Increased or decreased if heart is failing |
| Skin | Dry, less elastic | Edematous |
| Saliva | Thick, viscous | Copious, frothy |
| Tongue | Dry, coated | Moist |
| Thirst | Present | No disturbance |
| Face | Sunken eyes | Periorbital edema |
| Temperature | May be raised | No disturbance |

❖ If the condition is very severe, intravenous infusion of fluids (normal saline) is required.

## Water Excess (Hypervolemia)

It is a condition in which the body water content is excessive as shown.

### Causes

❖ Hypersecretion of ADH following the administration of anesthetics. This effect occurs for about 12–36 hours after the surgery.
❖ Renal failure
❖ SIADH syndrome (inappropriate ADH secretion).

Here hypersecretion of ADH occurs.

*Causes for SIADH:* Some malignant conditions, disease of CNS, and side effects of certain drugs.

Overhydration can occur alone or in conjunction with excess blood volume. Distinguishing between the two conditions may be quite complicated. Overhydration induces water accumulation within and around the cells but does not typically show symptoms of fluid accumulation. On the other hand, with excess blood volume, there is an accumulation of sodium and the body cannot transfer water into the reservoir within cells. Conditions such as **heart failure** and liver cirrhosis may induce volume overload, whereby fluid accumulates around cells in the abdomen, chest, and lower legs.

### Features

❖ Mental confusion, incoordination, muscular weakness, nausea.
❖ Decreased PCV
❖ Decreased plasma electrolytes, plasma osmolality, increased urine osmolality and increased blood pressure. When there is increased ADH secretion, more $H_2O$ is absorbed from the renal tubules. As the volume of fluid, increases, the salts get diluted. Hence, the plasma osmolality decreases.

### Treatment

❖ Withdrawal of fluids
❖ Administration of diuretics

## Electrolyte Balance

### Introduction

The electrolytes, anions, or cations which are present either in ECF or ICF should be maintained in balance, otherwise the human body has to face several serious problems.

**Explain the distribution of electrolytes in ICF and ECF.**

## Distribution of Electrolytes

| Solutes | Plasma (mEq/L) | |
|---|---|---|
| | ECF | ICF |
| Cations | | |
| $Na^+$ | 142 | 10 |
| $K^+$ | 5 | 148 |
| $Ca^{2+}$ | 5 | 2 |
| $Mg^{2+}$ | 3 | 40 |
| Anions | | |
| $Cl^-$ | 103 | |
| $HCO_3^-$ | 24 | 8 |
| $HPO_4^{2-}$ | 2 | 136 |
| $SO_4^{2-}$ | 1 | |
| Protein | 15 | 56 |
| Organic ions | 10 | |

(ECF: extracellular fluid; ICF: intracellular fluid)

* The sum of *cations* must be equal to the sum of *anions* to maintain electrical neutrality.
* Electrolyte composition of other ECF is similar to that of plasma except that of proteins. Protein concentration is higher in plasma than other ECF.
* *Sodium* is the major cation of plasma.
* *Chloride* and *bicarbonate* are the major anions of plasma.
* The total electrolyte concentration in ICF is higher than in ECF.
* The major cations in ICF are $K^+$ and $Mg^{2+}$ and these are balanced mainly by the anions $PO_4^{2-}$ and proteins.

**Briefly explain the importance of serum (ECF) and urine osmolality.**

**Serum osmolality:** Serum osmolality is a useful preliminary investigation for identifying the cause of hyponatremia. If a patient with significant hyponatremia (serum sodium <130 mmol/L) has a normal plasma osmolality, the patient may have pseudohyponatremia due to excess lipids or proteins, or the sample may have been collected from a drip arm containing dextrose. If the patient has an increased osmolality, it is likely the patient has reactive hyponatremia due to an excess of solute pulling water out of cells. Examples of this include glucose in diabetes mellitus or hyperglycinemia after trans-urethral resection of the prostate.

**Urine osmolality:** Urine osmolality is an important test for the concentrating ability of the kidney. Interpretation of urine osmolality must always be made in the light of the appropriate physiological response to the state of hydration of the patient. The test is useful in the following areas:

* For determining the differential diagnosis of hyper- or hyponatremia
* For identifying SIADH (urine osmolality >200 mmol/kg, urine sodium >20 mmol/L, low serum sodium, patient not dehydrated and no renal, adrenal, thyroid, cardiac or liver disease or interfering drugs).
* For differentiating prerenal from renal kidney failure (high urine osmolality is consistent with prerenal impairment, in renal damage the urine osmolality is similar to plasma osmolality).
* For identifying and diagnosing diabetes insipidus.

## Sodium Balance

* Kidney is the only organ involved in the excretion of sodium and helps to regulate the body $Na^+$ content.
* The filtered $Na^+$ in the glomerular filtrate is reabsorbed in the distal tubule.
* A hormone, namely, *aldosterone* secreted by the adrenal cortex is involved in the regulation of sodium reabsorption in the renal tubules.
* Aldosterone increases the reabsorption of $Na^+$ whenever the plasma $Na^+$ is low.
* Along with $Na^+$, $Cl^-$ is also reabsorbed.
* Absorption of $Na^+$ takes place in exchange for $K^+$.

- Aldosterone secretion is controlled by the volume of ECF and its $Na^+$ concentration.

**Describe in detail how sodium is balanced maintained in the human body.**

- In addition to regulating total volume, the *osmolality* of body fluids is also highly regulated.
- Extreme variation in osmolality causes cells to shrink or swell, damaging or destroying cellular structure and disrupting normal cellular function.
- Regulation of osmolality is achieved by balancing the intake and excretion of sodium with that of water.
- Sodium is the major solute in ECFs, so it effectively determines the osmolality of ECFs.
- An important concept is that regulation of osmolality must be integrated with regulation of volume, because changes in water volume alone have diluting or concentrating effects on a bodily fluid.
- For example: when a person becomes dehydrated, they lose more water than sodium. Then, the osmolality of bodily fluids increases. In this situation, the body tries to conserve water but not sodium, thus stemming the rise in osmolality.
- When a person loses a large amount of blood from trauma or surgery, the losses of sodium and water are proportionate to the composition of bodily fluids. In this situation, the body should conserve both water and sodium.
- As discussed in the previous unit, ADH plays a role in lowering osmolality by increasing water reabsorption in the kidneys, thus helping to dilute bodily fluids. To prevent osmolality from decreasing below normal, the kidneys also have a regulated mechanism for reabsorbing sodium in the distal nephron. This mechanism is controlled by *aldosterone*, a steroid hormone produced by the adrenal cortex.

- Aldosterone secretion is controlled in two ways:
  1. When the osmolality increases above normal, aldosterone secretion is inhibited.
     - The lack of aldosterone causes less sodium to be reabsorbed in the distal tubule.
     - ADH secretion will increase to conserve water, thus complementing the effect of low aldosterone levels to decrease the osmolality of bodily fluids.
     - The net effect on urine excretion is a decrease in the amount of urine excreted, with an increase in the osmolality of the urine.
  2. The kidneys sense low blood pressure.
     - This triggers a complex response to raise blood pressure and *conserve volume*. Specialized cells in the afferent and efferent arterioles produce *renin*, a peptide hormone that initiates a hormonal cascade that ultimately produces *angiotensin II*.
     - Angiotensin II stimulates the adrenal cortex to produce aldosterone.

**Explain the causes and symptoms of different types of hyponatremia and hypernatremia**

## Hyponatremia

Hyponatremia refers to a lower-than-normal level of sodium in the blood.

*Causes:* Imbalance of water and sodium. Most frequently it occurs when excessive water dilutes the amount of sodium in the body or when not enough total sodium is present in the body. A common classification of hyponatremia is based on the amount of total body water that is present.

- Decrease in plasma sodium may be due to defect in kidneys or adrenal cortex.
- Sweating, burns, vomiting or diarrhea which can cause loss of sodium-containing fluids.

- In adrenocortical insufficiency (Addison's disease), decrease of serum sodium and increase in sodium excretion are seen.

### Normal Volume (Euvolemic) Hyponatremia

The amount of water in the body is normal, but an ADH is being inappropriately secreted SIADH = syndrome of inappropriate ADH secretion) from the pituitary gland. This may be seen in patients with pneumonia, small cell lung cancer, bleeding in the brain, or brain tumors.

### Excess Volume (Hypervolemic) Hyponatremia

Too much total body water dilutes the amount of sodium contained in the body. This can be seen in heart failure, kidney failure, and liver diseases such as cirrhosis.

### Inadequate Volume (Hypovolemic) Hyponatremia

The amount of water in the body is too low as can occur in dehydration. The ADH is stimulated, causing the kidneys to make very concentrated urine and hold onto water. This may be seen with excessive sweating and exercising in a hot environment. It can also occur in patients with excess fluid loss due to vomiting and diarrhea, pancreatitis, and burns.

*Symptoms*
- Confusion
- Nausea and fatigue
- Seizures
- Some individuals do not show any symptoms

## Hypernatremia

It is an electrolyte disturbance with elevated sodium level in the blood.

Hypernatremia is generally not caused by an excess of sodium, but rather by a relative deficit of free water in the body. Water is lost from the body in a variety of ways, including perspiration, imperceptible losses from breathing, and in the feces and urine. If the amount of water ingested consistently falls below the amount of water lost, the serum sodium level will begin to rise, leading to hypernatremia. Rarely, hypernatremia can result from massive salt ingestion.

Even a small rise in the serum sodium concentration above the normal range results in a strong sensation of thirst, an increase in free water intake, and correction of the abnormality. Therefore, hypernatremia most often occurs in people such as infants, those with impaired mental status, or the elderly, who may have an intact thirst mechanism but are unable to ask for or obtain water.

Common causes include:
- *Hypovolemic*
  - Inadequate intake of water typically in elderly or otherwise disabled (common cause).
  - Excessive losses of water from the urinary tract, which may be caused by glycosuria.
  - Extreme sweating
  - Severe watery diarrhea
- *Euvolemic*
  - Excessive excretion of water from the kidneys caused by diabetes insipidus, which involves either inadequate production of the hormone, vasopressin (ADH), from the pituitary gland or impaired responsiveness of the kidneys to vasopressin.
- *Hypervolemic*
  - Intake of a hypertonic fluid (a fluid with a higher concentration of solutes than the remainder of the body). This is relatively uncommon.
  - Mineralocorticoid excess due to a disease state such as Conn's syndrome or Cushing's disease.

## Signs and Symptoms

- Lethargy
- Restlessness
- Spasticity

- Edema
- Seizures

## Potassium (K⁺)

- Potassium (K⁺) is the most important cation of ICF.
- Average concentration in the ICF is 150 mEq/L.
- **Extracellular** potassium concentration is normally kept within a tight range of **3.5–5.0 mEq/L**.
- **Extracellular** potassium is important for its controlling influence upon neuromuscular irritability, cardiac muscle (a proper balance between potassium and calcium is essential for the contraction of heart muscle) and the operation of Na⁺/K⁺-ATPase (Na⁺ pump) against the concentration gradient.

## Hypokalemia

It is a metabolic disorder that occurs when potassium level in the blood drops too low.

It is the condition in which **serum potassium is reduced**.

This decreases the heartbeat and interferes with vital muscles such as those involved in respiration.

Possible causes of hypokalemia include:
- Antibiotics (penicillin, nafcillin, carbenicillin, gentamicin, amphotericin B, foscarnet)
- Diarrhea
  - Gastrointestinal loss: A more common cause is excessive loss of potassium, often associated with heavy fluid losses that "flush" potassium out of the body. Typically, this is a consequence of diarrhea, excessive perspiration, or losses associated with surgical procedures. Vomiting can also cause hypokalemia, although not much potassium is lost from the vomitus. Rather, there are heavy urinary losses of K⁺ in the setting of postemetic bicarbonaturia that force urinary potassium excretion. Other GI causes include pancreatic fistulae and the presence of adenoma.
- Diseases that affect the kidneys' ability to retain potassium (Liddle syndrome, Cushing syndrome, hyperaldosteronism, Bartter syndrome, Fanconi syndrome).
- Diuretic medications, which can cause excess urination.
- Eating disorders (such as bulimia).
- Magnesium deficiency
  - Magnesium is required for adequate processing of potassium. This may become evident when hypokalemia persists despite potassium supplementation. Other electrolyte abnormalities may also be present.
- Sweating
- Vomiting
- Since aldosterone increases the excretion of potassium or administration of cortisone leads to hypokalemia.
- Certain diuretics increase the excretion of potassium. It is, therefore, important to supplement enough potassium when these diuretics are used.
- Reduced intake of potassium may cause hypokalemia but it is rare. Renal retention of potassium in response to reduced intake ensures that hypokalemia occurs only when intake is severely restricted.

## Pseudohypokalemia

Pseudohypokalemia is a decrease in the amount of potassium that occurs due to excessive uptake of potassium by metabolically active cells in a blood sample after it has been drawn. It is a laboratory artifact that may occur when blood samples remain in warm conditions for several hours before processing.

### Symptoms

A small drop in potassium usually does not cause symptoms. However, a big drop in the level can be life threatening.

Symptoms of hypokalemia include:
- Abnormal heart rhythms (dysrhythmias), especially in people with heart disease.
- Constipation
- Fatigue
- Muscle damage (rhabdomyolysis)
- Muscle weakness or spasms
- Paralysis (which can include the lungs)

## Tests

- Serum potassium determination
- Arterial blood gas

## Treatment

Mild hypokalemia can be treated by taking potassium supplements by mouth. Persons with more severe cases may need to get potassium through a vein (intravenously).

# Hyperkalemia

- Elevated plasma potassium concentration.
- It occurs in Addison's disease and in intravenous infusion of potassium at a rate excess of 25 mmol/h.
- Treatment using concentrated potassium solutions.

## Causes

- Renal insufficiency (renal failure).
- Medication that interferes with urinary excretion:
  - ACE inhibitors and angiotensin receptor blockers.
  - Potassium-sparing diuretics (e.g., amiloride and spironolactone).
  - NSAIDs such as ibuprofen, naproxen, or celecoxib
  - The calcineurin inhibitor immunosuppressants ciclosporin and tacrolimus
  - The antibiotic trimethoprim
  - The antiparasitic drug pentamidine
- Mineralocorticoid deficiency or resistance, such as:
  - Addison's disease
  - Aldosterone deficiency
  - Some forms of congenital adrenal hyperplasia.
  - Type IV renal tubular acidosis (resistance of renal tubules to aldosterone).
- Gordon's syndrome (pseudohypoaldosteronism type II), a rare genetic disorder caused by defective modulators of salt transporters, including the thiazide-sensitive Na$^-$Cl cotransporter.
- Excessive release from cells.
  - Rhabdomyolysis, burns, or any cause of rapid tissue necrosis, including tumor lysis syndrome.
  - Massive blood transfusion or massive hemolysis.
  - Shifts/transport out of cells caused by acidosis, low insulin levels, beta-blocker therapy, digoxin overdose, or the paralyzing agent succinylcholine.
- **Excessive intake:** Excess intake with salt-substitute, potassium-containing dietary supplements, or potassium chloride (KCl) infusion.
- **Pseudohyperkalemia:** Pseudohyperkalemia is a rise in the amount of potassium that occurs due to excessive leakage of potassium from cells, during or after blood is drawn. Pseudohyperkalemia is typically caused by hemolysis during venipuncture.
- Tissue trauma causing the cells to release potassium into the ECF includes burns, traumatic injury, and intestinal bleeding.

## Signs and Symptoms

- Fatigue
- Weakness
- Tingling
- Numbness
- Paralysis
- Palpitations and difficulty in breathing.

## Chloride (Cl⁻)

- Chloride (Cl⁻) is the major extracellular anion.
- Its average serum concentration is 105 mEq/L.

### Functions

- It is involved in maintaining osmotic pressure, proper body hydration, and electric neutrality.
- Dietary Cl⁻ is almost completely absorbed by the intestine.
- It is filtered out by the glomerulus and passively reabsorbed in conjunction with Na⁺ by the proximal tubules.
- Excess Cl⁻ is excreted in urine and through sweating.
- Excessive sweating stimulates aldosterone secretion, which acts on the sweat glands to conserve Na⁺ and Cl⁻.

The normal level is between 94 and 111 mEq/L.

## Hypochloremia

A low serum Cl⁻ is associated with loss of gastric HCl due to prolonged vomiting, salt-losing renal disease, in metabolic acidosis, etc.

### Causes

- Diarrhea
- Congestive heart failure
- Pyloric obstruction
- Uremia
- Addison's disease
- Pulmonary emphysema
- Diabetic acidosis

## Hyperchloremia

High serum Cl⁻ is seen in dehydration and decreased renal blood flow.

### Causes

- Dehydration
- Acute renal failure

---

## SUMMARY

**Water balance** is the concept of human homeostasis that the amount of fluid lost from the body is equal to the amount of fluid taken in. Water constitutes 60% of the body weight. Thirst center and ADH mechanisms help in the regulation of water balance in the body. Loss of water from the body leads to dehydration, which will become the cause for hypovolemia. Excess accumulation of water in the body leads to hypervolemia. Along with sodium, water also has the effect on serum and urine osmolality. Serum osmolality is a useful preliminary investigation for identifying the cause of hyponatremia. Kidney is the only organ involved in the excretion of sodium and helps to regulate the body Na⁺ content. The filtered Na⁺ in the glomerular filtrate is reabsorbed in the distal tubule. A hormone namely aldosterone secreted by the adrenal cortex is involved in the regulation of sodium reabsorption in the renal tubules. Aldosterone increases the reabsorption of Na⁺ whenever the plasma Na⁺ is low. Maintenance of electrolyte balance is equally important as water balance for the normal functioning of the body. Sodium is the major extracellular cation. Loss of sodium results in hyponatremia and more sodium level in the blood causes hypernatremia. Potassium is the major cation of ICF and its low level in the blood causes hypokalemia. High blood level of sodium causes hyperkalemia. Chloride is the extracellular anion. Low and high level of blood chloride results in hypo- and hyperchloremia, respectively.

## SELF-ASSESSMENT QUESTIONS

1. Briefly discuss the regulation of fluid balance in the human body.
2. Give the causes and features of hypovolemia.
3. Write the causes of hypervolemia.
4. How does the thirst mechanism help to gain water?
5. Give the normal serum value of chloride.
6. What are the methods available to determine the concentration of sodium and potassium?
7. Name the method used to determine the CSF chloride.
8. State the conditions in which serum calcium increases.
9. Explain the clinical significance of serum inorganic phosphorous estimation.

## MULTIPLE CHOICE QUESTIONS

1. **The regulation of fluid balance is by:**
   - (a) Antidiuretic hormone
   - (b) Thyroid hormone
   - (c) Insulin
   - (d) Oxytocin
2. **All the following are the causes for hypervolemia, *except*:**
   - (a) Renal failure
   - (b) SIADH syndrome
   - (c) Hypersecretion of ADH
   - (d) Diabetes insipidus
3. **The concentration of sodium in the serum is:**
   - (a) 130–150 mEq/L
   - (b) 135–140 mEq/L
   - (c) 100–120 mEq/L
   - (d) 150–160 mEq/L
4. **The major extracellular anion is:**
   - (a) Potassium
   - (b) Chloride
   - (c) Sodium
   - (d) Bicarbonate
5. **Reduced calcium levels are seen in all the following conditions, *except*:**
   - (a) Tetany
   - (b) Hypoparathyroidism
   - (c) Acidosis
   - (d) Childhood rickets
6. **Elevated calcium levels are seen in all the following conditions, *except*:**
   - (a) Primary hyperparathyroidism
   - (b) Vitamin D overdosage
   - (c) Bone tumors
   - (d) Liver disease
7. **Elevated phosphorous levels are seen in:**
   - (a) Renal failure
   - (b) Vitamin D overdosage
   - (c) Pancreatitis
   - (d) Liver disease

### ANSWERS
1. a  2. d  3. b  4. b  5. c  6. d  7. a

# Chapter 20

# Nutrition and Dietetics

## LEARNING OBJECTIVES

*At the end of this chapter students should be able to:*
- Understand the importance of macro and micronutrients and disorders associated with their deficiency
- Explain the basal metabolic rate and the factors affecting it
- Calculate the calorie requirement for different types of work
- Describe the protein-calorie malnutrition and protein-energy malnutrition
- Know the dietary requirement for people with diabetes, cardiovascular disease and pregnancy

## Introduction

Nutrition is a process of intake of nutrients and its utilization by the organism to maintain growth and daily activities. The diet, what we eat, is determined by the quality and quantity of foods. A healthy diet has many good impacts on health status of an organism. A poor diet causes many deficiency diseases such as anemia, beriberi, scurvy, and kwashiorkor and also life-threatening conditions such as obesity, metabolic syndrome diabetes, and cardiovascular diseases.

There are seven major classes of nutrients such as carbohydrates, fats, fiber, minerals, proteins, vitamins, and water. These nutrients classes can be categorized into macro- and micronutrients. Macronutrients are required in large amounts whereas micronutrients in smaller quantities. The macronutrients are carbohydrates, fats, fiber, proteins, and water. The micronutrients are minerals and vitamins.

## Calorie

- A measurement of energy in a bomb calorimeter.
- The amount of heat it takes to raise the temperature of 1 g of water by 1°C.
- Food is measured in kilocalories (kcal) "Calories" with a large "C" on nutrition label are in kcal.

## Caloric Values of Carbohydrate, Fat, and Protein

Caloric value: It is the amount of heat obtained when 1 g of substance is completely oxidized.

Energy = Calories in nutrition
- When 1 g of carbohydrate is oxidized in the body, 4 calories are formed.
- When 1 g of protein is oxidized in the body, 4 calories are formed.
- When 1 g of fat is oxidized in the body, 9 calories are formed (**Fig. 20.1**).

## Respiratory Quotient of Food Stuffs

The respiratory quotient (RQ) is the volume of $CO_2$ produced divided by the volume of $O_2$ consumed at the whole-body level. Because of inherent chemical differences in the composition of carbohydrates, fats, and proteins, different amounts of oxygen are required to completely oxidize the carbon and hydrogen atoms in carbohydrates, fats, and protein into

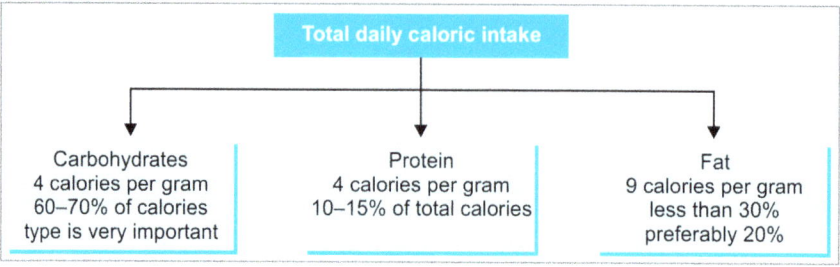

**Fig. 20.1:** Energy nutrients (energy = calories in nutrition).

carbon dioxide and water. Thus the quantity of carbon dioxide produced relative to the oxygen consumed will vary depending on the proportional mix of energy nutrients (carbohydrate, fat, protein) metabolized.

$$RQ = \frac{\text{Volume of } CO_2}{\text{Volume of } CO_2 \text{ utilized}}$$

$$RQ = \frac{VCO_2}{VO_2}$$

## Carbohydrates

When carbohydrates are completely oxidized, their RQ is:

$C_6H_{12}O_6$ (glucose) $+ 6O_2 \rightarrow 6CO_2 + 6H_2O$
$VCO_2$ produced $= 6$
$VO_2$ utilized $6 = 1$

## Fats

When palmitic acid is completely oxidized, their RQ is:

$C_{15}H_{32}COOH$ (palmitic acid) $+ 23O_2 \rightarrow 16CO_2 + 16H_2O$
$VCO_2$ produced $= 16$
$VO_2$ utilized $= 23$
$= 16/23 = 0.7$

This reaction shows fats have relatively low RQ, since they have low oxygen content.

## Proteins

The protein is not completely oxidized to $CO_2$ and cannot be represented by the formula.

For example, the protein albumin is oxidized as follows:

$C_{72}H_{112}N_2O_{22}S + 77O_2 \rightarrow 63CO_2 + 38H_2O + SO_3 + 9CO(NH_2)_2$

$VCO_2$ produced $= 63$
$VO_2$ utilized $= 77$
$= 63/77 = 0.818$

The RQ for protein is 0.82 (indirect measurements).

The RQ of a mixed diet is 0.8.

The "RQ" value is important not only in determining the body's rate of energy expenditure, but it also enables the investigator to determine the nutrient mixture being metabolized during rest or exercise.

The RQ is very helpful in understanding the kind of food which is predominantly oxidized at any time.

## Importance of Carbohydrates, Proteins, and Fats

### Carbohydrates

The role of carbohydrates is as follows:
- The cells of the nervous system and the brain almost exclusively use glucose for energy.
- Simple carbohydrates are monosaccharides (glucose, fructose, galactose) and disaccharides (maltose, sucrose, lactose).
- Complex carbohydrates (glycogen, starches, and fiber): Foods rich in complex carbohydrates tend to be low in fat and sugar and can, therefore, add bulk to meals.
- Glycogen is not a significant food source of carbohydrate. However, the body stores much of its glucose as glycogen. Glycogen is released when the body needs glucose for energy.
- Starch: Plants store starch like human bodies store glycogen, and when we eat

the plant, our body hydrolyzes the starch to glucose. Grains are the richest food source of starch and provide much of the food energy. Some examples of starches are rice, corn, rye, barley, and oats.
- Fibers are different than starches in that they cannot be broken down by the digestive system, and therefore they provide little or no energy for the body. Fiber has been shown to protect against heart disease and diabetes by lowering cholesterol and glucose levels. Fiber has also been shown to help provide a feeling of fullness and promote proper bowel function. Some examples of good sources of fiber are bran cereals, okra, butter beans, kidney beans, navy beans, sweet potatoes, and pears.

## Protein
The role of proteins in the body is many.
- Proteins are essential for our body growth, repairing or replacing tissue.
- Proteins form the building blocks of bones, teeth, muscles, skin, and blood.
- In addition, proteins help to regulate fluid balance; act as enzymes, and act as transporters, and some hormones are proteins as well.
- As antibodies, proteins also help with the body's defense against disease.
- Proteins can also be used as a source of energy if needed.
- Proteins help in the transportation of various substances in the body.

*Complete and Incomplete Proteins*
- **Complete proteins** contain all of the essential amino acids needed for growth.
- Essential amino acids must be acquired in the diet. Foods derived from animals such as meat, fish, poultry, cheese, eggs, yogurt, and milk generally provide complete proteins.
- Sources: Milk, fish, poultry, cheese, eggs, yogurt.
- **Incomplete proteins** are missing one or more essential amino acids needed for growth. Incomplete proteins are found in the plant form.
- Sources: Vegetables, seeds, nuts, grains, and legumes.

**Complementary proteins**: Two or more dietary proteins whose amino acid composition complement each other in such a way that the essential amino acids missing from one are supplied by the other. By combining two or more plant proteins, we can consume all of the essential amino acids needed to support growth. We can receive all of the amino acids we need over the course of a day by choosing a variety of grains, legumes, seeds, nuts, and vegetables.

*Protein and Weight Gain*
- Ideally, protein should contribute to 10-35% of energy intake.
- Protein-rich foods are often higher in fat, which can contribute to weight gain.
- In order to prevent weight gain, choose lean cuts of meat and trim away visible fat from meats and poultry before cooking.
- Broil or grill meat instead of frying.

*Protein and Weight Loss*
- It is generally not advisable to use a high protein diet to lose weight.
- High protein diets can be effective in weight loss. However, the reason high protein diets work is because they increase the feeling of satiety and are lower in calories.
- Eating excess protein may trouble the kidney with extra work. As the kidneys work to eliminate the excess protein, they also excrete a lot of water out of our system.
- It is generally wise to consume extra amounts of water if eating extra protein.

*Recommended Daily Allowance for Protein*
The recommended daily allowance (RDA) for adults is 0.8 g protein/kg/body weight/day.

## Fats
The role of fats is as follows:
- Fat provides us 60% of our energy needs at rest, it spares protein, insulates our bodies against extreme temperatures, and protects us against shock by providing a cushion for bones and vital organs.

- Fat also helps to maintain cell membranes and aids in the absorption of vitamins A, D, E, and K.
- As a food ingredient, fat provides flavor, consistency, stability, and satiety.

**Unsaturated fats:** The most effective dietary strategy in preventing heart disease may be replacing saturated fats in the diet with mono-unsaturated and polyunsaturated fats.
- *Sources of monounsaturated fats*: Olive oil, canola oil, peanut oil, and avocados.
- *Sources of polyunsaturated fats*: Vegetable oils (safflower, sesame, soy, corn, and sunflower), nuts, and seeds.

**Essential fatty acids:** The body can make all except two—linoleic and linolenic acids. These two acids must be supplied by our diet.
1. Linoleic acid sources: Sunflower, safflower, corn, and soybean oils.
2. Linolenic acid sources: Soybean and canola oils, walnuts, and salmon.

## Saturated Fats and its Risks

*Main sources* come from animal sources such as whole milk, cream, butter, cheese, and fatty cuts of beef and pork. Coconut, palm and palm kernel oils, and the products containing them (pastries, pies, doughnuts and cookies, and the like) are also sources of saturated fat.
- Saturated fat is implicated in raising low-density lipoprotein (LDL) cholesterol.
- LDL cholesterol raises risk of heart disease.

**Trans fat:** The majority of trans fats are formed when liquid oils are made into solid fats such as hard margarine. However, it is found naturally in some animal-based foods as well. Trans fat is made when hydrogen is added to an unsaturated fat such as vegetable oil, in a process called hydrogenation. Hydrogenation increases the shelf life of products containing these fats.

Found in deep-fried foods, cakes, cookies, margarine, meat, and dairy products. Partially hydrogenated oils are the main dietary source of trans fats.

*Trans fat risks:* Trans fats, such as saturated fats, can increase the LDL blood cholesterol levels and increase the risk of heart disease.

## Dietary Fiber

- Dietary fiber is a complex mixture of plant materials that are resistant to breakdown (digestion) by the human digestive enzymes.
- There are two major kinds of dietary fiber: insoluble (cellulose, hemicellulose, and lignin)—found in whole-grain products such as whole-wheat bread—and soluble (gums, mucilages, pectins) fibers—found in fruits, vegetables, dry beans and peas, and some cereals such as oats.
- Insoluble fiber promotes normal elimination by providing bulk for stool formation and thus hastening the passage of the stool through the colon. Insoluble fiber also helps to satisfy appetite by creating a full feeling. Some studies indicate that soluble fibers may play a role in reducing the level of cholesterol in the blood.
- Eating a variety of foods that contain dietary fiber is the best way to get an adequate amount. Healthy individuals who eat a balanced diet rarely need supplements.
- Breads, cereals, other grain products, fruits, vegetables, meat, poultry, fish. and alternates are the sources.

## Importance

### The Use of Fiber in the Irritable Bowel

Irritable bowel syndrome (IBS) is one of the most common disorders of the lower digestive tract.
- It creates bothersome symptoms such as altered bowel habits, constipation, diarrhea, or both alternately.
- There may also be bloating, abdominal pain, cramping, and spasm. An attack of IBS can be triggered by emotional tension and anxiety, poor dietary habits, and certain medications.

- Increased amounts of fiber in the diet can help to relieve the symptoms of IBS by producing soft, bulky stools.
- This helps to normalize the time it takes for the stool to pass through the colon.
- Liquids help to soften the stool.
- IBS, if left untreated, may lead to diverticulosis of the colon.

## Fiber and Colon Polyps/Cancer

Colon cancer is a major health problem and is most common in western cultures.
- Most colon cancer starts out as a colon polyp, a benign mushroom-shaped growth.
- In time, it grows, and in some people, it becomes cancerous.
- Colon cancer is usually always curable, if polyps are removed when found or if surgery is performed at an early stage.
- It is now known that people can inherit the risk of developing colon cancer, but diet may be important, too.
- There is a very low rate of colon cancer in residents of countries where grains are unprocessed and retain their fiber.
- The theory is that in the Western world, cancer-containing agents (carcinogens) remain in contact with the colon wall for a longer time and in higher concentrations. So, a large bulky stool may act to dilute these carcinogens by moving them through the bowel more quickly.
- Less carcinogenic exposure to the colon may mean fewer colon polyps and less cancer.

## Fiber and Diverticulosis

Prolonged, vigorous contraction of the colon, usually in the left lower side, may result in diverticulosis.
- This increases pressure causing small and eventually larger ballooning pockets to form. These pockets usually cause no problems.
- However, sometimes they can become infected (diverticulitis) or even break open (perforate) causing pockets of infection or inflammation of the sac lining the abdomen (peritonitis).
- A high-fiber diet may increase the bulk in the stool and thereby reduce the pressure within the colon.
- The formation of pockets is reduced or possibly even stopped.

## Fiber, Cholesterol, and Gas

*Insoluble fiber* is found in wheat, rye, bran, and other grains.
- It does not dissolve in water.
- It also cannot be used by intestinal-colon bacteria as a food source, so these beneficial bacteria generally do not grow and produce intestinal gas.
- Soluble fiber, on the other hand, does dissolve in water forming a gelatinous substance in the bowel.
- Soluble fiber is found in oatmeal, oat bran, fruit, barley, and legumes.
- Soluble fiber, among its other benefits, seems to bind up cholesterol allowing it to be eliminated with the stool (10–15%).
- The downside of soluble fiber is that it can be metabolized by gas-forming bacteria in the colon.
- These bacteria are harmless but for those who have an intestinal gas or flatus problem are probably best to avoid or carefully test soluble fibers to see if they are contributing to intestinal gas.
- Whenever possible, both soluble and insoluble fiber should be eaten on a daily basis.

## Basal Metabolic Rate

- Basal metabolic rate (BMR) is defined as the minimum amount of energy required by the body to maintain life at complete physical and mental rest in the postabsorptive period (12 hours after the intake of last meal).
- BMR includes the energy expended in ventilation, blood circulation, intestinal

contraction, the activities of internal organs, and maintenance of thermal equilibrium. Stringent measurement of BMR requires that the subject be in a fasting (minimum of 12 hours), well-rested state having not exercised for the previous 12 hours and being in a supine position within a nonstressful, controlled environment for a minimum of 30 minutes prior to measurement.

- BMR is expressed as $C/m^2$ body surface/hour.

*Resting metabolic rate* (RMR) is the energy expended while an individual is resting quietly in a supine position.

RMR and BMR are sometimes used interchangeably but there are some small differences.

RMR includes the thermal effect of substrate metabolism and heightened metabolic activity due to prior physical or mental activity. These factors, collectively known as facultative thermogenesis, may be thought of as components of a person's *RMR* and are not part of the BMR.

## Measurement of Metabolic Rate or Energy Expenditure

- Energy expenditure can be measured in two different ways.
- The determination of energy expenditure by measuring the amount of heat produced over a period of time is called direct calorimetry.
- The determination of energy expenditure by measuring the amount of carbon dioxide consumed over a period of time is called indirect calorimetry.
- Two procedures of indirect calorimetry are closed-circuit and open-circuit spirometry (Douglas bag).
- During metabolic energy transformations, oxygen is consumed and heat is produced. Either of these variables can, therefore, be used to estimate energy expenditure.
- Using the fact that 1 L of oxygen liberates 4.82 kcal of heat energy when a mixture of carbohydrate, fat, and protein is burned in a bomb calorimeter; a highly accurate indirect measure of energy production is possible.

## Factors that Affect Basal Metabolic Rate

Factors that affect basal metabolic rate are as follows:

1. *Body surface area*:
   - This is a reflection of height and weight.
   - The greater the body surface area factor, the higher the BMR.
   - Tall, thin people have higher BMRs. If we compare a tall person with a short person of equal weight, then if they both follow a diet calorie-controlled to maintain the weight of the taller person, the shorter person may gain up to 15 lb in a year.
2. *Sex*: Males average a higher BMR because of a greater proportion of lean body mass.
3. *Body temperature*: Fever, for example, increases BMR.
4. *Hormones*: Thyroid hormones have a stimulatory effect on the metabolism of the body and, therefore, BMR. Thus BMR is raised in hyperthyroidism and reduced in hypothyroidism.
5. *Age*: Metabolic rate declines with age. In infants and children, BMR is higher and in adults it is less.
6. *Diet*: Starvation or serious abrupt calorie-reduction can dramatically reduce BMR (30%). Restrictive low-calorie weight-loss diets may cause BMR to drop as much as 20%.
7. *Pregnancy/breastfeeding*: These increase metabolic rate.
8. *Environment*: In cold climates, the BMR is higher compared to warm climates.
9. *Rapid growth and/or development*: Infancy, growth spurts, healing after illness or injury.

10. *Disease states*: BMR is higher in cardiac failure, leukemias, and hypertension. It is marginally lowered in Addison's disease.
11. *Weight*: Heavier the weight, the higher BMR.
    *Example*: The metabolic rate of obese women is 25% higher than the metabolic rate of thin women.
12. *Exercise*: Physical exercise not only influences body weight by burning calories, but it also helps to raise our BMR by building extralean tissue (Lean tissue is more metabolically demanding than fat tissue). So, we burn more calories even when sleeping.
13. *Amount of lean body mass*: Muscle, liver, brain, kidney all metabolize at a high rate at rest and have high energy needs when more active.

## Calculation of Basal Metabolic Rate

The first step in designing a personal nutrition plan for ourselves is to calculate how many calories we burn in a day; our total daily energy expenditure (TDEE). TDEE is the total number of calories that our body expends in 24 hours, including all activities.

## Methods of Determining Caloric Needs

Quick method (based on total bodyweight).

*Equations based on BMR*: A much more accurate method for calculating TDEE is to determine BMR using multiple factors, including height, weight, age, and sex, then multiply the BMR by an activity factor to determine TDEE. BMR is the total number of calories our body requires for normal bodily functions. BMR usually accounts for about two thirds of TDEE. BMR may vary dramatically from person-to-person depending on genetic factors.

*The Harris-Benedict formula (BMR based on total body weight)*: The Harris-Benedict equation is a calorie formula using the factors of height, weight, age, and sex to determine BMR. This makes it more accurate than determining calorie needs based on total bodyweight alone. The only variable it does not take into consideration is lean body mass. Therefore, this equation will be very accurate in all but the extremely muscular and the extremely over fat.

*Men*: BMR = 66 + (13.7 × wt in kg) + (5 × height in cm) − (6.8 × age in years)

*Women*: BMR = 655 + (9.6 × wt in kg) + (1.8 × ht in cm) − (4.7 × age in years)

Note: 1 inch = 2.54 cm

1 kg = 2.2 lb

*Example:* Female, 30 years old, 5′ 6″ tall (167.6 cm), weighing 120 lb (54.5 kg).

BMR = 655 + 523 + 302 −141 = 1,339 cal/day

To determine TDEE from BMR, simply multiply BMR by the activity multiplier:

## Activity Multiplier

Sedentary = BMR × 1.2 (little or no exercise, desk job).

Lightly active = BMR × 1.375 (light exercise/sports 1–3 days/week).

Moderately active = BMR × 1.55 (moderate exercise/sports 3–5 days/week).

Very active = BMR × 1.725 (hard exercise/sports 6–7 days/week).

Extraactive = BMR × 1.9 (hard daily exercise/sports and physical job or 2 × day training, i.e.,

- Your BMR is 1,339 cal/day.
- Your activity level is moderately active (work out 3–4 times per week).
- Your activity factor is 1.55
- Your TDEE = 1.55 × 1,339 = 2,075 cal/day

## Specific Dynamic Action

- Ingestion of food is accompanied by an increased rate of heat production. The extraheat production by the body, over and above the calculated caloric value, when a given food is metabolized by the body, is called specific dynamic action (SDA). Various names for this effect have been suggested, including SDA, specific dynamic effect, heat increment of a feeding, calorigenic effect of foods, and thermogenic effect.

* Imagine that a man requires 1,800 cal/day to maintain his basal metabolic requirement. His heat output may exceed 1,800 cal (by about 180 cal) after eating a food. This means that the excess Calories would have to come from his own tissues, and maintain his weight, he has to take about 2,000 [1,800 + extra 10% (180)] cal. If he continues with 1,800 cal, he would lose weight.
* The SDA values vary according to the type of food taken. If he eats 25 g of protein, we expect his heat output is 100 cal (25 × 4 cal, a caloric value of protein). But his actual heat output is 130 cal (a rise of 30%). So, the SDA for protein is 30%.
* The SDA value for carbohydrate is 5% (After he consumes 25 g carbohydrate, the heat output is 105 cal instead of 100 cal).
* The SDA value for fat is 12%. (After he consumes 11 g fat, the heat output is 112 cal instead of 100 cal) (11 × 9 + 12).
* For a mixed diet, the SDA is 10%. This is because of the presence of carbohydrates and fats which reduces the SDA of protein.
* The significance of SDA of a protein is the maintenance of body temperature in cold climate. The higher SDA for protein indicates that it is not a good source of energy.

*The energy requirement of a man (age 20 years, BMR = 42 cal/$m^2$ body surface/h, body surface area = 1.7 $m^2$) engaged in light work:*

The energy demand depends on three important factors:
1. BMR
2. Physical activity
3. SDA.

The food provides energy for:
* Basal metabolism (8 hours)
* Simple activities: Standing, sitting, walking, dressing, and writing (8 hours).
  ■ Professional work: (1) light work, (2) moderate work, (3) heavy work, and (4) very heavy work.
  ■ Other 10% as SDA.

The daily energy requirement is variable which depends on age, sex, and body size.
* Sleep-basal level (8 hours) BMR × body surface area × 8 hours = 42 × 1.7 × 8 = 571 cal.
* Simple activities (8 hours) at basal level = 571 cal

For simple activities at 25 cal/h over basal level 25 × 8 = 200 cal.
* For professional work (light work) at basal level = 571 cal

For professional work at 60 cal/h over basal level 55 × 8 = 440 cal
Subtotal = 2,353
Extra 10% for SDA = 235 cal
Total = 2,588 cal/day

*The energy requirement of dental student (age 18 years, BMR = 40 cal/$m^2$ body surface/h, body surface area = 1.7$m^2$) engaged in moderate work:*
* Sleep-basal level (8 hours) BMR × body surface area × 8 hours = 40 × 1.7 × 8 = 544 cal.
* Simple activities (8 hours) at basal level = 544 cal

For simple activities at 25 cal/h over basal level 25 × 8 = 200 cal
For professional work (light work) at basal level = 544 cal
For professional work at 75 cal/h over basal level 75 × 8 = 600 cal
Subtotal = 2,432
Extra 10% for SDA = 243 cal
Total = 2,675 cal/day

*The energy requirement of men (age 25 years, BMR = 40 cal/$m^2$ body surface/h, body surface area = 1.7 $m^2$) engaged in heavy work:*
* Sleep-basal level (8 hours) BMR × body surface area × 8 hours = 40 × 1.7 × 8 = 544 cal.
* Simple activities (8 hours) at basal level = 544 cal

For simple activities at 25 cal/h over basal level 25 × 8 = 200 cal
* For professional work (heavy work) at basal level = 544 cal

For professional work at 150 cal/h over basal level 75 × 8 = 1,200 cal

Subtotal = 3,032

Extra 10% for SDA = 303 cal

Total = 3,335 cal/day

*From the above calculations, the reference ranges of caloric requirements of various types of work for an adult per day is as follows:*

* Light work 2,100–2,600
* Moderate work 2,500–3,000
* Heavy work 3,000–3,500
* Very heavy work 3,500–4,000

## Biological Value of a Protein

It is a measurement of protein quality expressing the rate of efficiency with which protein is used for growth. A protein with high BV has all the essential amino acids in the right proportion. The BVP can be calculated by using a formula.

Egg contains the highest quality food protein known. It is so nearly perfect, in fact, that egg protein is often the standard by which all other proteins are judged. Based on the essential amino acids it provides, egg protein is second only to mother's milk for human nutrition. On a scale with 100 representing top efficiency, these are the biological values of proteins in several foods.

* Whole egg—93.7
* Milk—84.5
* Fish—76.0
* Beef—74.3
* Soybeans—72.8
* Rice, polished—64.0
* Wheat, whole—64.0
* Corn—60.0
* Beans, dry—58.0

Protein from animal sources (meat, fish, dairy products, egg white) is considered high biological value protein or a "complete" protein because all nine essential amino acids are present in these proteins. An exception to this rule is collagen-derived gelatin which is lacking in tryptophan.

## Nitrogen Balance

* This is when a person's daily intake of nitrogen from proteins equals the daily excretion of nitrogens.
* If a person excretes more nitrogen than he consumes, his body will breakdown muscle tissue to get the nitrogen it needs (**negative nitrogen state**). Muscle loss occurs.
* If a person consumes more nitrogen than he excretes, he will be in an anabolic—muscle building—state (**positive nitrogen state**).

# Nutrition-related Diseases

## Protein-Calorie Malnutrition and Protein-Energy Malnutrition

Protein–calorie malnutrition is present when sufficient energy and/or protein is not available to meet metabolic demands, leading to impairment in normal physiologic processes.

* **Kwashiorkor (Protein-calorie malnutrition)** is a condition that develops when there is gross protein deficiency though nonprotein calorie intake may be adequate.
* **Marasmus (Protein-energy malnutrition)** occurs with a deficiency of both protein and calories.

## Causes

* Inadequate dietary intake
* Poor quality dietary protein
* Increased metabolic demands
* Increased nutrient losses.

## Kwashiorkor

It is caused by diet deficient in protein and high in carbohydrate. It is a high mortality deficiency disease known as kwashiorkor meaning red boy. The name comes from the odd reddish-orange color of the hair, as well as from the skin rash, characteristic of the disease. Moderate-to-severe growth failure is present in kwashiorkor.

For the first few months of life, the breast-fed infant in the developing countries grows at a rate that is comparable to that of well-fed infants, but thereafter, symptoms start occurring of a kwashiorkor child if the nutrition is not adequate.

## Symptoms

The symptoms of kwashiorkor are as follows:
- The increase in stature and retarded tissue development **(Fig. 20.2)**.
- Poorly developed muscle and lack tone.
- Severe edema.
- Potbelly (protruding of the stomach).
- Swollen legs and face.
- Anorexia and diarrhea are common. Poor sanitation is cause of diarrhea.
- Whimpering, but does not cry or scream.
- The child is not interested in or curious about his surrounding but remains seated whenever he is put down.

## Pathologic and Biochemical Changes

The pathologic and biochemical changes of kwashiorkor are as follows:
- Fatty infiltration of the liver.
- Decreased serum levels of triglycerides, phospholipids, and cholesterol.
- Reduced amylase, lipase, and trypsin.
- Serum proteins and albumin fractions are markedly reduced.
- Low Hb levels, especially if parasite infestation is also present.
- Vitamin A levels are usually reduced. This could be a serious complication leading to blindness and death in some children.

## Marasmus

It is a protein–calorie malnutrition caused by a diet deficient in both protein and carbohydrates **(Fig. 20.3)**.

Severe growth failure and emaciation are the most striking characteristics of the marasmic infant. Marasmus differs from kwashiorkor in several important aspects **(Table 20.1)**.

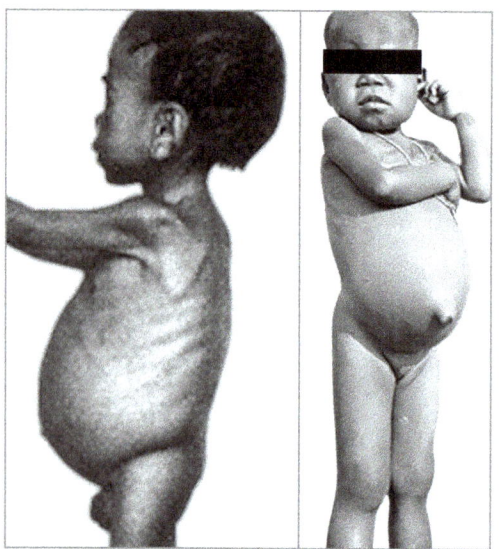

**Fig. 20.2:** Symptoms of kwashiorkor.

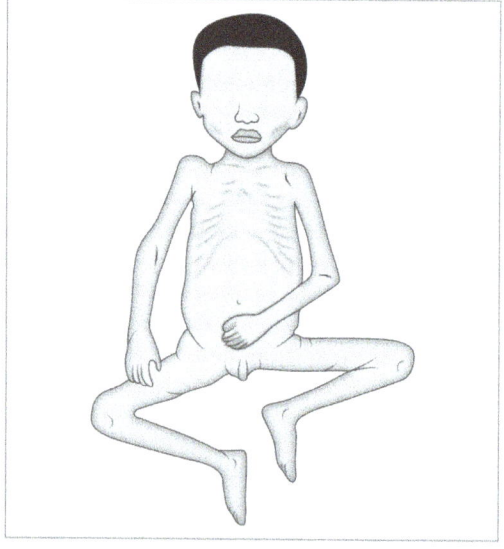

**Fig. 20.3:** Features of marasmus.

# CHAPTER 20: Nutrition and Dietetics

**Table 20.1:** Differences between marasmus and kwashiorkor.

| Marasmus | Kwashiorkor |
| --- | --- |
| 1. Onset is earlier, usually in the first year of life | Onset is later, after the breastfeeding is stopped |
| 2. Growth failure is more pronounced | Not very pronounced |
| 3. There is no edema | Edema present |
| 4. Blood protein concentration is reduced | Blood protein concentration is reduced very much |
| 5. Skin changes are seen less frequently | Red boils and patches are classic symptoms |
| 6. Liver is not infiltrated with fat | Fatty liver is seen |
| 7. Recovery is much longer | Recovery period is short |

## Anemia

Vitamin $B_{12}$ deficiency and folate (folic acid) deficiency cause megaloblastic anemia.

The bone marrow produces large and abnormal red cells (megaloblasts).

### Symptoms

The symptoms of anemia re as follows:
* People may be weak, short of breath, and pale.
* Nerves may also malfunction.
* Blood tests can detect abnormal cells that indicate vitamin-deficiency anemia.

Iron-deficiency anemia, often caused by insufficient iron intake, is the major cause of anemia in childhood.

## Iron-deficiency Anemia

### Causes

The causes of iron-deficiency anemia are as follows:
* Insufficient iron in the diet.
* Poor absorption of iron by the body.
* Ongoing blood loss, most commonly from menstruation or from gradual blood loss in the intestinal tract.
* Periods of rapid growth.

### Symptoms

The symptoms of iron-deficiency anemia are as follows:
* Fatigue and weakness
* Pale skin and mucous membranes
* Rapid heartbeat or a new heart murmur
* Irritability
* Decreased appetite
* Dizziness or a feeling of being light-headed.

## Clinical Signs of Nutritional Deficiency

Refer **Table 20.2**.

## Assessing Nutritional Status

* The nutritional status of an individual is the result of many interrelated factors.
* It is influenced by food intake, quality, quantity, and physical health.
* The spectrum of nutritional status spread from obesity to malnutrition.

### Why Nutritional Assessment Required

It is required to:
* Develop health care programs which meet the community needs which are defined by the assessment.
* Measure the effectiveness of the nutritional programs and intervention once initiated.

### Methods of Nutritional Assessment

It is assessed by direct and indirect methods.

### The Direct Method

Deal with the individual and measure objective criteria.

Summarized as ABCD:
* Anthropometric methods
* Biochemical, laboratory methods
* Clinical methods
* Dietary evaluation methods

**Table 20.2:** Clinical signs of nutritional deficiency.

**Hair**
- Spare and thin
- Easy to pull out
- Corkscrew coiled hair

- Due to protein, zinc or biotin deficiency
- Protein deficiency
- Vitamin C and A deficiency

**Mouth**
- Glossitis
- Angular stomatitis cheilosis and fissured tongue:
- Bleeding and spongy gums
- Leukoplakia
- Sore mouth and tongue

- Riboflavin, niacin and folic acid
- Riboflavin, pyridoxine and niacin deficiency
- Vitamin C deficiency
- Vitamin A, $B_{12}$, folic acid and niacin deficiency
- Vitamin $B_6$, niacin and iron deficiency

**Eyes**
- Night blindness and exophthalmia
- Photophobia, blurring and conjunctival inflammation

- Vitamin A deficiency
- Vitamin A deficiency

**Nails**
- Spooning
- Transverse lines

- Iron deficiency
- Protein deficiency

**Skin**
- Pallor
- Follicular hyperkeratosis
- Flaking dermatitis
- Pigmentation and desquamation
- Bruising purpura

- Folic acid, iron $B_{12}$ deficiency
- Vitamin B and C deficiency
- Vitamin $B_{12}$, A, PEM, zinc and niacin deficiency
- Niacin and PEM
- Vitamin K, C and folic acid deficiency

**Thyroid gland**
- Goiter (**Fig. 20.4**)

- Iodine deficiency

**Bones and joints**
- Rickets (**Fig. 20.4**)
- Scurvy

- Vitamin D deficiency
- Vitamin C deficiency

(PEM: protein–energy malnutrition)

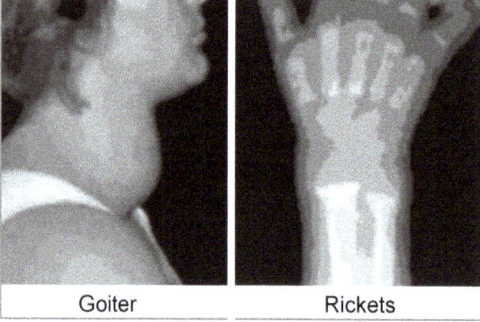

Fig. 20.4: Signs of iodine and vitamin D deficiency.

## Indirect Methods of Nutritional Assessments

Uses community health indices that reflect nutritional influences.

These include:
- Ecological variables including crop production.
- Economic factors, e.g. per capita income, population density, and social habits.
- Vital health statistics particularly infant under five mortality and fertility index.

## Clinical Assessment Method

- It is an essential feature of all nutritional surveys.
- It is the simplest and most practical method of ascertaining the nutritional status of a group of individuals.
- It utilizes a number of physical signs that are known to be associated with

malnutrition and deficiency of vitamins and micronutrients.
- Good nutritional history should be obtained.
- General clinical examinations, with special attention to organs, such as hair, nails, skin, gums, eyes, muscles tongue, angles of mouth, and thyroid gland.
- Detection of relevant signs helps in establishing the nutritional diagnosis.

## Advantages of Clinical Assessment

The advantages of clinical assessment are as follows:
- Fast and easy to perform
- Inexpensive
- Noninvasive

## Limitations

May not detect the early stages.

## Anthropometric Measurements

- Anthropometry is the measurement of body weight and proportions.
- It is an essential part of clinical examination of infants, children, and pregnant woman.
- It is also used to evaluate both under and over nutrition.
- The measured values reflect the current nutritional status.

## Other Anthropometric Measurements

- Mid upper arm circumference
- Head circumference
- Skinfold thickness
- Head/chest ratio
- Hip/waist ratio

## Anthropometry for Children

Accurate measurement of height and weight is necessary to evaluate the physical growth of the child.

### Height/Age

Height of index child compared with the expected weight of a healthy child of the same age.

It helps in measuring long-term nutritional status or stunting.

### Weight/Height

It measures wasting, i.e., appropriate weight for given height.

### Mid Upper Arm Circumference

Measured half-way between the acromion process of the scapula and the tip of the elbow (ulnar) with the arm hanging vertically and forearm supinated.

It provides an estimate of arm muscle area: reflects skeletal protein reserves–lean body mass useful in monitoring vulnerable groups, especially children.

### Head Circumference

It is useful in children under the age of 3 and is an indicator of nonnutritional abnormalities. Undernutrition must be severe to affect head circumference.

## Anthropometry for Adults

### Height Measurement

The subject stands erect and barefooted on a stadiometer with a movable headpiece is leveled with skull vault and height is recorded to the nearest 0.5 cm.

### Weight Measurement

Use of regularly calibrated electronic or balanced-beam scale is suggested to measure the weight.

During weight measurement wearing light clothes without shoes is suggested.

It reads to the nearest 100 g.

### Skinfolds

Triceps, biceps, subscapular, suprailiac—used in combination to obtain body fat **(Figs. 20.5A and B)**.

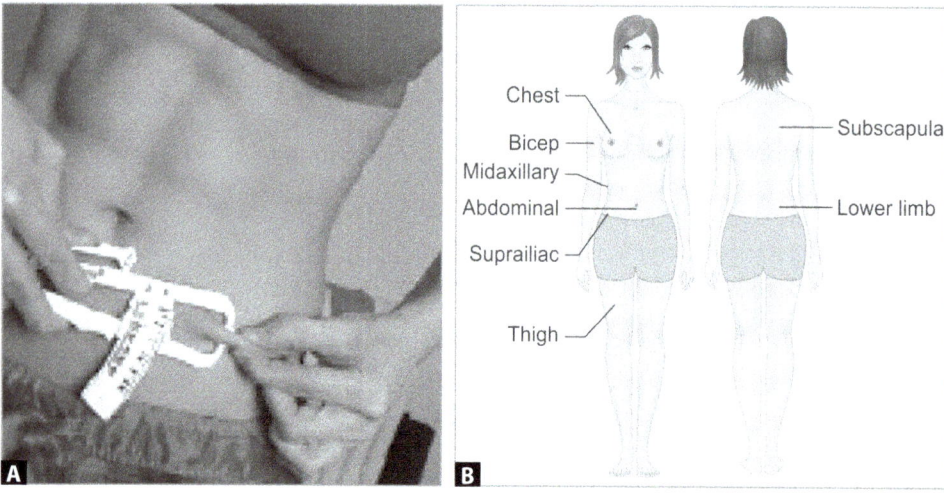

**Figs. 20.5A and B:** Skinfolds to obtain body fat.

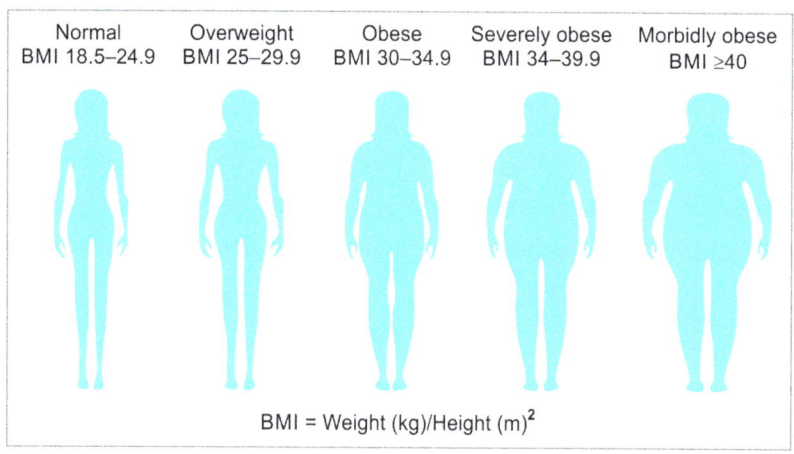

**Fig. 20.6:** Categories of weight.
(BMI: body mass index)

## Nutritional Indices in Adults

The international standard for assessing body size in adults is the body mass index (BMI).

BMI is computed using the following formula.

$$BMI = \frac{Weight\,(kg)\,kg/mg^2}{Height\,(m)^2}$$

| | |
|---|---|
| <18.5 | = Underweight |
| 18.5–24.9 | = Normal weight |
| 25–29.9 | = Overweight |
| 30–34.9 | = Moderate obese (class 1) |
| 35–39.9 | = Severely obese (class 2) |
| ≥40 | = Extreme obesity |

$$BMI = \frac{Weight\,(lbs)}{Height\,(in)^2} \times 703$$

| | |
|---|---|
| <18.5 | = Underweight |
| 18.5–24.9 | = Normal weight |
| 25–29.9 | = Overweight |
| 30–34.9 | = Moderate obese (class 1) |
| 35–39.9 | = Severely obese (class 2) |
| ≥40 | = Extreme obesity (class 3) |

High BMI (obesity level) is associated with type 2 diabetes and high risk of cardiovascular morbidity and mortality (**Fig. 20.6**).

## Waist/Hip Ratio

- Waist circumference is measured at the level of the umbilicus to the nearest 0.5 cm.
- The subject stands erect with relaxed abdominal muscles, arms at the side, and feet together.
- The measurement should be taken at the end of a normal expiration.

## Waist Circumference

- Waist circumference predicts mortality better than any other anthropometric measurement.
- It has been waist circumference alone can be used to assess obesity and two levels of risks have been identified.

|  | Males (cm) | Females (cm) |
| --- | --- | --- |
| Level 1 | >94 | >80 |
| Level 2 | >102 | >88 |

- Level 1 is the maximum acceptable waist circumference irrespective of the adult age, and there should be no further weight gain.
- Level 2 detects the obesity and requires weight management to reduce the risk of type 2 diabetes and cardiovascular complications.

## Hip Circumference

- It is measured at the point of greatest circumference around hips and buttocks to the nearest 0.5 cm.
- The subject should be standing and the measurer should squat beside him.
- Both measurement should be taken with a flexible, nonstretchable tape in close contact with the skin, but without indenting the soft tissue.

## Interpretation of Waist/Hip Ratio

High-risk waist/hip ratio (WHR) ≥0.80 for females and >0.95 for males, i.e., waist measurement >80% of hip measurement for women and 95% for men indicates central obesity and is considered high risk for diabetes and cardiovascular disorders.

A WHR below these cut-off levels considered low risk.

## Advantages of Anthropometry

The advantages of anthropometry are as follows:
- Simple, noninvasive.
- Equipment is inexpensive, portable.
- Relatively unskilled personnel can perform measurements.
- Methods are reproducible.
- Measures long-term nutritional history.
- Quickly identifies mild-to-moderate malnutrition.
- Measures many variable of nutritional significance such as height weight, skinfold thickness, head circumference waist and hip ratio, and BMI.

## Disadvantages of Anthropometry

The disadvantages of anthropometry are as follows:
- Relatively insensitive to short-term nutritional status.
- Cannot identify specific nutrient deficiencies.
- Unable to distinguish disturbances in growth or body composition induced by nutrient deficiencies.
- Measurements: Skinfolds difficult to carry out in obese people.
- Ethnic differences in fat deposition.

## Biochemical and Other Laboratory Measurements

- Blood: Accessible, relatively noninvasive reflect recent dietary intakes but influenced by diet, drugs, infection, stress.
- Samples collected under controlled and standardized conditions: Hormones; trace elements; processing time; hemolysis.
- Hemoglobin is the most important test and useful index of the overall state of nutrition. Beside anemia, it also gives an idea about protein and trace element nutrition.
- Stool examination: To detect the presence of ova and intestinal parasites.
- Urine examination: Albumin, sugar, and blood.
- RBC vs. WBC: Gives an idea about long/short-term nutrient status.
- Analysis of hair nails and skin for micronutrients (Cu, Se, Zn, Hg, etc.).
- Detection of abnormal amount of metabolites in the urine (creatinine/hydroxyproline ratio).
- Functional tests done to study the metabolic pathways.

## Advantages of Biochemical Measurements

The advantages of biochemical measurements are as follows:
- It is useful in detecting early changes in body metabolism and nutrition before the appearance of overt clinical signs.
- It is precise, accurate, and reproducible.
- Useful to validate data obtained from dietary methods (e.g., comparing salt intake with 24-hour urinary excretion.

## Disadvantages of Biochemical Measurements

The disadvantages of biochemical measurements are as follows:
- Expensive
- Time consuming
- Needs trained personal and facilities.

## Dietary Assessment

Nutritional intake of humans is assessed by five different methods:
- 24-hour dietary recall
- Food frequency questionnaire
- Dietary history from the beginning
- Food dairy technique
- Observed food consumption.

## 24-hour Dietary Recall

- A trained interviewer asks the subject to recall all food and drink taken in the previous 24 hours.
- It is quick, easy, and depends on short-term memory but may not be truly representative of the person's usual intake.

## Food Frequency Questionnaire

- The subject is given a list of around 100 food items to indicate his or her intake (frequency and quantity) per day, per week, and per month.
- It is inexpensive, more representative and easy to use.

## Limitations

- Long questionnaire
- Errors with estimating size
- Needs updating with new food commercial food products to keep pace with changing dietary habits.

## Dietary History

- It is an accurate method for assessing the nutritional status.
- The information should be collected by a trained interviewer.
- Details about the usual intake, types, amount, frequency and timing need to be obtained.
- Cross-checking to verify data is very important.

## Food Diary
- Food intake (types and amounts) should be recorded by the subject at the time of consumption.
- The length of the collection period range between 1 and 7 days.
- It is reliable but difficult to maintain.

## Observed Food Consumption
- The most unused method in clinical practice (must for research).
- The meal eaten by the individual is weighed and contents are to be calculated exactly.
- High degree of accuracy but expensive and needs more time and efforts.

## Interpretation of Dietary Data
1. *Qualitative method*
   - Using the food pyramid and the basic food groups method.
   - Different nutrients are classified into five groups (fats and oils, bread and cereals, milk products, meat–fish–poultry, vegetables, and fruits).
   - Determine the number of serving from each group and compare it with minimum requirement.
2. *Quantitative method*
   - The amount of energy and specific nutrients in each food consumed can be calculated using food composition tables and then compare it with the recommended daily intake.
   - Evaluation by this method is expensive and time consuming, unless computing facilities are available.

## Cookery Rules and Preservation of Nutrients

**What is cooking?**
It is art, technology, and craft of preparing food with heat or fire.

**What are the principles of cooking?**
- Conduction
- Convection
- Radiation

**Conduction**: Metals are good conductors of heat. For example, heating pan-transfer of heat occurs through direct physical contact.

**Convection and radiation**: Boiling water is the best example of convection. As heat water at the bottom moves up due to less density and cold water moves down due to high density when heat is radiated it travels in straight lines and object in its path becomes heated. For example, Grilling.

**Why cooking is done?**
Tastes better, makes food easier to chew, makes digestion more efficient, takes less time to digest, improves nutritional quality, kills microorganisms, inactivates enzymes, improves absorption, appears better, and lasts longer.

**What are the methods of cooking and serving?**
Moist heat, dry heat, and combination.

**Moist heat method includes**: Poaching (water or liquid), simmering, boiling, and steaming.

**Dry heat methods cooking includes**: Broiling, grilling, roasting, and baking (air).
Pan frying, deep frying (fat).

**Combination methods include**: Braising (fat then liquid) and stewing (fat then liquid).

*Poaching:* It is a method of cooking technique that involves cooking by submerging food in water at low temperature. For example, boiling eggs.

*Simmering:* It is method of cooking in water at temperature below boiling point and above poaching temperature.

*Boiling:* Cooking food in liquid at 1,000 degrees of temperature. Food gets cooked properly when its bubble vigorously.

*Steaming:* Food is being cooked with the help of steam or water vapor produced by boiling water.

*Braising:* It is a method of cooking in which first food is browned using fat and then liquid is added and simmered.

*Stewing:* Similar to braising but generally used to cook smaller pieces of meat in less time.

## Serving Food

Never leave meat, poultry, eggs, fishes either raw or cooked at room temperature for more than an hour. It is always safe to preserve in the refrigerator within 1 hour.

- Do not reheat food that is contaminated. Reheating doesn't make it safe.
- If you not sure whether a food is safe, discard it out.
- If you not sure how long food has been in the refrigerator, throw it out.
- Always clean the utensils properly.
- Use the hotboxes to pack the food to keep it fresh for few hours.

## Safe Food Handling, Storage of Food

- Always buy the whole vegetables. Leaving leaves on and stalks in allows vitamin C to migrate to the edible parts of the plant.
- Cook foods in the minimum of water, or steam them.
- Avoid high cooking temperature and exposure to long heat.
- Never allow food to stand for long periods at room temperature and do not store food in warm places.
- Do not soak vegetables in water for longer time.
- Do not peel vegetables and fruits.

## Preserving the Nutrients of Food with Proper Care

Parboiled rice is more nutritious than regular white rice.

Dark green leafy vegetables and deep-yellow vegetables have more vitamin A than light-colored ones.

Cooked vegetables that are reheated after being kept in the refrigerator for 3 days lose more than 50% of their vitamin C.

Except for pineapples, fruits ripened on the plant and in the sun have more vitamin C than those picked green.

Orange juice in a covered container can be kept in a refrigerator for many days to preserve vitamin C.

The **nutrient preservation** is to reduce the amount of water used in cooking, reduce the cooking time, and reduce the surface area of the food that is exposed.

Waterless cooking, pressure cooking, steaming, stir-frying, and microwaving are the least destructive of nutrients. If food cooked in water, add it to a small amount of boiling water, cover the pot, and cook it rapidly.

## Safe Food Handling

Do not wash rice before cooking it.

The smaller the pieces' food is cut into, the greater the chances of losing nutrients. That means smaller pieces go for faster cooking.

Do not cook green vegetables with baking soda because it destroys thiamin and vitamin C.

Cooking in iron pots can destroy some vitamin C, but it can also add iron to the food, if the food is acidic.

Cooking utensils made **of glass, stainless steel, aluminum, or enamel or lined with a nonstick coating have no** effect on nutrient content.

More thiamine we lose when we roast the meat for a longer time.

## Food Poisoning or Toxicity

This will occur when we do not cook food thoroughly, stored the food in an improper way. Keeping foods unrefrigerated for longer time and contamination of food (touched by sick people).

## Food Preservation and its Methods

Food preservation is done mainly to prevent the growth of fungi, bacteria, and microorganisms as well as slowing the oxidation of fats that cause rancidity.

**Modern methods to preserve** the food are pasteurization, vacuum packing, irradiation, biopreservation, and cryopreservation.

**Traditional methods to preserve** the food are drying, cooling, boiling, salting, sugaring, smoking, pickling, jellying, jugging and burial:

**Drying:** Vegetables and fruits are naturally dried by the sun, and this will prevent decomposition of fruits and vegetables.

**Cooling:** Preserves food by slowing down the growth and reproduction of microorganisms and the action of enzymes that causes the food to rot.

**Boiling:** Boiling liquid food items can kill any existing microorganisms. Water and milk are often boiled to kill any harmful microorganisms if present in them.

**Salting:** Salting or curing takes out moisture from a substance by osmosis.

**Sugaring:** Sugar is used to preserve fruits, either in antimicrobial syrup with fruit such as apples, pears, peaches, apricots, and plums, or in a crystallized form where the preserved material is cooked in sugar to the point of crystallization and the resultant product is then stored dry. Sugar dehydrates the microbes.

**Smoking**: It is used to prolong the shelf-life period of perishable food items. It is achieved by exposing food to smoke by burying the plant materials.

**Pickling**: It is a method of preserving food in an edible, antimicrobial liquid. The food is placed in an edible liquid that inhibits or kills bacteria and other microorganisms.

**Canning:** It involves cooking food, sealing it in sterile cans or jars and boiling the containers to kill or weaken any remaining bacteria as a form of sterilization.

**Jellying:** Food may be preserved by cooking in gelatin, agar, maize flour that solidifies to form a gel.

**Jugging**: It is the process of stewing the meat in a covered casserole.

**Burial:** Foods can be preserved in soil that is very dry and salty due to variety of factors: lack of light, lack of oxygen, and cool temperature.

**Pasteurization:** It is a process for preservation of liquid food applied to dairy products. Milk is heated to 70°C for 30 seconds to kill the bacteria present in it and cooling it immediately to 10°C to prevent the remaining bacteria from growing.

**Vacuum packing:** Storing food in an air-tight bag or bottle, commonly used for storing nuts to reduce loss of flavor from oxidization.

**Irradiation:** Exposure of foods to ionizing radiation (alpha and beta) kills bacteria, insects, and reducing the ripening and spoiling of fruits.

## Food Additives

These are the substance added to food to preserve flavor or enhance its taste and appearance.

**The food additives:**
- Maintains quality and freshness.
- Prolong shelf-life period.
- Compensate vitamin, mineral deficiency and provide nutrition.
- Aids in processing and preparation of foods.
- Some people are allergic to these food additives.

## Acidulants

Acidulants confer acidic taste. It includes vinegar, citric acid, and tartaric acid.

**Acidity regulators:** These are used for controlling the pH of foods for stability.

**Anticaking agents:** These prevent powders such as milk powder from caking.

**Antifoaming agents:** These prevent foaming in foods.

**Antioxidants:** Vitamin C is a preservative it inhibits the degradation of food by oxygen.

**Food coloring:** These are added to replace colors lost or to make food look more attractive.

**Emulsifiers:** These allow water and oils to remain mixed together in an emulsion.

**Flavors:** These five foods a particular taste or smell.

**Glazing agents:** These provide a shiny appearance or protective coating to foods.

**Sweeteners:** These are added to foods for flavoring to keep the calories low.

## Facts about Food Additives

Artificial food color is suspected of causing increased hyperactivity in children

Dye yellow No. 5 has been though to worsen asthma symptoms.

## Food Adulteration

Examples: Milk which contains added water, ghee which contains any added matter not exclusively derived from milk fat, mixture of 2–3 edible oils as edible oil, any article of food which contains any artificial sweetener beyond the prescribed limit and milk or milk products containing other than milk.

Adulterated food is impure and unsafe food.

Adulteration is a mixing of other matters of an inferior and sometimes harmful quality with food or drink intended to be sold and this will become unfit for human consumptions. The sellers do these adulterations to make the profit, to earn money in a less time and to look food make attractive.

## Prevention of Food Adulteration Act, 1954

**Objective:** To protect public from poisonous and harmful tools.

**Functions:** To analyze the samples of food sent by any authorized officer.

**Penalties:** Guilty will be punished with imprisonment for a minimum term of 6 months to a maximum of 3 years or with fine up to 1,000 rupees.

## Preparation of Beverages

**Mango cocktail:** Ingredients: 60 mL vodka + 60 g fresh mangoes + 8 fresh mint leaves + 20 mL sweet + 1 inch ginger + sour syrup + 15 mL lime juice + 1 mint sprig to garnish.

Add vodka, mangoes, mint leaves, sweet, ginger, lime juice, and sour syrup along with few ice cubes in a blender. Blend all together until well combined. Pour it in a margarita glass and serve frozen garnished with a mint sprig.

**What is a balanced diet?**

## ▪ Balanced Diet

A diet is all that we consume in a day. And a balanced diet is a diet that contains an adequate quantity of the nutrients that we require in a day. A balanced diet includes six main nutrients, i.e., fats, protein, carbohydrates, fiber, vitamins, and minerals.

To get the proper nutrition from your diet, you should consume the majority of your daily calories in:

- Fresh fruits
- Fresh vegetables
- Whole grains
- Legumes
- Nuts
- Lean proteins

A balanced diet includes a variety of foods from all five food groups (carbohydrates, proteins, fats, vitamins, and minerals). It should provide enough calories to ensure a desirable eight and should include all the necessary daily nutrients.

The healthiest combination for a balanced diet is *low fat, low refined carbohydrates + healthy carbohydrates + moderate protein*. For example, as a general rule:
- About 50% of our calories should come from complex carbohydrates.
- About 20% should come from protein.
- About 30% should come from all fat (Of this, a max of one third may be saturated fat).

**What are the daily nutritional requirements for adults?**

Daily reference intakes for adults are:
- Energy: 8,400 kJ/2,000 kcal.
- Total fat: <70 g.
- Saturates: <20 g.
- Carbohydrate: At least 260 g.
- Total sugars: 90 g.
- Protein: 50 g.
- Salt: <6 g.

All these nutrients are present in the foods that we eat. Different food items have different proportions of nutrients present in them. The requirements of the nutrients depend on the age, gender, and health of a person.

## Components of a Balanced Diet

Some components of a balanced diet are as follows:

### Fats

Some part of our energy requirement is fulfilled by fats. Fats can be found in fatty foods such as butter, ghee, oil, cheese, etc.

### Proteins

We need proteins for growth purposes and to repair the wear and tear of the body. Protein also helps in building muscle. It is found in dairy products, sprouts, meat, eggs, chicken, etc.

### Carbohydrates

We need the energy to process and it is fulfilled by carbohydrates. Carbs provide us energy. Carbohydrates can be found in rice, wheat, chapati, bread, etc. Cereals are our staple food.

### Minerals and Vitamins

Vitamins, minerals, and fibers improve the body's resistance to disease. We mainly obtain it from vegetables and fruits. Deficiency diseases such as anemia and goiter can be caused due to lack of mineral in the body.

**Why a balanced diet is important?**

A balanced diet is important because your organs and tissues need proper nutrition to work effectively. Without good nutrition, your body is more prone to disease, infection, fatigue, and poor performance. Children with a poor diet run the risk of growth and developmental problems and poor academic performance, and bad eating habits can persist for the rest of their lives. Learn more about healthy meal plans for kids.

Rising levels of obesity and diabetes in America are prime examples of the effects of a poor diet and a lack of exercise. The Center for Science in the Public Interest reports that 4 of the top 10 leading causes of death in the United States are directly influenced by diet:
- Heart disease
- Cancer
- Stroke
- Diabetes

## Meal Planning (Fig. 20.7)

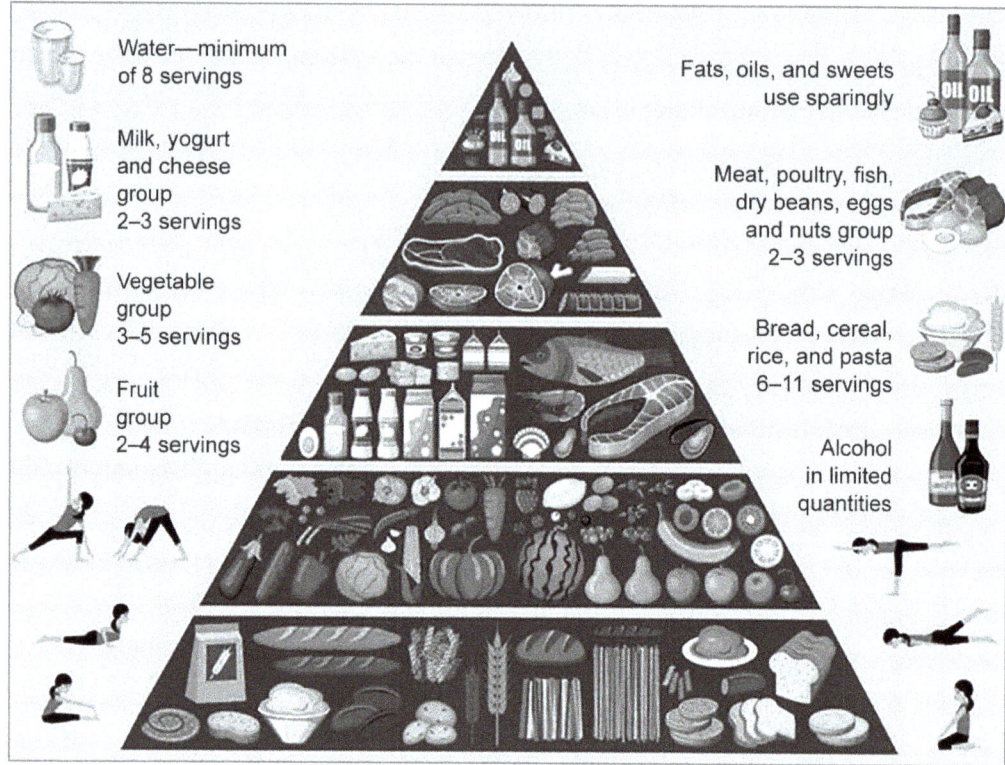

**Fig. 20.7:** Meal planning.

### Sample Menu

*Snack*

- Bran muffin or one slice bread **(Table 20.3)**
- Orange or apple juice 1/2 cup

*This sample diet may provide:*

| Calories | 2,491 | Fat 89 g |
|---|---|---|
| Protein | 121 g | Sodium 3,585 mg |
| Carbohydrates | 318 g | Fiber 38 g |

**Table 20.3:** Sample healthy diet.

| Breakfast | Lunch | Dinner |
|---|---|---|
| • Grapefruit 1/2<br>• Oatmeal 3/4 cup<br>• Raisins 2 tbsp<br>• Whole wheat toast 2 slices<br>• Margarine 2 tbsp<br>• Jelly/jam<br>• Skim milk 1 cup<br>• Coffee 3/4 cup or<br>• Tea 3/4 cup | • Vegetable soup 1 cup<br>• Hamburger patty 3 oz<br>• Bun 1<br>• Tomato 1 small<br>• Lettuce<br>• Baked beans 1/2 cup<br>• Apple 1<br>• Rice 1/2 cup<br>• Yogurt 1/2 cup | • Garden salad: lettuce 1 cucumber 1/6 tomato 1/2 med bean sprouts 1/6 cup salad dressing 2 tbsp<br>• Broiled chicken 3 oz (fat trimmed)<br>• Brown rice 1/2 cup<br>• Broccoli with cheese sauce 1/2 cup<br>• Strawberries 1/2 cup with plain low-fat<br>• Skim milk 1 cup |

# Food Group

The group into which several foods may be placed according to the type of nourishment they supply, such as carbohydrates or proteins.

## Classification

Popular types of food groups are two—five food groups and eleven food groups.

**Five-food group plans—Indian Council of Medical Research (ICMR):** India has given five-food group plans. This counts the food stuffs from all the five food groups, which is required to build a meal balanced.

**Group I**: Cereals, roots, and tubers
All these primarily supply energy.
- This group comprises foods like wheat, jowar, bajra, ragi, and other cereals. Tapioca, potato, sweet potato and yam come under roots and tubers.
- This group supply calories, protein, iron, and vitamins.
- These foods are low-priced and are taken in large amounts by the low-income groups.
- This group also provides thiamine and niacin.

**Group II:** Protein giving foods.
- All these primarily supply protein.
- It supplies protein both from the vegetable and animal source. The foods in this group are chiefly sources of protein though cereals also furnish protein.
- Dals, grains, peas, beans, groundnuts, cashew nuts, almonds, coconut, milk, curd, butter-milk, paneer (Cottage cheese) khoya, eggs, fish, mutton, chicken, pork, and other flesh foods come under this group.
- Milk and dairy products also provide calcium and riboflavin.
- Meat fish and eggs are good sources of protein, iron, and niacin.

**Group III:** Fats/oils, sugar/jaggery
- All these food stuffs are intense sources of energy.
- These include—vegetable oils, vanaspati, ghee, butter, cream, sugar and jaggery.
- This group constitutes about one sixth of the energy value of the diet.
- Butter is also a good source of vitamin A and D.
- Vegetable oils are a good source of essential fatty acids.

**Group IV**: Protective—vegetables and fruits
- These are rich sources of minerals and vitamins.
- These include green leafy vegetables, yellow or orange colored fruits and vegetables and citrus fruits.

**Group V**: Other vegetables.
These provide a combination in taste and texture and furnish roughage in the diet.

## Eleven Food Group Plans

These include fruits, stems, leaves and flowers of plants, ladies fingers, brinjals, bitter guards, cauliflower, etc. **(Table 20.4)**.
They are fair sources of certain vitamins and minerals.

**Significance:** Every 5 years—the dietary Guidelines for Americans are publishing an advice to Americans aged 2 years and older to promote good eating habits. The guidelines provide recommendations for use of all food groups, with grains, vegetables, fruits, milk, meat and beans, and fats. Foods are grouped jointly because they have similar nutritional properties. It is essential to consume foods from each group to get the nutrition your body needs for most favorable health.

**What is the nutritive value of food?**

## Nutritive Value of Food

Nutritional **value**: Nutritional **value** refers to contents of **food** and the impact of constituents on body. It relates to carbohydrates, fats, proteins, minerals, additives, enzymes, vitamins, sugar intake, cholesterol, fat, and salt intake.

**Table 20.4:** Eleven food groups plan.

| Food group | Main nutrients contributed |
|---|---|
| 1. a. Milk and cheese | Calcium, phosphorous, vitamin and proteins |
|    b. Ice creams | Fats and carbohydrate |
| 2. Meat, poultry, and fish | Proteins, phosphorous, iron, and vitamin B |
| 3. Eggs | Fats, protein, phosphorous, iron and vitamin |
| 4. Dry beans, peas, and nuts | Proteins and vitamin B |
| 5. Flour, cereals, and baked products | Thiamin, niacin, riboflavin, iron, carbohydrate, and cellulose |
| 6. Citrus fruits and tomatoes | Ascorbic acid and vitamin K |
| 7. Dark green and deep yellow vegetables | Provitamin A, ascorbic, and iron |
| 8. Potatoes | Carbohydrate and ascorbic acid |
| 9. Other vegetables and fruits | Ascorbic acid and cellulose |
| 10. Fats and oils | Essential fatty acid and vitamin E |
| 11. Sugar, syrup, and preservatives | Carbohydrate |

a. **Cereals and millets:** They are the most important group of food stuffs. They contain about 6–12% proteins and are good sources of some vitamin B, such as thiamine, niacin, and pantothenic acid; vitamin $B_6$; and minerals such as phosphorous and iron. Hence, they provide about 70–80% of the calories, proteins, and other nutrients. Ragi is one of the richest sources of calcium.

b. **Pluses:** Dried pulses are rich in proteins contains about 19–24%. They are good sources of many vitamin B and minerals.

c. **Nuts and oilseeds:** They are rich sources of proteins, containing about 18–40%. Soybean is the richest in proteins containing about 40%. They are also rich sources of fat and good sources of vitamin B and E with minerals such as phosphorous and iron.

d. **Vegetables:** The green leafy vegetables are rich sources of carotene. They are good sources of calcium, riboflavin, folic acid, and vitamin C. Sweet potato, tapioca, carrot, elephant yam, and *Colocasia* are the roots and tubers which are good sources of carbohydrate. Carrot and yellow flesh variety of potato are good sources of carotene.

e. **Fruits:** Most of them are good sources of vitamin C. Mango and papaya are fair sources of carotene. Indian gooseberry is a rich source of vitamin C.

f. **Milk and milk products:** The sole food of infants and supplement diets of children and adults. It is considered as a complete food except for deficiencies of iron and vitamin C and D. In addition to protein, fat, $Ca^{2+}$, riboflavin, vitamin A, and substantial amounts of vitamin B.

g. **Eggs:** Hens' egg contains about 13% proteins and 13% fat, rich source of vitamin A and some vitamin B.
- Meat, fish, and other foods.
- Meat: Rich in proteins 18–22%. It is a fair source of B-vitamins.
- Fish: Rich in proteins 18–22%. It is a fair source of B-vitamins. Fatty fish contains some vitamin A and D. Large fish are rich in phosphorus but are deficient in calcium. Small fish eaten with bones are good sources of calcium.
- Liver: Liver is rich in proteins. It is a fair source of A and rich sources of vitamins B12, 18–22%.

h. **Fats and oils:** They serve mainly as source of energy and provide essential fatty acids. Butter, vanaspati, and ghee are good sources of vitamin A. Many of them are good sources of vitamin E.

i. **Sugar and other carbohydrate foods:** Commonly used are cane sugar, jaggery, glucose, honey, syrup, custard powder, arrowroot flour, and sago. They serve mainly as a source of energy. Honey and jiggery contain small quantities of minerals and vitamins.

**CHAPTER 20: Nutrition and Dietetics**

j. **Condiments and spices:** These are used mainly for enhancing the palatability of the diet. The essential oils present in them help to improve the flavors and acceptability of food preparations.

**Serving and serving sizes or portion and portion sizes:** A serving is a defined quantity of a particular food with desired nutritional values. Serving is a tool used in nutrition for easy comparison of foods and to help in formulating balanced diet. Balanced-diet formulations based on serving sizes can be easily followed compared to nutrition composition tables.

Two different tools in serving sizes.

**Serving based as per the nutrition fact label of the food container:** A nutritional food label on a container displays the serving size, the nutritional values of each serving, and the number of total serving per container.

Significance:
* Gives the nutritional information
* For easy comparison with other similar foods
* Letting you know the calories and nutrients in a certain amount of food.

**Serving size of the foods in food exchange lists used in food pyramids:** It is based on the specific amount of food that provides approximately the same amount of calorie and carbohydrate as other similar foods within the exchange list.

Significance:
* Lists all the food of the food exchange system
* Useful in preparation of balance diets
* Helps in selecting food in familiar measures like cups, tablespoons, teaspoons, etc.
* Easily followed compared to nutrition composition tables.

Portion size and serving size:
* A serving size is the amount of food listed on a nutrition facts label and a pyramid.
* A portion is how much food you choose to eat at one time.

**Food pyramid:** It is a graphical representation of amounts and types of food required for a balanced diet. This gives guidelines that can be easily understood in graphical representation. It represents the amounts and types of food to be included in the daily diet (**Fig. 20.8**).

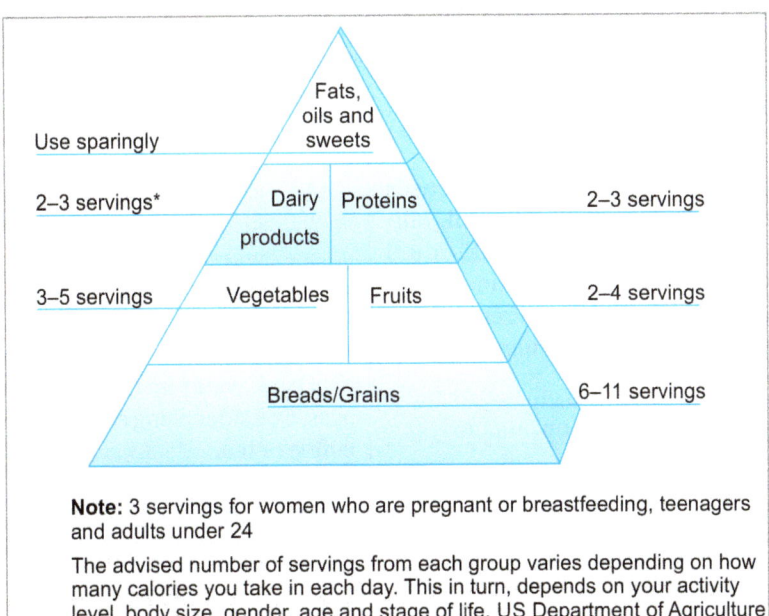

**Fig. 20.8:** Food pyramid.

## Budgeting of Food

Expenditure on food is an important and often the largest part of the family's budget. Higher budget will go on protective foods such as milk, vegetables, and fruits. We have to plan the expenditure of food and buy wisely so that the maximum nutrition can be achieved by the money spent. For example, as a source of protein, pulses are cheaper than animal foods. The fruits and vegetables are relatively cheaper than animal foods. The economy spent on food purchasing can be regularized in good measure by bulk purchase of foods, especially pulses and cereals.

## Introduction to Therapeutic Diets: Naturopathy Diet

Therapeutic diets are planned to maintain good nutrition in patient. In most cases, the therapeutic diets are used to supplement the medical or surgical treatment of the patient, while in some instances such as diabetes mellitus and cardiovascular diseases, a therapeutic diet is the most important aspect of the patient's treatment rather than medical therapy. Diet therapy is concerned with recovery from illness and prevention of diseases.

## Nutrition for Cardiovascular Diseases

**The people with cardiovascular diseases should not eat:** Red meat, coconut oil, butter, cheese, and whole and 2% milk. You'll also want to skip foods that contain cholesterol-raising trans fats, such as French fries, doughnuts, creamer, and stick margarine.

**Foods to eat are:** Oats, beans, olive and canola oils, nuts and fatty fish (salmon, anchovies).

## Nutrition for People with Diabetes

### Vegetables

- **Nonstarchy:** Includes broccoli, carrots, greens, peppers, and tomatoes.
- **Starchy:** Includes potatoes, corn, and green peas.
- **Fruits:** Includes oranges, melon, berries, apples, bananas, and grapes.
- **Grains:** At least half of the grains for the day should be whole grains.
  - Includes wheat, rice, oats, cornmeal, barley, and quinoa
  - Examples: Bread, pasta, cereal, and tortillas.

### Protein

- Lean meat
- Chicken or turkey without the skin
- Fish
- Eggs
- Nuts and peanuts
- Dried beans and certain peas, such as chickpeas and split peas.
- Meat substitutes, such as tofu.

### Dairy—Nonfat or Low Fat

- Milk or lactose-free milk if you have lactose intolerance.
- Yogurt
- Cheese

### Avoid Eating

Foods and drinks to limit include:
- Fried foods and other foods high in saturated fat and trans fat.
- Foods high in salt, also called sodium.
- Sweets, such as baked goods, candy, and ice cream.
- Beverages with added sugars, such as juice, regular soda, and regular sports or energy drinks.

Drink water instead of sweetened beverages. Consider using a sugar substitute in your coffee or tea.

## Dietary Requirements During Pregnancy and Lactation

The pregnant/lactating woman should eat a wide variety of foods to make sure that her own nutritional needs as well as those of her growing fetus are met.

Approximately 300 extra calories are needed daily to maintain a healthy pregnancy. These calories should come from a balanced diet of protein, fruits, vegetables, and whole grains, with sweets and fats kept to a minimum. A healthy, well-balanced diet during pregnancy can also help to minimize some pregnancy symptoms such as nausea and constipation.

The Academy of Nutrition and Dietetics recommends the following key components of a healthy lifestyle during pregnancy: appropriate weight gain, eating a balanced diet, exercising regularly, and appropriate and timely vitamin and mineral supplementation.

**Fluid intake** is also an important part of healthy pregnancy nutrition. Women can take in enough fluids by drinking several glasses of water each day, in addition to the fluids in juices and soups. All alcohol should be avoided in pregnancy.

It is better for all women of childbearing age consume 400 micrograms (0.4 mg) of **folic acid** each day. This folic acid is present in some green leafy vegetables, most berries, nuts, beans, citrus fruits, fortified breakfast cereals, and some vitamin supplements can help reduce the risk for birth defects of the brain and spinal cord (called neural tube defects).

Folic acid is most beneficial during the first 28 days after conception, when most neural tube defects occur. Unfortunately, many women do not realize they are pregnant before 28 days. Therefore, folic acid intake should begin prior to conception and continue through pregnancy.

**Iron** is needed for haemoglobin synthesis, mental function and to provide immunity against diseases.

Deficiency of iron leads to anaemia. Iron deficiency is common particularly in women of reproductive age and children.

Iron deficiency during pregnancy increases maternal mortality and low birth weight infants.

In children, it increases susceptibility to infection and impairs learning ability.

Plant foods like green leafy vegetables, legumes and dry fruits contain iron.

Iron is also obtained through meat, fish and poultry products.

Vitamin C rich fruits like gooseberries (Amla), guava and citrus improve iron absorption from plant foods

Commonly consumed plant based diets provide around 18 mg of iron as against recommended intake of 35 mg per day. Therefore, supplementation of iron (100 mg elemental iron, 0.5 mg folic acid) is recommended for 100 days during pregnancy from 16th week onwards to meet the demands of pregnancy Consume the following during pregnancy.

**Vegetables:** Carrots, sweet potatoes, pumpkin, spinach, cooked greens, tomatoes and red sweet peppers (for vitamin A and potassium).

**Fruits:** Cantaloupe, honeydew, mangoes, prunes, bananas, apricots, oranges, and red or pink grapefruit (for potassium).

**Dairy:** Fat-free or low-fat yogurt, skim or 1% milk, soymilk (for calcium, potassium, vitamins A and D)

**Grains:** Ready-to-eat cereals/cooked cereals (for iron and folic acid).

**Proteins:** Beans and peas; nuts and seeds; lean meats; salmon, trout, herring, sardines and Pollock.

Avoid the following during pregnancy:
- Unpasteurized milk and foods made with unpasteurized milk (soft cheeses)
- Hot dogs and luncheon meats (unless they are heated until steaming hot before serving)
- Raw and undercooked seafood, eggs and meat. Do not eat sushi made with raw fish (cooked sushi is safe).
- Refrigerated pâté and meat spreads
- Refrigerated smoked seafood

Nutrient needs during lactation depend primarily on the volume and composition of milk produced and on the mother's initial nutrient needs and nutritional status. Among women exclusively breastfeeding their infants, the energy demands of lactation exceed pre-pregnancy demands by approximately 640 kcal/day during the first 6 months postpartum compared with 300 kcal/day during the last two trimesters of pregnancy.

## National Nutritional Programs

**Introduction:** Undernutrition is the most important cause of illness and death globally. Nearly 12% of all deaths and 16% of disability are due to this. Low weight in accordance with age is the associated with more than half of all deaths in young children, accounting for more than 6 million deaths per year.

Programs: Broadly classified into two types:
1. Direct programs are:
   - Integrated Child Development Services (ICDS) Scheme
   - Nutrition Programs for Adolescent Girls
   - Nutrition Advocacy and Awareness General Programs for Food and Nutrition Board
   - Follow-Up Action for National Nutrition Policy, 1993
   - Ministry of Health and Family Welfare.
     - Iron and Folic Acid Supplementation of Pregnant Women.
     - Vitamin A Supplementation of Children of 9–36 Months Age Group
     - National Iodine Deficiency Disorder Control Program
     - Department of Elementary School and Literacy
     - Midday Meal for Primary School Children.
2. Indirect programs are:
   - Food and Public Distribution: This targets public distribution system such as Antyodaya Anna Yojana and Annapurna Scheme.
   - Department of Agriculture and Cooperation helps in increasing the food production and horticulture interventions.
   - Department of Education and Literacy through Sarva Shiksha Abhiyan, Adult Literacy Program.
   - Department of Women and Child Development as Various Women's Welfare and Support Program.
   - Rural and Urban Development through Food for Work Program, Safe Drinking Water and Alleviation Program, National Rural Employment Guarantee Scheme, etc.

*Special Nutrition Program:* The program was launched in the country in 1970–1971. It provided supplementary feeding of about 300 cal and 10 g of proteins to preschool children and about 500 cal and 25 g of proteins to expectant and nursing mothers for 6 days a week. This program was operated as under Minimum Needs Program Fund for nutrition component of ICDS program and was shared with Scottish National Party (SNP) budget.

*Balwadi Nutrition Program:* This program was launched by the Ministry of Social Welfare in 1970. This program is for the welfare of children in the age group of 3–6 years in rural areas. The children are given preschool education, diet supplementation by providing 30 kcal, and 10 g of protein per day per child for 270 days a year and care for their psychosocial development.

Integrated Child Development Services (ICDS) Scheme was launched on October 2, 1975 (fifth 5-year plan) in pursuance of the National Policy for children. This is mainly a health intervention that adopts a holistic approach aimed at improving both the pre- and postnatal environment of the child. It is a centrally-sponsored, state-administered scheme consisting of maternal health care in pregnancy and growth monitoring and nutritional supplements for children—services received at community centers or anganwadis.

Main objectives are:
- To improve the nutrition and health status of children aged 0–6 years.

- To lay the foundations for proper psychological, physical, and social development of the child.
- To reduce the incidence of mortality, morbidity, malnutrition, and school drop-out.
- To achieve effective coordinated policy and its implementation amongst the various departments to promote child development.
- To enhance the capability of the mother to look after the normal health and nutritional needs of the child through proper nutrition and health education in which children below 6 years, pregnant and lactating women, women in the age group of 15–45 years, and adolescent girls are included.

Programs to Prevent Specific Deficiency States Vitamin A Prophylaxis Program: This program is one of the components of National Programs for Control of Blindness. This includes administration of 200,000 IU of vitamin A orally to all preschool children every 6 months. The program was launched in 1970 by the Ministry of Health and Family Welfare: maternal and child health (MCH) centers in urban areas, primary health care (PHC) in rural areas, and ICDS projects are engaged in the implementation of the program.

**Prophylaxis against Nutritional Anemia:** The program was started by the Ministry of Health and Family Welfare during the fourth 5-year plan to prevent nutritional anemia. The program envisages distribution of iron and folic acid to young children and expectant mothers through MCH centers in urban areas, PHC/subcenter (SC) in rural areas, and Anganwadis in project areas. The commercial production of iron fortified common salt was started in 1985.

**Control of Iodine Deficiency Disorder:** The National Goiter Control Program was launched by the Government of India in 1962 in the Goiter belt in the Himalayan region, and iodized salt was supplied in Goiter endemic areas. Later on in 1986, this program was changed to National Iodine Deficiency.

**Disorders Control Program:** The program was conducted because the problem was found to be widespread and more than the problem of Goiter.

**Pilot Project on Program against Micronutrient Malnutrition:** The Pilot Project Program against Micronutrient Malnutrition was implemented in Assam along with four other states, namely, Bihar, Odisha, West Bengal, and Gujarat. The program was launched in the year 1995. The objectives of the programs are:
- To assess the and improve iron and vitamin A status in school-going children, adolescent boys and girls, nonpregnant women, adult males, and geriatric population.
- To assess the magnitude of fluorosis and dental caries.
- To launch extensive information, education and communication strategies through mass media to improve the dietary habits of the population.
- To study zinc level in various food products and soil.

The program was implemented in one district from each of the five states. The following activities were undertaken:
- Advocacy and sensitization meetings with people involved in policymaking with elected members, teachers, social workers, etc.
- A baseline survey was conducted to assess the socioeconomic status, food intake pattern, estimation of Hb, soil, zinc, fluorine in drinking water, etc.
- Training was also organized at block level, prior to field activity surveys.

**World Food Program (WFP):** World Food Program is the world's largest international food aid organization, serving in 84 counties with a goal of achieving "a world in which every man, woman, and child can have an access to food at all times. There can be no sustainable peace, no democracy, and no development when there is lack of food."

Founded in 1963 as the food aid arm of United Nation after the Rome Declaration on World Food Security day in 1996. WFP is committed to achieve a goal of reducing half the number who have adequate access to food by 2015.

## Infant and Young Child Feeding (IYCF) Guidelines—Breastfeeding and Infant Foods

Infant and young child feeding (IYCF) is a set of common recommendations for appropriate feeding of newborn and children under two years of age.

## Importance

- Protection and promotion of appropriate infant and young child feeding (IYCF) in emergencies helps to save the lives of the most vulnerable infants and young children.
- It plays a key role in preventing malnutrition and micronutrient deficiencies.

**There are three components of IYCF:**
1. Initial breastfeeding.
2. Exclusive breastfeeding.
3. Complementary feeding.
   Breastfeeding is unequalled way of providing ideal food for the healthy growth and the development of infants. It is also an integral part of the reproductive process with important implications for the health of mothers.

**Infant and young child feeding includes the following care practices:**
a. Early initiation of breastfeeding; is extremely important for establishing successful lactation as well as for providing colostrum (mothers first milk). The baby should receive the first breastfeed as soon as possible and preferably within one hour of birth.
b. Exclusive breastfeeding for the first six months of life (180 days): It means that babies are given only breast milk and nothing else—no other milk, food, drinks and not even water.
c. Timely introduction of complementary foods (solid, semisolid or soft foods) after the age of six months.
d. Continued breastfeeding for 2 years or beyond
e. Age appropriate complementary feeding for children 6–23 months, while continuing breastfeeding. Children should receive food from 4 or more food groups
   - Grains, roots and tubers, legumes and nuts
   - Dairy products
   - Flesh foods (meat fish, poultry)
   - Eggs
   - Vitamin A rich fruits and vegetables
   - Fruits and vegetables
     These can be fed for a minimum number of times (2 times for breasted infants 6–8 months; 3 times for breastfed children 9–23 months; 4 times for non-breastfed children 6–23 months)
f. Active feeding for children during and after any illness

## Supplementary/Complementary Foods

Foods that are regularly fed to the infant, in addition to breast-milk, providing sufficient nutrients are known as supplementary or complementary foods.

Complementary feeding is defined as the process starting when breast milk alone is no longer sufficient to meet the nutritional requirements of infants, and therefore other foods and liquids are needed, along with breast milk.

## RDA

**Recommended Dietary Allowance (RDA):** The RDA is the average daily level of intake sufficient to meet the nutrient requirements.

# CHAPTER 20: Nutrition and Dietetics

The RDA is the value to be used in guiding individuals to achieve adequate nutrient intake. RDAs are given separately for specified life stage groups and by gender if applicable; they are intended to apply to healthy individuals.

Recommended dietary allowance are applied to vitamins and minerals from food and daily supplements. The purpose of these guidelines is to inform how much of a specific nutrient the human body needs on a daily basis. It is important to meet bodies daily recommended dietary allowances so that our body gets everything it needs to function.

## Recommended Dietary Allowances for Different Age Groups

**Recommended dietary allowance:** For 0 to 6 months
Energy 110 to 140 kcal/kg
Protein requirement is about 2 g/kg
Calcium 500 mg/day
Best food for the neonate is mother's milk

**Recommended dietary allowance:** For 6 to 12 months
| | |
|---|---|
| Energy: | 98 kcal/kg |
| Protein: | 1. 65 g/kg |
| Calcium: | 500 mg/kg |
| Vitamin: | A 1550 µg/d |
| Vitamin: | B 1–50 µg/kg, B 2 65 µg/kg |
| Vitamin: | C 25 mg/d |

**Recommended dietary allowance:** For 1 to 3 and 4 to 6 years
| | |
|---|---|
| Energy: | 1240 kcal/d, 1690 kcal/d |
| Protein: | 22 g/d, 30 g/d |
| Fat: | 25 g/d |
| Calcium: | 400 mg/d |
| Iron: | 12 mg/d, 18 mg/d |

**Limitations**

- The amounts are intended to prevent disease, not to promote optimal health.
- The amounts group all adults into the same recommendations.
- The recommendations are not considering the interaction of other nutrients.

## Types of Infant Feeding

**Infant feeding may consist of**
- Direct breastfeeding (DBF)
- Pumping and bottle feeding (P&F)
- Formula feeding (FF)
- Solid food feeding (SFF)
- And any combination

## Feeding Techniques

- Stick with breast milk or formula
- Feed the newborn on cue
- Consider vitamin D supplements
- Expect variations in the newborn's eating patterns
- Consider each feeding a time to bond with the newborn
- Keep feedings consistent

## Alternative Feeding Methods

There are some alternative methods of feeding which are:
- Bottle feeding
- Cup feeding
- Spoon feeding
- Syringe or eye dropper feeding
- Finger feeding

## Effective Positions of Breastfeeding

- *Cradle hold:* In the cradle hold, mother hold her baby's body with the arm nearest to the breast, she is nursing from. So, if they are nursing on your left breast, she will hold their body with her left arm. Gently cradle their back with her forearm, and make sure they are tummy to tummy with her, their head turned toward her chest. She can use her free arm to support her breast or shape her nipple so it is easier for baby to latch.
- *Cross-cradle hold:* This looks similar to the cradle hold but mother arms switch roles so her baby's body lies along her

opposite forearm. The aim is to support her baby around his neck and shoulders to allow him to tilt his head prior to latch.
- Football hold
- Football hold for twins
- Side-lying position
- Laid-back breastfeeding
- Upright breastfeeding
- Dangle feeding
- Lying down with twins
- Breastfeeding in a baby carrier

## Diet for Obesity

Reducing calories and practicing healthier eating habits are vital to overcoming obesity.

It is essential to strictly follow a food list for obesity. A low fat diet, is a dietary pattern that limits the fat intake at about 1/3 of the total daily calories consumed and hence an ideal diet for obesity. It consists of little fat, particularly saturated fats and cholesterol which lead to increased blood cholesterol levels and heart attack. This type of diet plans to reduce obesity focuses on foods that contain whole grains, fruits and vegetables. It is directed towards weight loss and treatment of certain diseases by offering 20 to 30 percent of total daily calories from fat. Plenty of vegetables and proteins in a typical low fat diet supply the body with energy but very little fats. However, fats should not be eliminated entirely as some dietary fat is needed for good health, supplying energy and fat soluble vitamins, such as A, D, E and K. Studies have revealed that the right kinds of fats can actually help in losing weight. Hence, the prime focus of healthy diet plan for obesity is on limiting the unhealthy fats and consumption of right amounts of fats.

## Diet for Liver Disease

The most common liver disease is non-alcoholic fatty liver (NAFL). the diet should provide the right amount of calories, nutrients, and liquids that need to manage liver disease. It is essential to strictly follow a food list for hepatic disease. The first line of treatment for NAFLD is weight loss, through a combination of calorie reduction, exercise, and healthy eating. In general, the diet for fatty liver disease includes: fruits and vegetables, high-fiber plants, such as legumes and whole grains, significantly reducing intake of certain foods and beverages including those high in added sugar, salt, refined carbohydrates, and saturated fat and no alcohol.

## Diet for Underweight

Just like obesity causes health concerns, having less weight than the normal also poses health issues. Being underweight can be result of poor nutrition and should be a matter of concern. If the body does not receive adequate amounts of nutrients, the body fails to function to its utmost. Underweight should include this in the diet plan:
- Heavy food items that are more in calories.
- Frequent consumption of food items which are rich in nutrients, it could be snacks, shakes or juices, or proper meals.
- Adding extra ingredients that are high in calories to regular diet, for example, including eggs and bananas in morning breakfast, etc., can help in increasing the weight.
- Consume protein supplements along with adequate amount of vegetables and fruits.
- Eating calorie dense food and maintaining a balanced diet will help in gaining the weight.
- However, the diet should not be started drastically and instead, should be implemented gradually so that the body is accustomed with it.

## Diet for Renal Disease

The diet plan should be such that it should minimize buildup of waste product and fluid. The DASH (Dietary Approaches to Stop Hypertension) diet is a recognized treatment for hypertension, heart disease, and kidney disease. The DASH diet can slow the progression of both heart disease and kidney disease. It includes more fruits, vegetables, and low-fat dairy foods. To cut back on foods that are high in saturated fat, cholesterol, and trans fats. To eat more whole-grain foods, fish, poultry, and nuts and to limit sodium, sweets, sugary drinks, and red meats.

## Diet for Pre- and Postoperative Period

It is recommended to maintain a clear liquid diet the day before the surgery and hence more liquid food, such as water, clear broths (vegetable or chicken or beef) juices (apple or cider) is preferred.

After the surgery, your body should be ready for blended or puréed foods. At this stage, you can eat lean meats, vegetables and fruits as long as they are in liquid form. However, you should avoid raw fruits or vegetables. Canned or cooked fruits and vegetables that are puréed are acceptable. Avoid fried food, cheese and alcohol.

## SUMMARY

Intake of nutrients and its utilization by the organism are essential to maintain growth and perform daily activities. The diet, what we eat, is determined by the quality and quantity of foods. A healthy diet has many good impacts on health status of an organism. A poor diet causes many deficiency diseases such as anemia, beriberi, scurvy, and kwashiorkor and also life-threatening conditions such as obesity, metabolic syndrome diabetes, and cardiovascular diseases. There are seven major classes of nutrients such as carbohydrates, fats, fiber, minerals, proteins, vitamin, and water. A gram of carbohydrate, protein, and fat give 4, 4, and 9 cal, respectively, on oxidation. Carbohydrates, proteins, and fats have their own respiratory quotient. The respiratory quotient is the volume of $CO_2$ produced divided by the volume of $O_2$ consumed at the whole-body level. The carbohydrate, proteins, and fats are essential for us to perform various functions. Dietary fiber is a complex mixture of plant materials that are resistant to breakdown (digestion) by the human digestive. Consuming fiber along with other nutrients will help in the digestion as well as in the prevention of cancer. BMR is defined as the minimum amount of energy required by the body to maintain life at complete physical and mental rest in the postabsorptive period. There are several factors that affect BMR. The protein–calorie malnutrition results in kwashiorkor and marasmus. Vitamin $B_{12}$, iron, and folate deficiency results in anemia. Vitamin D deficiency causes rickets in children and osteomalacia in adults. There are different methods to assess nutrition requirement—direct and indirect. Anthropometric methods, biochemical, laboratory methods, clinical methods, and dietary evaluation methods are the direct methods to assess nutritional requirement.

## SELF-ASSESSMENT QUESTIONS

1. Mention the caloric values for proteins, carbohydrates, and fats.
2. What is respiratory quotient and mention its significance?
3. What are complete and incomplete proteins?
4. How do you explain protein and weight gain?
5. Add a note on protein and weight loss.
6. Write the importance of carbohydrates.
7. Briefly discuss the dietary fiber and its importance.
8. What is protein–calorie malnutrition?
9. How do you differentiate kwashiorkor from marasmus?
10. Give the signs and symptoms of kwashiorkor.
11. What is biological value of protein and write the formula to calculate it?

12. Discuss the components of balanced diet.
13. What is specific dynamic action and mention its importance?
14. Define BMR and mention the factors affecting BMR.
15. Briefly discuss the negative and positive nitrogen balance.
16. Calculate the energy requirement of allied health student (age 18 years, BMR = 40 cal/m² body surface/h, body surface area = 1.7 m²) engaged in moderate work.
17. What is resting metabolic rate?
18. How do you differentiate soluble fiber from insoluble fiber?

## MULTIPLE CHOICE QUESTIONS

1. **The caloric value for a gram of fat is:**
   (a) 9
   (b) 6
   (c) 3
   (d) 4

2. **The respiratory quotient for carbohydrate is:**
   (a) 0.8
   (b) 1.0
   (c) 2.0
   (d) 0.7

3. **All the following foods give complete proteins, *except*:**
   (a) Meat
   (b) Fish
   (c) Legumes
   (d) Cheese

4. **Concerning fats, one of the following statements is incorrect:**
   (a) It provides us 60% our energy needs
   (b) It helps to maintain cell membrane structure
   (c) It helps in the absorption of vitamins A and D
   (d) Protein-rich foods are deficient in fat

5. **Trans fat:**
   (a) Increases blood glucose
   (b) Increases blood IDI
   (c) Increases blood HDI
   (d) Increases blood chylomicron

6. **Concerning the dietary fiber, all the following statements are true, *except*:**
   (a) They are resistant to breakdown by the human digestive enzymes
   (b) Insoluble fiber promotes normal elimination by providing bulk for stool formation
   (c) Increased amounts of fiber in the diet is the reason for irritable bowel syndrome
   (d) Fruits and vegetables are rich in soluble fiber

7. **Concerning BMR, one of the following statements is incorrect:**
   (a) It is expressed as cal/m² body surface/hour
   (b) Age and sex may affect the BMR
   (c) The Harris–Benedict formula may be used to calculate the BMR
   (d) Hormones do not affect the BMR

8. **Negative nitrogen balance may result in:**
   (a) Unconsciousness
   (b) Muscle loss
   (c) Liver disorder
   (d) Amino acid degradation

9. All of the following are causes for protein–calorie malnutrition, *except*:
    (a) Increased carbohydrate
    (b) Inadequate dietary intake
    (c) Poor quality dietary protein
    (d) Increased metabolic demands
10. Which of the following is not a symptom of protein–calorie malnutrition?
    (a) Poorly developed muscle and lack tone
    (b) Severe edema
    (c) Potbelly
    (d) High serum vitamin A

## ANSWERS

1. a  2. b  3. d  4. b  5. c  6. d  7. d  8. b
9. a  10. d

# Chapter 21

# Organ Function Tests

## LEARNING OBJECTIVES

*At the end of this chapter students should be able to:*
- ❖ Explain the functions tests performed by liver, kidney, thyroid and adrenal gland
- ❖ Know about the list of biochemical tests performing to diagnose liver, kidney, thyroid and adrenal disorders

## Liver Function Tests

### Introduction

- ❖ Liver plays a major role in storing blood (acts as a reservoir of blood).
- ❖ The parenchymal cells of the liver are related to the breakdown of hemoglobin to bilirubin and the removal of pigments.
- ❖ It plays a central role in the metabolism:
  - Carbohydrates (glycogenesis, glycogenolysis, gluconeogenesis and alcohol metabolism).
  - Proteins (transamination, oxidative deamination of amino acids, urea synthesis and protein synthesis).
  - Lipids
  - Hormones
  - Vitamins
  - Bilirubin
  - Bile acids
- ❖ The hepatobiliary tree represents hepatic cells and biliary tract cells (**Fig. 21.1**).
- ❖ Inflammation of the hepatic cells results in elevation of alanine aminotransferase or alanine transaminase (ALT), aspartate aminotransferase or aspartate transaminase (AST) and possibly the bilirubin.
- ❖ Inflammation of the biliary tract cells results predominantly in an elevation of the alkaline phosphatase (ALP).

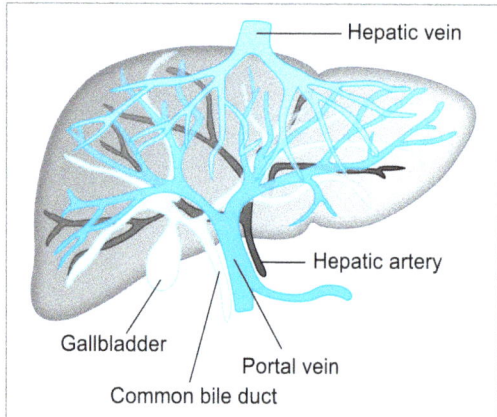

**Fig. 21.1:** Hepatobiliary tree representing hepatic cells and biliary tract cells.

- ❖ In liver disease there are crossover between purely biliary disease and hepatocellular disease.
- ❖ To interpret these, the physician will look at the entire picture of the hepatocellular and biliary tract disease to determine which one is the primary abnormality.

### Indications of Liver Function Test

- ❖ Liver functions tests (LFTs) are useful in the differential diagnosis of jaundice.
- ❖ Detection of liver diseases
- ❖ Assessment of severity and progress of liver disease.

# CHAPTER 21: Organ Function Tests

## Basic Processes in Liver Diseases

**Liver cell damage:** This may vary from areas of local damage to destruction of most of the liver cells leading to liver failure.

*Causes:* Acute hepatitis may be viral and chronic hepatitis is due to the continuing action of infective or toxic agents or that associated with autoimmune response.

- **Cirrhosis:** Destruction of hepatic cells.
- **Biliary tract involvement:** It is associated with obstruction to bile flow (cholestasis) and may present as obstructive jaundice.

There are two types of obstruction:
1. **Intrahepatic cholestasis:** Mainly arises with liver cell destruction.
   *Causes:* Viral hepatitis, use of steroids (during pregnancy or in the case of woman taking oral contraceptives).
2. **Extrahepatic cholestasis.**
   *Causes:* Gallstone in the common bile duct, carcinoma of the pancreas and cirrhosis of the bile duct.

The LFTs are considered under the following categories:
- Tests, which indicate the liver cell damage:
  - Aspartate transaminase
  - Alanine transaminase
- Tests indicating biliary tract involvement:
  - Alkaline phosphatase
  - Gamma-glutamyl transferase (GGT)
  - 5'-nucleotidase
- Tests indicating impaired function:
  - Serum proteins
  - Bilirubin

## Total Protein (Albumin and Globulin)

### Albumin

- Albumin is the major protein present within the blood.
- The liver synthesizes albumin.
- It represents a major synthetic protein and is a marker for the ability of the liver to synthesize proteins.
- It is one of the proteins synthesized by the liver. However, since it is easy to measure, it represents a reliable and inexpensive laboratory test for physicians to assess the degree of liver damage present in the particular patient. **Albumin level goes down when liver gets severely damaged.**
- Malnutrition can also cause low albumin with no associated liver disease.

### Serum Total Protein Estimation

- Albumin estimation
- Globulins estimation.

*Methods:* The serum proteins are estimated by differential precipitation of albumin and globulin fraction:
- Biuret method
- Albumin by dye-binding method

### Serum Protein Electrophoresis

- This is an evaluation of the types of proteins present in serum.
- With an electrophoresis, major proteins can be separated and this results in four major types of proteins:
  1. Albumin
  2. $\alpha$-globulins
  3. $\beta$-globulins
  4. $\gamma$-globulins
- Normal range:
  - Total protein: 5.0–7.5 g/dL
  - Albumin: 3.5–4.5 g/dL
  - Globulin: 2–3 g/dL
  - $\gamma$-globulin: 0.5–1.5 g/dL

## Prothrombin Time

- Liver synthesizes clotting factors such as prothrombin, fibrinogen, factor V, VII and X.
- The prothrombin time (PT) is prolonged in the cases of hepatocellular damage. The ability of the parenchymal cells to synthesize clotting factors is impaired.

## Jaundice

- Jaundice comes from French word jaune, which means yellow.
- Normal serum bilirubin is around 1.2 mg/100 mL.
- Whenever the level exceeds more than the normal range it diffuses into the tissues and the skin and sclera of the eye turns yellow. This condition is called jaundice (icterus).
- The yellowish coloration is caused by an excess amount of bilirubin in the skin. Bilirubin is a yellowish red pigment.
- Normally, small amounts of bilirubin are found in everyone's blood.
- When too much bilirubin is made, the excess is dumped into the bloodstream and is deposited in tissues for temporary storage.
- Jaundice in the infant appears first in the face and upper body and progresses downward towards the toes.

### Formation and Metabolism of Bilirubin (Fig. 21.2)

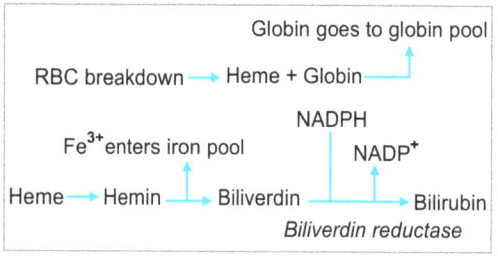

Fig. 21.2: Formation of bilirubin.

### Normal Values

- Total bilirubin = 0.2–1.0 mg%
- Direct bilirubin = 0–0.2 mg%
- Indirect bilirubin = 0–0.8 mg%

There are three different types of jaundice:
1. Hemolytic jaundice
2. Hepatic jaundice
3. Obstructive or posthepatic jaundice

Causes and biochemical findings of different types of jaundice are given in the **Table 21.1**.

### Van den Bergh's Reaction

#### Direct van den Bergh's Test

The conjugated water-soluble bilirubin when treated with diazo reagent [sodium nitrate ($NaNO_3$) + sulfanilic acid] gives red color immediately. This is called direct van den Bergh's test. The bilirubin reacting directly is also called direct bilirubin.

#### Indirect van den Bergh's Test

The water-insoluble unconjugated bilirubin gives a positive van den Bergh's test only if methanol is added to the serum. This is indirect van den Bergh's test. This is also called indirect bilirubin.

### Urobilinogen in Urine and Feces

- The presence of urobilinogen in a test sample can be shown by a test based on the production of red color when urobilinogen reacts with Ehrlich's aldehyde reagent.
- In hemolytic jaundice, there is increased formation of bilirubin, excretion into the intestine through the bile; therefore, there will be increased formation of urobilinogen in the intestine and increased level in the urine, and feces.

### Serum Enzymes in Liver Disease

The assay of serum enzymes is very useful in the differential diagnosis and monitoring of various hepatobiliary disorders.

- Enzymes, which are normally present inside the hepatocytes, released into the blood when there is hepatocellular damage—markers for hepatocellular damage (viral hepatitis, cirrhosis of the liver).
- Enzymes, which are primarily membrane bound (plasma membrane or side of hepatocytes)—marker for cholestasis.

# CHAPTER 21: Organ Function Tests

**Table 21.1:** Causes and biochemical findings of different types of jaundice.

| Features | Prehepatic/Hemolytic | Hepatic | Posthepatic/Obstructive |
|---|---|---|---|
| Causes | Abnormal red cells, antibodies, abnormal hemoglobin | Viral hepatitis, toxic hepatitis, intrahepatic cholestasis of bile duct, drugs and toxins | Extrahepatic cholestasis, gallstones, tumor of bile duct, carcinoma of pancreas |
| **Blood** | | | |
| Unconjugated bilirubin | Present (++) | Present (++) | Normal |
| Conjugated bilirubin | Normal | Increases in early phase and later decreases | Present (++) |
| **Urine** | | | |
| Urine bile salt (Hay's test) | Absent | Absent | Present |
| Conjugated bilirubin (Fouchet's test) | Absent | Present | Present |
| Urobilinogen (Ehrlich' test) | Present (+++) | Increases in early phase | Absent |
| **Feces** | | | |
| Urobilins | Present (++) | In intrahepatic cholestasis decreases | Clay colored |
| **Serum enzymes** | | | |
| Alkaline phosphatase (ALP) | Normal | Moderately increased | Increased markedly |
| Alanine aminotransferase or alanine transaminase (ALT) | Normal | Increased markedly | Moderately increased |
| Aspartate aminotransferase or aspartate transaminase (AST) | Normal | Increased markedly | Moderately increased |
| Gamma-glutamyl transpeptidase (GGT) | Normal | Moderately increased | Increased markedly |

## Serum Transaminases: AST and ALT

❖ The ALT is specific for liver.
❖ Its level increases more than the normal in liver diseases (viral hepatitis, cirrhosis of the liver).
❖ But AST is not specific to liver, its level varies in other forms of tissue damage such as myocardial infarction, muscle necrosis and renal disorders.

## Alkaline Phosphatase

❖ The serum ALP estimation is the most widely used biochemical test to put in evidence for cholestasis of intrahepatic or extrahepatic origin.

❖ Normal level = 4–13 kA units or 40–140 IU/L.
❖ Increase in serum level of alkaline phosphatase from liver is a very sensitive indicator of cholestasis.
❖ Increased ALP level in cholestasis may be due to two features:
  1. Regurgitation of ALP from bile to blood.
  2. Increased synthesis from the cells lining the biliary canaliculi.

## Gamma-glutamyl Transferase Estimation

❖ The GGT enzyme catalyzes the transfer of γ-glutamyl group from glutamyl peptides to another peptide or an amino acid.

- It is a marker of cholestasis.
- The GGT level increases both in liver disease and in cholestasis, but it is very high in cholestasis.
- It is also considered as a marker enzyme in the patients of cirrhosis in chronic alcoholics. Normal value is 10–30 U/L.

## Different Types of Viral Hepatitis

1. Hepatitis A caused by hepatitis A virus (HAV).
   *Markers:* HAV antigen (Ag), HAV antibody (Ab) and HAV immunoglobulin M (IgM).
2. Hepatitis B caused by hepatitis B virus (HBV).
   *Markers:* HBV deoxyribonucleic acid (DNA), hepatitis B surface antigen (HBsAg), hepatitis Be antigen (HBeAg), hepatitis B core antigen (HBcAg), antibody to HBsAg (anti-HBs), antibody to HBeAg (anti-HBe), HBc IgM and HBc immunoglobulin G (IgG).
3. Hepatitis C caused by hepatitis C virus (HCV).
   *Markers:* HCV ribonucleic acid (RNA) qualitative, HCV RNA quantitative and anti-HCV.
4. Hepatitis D caused by hepatitis delta virus (HDV).
   *Markers:* HDV Ag, HDV RNA [polymerase chain reaction (PCR)], HDV IgG, HDV IgM and HDV total (IgG + IgM).
5. Hepatitis E caused by hepatitis E virus (HEV).
   *Markers:* HEV Ag, HEV IgG, HEV IgM and HEV Ab (total).

## Renal Function Tests

- Kidneys are the very important and vital organ.
- They perform many important functions to regulate the internal environment of the human body.
- It is the main regulator of all the substances of body fluids and responsible for maintaining homeostasis.

## Functions of Kidney

The functional unit of a kidney is nephron (**Fig. 21.3**). Kidney has five important functions:
1. Urine formation
2. Regulation of fluid and electrolyte balance.
3. Regulation of acid-base balance
4. Hormonal function
5. Excretion of non-protein nitrogen (NPN) substances.

Kidney function tests are grouped under two headings:
1. The tests measuring glomerular filtration rate (GFR).
2. Creatinine clearance test
   It is the volume of plasma completely cleared off creatinine, which is excreted in the urine:

$$\text{Creatinine clearance} = \frac{U \times V}{P} \text{ or } \frac{U \times V \times 1.73/A}{P}$$

Where,
U = Urine creatinine
P = Plasma creatinine
1.73 = Generally accepted body surface area
A = Body surface area of the patient under investigation

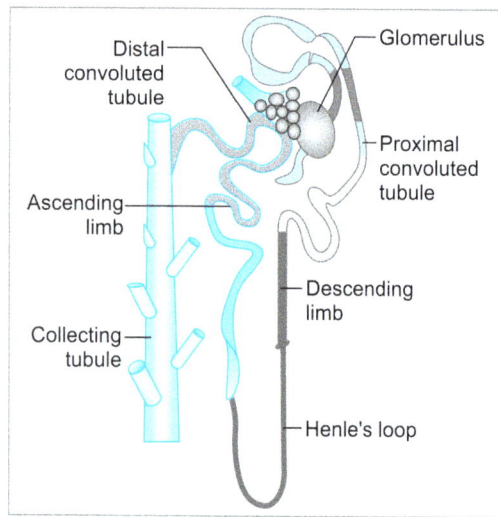

**Fig. 21.3:** Structure of nephron.

- The creatinine clearance is very convenient to measure GFR.
- It is fulfilling all the requirement of the substance, which is ideal for measuring GFR.
- The amount of creatinine produced is relatively constant and also it is not affected by the dietary intake.

*Normal Values*
- Male: 105 + 20 mL/min
- Female: 95 + 20 mL/min

*Clinical Significance*
Abnormal results are lower than normal GFR measurements and they indicate:
- Acute tubular necrosis
- Congestive heart failure
- Dehydration
- Glomerulonephritis
- Shock
- Acute nephrotic syndrome
- Acute and chronic renal failure

## Study of Elimination of NPN Substances

### Study of Elimination of NPN Substances

Tests measuring the retention of NPN substances in serum such as determination of urea, uric acid, creatinine, amino acids and ammonia.

*Urea*
- Urea constitutes about 45% of NPN substances.
- Study of their elimination can be done with blood and urine.
- One of the methods available for the determination of urea is diacetyl monoxime (DAM) method.

Normal values
Serum/Plasma urea:
- 15–45 mg/dL
- 2.49–7.47 mmol/dL
- Blood urea nitrogen (BUN): 7–21 mg/dL

Clinical significance
Causes for urea increase are:
- Prerenal causes:
  - Cardiac decompensation
  - Water depletion due to decreased intake or excessive loss.
  - Increased protein breakdown
- Renal causes are acute glomerulonephritis:
  - Chronic nephritis
  - Polycystic kidney
  - Nephrosclerosis
  - Tubular necrosis
- Post-renal causes:
  - Any obstruction to urine flow (stone, tumor, enlarged prostate).

*Creatinine*
- Creatinine is a breakdown product of creatine, which is an important part of muscle.
- The most important source of energy inside cells is the adenosine triphosphate (ATP) molecule, with its high-energy phosphate bonds.
- When one of these bonds is broken, energy is released and ATP becomes adenosine diphosphate (ADP).
- Creatine phosphate represents a back-up energy source for ATP because it can quickly reconvert ADP back to ATP.
- Overtime, the creatine molecule gradually degrades to creatinine.
- Creatinine is a waste product, i.e., it cannot be used by cells for any constructive purpose.
- The daily production of creatine and subsequently creatinine, depends on muscle mass, which fluctuates little in most normal people over long periods of time.
- Creatinine is excreted from the body entirely by the kidneys.

- With normal kidney function, the serum creatinine level should remain constant and normal.

Normal value
- 0.8–1.4 mg/dL
- Normal value ranges may vary slightly among different laboratories.

Clinical significance
- Higher than normal levels may indicate:
  - Nephrotic syndrome
  - Chronic glomerulonephritis
  - Acute tubular necrosis
  - Dehydration
  - Diabetic nephropathy
  - Reduced renal blood flow
  - Pyelonephritis
  - Renal failure
  - Urinary tract obstruction
- Lower than normal levels may indicate:
  - Muscular dystrophy (late stage)
  - Myasthenia gravis

*Uric Acid*

Normal value
The normal value of uric acid is 2.5–7 mg%.

Clinical significance
Value increases in:
- Renal failure
- Acute gout
- Pneumonia
- Sepsis
- Leukemia
- Polycythemia vera
- Anemia
- Value decreases in acromegaly

*Tests Measuring Tubular Function*
- Excretory function test
- Tests to measure the concentrating and diluting ability:
  - Specific gravity determination
  - Osmolality determination

*Calcium and phosphorus*
In chronic renal failure, there is impaired excretion of phosphate and progressive hyperphosphatemia occurs. This result in the decreased plasma calcium concentration giving rise to secondary hyperparathyroidism.

## Determination of Amino Acids

- Amino acids are a part of NPN.
- Their determination is helpful only in some congenital renal disorders.
- If there is defect in reabsorption more amino acid will appear in the urine, this condition is called aminoaciduria, e.g., cystinuria and homocystinuria.

*Aminoaciduria*

Aminoaciduria may be two types:
1. Primary aminoaciduria is due to an inherited enzyme deficiency, this is also called inborn error of metabolism. The defect is located in the pathway by which amino acid is metabolized or in the renal tubular system by which the amino acid is absorbed.
2. Secondary aminoaciduria may be due to disease of the liver or renal tubular dysfunction, or protein energy malnutrition. In both the conditions metabolites of amino acids accumulated in the blood are excreted in the urine. There are several tests to detect these amino acids and their metabolites in the urine.

## Pathological Conditions of the Kidney

*Acute Glomerulonephritis*

Acute glomerulonephritis (AGN) is an acute inflammation of the glomeruli, which results in:
- Oliguria
- Hematuria
- Proteinuria
- Anemia
- Increased blood urea and creatinine
- Decreased GFR

The presence of red blood cells (RBCs) in the urine is an insufficient evidence for AGN. Because of the appearance of blood may be from urinary tract.

## Nephrotic Syndrome

* It is a clinical entity characterized by massive proteinuria, edema, hypoalbuminemia, hyperlipidemia and lipiduria.
* The syndrome is having multiple causes.
* Increased membrane permeability leads to massive proteinuria (mainly albumin loss). There will be reduction in plasma osmotic pressure and the fluid movement from vascular to interstitial space that leads to edema.

## Tubular Disease

* Proximal renal tubular acidosis [reduced proximal tubular bicarbonate ($HCO_3^-$) reabsorption].
* Distal renal tubular acidosis (DRTA); there is an inability of tubular cells to create and maintain the usual pH difference between tubular, and blood.

## Urinary Tract Infection

* Infection may occur in the bladder (cystitis) or it may involve the kidneys.
* Diagnosis is made by the presence of bacterial concentration of more than 1 lakh colonies/mL of urine.

## ■ Thyroid Function Tests

The function of the thyroid gland is to take iodine found in many foods and convert it into thyroid hormones, i.e., thyroxine (T4), and triiodothyronine (T3).

Thyroid cells are the only cells in the body, which can absorb iodine. These cells combine iodine and the amino acid tyrosine to make T3, and T4. Then the T3 and T4 are released into the bloodstream, and are transported throughout the body where they control metabolism. Most of the cells in the body depend upon thyroid hormones for regulation of their metabolism:

* The hypothalamus, pituitary gland and the thyroid all play a part in the feedback and regulatory mechanisms involved in the production of T4, and T3 from the thyroid gland.
* Thyroid-releasing hormone (TRH) is secreted by the hypothalamus and stimulates the production of the polypeptide thyroid-stimulating hormone (TSH) from the anterior pituitary.
* The TSH then stimulates the production and release of T4, and T3 from the thyroid.
* Once released, T4 and T3 then exert a negative feedback mechanism on TSH production.
* T4 is the main hormone produced by the thyroid.
* T3 is mainly produced by peripheral conversion of T4.
* T3 and T4 both act via nuclear receptors to increase cell metabolism.
* The normal thyroid gland produces about 80% T4 and about 20% T3; however, T3 possesses about four times the hormone 'strength' as T.
* The 70–80% of T3 and T4 are transported in plasma by a thyroid-binding globulin (TBG), a plasma protein.
* The remaining 20–30% of T3 and T4 is transported by thyroxine-binding pre-albumin (TBPA) and albumin.
* Only the unbound or 'free' portion (FT3, FT4) is active.
* It is the free portion of the thyroid hormones is the true determinant of the thyroid status of the patient.
* The evaluation of the thyroid status is not a simple procedure because it does not depend mainly on the measurement of circulating thyroid hormones.

- The one or more factors may be abnormal and they are:
  - The TBG concentration and its degree of saturation with T3 and T4.
  - Concentration of free T3 and T4.
  - The state of the hypothalamus and anterior pituitary with their respective outputs of TRH and TSH.
  - The response of pituitary to TRH and response of the thyroid gland.

Thyroid disease is common, presents with many nonspecific symptoms so needs to be considered in many differentials and once diagnosed, needs to be regularly monitored for therapy. As a consequence, TFTs are the most commonly used endocrine test. Therefore, laboratory investigations of thyroid functions are useful in distinguishing patients with euthyroidism from those with hyperthyroidism and hypothyroidism.

## Common Thyroid Problems

- **Goiters:** A thyroid goiter is a enlargement of the thyroid gland. Goiters are often removed because of cosmetic reasons or more commonly because they compress other vital structures of the neck include the trachea and the esophagus making breathing and swallowing difficult. Sometimes goiters will actually grow into the chest, where they can cause trouble as well.
- **Thyroid cancer:** It is a fairly common malignancy; however, the vast majorities have excellent long-term survival.
- **Solitary thyroid nodules:** There are several characteristics of solitary nodules of the thyroid, which make them suspicious for malignancy. Although as many as 50% of the population will have a nodule somewhere in their thyroid, the overwhelming majority of these are benign. Occasionally, thyroid nodules can take on characteristics of malignancy and require either a needle biopsy or surgical excision.
- **Hyperthyroidism:** It means too much thyroid hormone. Current methods used for treating a hyperthyroid patient are radioactive iodine, anti-thyroid drugs, or surgery. Each method has advantages and disadvantages and is selected for individual patients.
- **Hypothyroidism:** It means too little thyroid hormone and is a common problem. In fact, hypothyroidism is often present for a number of years before it is recognized and treated. Hypothyroidism can even be associated with pregnancy.
- **Thyroiditis:** It is an inflammatory process ongoing within the thyroid gland. Thyroiditis can present with a number of symptoms such as fever and pain, but it can also present as subtle findings of hypo- or hyperthyroidism.

## Tests for Thyroid Function

The thyroid function tests are grouped into two types:
1. The in vitro tests are:
   - Total serum T3 and T4
   - Free serum T3 and T4
   - Blood TBG
   - Resin uptake test
   - Serum TSH
   - Thyroid autoantibodies
2. In vivo tests are:
   - Thyroid iodine uptake
   - TRH stimulation test
   - TSH stimulation test

### *Total Serum T3 and T4 Determination by Immunoassay (RIA or ELISA) and Chemiluminescence Method*

Immunoassay and chemiluminescence method are direct measurements of the total T3 and T4 in the blood. The serum T4 assays are more reliable than T3, because it is the major secretory product of thyroid gland. The majority of the T3 comes from peripheral de-iodination of T4. This test mainly helps to rule out hyperthyroidism and hypothyroidism. Radioimmunoassay (RIA) or enzyme-linked immunosorbent assay (ELISA) is the choice.

*Normal range*
- $T4 = 5\text{--}12.5\ \mu g/dL$
- $T3 = 80\text{--}180\ ng/dL$

*Clinical significance*
- Value increased in hyperthyroidism and decreased in hypothyroidism.
- The values also decreased in when TBG concentration goes down due to loss in urine and liver disease.

## Free T3 and T4 Determination

This is a measure of circulatory T4 and T3 that exists in the free form in the blood. The free thyroid hormone concentration is independent of changes in the concentration and affinity of thyroid-binding proteins and provides more reliable means of diagnosing thyroid dysfunction than measurement of total T3 and T4 hormones.

*Normal values*
- Free T4 = 10–27 pmol/L
- Free T3 = 3–9 pmol/L

*Clinical significance*
Value increased in hyperthyroidism and thyrotoxicosis and decreased in hypothyroidism.

## Hyperthyroidism

Hyperthyroidism occurs as a consequence of excessive thyroid hormone activity. Common causes in include thyroiditis, Graves' disease and toxic nodular goiter.

## Diagnosis

- The initial laboratory investigation with a possible diagnosis of hyperthyroidism should be a sensitive serum TSH assay, which will show reduced circulating levels of TSH.
- Low serum TSH is not specific for hyperthyroidism. It may also occur with 'non-thyroidal illness' or with the use of some commonly prescribed drugs.
- Patients who have a low TSH may then go on to have further investigations such as **(Table 21.2)**:
  - Free T4 and T3 assays: A subnormal TSH should trigger the measurement of FT4. If this is not elevated, FT3 should be measured to identify cases of T3-thyrotoxicosis.
  - Thyroid autoantibodies, e.g., thyroid peroxidase antibodies (TPOAb), TSH receptor antibodies (TRAb).
  - Radioactive iodine uptake: Thyroid scanning with either iodine-131 (most frequent) or $^{99m}Tc$ helps to determine cause of hypothyroidism, e.g., diffuse pattern of uptake in Graves' disease compared to one or more 'hot' nodules in toxic nodular hyperthyroidism.

## Hypothyroidism

- Primary hypothyroidism occurs as a result of under secretion of thyroid hormone from the thyroid gland.
- Causes include as Hashimoto's thyroiditis, irradiation and drugs such as lithium.

## Diagnosis

- To diagnose primary hypothyroidism, needs to measure both TSH and FT4. Where TSH is more than 10 mU/L and FT4 below reference range, the diagnosis is overt primary hypothyroidism and the patient needs treatment with thyroid replacement therapy.
- Secondary hypothyroidism is suggested by low within or mildly elevated TSH combined with a low FT4. Differentiating this from non-thyroidal illness can be difficult and clinical history, FT3 and sometimes anterior pituitary hormone tests are necessary.

**Table 21.2:** Differentiating causes of reduced thyroid-stimulating hormone (TSH) or raised free thyroxine (FT4) or triiodothyronine (FT3).

| Conditions | TSH | Free T4 | Free T3 | Other investigations |
|---|---|---|---|---|
| Graves' disease | Reduced ++ | Usually raised | Usually raised | Thyroid scan: Diffuse isotope uptake<br>Thyroid peroxidase antibodies |
| Toxic multinodular goiter | Reduced | Raised or normal | Raised or normal | Thyroid scan: Functioning nodule with suppression of other tissue |
| Thyroiditis | Reduced<br>Increased | Increased | Increased | Thyroid scan: Low radioiodine uptake<br>Thyroglobulin level, markedly raised erythrocyte sedimentation rate (ESR); often raised |
| Pregnancy | Normal | Raised total T4<br>Normal FT4 | Raised total T3<br>Normal FT3 | Positive pregnancy test |
| Thyroxine-induced hyperthyroidism | Reduced | Raised | Raised or normal | Thyroid scan: Low radioiodine uptake<br>Thyroglobulin levels absent |

Secondary hypothyroidism may occur as a result of damage or disease of the pituitary or hypothalamus.

- Additional diagnostic tests may include:
  - Thyroid autoantibodies—antithyroid peroxidase and antithyroglobulin antibodies.
  - Thyroid scan

## Subclinical Disease

Subclinical thyroid disease is common in American population. Diagnosis is based solely on test results when to treat subclinical disease is contentious.

## Subclinical Hyperthyroidism

- It is diagnosed by low serum TSH, normal FT4 and FT3, in the absence of non-thyroidal illness or relevant drug therapy **(Table 21.3)**.
- May increases risk of developing atrial fibrillation (AF) and cardiovascular disease (CVD).
- The TFTs should be repeated at 3–6 months or earlier if elderly, or if patient has pre-existing CVD, to determine whether full blown hyperthyroidism has developed or if the subclinical picture has persisted.

## Subclinical Hypothyroidism

- Occurs where TSH is above reference range with a normal FT4.
- Diagnosis should be confirmed with repeat TFTs after 3–6 months.
- Where TSH is less than 10 mU/L, there is no consistent evidence of association with symptoms, hyperlipidemias or increased risk of CVD. Above this level, there is more evidence of progression to overt thyroid disease and worsening hyperlipidemia.
- Thyroxin therapy is not recommended unless TSH more than 10 mU/L or, below this, if patients are pregnant, have a goiter or are trying to conceive.

## Thyroid-binding Globulin

- Most of the thyroid hormones in the blood are attached to a protein called thyroid-binding globulin. If there is an excess or deficiency of this protein it alters the T4 or

**Table 21.3:** Differentiating causes of raised thyroid-stimulating hormone (TSH) or raised free thyroxine (FT4) or triiodothyronine (FT3).

| Conditions | TSH | Free T4 | Free T3 | Other investigations |
|---|---|---|---|---|
| Chronic thyroiditis | Normal or raised | Normal or reduced | Normal or reduced | Thyroid nodules occur relatively frequently with this condition and have a 5% risk of malignancy |
| Hashimoto's thyroiditis | Usually raised | Normal or reduced | Normal or reduced | High titers of autoantibodies in 95% |
| Sick euthyroid syndrome | Normal or low | Reduced | Normal or reduced | Autoantibodies not present |

T3 measurement, but does not affect the action of the hormone. If a patient appears to have normal thyroid function, but an unexplained high or low T4, or T3, it may be due to an increase or decrease of TBG. Direct measurement of TBG can be done and will explain the abnormal value. Excess TBG or low levels of TBG are found in some families as a hereditary trait. These people are frequently misdiagnosed as being hyperthyroid or hypothyroid, but they have no thyroid problem and need no treatment.

* Normal value: 12–28 µg/mL.
* TBG value increased in hypothyroidism, pregnancy and estrogen therapy.
* TBG value decreased in hyperthyroidism, nephrotic syndrome and liver disease.

## Measurement of Pituitary Production of TSH

* Pituitary production of TSH is measured by a method referred to as RIA.
* Normally, low levels (<5 U) of TSH are sufficient to keep the normal thyroid gland functioning properly.
* When the thyroid gland becomes inefficient such as in early hypothyroidism, the TSH becomes elevated even though the T4 and T3 may still be within the 'normal' range.
* This rise in TSH represents the pituitary glands response to a drop in circulating thyroid hormone; it is usually the first indication of thyroid gland failure. Since TSH is normally low when the thyroid gland is functioning properly, the failure of TSH to rise when circulating thyroid hormones are low is an indication of impaired pituitary function.
* The new 'sensitive' TSH test will show very low levels of TSH when the thyroid is overactive (as a normal response of the pituitary to try to decrease thyroid stimulation). Interpretations of the TSH level depend upon the level of thyroid hormone; therefore, the TSH is usually used in combination with other thyroid tests such as the T4 RIA and T3 RIA.

## Thyroid-releasing Hormone Test

* In normal people, TSH secretion from the pituitary can be increased by giving a shot containing TRH.
* A baseline TSH of five or less usually goes up to 10–20 after giving an injection of TRH. Patients with too much thyroid hormone (thyroxine or triiodothyronine) will not show a rise in TSH when given TRH.
* This 'TRH test' is presently the most sensitive test in detecting early hyperthyroidism. Patients who show too much response to TRH (TSH rises greater than 40) may be hypothyroid.
* This test is also used in cancer patients who are taking thyroid replacement to see

if they are on sufficient medication. It is sometimes used to measure if the pituitary gland is functioning.

* The new 'sensitive' TSH test (above) has eliminated the necessity of performing a TRH test in most clinical situations.

## Thyroid Iodine Uptake Scan

A means of measuring thyroid function is to measure how much iodine is taken up by the thyroid gland. Remember, cells of the thyroid normally absorb iodine from our bloodstream (obtained from foods we eat) and use it to make thyroid hormone. Hypothyroid patients usually take up too little iodine and hyperthyroid patients take up too much iodine. The test is performed by giving a dose of radioactive iodine on an empty stomach. The iodine is concentrated in the thyroid gland or excreted in the urine over the next few hours. The amount of iodine that goes into the thyroid gland can be measured by a 'thyroid uptake.' At other times the gland will concentrate iodine normally, but will be unable to convert the iodine into thyroid hormone; therefore, interpretation of the iodine uptake is usually done in conjunction with blood tests.

## Thyroid Scan

Taking a 'picture' of how well the thyroid gland is functioning requires giving a radioisotope to the patient and letting the thyroid gland concentrate the isotope. Therefore, it is usually done at the same time that the iodine uptake test is performed. Although other isotopes such as technetium will be concentrated by the thyroid gland; these isotopes will not measure iodine uptake, which is what we really want to know because the production of thyroid hormone is dependent upon absorbing iodine. All scans are now done with radioactive iodine. Pregnant women should not have thyroid scans performed because the iodine can cause development troubles within the baby's thyroid gland.

## Adrenal Gland

The adrenal gland comprises cortex and Medulla.

Cortex has again three zones **(Fig. 21.4)**:
1. Zona glomerulosa → produces mineralocorticoids.
2. Zona fasciculata → produces glucocorticoids.
3. Zona reticularis → secretes sex steroids like androgens and estrogens.

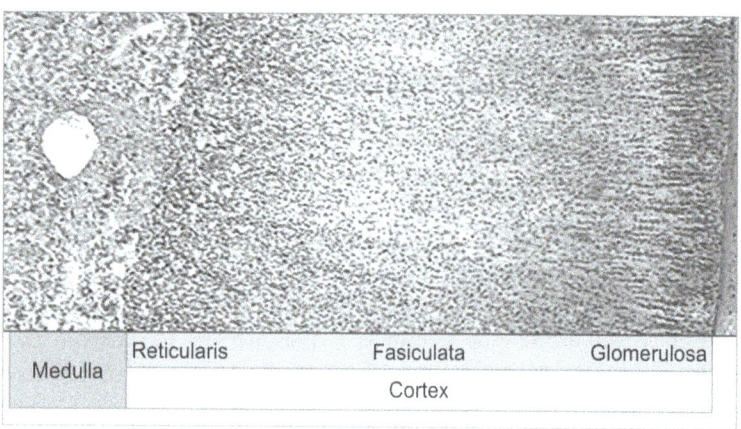

**Fig. 21.4:** Histology of adrenal gland.

## Assessment of Glucocorticoid Secretion

The plasma or serum cortisol level determination is one of the methods for assessing the secretion of glucocorticoids.

*Normal value*
* 8-26 mg/dL at AM (250-850 nmol/L)
* 5-18 mg/dL at PM (110-390 nmol/L)

## Control of Cortisol Secretion

Cortisol and other glucocorticoids are secreted in response to a single stimulator—adrenocorticotropic hormone (ACTH) from the anterior pituitary. ACTH is itself secreted under control of the hypothalamic peptide corticotropin-releasing hormone (CRH). The central nervous system is thus the commander and chief of glucocorticoid responses, providing an excellent example of close integration between the nervous and endocrine systems **(Fig. 21.5)**.

*Pathophysiology:*
Addison's disease (Adrenal insufficiency):
* Addison's disease is a rare endocrine or hormonal disorder that occurs in all age groups

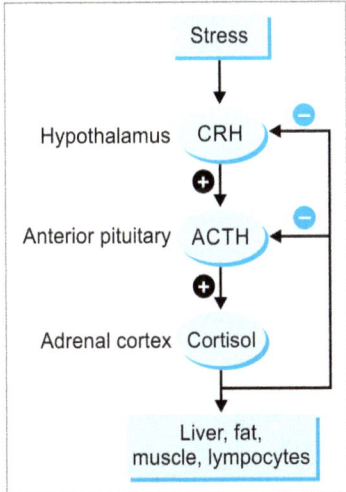

**Fig. 21.5:** Synthesis of cortisol.
(CRH: corticotropin-releasing hormone; ACTH adrenocorticotropic hormone)

* In this condition the adrenal gland reduces insufficient amounts of steroid hormones (glucocorticoids and often mineralocorticoids
* The disease is also called adrenal insufficiency, or hypocortisolism.

*Causes:*
* Failure to produce adequate levels of cortisol can occur for different reasons. The problem may be due to a disorder of the adrenal glands themselves (primary adrenal insufficiency)
  * Destruction of the adrenal glands by infection.
  * Their destruction by an autoimmune attack.
* Inadequate secretion of ACTH by the pituitary gland (secondary adrenal insufficiency).

*Adrenocorticotropic Hormone Stimulation Test*
This is the most specific test for diagnosing Addison's disease. In this test, blood cortisol, urine cortisol, or both are measured before and after a synthetic form of ACTH is given by injection. In the so-called short, or rapid, ACTH test, measurement of cortisol in blood is repeated 30-60 minutes after an intravenous ACTH injection. The normal response after an injection of ACTH is a rise in blood and urine cortisol levels. Patients with either form of adrenal insufficiency respond poorly or do not respond at all.

*Cushing's syndrome*
* Cushing's syndrome is a hormonal disorder caused by prolonged exposure of the body's tissues to high levels of the hormone cortisol.
* In Cushing's syndrome, the level of adrenal hormones, especially of the glucocorticoids (cortisol) is too high.

*Cause:*
* Excessive production of ACTH by the anterior lobe of the pituitary.
* Excessive production of adrenal hormones themselves (e.g., because of a tumor).

- **Ectopic ACTH syndrome:** Some benign or malignant tumors that arise outside the pituitary can produce ACTH. This condition is known as ectopic ACTH syndrome. Lung tumors cause over 50% of these cases.
- As a result of glucocorticoid therapy for some other disorder such as rheumatoid arthritis or Decreased glucocorticoid hormone synthesis.

*Symptoms:*
- Hyperglycemia
- High blood pressure
- Severe protein catabolism results in thinning of skin, muscle wasting, osteoporosis and negative nitrogen balance.
- There is a peculiar redistribution of fat in trunks.
- Moon face
- Central obesity and typical buffalo hump.
- Resistant to infection and inflammatory response is impaired.
- Facial hair growth

*24-hour Urinary Free Cortisol Level*
This is the most specific diagnostic test. The patient's urine is collected over a 24-hour period and tested for the amount of cortisol. If the cortisol level is higher than 50–100 µg a day for an adult suggests Cushing's syndrome. The normal range may vary from laboratory to laboratory depending on the techniques they use.

*Dexamethasone Suppression Test*
This test is used to distinguish patients with excess production of ACTH due to pituitary adenomas from those with ectopic ACTH-producing tumors. Patients are given dexamethasone, a synthetic glucocorticoid, by mouth every 6 hours for 4 days. For the first 2 days, low doses of dexamethasone are given, and for the last 2 days, higher doses are given. 24-hour urine sample collections are made before dexamethasone is administered and on each day of the test. Since cortisol and other glucocorticoids signal the pituitary to lower secretion of ACTH, the normal response after taking dexamethasone is a drop in blood and urine cortisol levels. Different responses of cortisol to dexamethasone are obtained depending on whether the cause of Cushing's syndrome is a pituitary adenoma or an ectopic ACTH-producing tumor.

The dexamethasone suppression test can produce false-positive results in patients with depression, alcohol abuse, high estrogen levels, acute illness, and stress. Conversely, drugs such as phenytoin and phenobarbital may cause false-negative results in response to dexamethasone suppression. For this reason, patients are usually advised by their physicians to stop taking these drugs at least one week before the test.

*CRH Stimulation Test*
This test helps to distinguish between patients with pituitary adenomas and those with ectopic ACTH syndrome or cortisol-secreting adrenal tumors. Patients are given an injection of CRH, the corticotropin-releasing hormone which causes the pituitary to secrete ACTH. Patients with pituitary adenomas usually experience a rise in blood levels of ACTH and cortisol. This response is rarely seen in patients with ectopic ACTH syndrome and practically never in patients with cortisol-secreting adrenal tumors.

*Mineralocorticoids*
- It is a steroid hormone and mainly derived from the cholesterol.
- The mineralocorticoids get their name from their effect on mineral metabolism. The most important of them is the steroid **aldosterone**.
- Aldosterone acts on the kidney promoting the reabsorption of sodium ions ($Na^+$) into the blood.
- Water follows the salt and this helps maintain normal blood pressure.
- Aldosterone also acts on sweat glands to reduce the loss of sodium in perspiration.

- Acts on taste cells to increase the sensitivity of the taste buds to sources of sodium.
- The secretion of aldosterone is stimulated by:
    - A drop in the level of sodium ions in the blood.
    - A rise in the level of potassium ions in the blood.
    - Angiotensin II
    - Adrenocortocotropic hormone

*Primary aldosteronism or Cohn's syndrome:*
- Results from an aldosterone-secreting tumor which leads to elevated levels of plasma aldosterone.
- The plasma pH in this condition increases because of hypokalemic alkalosis and the plasma osmolality also increases.

*Adrenal medulla:*
*Secretes*
- Dopamine
- Adrenaline (epinephrine)
- Noradrenaline (norepinephrine)

*Functions*
- The adrenal medulla consists of masses of neurons that are part of the sympathetic branch of the autonomic nervous system.
- Instead of releasing their neurotransmitters at a synapse, these neurons release them into the blood. Thus, although part of the nervous system, the adrenal medulla functions as an endocrine gland.

## SUMMARY

This chapter deals with the liver function, renal function and thyroid function tests. Liver plays a major role in the metabolism. There is no single test to detect the abnormality of the liver because of the variety of the functions performed by the liver. Therefore, there are group of tests available to detect the abnormality of the liver. Detection of total protein, albumin, AST, ALT, bilirubin and GGT helps in the diagnosis of liver diseases and to diagnose the jaundice. Renal function tests performed to detect the diseases of the kidney. The kidneys perform many important functions to regulate the internal environment of the human body. It is the main regulator of all the substances of body fluids and responsible for maintaining homeostasis. The major functions of the kidney are urine formation, regulation of fluid and electrolyte balance, regulation of acid–base balance, hormonal function and excretion of non-protein nitrogen (NPN) substances. The serum urea and creatinine determination helps to detect the abnormal function of the kidneys. Thyroid function tests help to diagnose the thyroid disorders. Thyroid gland secretes T3 and T4 upon stimulation by TSH. The reduced level of thyroid hormones is called hypothyroidism (goiter, Hashimoto's thyroiditis). The high level of thyroid hormones (hyperthyroidism) seen in Graves' disease, thyroiditis and toxic multinodular goiter. Thyroid iodine uptake scan will be done to measure how much iodine is taken up by the thyroid gland. Adrenal gland comprises medulla and cortex. The cortex has three regions such as zona glomerulosa which secretes mineralocorticoids (aldosterone), zona fasciculata secretes glucocorticoids and zona reticularis secretes sex steroids. Adrenal medulla secretes dopamine, epinephrine and norepinephrine. There are several tests done to detect the functions of adrenal gland for example ACTH stimulation and dexamethasone suppression test. Elevated level glucocorticoids result in Cushing's syndrome and reduced level leads to Addison's disease.

## SELF-ASSESSMENT QUESTIONS

1. List the tests under liver function test (LFT) panel.
2. What are the indications of LFT?
3. What are the functions performed by the liver?
4. Name the tests related to protein metabolism.
5. Give the normal values for:
    (a) Total protein.
    (b) Albumin.
    (c) Alanine transaminase.
    (d) Aspartate transaminase.
    (e) Total bilirubin.
    (f) Direct bilirubin.
6. Write the flow chart to show the formation of bilirubin from the red blood cell (RBC).
7. What are the steps involved during the bilirubin excretion?
8. Mention the conditions in which bilirubin metabolism and excretion is disturbed.
9. Define jaundice.
10. What are the different types of jaundice?
11. Write the biochemical findings of any two types of jaundice.
12. What is direct and indirect van den Bergh test?
13. Which test is used to find the bilirubin in the urine and write its procedure?
14. Why bile salts sinks to the bottom of the solution if it is present in the urine?
15. Which enzymes are considered as marker enzymes for hepatocellular damage?
16. Mention the enzymes, which are used as marker enzymes to detect the cholestasis.
17. How many isoenzyme forms of alkaline phosphatase (ALP) are there?
18. Give the normal value of ALP.
19. Name the functions performed by the kidney.
20. List the tests under renal function test (RFT).
21. Define creatinine clearance.
22. Give the formula to calculate creatinine clearance.
23. Give the procedure for performing creatinine clearance.
24. Why creatinine is selected for measuring glomerular filtration rate (GFR)?
25. Mention the conditions in which creatinine clearance decreases.
26. Write the normal values for the following:
    (a) Urea.
    (b) Creatinine.
    (c) Uric acid.
27. Mention the causes in which urea level decreases.
28. Write short notes on:
    (a) Nephrotic syndrome.
    (b) Glomerulonephritis.
29. Which tests are used to identify the amino acids?
30. Give the normal creatinine clearance value.

## Case Studies

1. A 30-year-old man was admitted to a hospital following episodes of nausea, vomiting, and abdominal pain. Upon examination it was discovered that his kidneys were slightly enlarged. Then the physician requested his blood investigation. Following results were obtained from the clinical biochemistry laboratory:

   | Laboratory test | Result |
   | --- | --- |
   | Fasting blood sugar | 85 mg/dL |
   | Blood urea | 80 mg/dL |
   | Creatinine | 6.0 mg/dL |
   | Uric acid | 7.0 mg% |
   | Serum osmolality | 380 mOsm/kg |
   | Inorganic phosphorous | 3.5 mg% |
   | Potassium | 6.0 mEq/L |

   a. What is the most likely diagnosis?
   b. How would you make a definite diagnosis?
   c. Can the diagnosis made using the NPN substance values?

2. A 12-year-old female child was brought to the hospital with symptoms of vomiting, anorexia and a sign of swollen face. The pediatrician admitted the child and after physical examination requested for blood and urine tests. The laboratory revealed the following results:

   | Laboratory test | Result |
   | --- | --- |
   | Total serum protein | 5.0 g/dL |
   | Albumin | 2.5 g/dL |
   | Globulins | 3.0 g/dL |
   | Urine osmolality | 1200 mOsm/kg $H_2O$ |
   | Urine albumin | Very high |

   a. What is the probable diagnosis to be done with the available laboratory results?
   b. How would you make a definite diagnosis?
   c. What is the pathophysiology of this disorder?

3. A 70-year-old man who lived alone was discovered by his friend in a drowsy, confused state. On admission she was extremely dirty and her tongue was dry. Immediately he was given some saline through intravenously. After some time, the doctor requested for blood tests which revealed the following results:

   | Laboratory test | Result |
   | --- | --- |
   | Sodium | 141 mEq/L (normal) |
   | Potassium | 5.7 mEq/L (elevated) |
   | Chloride | 107 mEq/L (elevated) |
   | Creatinine clearance | 80 mL/min (reduced) |
   | Urea | 70 mg/dL (elevated) |
   | Creatinine | 4.0 mg/dL |

   a. What is the likely cause of her symptoms?
   b. What is the likely diagnosis?
   c. How would you make a definite diagnosis?

4. A 8 year old child was brought to the clinic by his parents. They explained that the child is not eating properly and complaining weakness. The physician examined and noticed swelling especially in face and extremities. He requested for RFT and LFT. The laboratory revealed the following results:

| Laboratory test | Result |
|---|---|
| Serum bilirubin | 1.2 mg% |
| Direct bilirubin | 0.2 mg% |
| Indirect bilirubin | 1.0 mg% |
| AST | 25 units/L |
| ALT | 20 units/L |
| Alkaline phosphatase | 40 units/L |
| Total protein | 4.5 g/dL |
| Albumin | 2.0 g/dL |
| Globulin | 2.5 g/dL |
| Urea | 30 mg% |
| Creatinine | 2.0 mg% |
| Urinary protein | 10 g/L |

  a. What diagnosis was made depending on the following blood results? Explain with specific reasons.
  b. What was the reason for swelling in face and extremities?

5. A 50-year-old Mr Joseph was brought to the Mount Hope Hospital with the symptoms of pain in the flanks, anorexia (loss of appetite for food) and severe vomiting. The physician admitted him to the ward examined him thoroughly. Physician asked the nurse to send his blood sample for sugar and RFT and urine sample for microalbumin. Results of laboratory test are as follows:

| Laboratory test | Result |
|---|---|
| Fasting blood sugar | 200 mg/dL |
| Urea | 70 mg/dL |
| Creatinine | 10.0 mg/dL |
| Microalbumin | 140 mg/L |

  a. What probable diagnosis can be made using the above-mentioned laboratory results?
  b. What is basis for the diagnosis made? Explain with reasons.
  c. Why microalbumin was high in urine sample?

6. Mr Joseph visited the physician at Mout Hope adults PCF with several health problems and he explained him that he is feeling tiredness and burning sensation at the feet and above the stomach. He also explained that he is passing urine very frequently. The physician examined him and requested his blood and urine test. The laboratory results showed the following results:

| Laboratory test | Result |
|---|---|
| TSH | 3.0 mIU/mL |
| T3 | 1.5 ng/mL |
| T4 | 6.0 µg/dL |
| FBS | 400 mg/dL |
| Urea | 20 mg/dL |
| Creatinine | 1.0 mg/dL |
| AST | 25 units/L |
| ALT | 20 units/L |
| Alkaline phosphatase | 40 units/L |
| Total protein | 7.5 g/dL |
| Blood pH | 7.0 |
| Plasma $HCO_3^-$ | 17 mEq/L |
| Benedicts test | Brick red color |
| Urine ketone bodies | Positive |

  a. What diagnosis made by the physician with the above results?
  b. How the physician explained about the case to 4th year MBBS students?

## CHAPTER 21: Organ Function Tests

7. Steve, a 40-year-old man was admitted to the hospital with the symptoms of anorexia (loss of appetite) vomiting, and diarrhea. He mentioned to the physician that his urine was dark in color and passed the light stools. Serum and blood analysis which was requested revealed the following results:

   | Laboratory test | Result |
   | --- | --- |
   | Serum bilirubin | 5.0 mg% |
   | Direct bilirubin | 3.6 mg% |
   | Indirect bilirubin | 1.4 mg% |
   | AST | 55 units/L |
   | ALT | 80 units/L |
   | Alkaline phosphatase | 100 units/L |
   | Protein | 7.5 g/dL |
   | Albumin | 4.5 g/dL |
   | Urine bile pigments | Negative |
   | Urine bile salts | Negative |
   | Urobilinogen | Trace |
   | Feces | Normal color |

   a. What diagnosis can be made with the available laboratory results?
   b. Give specific reasons for elevated bilirubin and transaminase enzymes?
   c. Why the protein value remains normal?

8. Mr Suresh, a 40-year-old man who travels lot and recently visited two countries. After a month of his return he started getting the symptoms of dark urine, abdominal swelling, pruritus (itching), complaining loss of appetite, unexplained weight loss or gain, and abdominal pain. His wife took him doctor. The physician examined him and noticed swelling in liver below the ribs. Then he requested for blood test. The laboratory revealed the following results:

   | Laboratory test | Result |
   | --- | --- |
   | Serum bilirubin | 10.0 mg% |
   | Direct bilirubin | 5.2 mg% |
   | Indirect bilirubin | 4.8 mg% |
   | AST | 200 units/L |
   | ALT | 800 units/L |
   | Alkaline phosphatase | 170 units/L |
   | HBSAg | Positive |
   | Prothrombin time | Delayed |

   a. What diagnosis made using the above laboratory results?
   b. Explain with reasons for your diagnosis and symptoms mentioned.

9. Mrs Sumathi, admitted at gynecology ward, where she delivered a baby after 3 days. The neonatologist examined the baby and noticed the yellowish skin and sclera of the of the eye. He asked house officer to put the baby in phototherapy treatment. Also, he requested him to send the blood sample to laboratory. The laboratory results appear as follows:

   | Laboratory test | Result |
   | --- | --- |
   | Serum bilirubin | 8.0 mg% |
   | Direct bilirubin | 0.2 mg% |
   | Indirect bilirubin | 4.8 mg% |
   | AST | 25 units/L |
   | ALT | 28 units/L |

   a. What type jaundice the baby has?
   b. Why phototherapy suggested?

10. Mr Mahesh, admitted to the adult priority care ward with symptoms of anorexia and abdominal pain. His wife took him to the doctor. The physician examined him and noticed yellowish discoloration of the skin and sclera of the eye. Then he requested for blood and urine test. The laboratory revealed the following results:

| Laboratory test | Result |
|---|---|
| Serum bilirubin | 12 mg% |
| Direct bilirubin | 11.6 mg% |
| Indirect bilirubin | 0.4 mg% |
| AST | 55 units/L |
| ALT | 60 units/L |
| Alkaline phosphatase | 300 units/L |
| Urine bile pigments | ++ |
| Urine bile salts | ++ |
| Urobilinogen | Negative |
| Feces—stercobilinogen | Negative |

   a. What diagnosis would be made using the laboratory results?
   b. Explain with reasons for the above-mentioned symptoms.

11. Mr David, a 40-year-old man who travels lot and recently visited two countries. After a month of his return he started getting the symptoms of dark urine, abdominal swelling, pruritus (itching), complaining loss of appetite, unexplained weight loss or gain, and abdominal pain. He rushed to physician and requested laboratory tests revealed the following results:

| Laboratory test | Result | |
|---|---|---|
| Serum bilirubin | 10.0 mg% | Elevated |
| Direct bilirubin | 5.2 mg% | Elevated |
| Indirect bilirubin | 4.8 mg% | Elevated |
| AST | 200 units/L | Elevated |
| ALT | 800 units/L | Elevated |
| Alkaline phosphatase | 170 units/L | Elevated |
| HBSAg | Positive | egative |
| Urea | 20 mg/dL | Normal |
| Creatinine | 0.8 mg/dL | Normal |
| Blood sugar | 80 mg/dL | Normal |

   a. Which tubes were used for collecting blood for analyzing the above parameters?
   b. What diagnosis can be made using the above laboratory results?
   c. What could be the cause for his elevated bilirubin and enzymes?
   d. Explain with reasons for your diagnosis and symptoms mentioned

12. A 30-year-old man reported in the emergency ward of Mount Hope Hospital with complaints of abdominal pain, muscle cramps and urinary discomfort. His requested laboratory tests revealed the following results:

| Laboratory test | Result | |
|---|---|---|
| Urea | 100 mg/dL | Increased |
| Creatinine | 12 mg/dL | Increased |
| $Na^+$ | 200 mEq/L | Increased |
| $K^+$ | 6.5 mEq/L | Increased |
| Chloride | 120 mEq/L | Increased |
| Phosphorous | 6.0 mEq/L | Increased |
| Serum bilirubin | 1.0 mg% | Normal |
| Direct bilirubin | 0.2 mg% | Normal |
| Indirect bilirubin | 0.8 mg% | Normal |

**CHAPTER 21:** Organ Function Tests

| | | |
|---|---|---|
| AST | 30 units/L | Normal |
| ALT | 25 units/L | Normal |
| Alkaline phosphatase | 80 units/L | Normal |

a. What could be the cause for elevated RFT and electrolytes?
b. List the preananlytical variable that could lead to elevated sodium.
c. Why Red top tube is preferred for sample collection for electrolyte analysis?
d. Which hormone helps to maintain fluid balance and explain?

## MULTIPLE CHOICE QUESTIONS

1. Which of the following enzyme elevated in obstructive jaundice?
   (a) AST
   (b) ALP
   (c) ALT
   (d) LDH
2. The electrophoresis of serum from liver cirrhosis shows:
   (a) Beta-gamma bridging
   (b) Presence of M band
   (c) Increased alpha-2 globulin and decreased albumin
   (d) Increased albumin and decreased alpha-1 globulin
3. All the following are the tests used to detect renal function, except:
   (a) Uric acid determination
   (b) Urea determination
   (c) Creatinine determination
   (d) Bilirubin determination
4. Which of the following is incorrect concerning renal failure:
   (a) The AST elevated
   (b) The serum creatinine elevated
   (c) Hyperphosphatemia seen
   (d) The serum protein decreased
5. Which of following is a best marker enzyme for alcoholic cirrhosis:
   (a) ALP
   (b) AST
   (c) GGT
   (d) ALT
6. Concerning nephrotic syndrome:
   (a) It is characterized by edema
   (b) Patient loses globulin in the urine
   (c) Patient serum will show very high protein
   (d) Patient does not show any symptoms
7. Which of the following will be elevated in liver disease?
   (a) ALP
   (b) Lipase
   (c) Amylase
   (d) AST
8. All the following are the symptoms of hyperthyroidism, except:
   (a) Rapid heart rate
   (b) Inability to sleep
   (c) Weight loss
   (d) Sensitivity to cold
9. Which of the following is not a biochemical finding of primary hypothyroidism?
   (a) Reduced TSH
   (b) Reduced T3
   (c) Reduced T4
   (d) Increased TSH
10. Which of the following elevated in the neonatal jaundice?
    (a) Indirect bilirubin
    (b) Direct bilirubin
    (c) ALP
    (d) AST

### ANSWERS

1. b  2. a  3. c  4. a  5. c  6. a  7. d  8. d
9. a  10. a

# Chapter 22: Laboratory Values

## ■ Blood

| Tests | Normal values | To diagnose |
|---|---|---|
| Fasting glucose | 60–110 mg/dL | Diabetes |
| Postprandial glucose | 90–140 mg/dL | Diabetes |
| Random glucose | 90–150 mg/dL | Diabetes |
| Urea (UN) | 8–40 mg/dL | Pre-renal and renal disorder |
| Blood urea nitrogen (BUN) | 7–25 mg/dL | Pre-renal and renal disorder |
| Creatinine | 0.6–1.4 mg/dL | Renal disease and muscle degeneration |
| Sodium | 130–143 mEq/L | Renal and cardiac disorder |
| Potassium | 3.5–5.0 mEq/L | Renal disorder |
| Chloride | 93–110 mEq/L | Renal disorder |
| Total $CO_2$ | 22–26 mEq/L | Renal and acid-base disorder |
| Anion gap | 10–20 | Acid-base disorder |
| Osmolality | 270–285 mOsm/kg | Renal disorder |
| Uric acid | 3–7 mg/dL | Renal disorder and gout |
| Calcium | 8.5–10.6 mg/dL<br>8.5–10.3 mEq/dL | Renal and bone disorder |
| Phosphate | 2.5–4.5 mg/dL | Renal disorder |
| Cholesterol | 170–200 mg/dL | Atherosclerosis, diabetes, and hypothyroidism |
| Triglycerides | 40–160 mg/dL | Atherosclerosis, hypothyroidism, liver disease, pancreatitis, myocardial infarction, metabolic disorders |
| High-density lipoprotein (HDL) cholesterol | 45–70 mg/dL | High value indicates healthy metabolic system, low in liver disease |
| Low-density lipoprotein (LDL) cholesterol | 60–130 mg/dL | Atherosclerosis |
| Total bilirubin | 0.2–1.2 mg/dL | Jaundice and liver disease |
| Direct bilirubin | 0–0.2 mg/dL | Jaundice and liver disease |
| Total protein | 6.0–8.0 g/dL | Liver disease, malabsorption, lupus, chronic infections, alcoholism, leukemia |

*Contd...*

*Contd...*

| | | |
|---|---|---|
| Albumin | 3.5–5.0 g/dL | Liver disorder, shock, multiple myeloma |
| Globulin | 1.8–3.4 g/dL | Liver disease and chronic infections, multiple myeloma, rheumatoid arthritis |

| Tests | Normal values | To diagnose |
|---|---|---|
| Albumin/globulin (A/G) ratio | 0.8–2.0 | Liver disease and chronic infections, multiple myeloma |
| Zinc turbidity | 2–8 U | Liver disorder |
| Serum glutamic oxaloacetic transaminase (aspartate transaminase) | 5–40 U/L | Liver and cardiac disease |
| Serum glutamic-pyruvic transaminase (alanine aminotransferase) | 5–40 U/L | Liver disease |
| Alkaline phosphatase (ALP) | 35–125 U/L | Obstructive jaundice and bone disorder |
| Gamma-glutamyl transferase (GGT) | 10–50 U/L | Liver disease, alcoholism, obstructive jaundice |
| Amylase | 80–240 U | Pancreatitis |
| Acid phosphatase | Up to 11 U/L | Carcinoma prostate |
| Lactate dehydrogenase (LDH) | 0–250 U/L | Myocardial infarction (MI) and heart disease |
| $LDH_1$ | Up to 175 U/L | MI and heart disease |
| $LDH_1$/LDH ratio | <0.4 | MI and heart disease |
| CK | 10–80 U/L | MI and heart disease |
| $T_3$ | 0.8–2.0 ng/mL | Thyroid disorder |
| $T_4$ | 4.5–12.0 µg/dL | Thyroid disorder |
| Thyroid-stimulating hormone (TSH) | 0.3–5.0 µIU/mL | Thyroid disorder |
| Ferritin | 27–300 ng/mL | Anemia |
| Cortisol | | |
| Morning: | 8–26 µg/dL | Cushing's disease |
| Evening: | 5–18 µg/dL | Addison disease |
| B-hCG | 0–5 mU/mL | Choriocarcinoma |
| Alpha fetoprotein (AFP) | 0–15 ng/mL | Carcinoma liver and neural tube defect |
| Carcinoembryonic antigen (CEA) | 0–4 ng/mL | Colon cancer |
| CA-125 | 0–35 U/mL | Ovarian cancer |
| Prostate-specific antigen (PSA) | 0–4 ng/mL | Carcinoma prostate |
| Follicle-stimulating hormone (FSH) | | |
| Men: | 1–12 mIU/mL | |
| Women: | | |
| Follicular: | 3–20 | |
| Midcycle: | 9–26 | Fertility workup |
| Luteal: | 1–12 | |
| Menopausal: | 18–153 | |

*Contd...*

Contd...

| | | |
|---|---|---|
| Luteinizing hormone (LH) | | |
| Men: | 2.0 mIU/mL | |
| Women: | | |
| Follicular: | 2–15 | Fertility workup |
| Luteal: | 0.6–19.0 | |
| Menopausal: | 16–64 | |
| Prolactin | | |
| Women: | | |
| Midcycle: | 5.4–22.5 ng/mL | Fertility workup |
| Menopausal: | 4.5–15 ng/mL | |
| Tests | Normal values | To diagnose |
| Testosterone | | |
| Men: | 2.8–8.2 ng/mL | Fertility workup |
| Women: | 0.1–4.0 ng/mL | |
| Progesterone | 1–20 ng/mL | Fertility workup |
| Estradiol | | |
| Men: | 2–50 ng/mL | |
| Women: | | |
| Follicular: | 23–145 | |
| Midcycle: | 112–443 | Fertility workup |
| Luteal: | 48–241 | |
| Menopausal: | 0–59 | |
| Immunoglobulin G (IgG) | 1,200–1,480 mg/dL | Immune disorder |
| Immunoglobulin A (IgA) | 200–280 mg/dL | Immune disorder |
| Immunoglobulin M (IgM) | 110–136 mg/dL | Immune disorder |
| C3 | 90–150 mg/dL | Immune disorder |
| C4 | 15–50 mg/dL | Immune disorder |
| α-1 Antitrypsin | 90–150 U/dL | Acute-phase reactant |
| α-1 Antichymotrypsin | 45–75 U/dL | Acute-phase reactant |
| C-reactive protein | Up to 6.0 mg/L | Immune disorder |
| Haptoglobin | 70–240 mg/dL | Immune disorder |
| Glu-6-$PO_4$ dehydrogenase | 8–18 U/g | Immune disorder |
| Antinuclear antibodies (ANA) | <20 –ve<br>> 160 +ve<br>120–160 borderline | Autoimmune disorder |
| Anti-ds-DNA antibodies | <50 –ve<br>>65 +ve<br>50–65 borderline | Autoimmune disorders |

Contd...

*Contd...*

| | | |
|---|---|---|
| Anticardiolipin Antibodies (ACA) | < 10 –ve >15 +ve | Autoimmune disorders |
| Antiphospholipid | 10–15 borderline | |

## ▮ Urine

| | |
|---|---|
| Calcium | 50–300 mg/24 h |
| Phosphorus | 400–1,300 mg/24 h |
| Uric acid | 200–500 mg/24 h |
| Oxalate | 17–53 mg/24 h |
| Magnesium | 60–120 mg/24 h |
| Citrate | 300–900 mg/24 h |
| Cystine | Negative |
| Xanthine | Negative |
| pH | 4.5–7.8 |
| Volume | 600–2,000 mL/24 h |
| Urea | 10–35 g/24 h |
| Creatinine | 800–1,500 mg/24 h |
| Creatinine clearance | 60–120 mL/min |
| Protein | 24–180 mg/24 h |
| Ammonia | 140–1,500 mEq/24 h |
| Sodium | 40–220 mEq/24 h |
| Potassium | 35–90 mEq/24 h |
| Chloride | 60–125 mEq/24 h |
| Osmolality | 50–1,400 mOsm/kg |
| Volume | 1,000–2,000 mL/24 h |
| Estriol | 4 mg/24 h |
| 17-ketosteroids | |
| Morning: | 8–20 mg/24 h |
| Evening: | 6–15 mg/24 h |
| Catecholamines | Up to 150 µg/24 h |
| Vanillylmandelic acid (VMA) | 2–8 mg/24 h |
| Homovanillic acid (HVA) | 3–28 mg/creatinine |
| 5-hydroxyindoleacetic acid (5-HIAA) | 1–10 mg/24 h |
| Cortisol | Up to 150 µg/24 h |
| Cerebrospinal fluid (CSF) glucose | 60 mg% | Meningitis |
| CSF protein | 5–40 mg% |
| Hematology values | Normal |

*Contd...*

*Contd...*

| | | |
|---|---|---|
| Hemoglobin (Hb) | 12–16 g/dL | |
| Hematocrit (HCT) | 37–47% | |
| Mean corpuscular hemoglobin (MCH) | 27–33 pg | |
| Mean corpuscular volume (MCV) | | 80–100 fL |
| Mean corpuscular hemoglobin concentration (MCHC) | 32–36% | |
| Red blood cell count (male) | 4.2–5.6 mill/µL | |
| Red blood cell count (female) | 3.9–5.2 mill/µL | |
| White blood cell count | 3.8–10.8 thous/µL | |
| Platelet count | 130–400 thous/µL | |
| Neutrophil count (adult) | 48–73% | High in infection |
| Neutrophil count (children) | 30–60% | |
| Lymphocyte count (adult) | 18–48% | High in viral infections |
| Lymphocyte count (children) | 25–50% | |
| Monocyte count | 0–9% | High in chronic infections, leukemia, carcinomas |
| Eosinophil count | 0–5% | High in allergic reactions |
| Basophil count | | |

# Index

Page numbers followed by *f* refer to figure and *t* refer to table.

## A

Acetic acid 137, 164
Acetoacetate 173
Acetyl CoA 53, 57
　promotes gluconeogenesis 58
Acetyl transferase 157
Acetylcholine 8
Acid 209
　phosphatase 9, 15, 24, 26, 387
Acid-base
　analysis, assessment of 216
　balance 209, 213
　disorder 213, 216, 386
　disturbances 216*t*
　metabolic 214*f*
　mixed 216
　regulation of 210, 212, 213*f*
　respiratory 215*f*
　　regulation of 212
　status, extracellular 217
Acidemia 213, 214
Acidosis 213
Acidulants 348
Acrodermatitis enteropathica 310
Acromegaly 74
Actin 270, 272
　structure of 271*f*
Active transport 6, 7, 7*f*
Acyl carrier protein 157
Addison's disease 237, 305, 320, 326, 377, 379, 387
Adenoma 235
Adenosine
　diphosphate 45, 48, 49, 181, 186, 187, 369
　monophosphate 185, 187
　synthetase 225
　triphosphate 45, 48, 49, 181, 186, 187, 230, 369
Adipocytes 231
Adiponectin 188
　functions 188
Adipose tissue 64, 142, 183, 151, 163
　hormones 188
　in starvation 184
Adrenal gland 64, 235, 376, 376*f*, 379
Adrenal hyperplasia, congenital 326
Adrenal insufficiency 377
　causes of primary 237
　secondary 237
Adrenal medulla 239, 379
　tumor of 239
Adrenaline 70, 239, 379
Adrenocorticotropic hormone 187, 231, 232, 236, 377
　stimulation test 237, 377
Aerobic glycolysis 47
Alanine 90
　aminotransferase 364, 367, 387

transaminase 24, 364, 365, 367
transferase 206
Albumin 96, 100, 365, 382, 383, 387
　action of 100
　buffering function 100
　estimation 365
　functions of 100
　nutritive function 100
　osmotic function 100
　transport function 100
Alcohol
　effects of 164*f*
　metabolism 163, 364
Alcoholism 386, 387
　effects 164
Aldehyde 33, 53
　oxidase 311
Aldohexose 33
Aldolase 67
　reductase 68
Aldopentose 33, 65
Aldosterone 76, 322, 323, 378, 379
　deficiency 305, 326
　secretion 323
Aldosteronism, primary 239, 379
Aldotetrose 33
Aldotriose 33
Alkalemia 213
Alkali denaturation test 200
Alkaline phosphatase 24, 25, 206, 310, 364, 365, 367, 382, 383, 387
Alkalosis 213, 215
　chronic 212
Alkaptonuria 121
　symptoms of 121
Allergic reactions 143
Allosteric enzymes 23
Allosteric regulation 62
Alpha helix structure 98*f*
Alpha-fetoprotein 387
Alpha-melanocyte-stimulating
　hormone 231
Alzheimer's disease 267
Amethopterin 21, 22
　action of 21*f*
Amine-derived hormones 229
Amino acid 70, 90, 94*f*, 95, 116, 118, 119, 124, 125, 125*t*, 162, 182, 223, 337
　absorption of 115
　analysis
　　C-terminal 106
　　N-terminal 104
　biosynthesis of nonessential 118
　carbon skeletons of 118*f*
　catabolism of 115
　chemical properties of 93
　chemistry of 90
　classification of 93, 93*f*
　composition 104
　degradation 182

deletion 198
determination of 370
essential 93
glucogenic 119
in human body 115
ketogenic 94, 94*t*, 119
metabolism of 114
neutral 93
nonessential 93, 93*t*
oxidative deamination of 364
paper chromatography of 105*f*
pool 116*f*
simplest 119
substitutions 198
toxic 153
Amino groups, removal of 115
Amino sugars 38
Amino transferase 70
Aminoaciduria 370
　primary 370
　secondary 370
Aminolevulinic acid 204, 283
Aminopeptidase 43
Aminopterin 21, 22
　action of 21*f*
Ammonia 389
　accumulation, symptoms of 117
　fates of 118
　intoxication 117
　metabolic fate of 116
Amniotic fluid 124
Amylase 24, 26, 43, 387
Amylo 1,6 glucosidase splits 61
Amyloidosis 237, 257
Amylopectin 35, 35*t*
Amylopectinosis 64
Amylose 35, 35*t*
Anaerobic glycolysis 47, 50, 53
Anaplerotic reactions 56, 56*f*
Andersen's disease 64
Anemia 329, 339, 370, 387
　symptoms 339
　variety of 201
Anesthesia 217
Angiopathy 74
Angiotensin converting enzyme 21
Aniline dyes 201
Animal liver 274
Anion 103
　gap 216, 386
Anomerism 36
Anomers 36*f*
Anorexia 281, 381, 382
　symptoms of 383, 384
Anterior pituitary hormones 186, 231
Anthropometry
　advantages of 343
　disadvantages of 343
Antibiotics 325
　amphotericin B 325

carbenicillin 325
foscarnet 325
gentamicin 325
nafcillin 325
penicillin 325
Antibody 253, 258
  containing gel 255
  mediated immunity 249
  method, single 254
  producing cell 253
  production, mechanism of 252, 253f
Antidiuretic hormone 233, 299, 320
Anti-EGG white injury factor 285
Antigen 250, 257
  complex 249
Anti-insulin hormone 240
Antiketogenic substances 162
Antioxidants 261, 263, 264, 267
  system of 261
Antioxidation, chain-breaking 265f
Antiphospholipid 389
Apoenzymes 13
Apoferritin 307
Apotransferrin 307
Appetite, loss of 383
Arabidopsis thaliana 264
Arachidonic acid 137, 138, 141, 143
Argentaffinoma 123
Arginase 90, 117
Argininosuccinase 117
Argininosuccinic acid synthetase 117
Ariboflavinosis 281, 282
  signs of 282f
  symptoms of 282f
Arterial blood 216
Artificial sweeteners 189
Ascorbic acid 279, 288
Asparagine 91
Aspartame 189
Aspartate
  aminotransferase 24, 25, 190, 364, 367
  transaminase 116, 364, 365, 367, 387
  transferase 206
Aspartic acid 91
Aspirin 142
Atherosclerosis 68, 75, 169, 386, 386
  risk factors for 170
Atrial natriuretic peptide 300
  deficiency 300
  role of 300f
Autoimmune diseases 249
Autoimmune disorders 388, 389
Autoimmune hepatitis, chronic active 256
Autoimmunity 249
Autosomal recessive disorder 206

## B

B cells 250
B complex 273
B lymphocytes 250
Balanced diet 348, 349
  components of 349
Balwadi Nutrition Program 356
Bartter syndrome 325

Basal metabolic rate 333
  calculation of 335
Basophil count 390
Bence-Jones protein 102, 257
Benedict's test 37, 382
Benzene 133
Beriberi 280, 329
  dry 280
    symptoms of 280f
  infantile 280
  types 280
  wet 280, 281
Beta-oxidation, regulation of 153
Beta-thalassemias, types of 198
Bicarbonate 322
  buffer system 210
Bile acid 64, 364
  synthesis 160
    significance of 160
Bile salts, enterohepatic circulation of 150
Biliary cirrhosis, primary 256
Biliary tract
  cells 364f
  involvement 365
Bilirubin 203, 266, 364, 365
  conjugated 205, 206
  fate of 203
  formation of 366, 366f
  metabolism of 366
  water-insoluble unconjugated 205
  water-soluble 204
Biochemical measurements
  advantages of 344
  disadvantages of 344
Biological oxidation 222
Biosynthesis 155
Biotin 14, 284, 289
  antagonists 285
  antivitamin 285
  deficiency 285
  sources 284
  symptoms 285
Biuret
  method 365
  reaction 107
Blood 367, 386
  buffer system 210
  calcium 235
  cholesterol, high 172
  glucose 57, 70, 71
    level 51
    regulation of 52f, 69
  heparinized 216
  pH 382
  plasma 299, 317
  pressure
    high 172, 378
    regulation of 142
  specimen 258
  sugar regulation 240
    fasting 69
    sugar, random 70
  transport in 309
  urea nitrogen 369, 386
Blurred vision 118

Body electrolyte 299
Body fluid 317
Body mass index 342
Body temperature 334
Bohr effect 197, 197f
Bone 234
  abnormalities 310
  disorder 24, 386, 387
  mature in 250
Bottle feeding 359
Brain 183, 309
  disorder 24
  natriuretic peptide 300, 300f
Branched chain amino acids
  catabolism of 124f
  metabolism of 124
Breastfeeding 358, 360
  direct 359
  effective positions of 359
  exclusive 358
Breathlessness 199
Bronze diabetes 309
Burns, severe 256
Butylatedhydroxy toluene 140
Butyric acid 137

## C

Calcitonin, action of 295
Calcium 294, 370, 386, 389
  absorption 295
  binding protein 276
  effect of 62
  functions 295
  homeostasis 234
  mobilization of 276
  reabsorption of 276
  regulation of 235f
  sources 294
Calmodulin 295
Cancer 266, 267, 333, 349
  cells 53, 237
    proliferation of 266
  chronic 267
  colon 387
Carbamoyl phosphate synthetase 117
Carbohydrate 6, 33, 38, 43, 79, 330, 349, 364
  absorption of 45f
  chemistry of 33
  complex 330
  digestion of 43, 44
  foods 352
  isomerism in 35
  metabolism 43, 46, 74, 182, 183, 184
    effects on 70
    hormonal regulation of 184
    regulation of 185
  special 38
Carbon atoms, number of 33
Carbon dioxide 181, 194, 195, 214
  binding of 195f
Carbon skeleton, catabolism of 118
Carbonate-bicarbonate buffer 217
Carbonic anhydrase 310
Carbonyl hemoglobin 201
Carboxy hemoglobin 200

# Index

Carboxyl group 103, 137
Carboxyl peptidase A 310
Carboxylation reactions 14
Carboxypeptidase 115
Carcinogenesis 266
Cardiac disease 387
Cardiac disorder 386
Cardiac enzymes 25, 25f, 189, 191
Cardiac troponin 190
Cardiolipins 135
Cardiovascular disease 171, 329
    nutrition for 354
    risk factors for 171, 171f
Carnitine acyltransferase 173
Carotenoid pigments 274
Catalase 9, 264, 307
Cataract 271
Catecholamines 76, 389
    formation of 121f
Cell 1, 4
    cone 274
    death 267
    exposed 262
    fractionation 8
    lung cancer, nonsmall 296
    nucleus 237
    organelles 1, 9
    proliferation 266
    secretions of 7
    structure of 1f
    subcellular fractionation of 8f
    typical 1
    white 258
Cellular metabolism 7
Cellulose 34, 45
    acetate electrophoresis 200f
    acetate strip 200
Central nervous system 209, 310
Centrioles 4
Cephalin 135
Ceramide 136
Cerebral beriberi 280, 281
Cerebrosides 136
Cerebrospinal fluid glucose 389
Ceruloplasmin 24, 101, 265
Chaulmoogric acid 139
Cheilosis 282, 284f
Chemiluminescence method 372
Chemiosmotic hypothesis 226f
Chemotaxis 251
Chitin 34
Chloride 306, 322, 327, 381, 386, 389
    functions 306, 327
    shift 197f
Chloroform 133
Cholecalciferol 275
Cholecystokinin 114, 148
Cholestasis
    extrahepatic 365
    intrahepatic 365
Cholesterol 6, 139, 143, 158, 160, 333, 386
    biosynthesis 159
    ester 150, 168
    estimation 171
    excess 169

    functions of 139
    metabolic fate of 160
    metabolism 158
        hormonal regulation of 186
    structure of 139f
    synthesis 64, 159f
        regulation of 159, 159f
Cholesteryl ester transfer protein 168
Cholinesterase 24, 26
Chondroitin sulfate 35
Choriocarcinoma 387
Christmas factor 22
Chromatography 104
    types of 105f
Chromium 312
    deficiency 312
    functions 312
    sources 312
    toxicity 312
Chylomicron 165
    composition 165f
    transport of 166f
Chymotrypsin 43, 114
Chymotrypsinogen 43
Cirrhosis 324, 365
    alcoholic 26
    of liver 309
Citrate 389
    synthase 55
Clathrin 167
Cobalamin 287
Cobalt 311
    deficiency 311
    functions 311
    sources 311
    toxicity 311
Cod liver oils 274
Coenzyme 14, 14t, 21, 126
    functions 14t
    Q 224
Cognitive function, impairment of 266
Cohn's syndrome 239, 379
Collagen 99f, 272
    structure of 269f
    synthesis 279
    types of 268
Colocasia 352
Colon polyps 333
Coma 320
Connective tissue diseases 256
Constipation 332
Cookery rules 345
Cooking 345
    methods of 345
    principles of 345
Copper 309
    functions 309
    sources 309
Coproporphyria, hereditary 204
Cori's cycle 59, 60f, 210
Cori's disease 64
Cornea 47, 309
Coronary artery 171
Coronary heart disease 169, 171, 172
Corticotropin-releasing hormone 236, 377

Cortisol 70, 229, 237387, 389
    control of 236
    inhibit 141
    regulation of 236
    secretion 236, 236f
        control of 377
    synthesis of 377f
Creatine
    kinase 99, 190
    phosphokinase 24
    synthesis of 126
Creatinine 369, 381, 382, 386, 389
    clearance 381, 389
    test 368
    excretion 126
    kinase 25
        myocardial band 25
Cretinism 233
Crigler-Najjar syndrome 206
Cristae 223
Cryoglobulin 257
Cryoglobulinemia 257
Cup feeding 359
Cushing's disease 237, 387
Cushing's syndrome 74, 302, 325, 237, 238f, 377-379
    causes 238
    symptoms 238
Cyanocobalamin 14
Cyanomethemoglobin 201
Cyclic adenosine monophosphate 185-187, 230
Cystathionine gamma-lyase 283
Cystathionine alpha-synthase 283
Cystathionuria 126
Cysteine 91
Cystitis 371
Cytochrome 225
    C oxidase 9
Cytoplasm 1, 2, 173
Cytosol 9
Cytosolic protein 295

## D

Dangle feeding 360
De Novo synthesis 155
Decarboxylases 283
Dehydration 320, 369, 370
    cause of 320
    features of 320
    treatment 320
Dehydrogenation 222
Dementia 282
Dental caries, deficiency causes 312
Deoxy sugar 38
Deoxyadenosylcobalamin 14
Deoxyhemoglobin 196, 200
    neutralizes carbonic acid 212
    polymerization of 199f
Deoxyribonucleic acid 230
Dermatan sulfate 35
Dermatitis 282
Dexamethasone 239
    suppression test 238, 378
Dextrin 34

Diabetes 349, 386
  causes of 73f
  complications of 74
  diagnose 73
  insipidus 233
  mellitus 72, 172, 320
  metabolic changes in 74
  noninsulin dependent 73
  nutrition for 354
  symptoms of 73f
  type 1 72, 214
  uncontrolled 161, 214
Diabetic ketoacidosis 75, 214
Diacylglycerol 134, 151
Diarrhea 282, 383
Diet, nonessential in 119
Dietary data, interpretation of 345
Dietary glycerophospholipids 149
Dietary iron
  absorption of 308f
  transport of 308f
Dietary proteins, digestion of 126
Digestion 43
Dihydroxyacetone 33
Diisopropylphosphofluoride 22
Dipeptidase 43
Dipeptide 95
Diphenylhydantoin 76
Direct bilirubin 382, 383, 386
Disaccharides 33, 34t
Disorders Control Program 357
Distal renal tubular acidosis 371
Distinct globin chains 202
Dopamine 127, 239, 379
  synthesis of 121
Double antibody method 254
Dubin-Johnson syndrome 206, 207
Ductless glands 231
Dye-binding method 365

# E

Edema 281
Edman degradation 105, 106
  reaction 106
Edward Jenner's pioneering 249
Ehrlich's aldehyde reagent 366
Ehrlich's test 367
Elastin 269, 272
Electrolyte
  balance 321
  distribution of 321, 322
Electron microscope 1
Electron transport chain 164
  complexes in 223f
  formation, reactions of 223
  with inhibitors 224f
Electrophoresis 103
Emphysema 101
Enantiomer 36
Endocrine
  glands location 230f
  systems 236
Endocytosis 6, 8, 167f
  process of 8f
  receptor-mediated 8
Endoplasmic reticulum 1, 2, 3f, 9

Energy formation 53
Energy nutrients 330f
Enzymatic antioxidants 264
Enzymatic reactions 209
Enzyme 13, 16, 27, 159, 264
  active site of 15
  activity 15f, 16f
  catalysis, mechanism of 16
  chemical nature of 13
  classification of 16, 17t
  concentration, effect of 16, 16f
  defect 204
  diagnostic 24
  ferrochelatase 201
  hydrolyzes fatty acids 151
  inhibition 20
  kinetics 18
  reaction, velocity of 16
  specificity 16, 17t
  synthesis of 202
  systems 264
Enzyme-linked immunosorbent assay 254
Enzyme-substrate complex 15
Eosinophil count 390
Eosinophilia 237
Epimerism 36
Epimers 37f
Epinephrine 121, 127, 185, 239, 379
Epithelial cells 312
Erythrocytes 47
  immature 203
Erythroid cells 202, 203
Erythropoietic porphyria, congenital 204
Erythropoietic protoporphyria 204
Erythrose 33
Estradiol 388
Estriol 389
Estrogen, levels of 241
Ethanol 214
Ethanolamine 135
Ethylene glycol 214
Eukaryotic cell 4, 5f
  cytoplasm of 5
Excretory function test 370
Exocytosis 6, 7
Extrahepatic tissues 143, 173
Eye, vertebrate 271

# F

Fanconi syndrome 325
Fasting glucose 386
Fat 133, 330, 331, 349
  and oils 352
  cells 231
  metabolism 74
    hormonal regulation of 185, 186
  role of 331
  unsaturated 332
Fat-soluble vitamins 273, 278, 278t
Fatty acid 64, 137, 138, 140, 143, 155, 182, 223, 263f
  activated 152
  alpha-oxidation of 155
  classification of 137
  components of 157

dietary regulation of 158
essential 138, 332
functions of 138
metabolism, regulation of 154f
numbering of 137
oxidation 151, 182
  promotes 70
  regulation of 153
synthase enzyme complex 156f
synthesis 13, 64, 155, 158
  steps of 157f
trans 138
unsaturated 134, 137
Fatty liver 143
Feces 367, 383
Feeding
  high fat diet 161
  techniques 359
Female sex hormones 240
  after childbirth 241
  infancy 240
  menopause 241
  pregnancy 241
  puberty 240
  stages of 240
Ferritin 265, 387
  and hemosiderin 307
Fetal hemoglobin 195
Fiber 333
  and diverticulosis 333
  dietary 332
  insoluble 333
Fibrinogen 101
Figlu excretion test 123
Finger feeding 359
Fish liver oils 274
Flavin adenine dinucleotide 14, 281
Flavin mononucleotide 14
  functions of 281
Flavoprotein 152, 224, 281
Fluid balance 317, 321t
  regulation of 317, 319f
Fluid input 319
Fluid intake 355
Fluid mosaic model 5
Fluid output 319f
Fluoride 311
  functions 312
  sources 311
Folacin 288
Folate trap 287
Folic acid 14, 285, 288, 355
  active form of 286
  deficiency of 286
  sources 286
Follicle stimulating hormone 231, 232, 387
Follicular hyperkeratosis 274, 274f
Food
  adulteration 348
  budgeting of 354
  consumption 182
  diary 345
  frequency questionnaire 344
  nutritive value of 351
  poisoning 346

preservation 347
products, digestion of 44f
pyramid 353, 353f
serving 346
stuffs, respiratory quotient of 329
Food additives 347
Food Adulteration Act, prevention of 348
Food group 351
   plans, eleven 351, 352t
   types of 351
Formaldehyde 214
Formiminoglutamic excretion test 286
Formula feeding 359
Formylmethionine 125
Fouchet's test 367
Free fatty acid 136, 187
Free radical and antioxidant 261f
Fructokinase 67
Fructose 33, 34, 46, 47, 330
   1,6-bisphosphatase 58
   2,6-bisphosphate, role of 52
   6-phosphate 47
   high content of 68
   intolerance 67
   metabolism 67, 68f
Fructosuria, essential 67
Fumarase catalyzes 55
Fused rocket immunoelectrophoresis 255

## G

G-actin 270
   molecules 270
Galactose 33-35, 47, 136, 330
   fate of 67
   metabolism 66, 67f
Galactosemia 66
Galactosyltransferase 9
Gamma carboxylation 277f
Gamma-globulins 250
Gamma-glutamyl
   transferase 26, 206, 365, 367, 387
   transpeptidase 367
Gangliosides 136
Gas 333
Gastric contents 148
Gastric juice 43
Gastric motility, decreases 148
Gastric ulcer, prevention of 142
Gastrin 114, 148
Gastrointestinal hormones 70
Gastrointestinal loss 325
Gastrointestinal tract 13, 14, 114, 234
   enzymes of 43
Gaucher's disease 136
Gel filtration 102
Gestational diabetes mellitus 74
Gilbert's syndrome 206
Glands manufacture hormones 229
Gliossitis 284f
Globin 194
   synthesis 202
Globular proteins 270
Globulins 96, 101, 365, 382, 387
   estimation 365
Glomerular filtration rate 368

Glomerulonephritis 369
   acute 370
   chronic 370
Glossitis 282
Glucagon 58, 70, 71, 185, 186, 240
   action of 72f
   inactivates pyruvate kinase 58
   increased secretion of 74
   mechanism of action of 72
Glucantransferase 61
Glucocorticoid 72, 163, 185, 186, 235-237
   hormones, functions of 235
   secretion, assessment of 377
Glucogenic amino acids 58, 94, 119
Glucokinase 50, 50t, 51, 60, 70, 185
Gluconeogenesis 46, 57, 57f, 58, 364
   process of 57
   promotes 70
   regulation of 58, 58f
   substrates for 58, 59f
Glucophage 214
Glucose 33, 34, 45-47, 183, 330
   6-phosphate dehydrogenase deficiency 66
   absorption in intestinal epithelial cells 7
   concentration of 69
   oxidation 51
   production, effect on 70
   synthesis of 58, 59
   lack of 163
   transporter type 45
   utilization, effect on 70
Glucose tolerance
   abnormal 76, 77, 77f
   curve, normal 76, 77f
   diminished 77
   tests 75
   types of 75
Glucose-6-phosphate 47, 58, 63, 60, 64
   dehydrogenase 9
Glucose-alanine cycle 58, 59
Glucuronic acid 35
Glutamate 120
   metabolic fate of 120
   oxaloacetate transaminase 24
   pyruvate transaminase 24
Glutamic acid 91, 120, 199
Glutamine 91
   formation of 118
Glutathione 95, 264, 265
   peroxidase 265
   system 265
Glycated hemoglobin testing 78
Glyceraldehyde 33
   3-phosphate 47
Glycerol 58, 139
Glycerophospholipids 135
Glycine 91, 119
   metabolic fate of 119
Glycochenodeoxycholic acid 160
Glycocholic acid 160
Glycogen 34, 330
   breakdown 61
   from glucose, synthesis of 60
   metabolism 60, 62, 185f
   regulation of 63f, 186f

   storage
      diseases 62
      disorders 62
   synthesis 61
   synthetase 70
Glycogenesis 46, 60, 62, 364
   regulation of 62
Glycogenolysis 46, 61, 62, 62f, 70, 364
   allosteric regulation of 62
   regulation of 62
Glycolipids 134, 136
Glycolysis 46, 47, 58, 70, 182
   promotes 70
   reactions of 48f, 49f
   regulation of 51
   types of 47
Glycoprotein 38, 251
   hormones 230
Glycosides 38
Glycosidic bond 37
Glycyl-glycine dipeptidase, cofactor for 311
Glyoxylate cycle 56
Goiter 234, 312, 313f, 372, 379
Golgi apparatus 3f
Golgi complex 3, 10
   functions 3
Golgi membrane 9
Gordon's syndrome 326
Gout 370, 386
Grabar-Williams method 255
Granulomatous diseases 297
Graves' disease 234, 374, 379
Growth hormone 70, 72, 231
   role of 231f
   signs of 231
   symptoms of 231
Guanosine triphosphate 187, 297

## H

Haplotypes 258
Haptoglobins 101, 388
Harris-Benedict formula 335
Hartnup's disease 123
Hashimoto's thyroiditis 234, 375, 379
Hay's test 367
Heart disease 171, 172, 267, 349, 387
   congestive 369
   family history of 172
   major 172
   risk of 172
Heart failure 321, 324
   congestive 122
Helper T cells 249
Hematocrit 390
Hematologic disorders 256
Hematologic malignancy 296
Hematuria 370
Heme biosynthesis, regulation of 202
Heme catabolism 203, 203f
Heme synthesis 201, 202f
Hemochromatosis 309
Hemoglobin 99, 194, 195, 195f, 196, 196f, 197f, 217, 390
   abnormal 197, 200f

buffer
   action of 212
   system 212f
catabolism, disorders of 205
compounds, derived 200
deoxygenated 212
detection of abnormal 200
electrophoresis of 200
glycosylated 78
in disease, role of 203
metabolism 194
normal 200f
quaternary structure of 99f
structure of 194, 194f
Hemoglobinopathy 198
   qualitative 198
   quantitative 198
Hemolytic anemia 66, 199
Hemosiderin 308
Henderson-Hasselbalch equation 209, 210
Heparan sulfate 35
Heparin 35
Hepatic cells 364f
   destruction of 365
Hepatic glucuronyl transferase enzyme 206
Hepatitis 26
Hepatobiliary tree 364f
Hers' disease 64
Heteropolysaccharides 34
Hexokinase 50, 50t
Hexose 33
   monophosphate pathway 181
   monophosphate shunt 47
   reactions of 65f
High-density lipoprotein 134, 136, 137, 160, 165, 168
   cholesterol 170, 386
Hip circumference 343
Histidine 91
   metabolism 123
   catabolism of 123, 123f
Histones 96
Holoenzyme 13
Homeostasis 181
Homocystinuria 125, 127
   signs 125
   symptoms 125
   treatment 125
   types of 126f
Homogentisate oxidase 121
Homogentisic acid 121
Homopolysaccharides 34, 34t
Homovanillic acid 389
Hormonal action, mechanism of 230, 230f
Hormonal influence 158
Hormonal regulation metabolism 184f
Hormone 151, 189, 229, 334, 364
   chemical classes of 229
   regulation by 70
   role of 70
   sensitive lipase, activation of 151f
   thyroxine 232
Human chorionic gonadotropin 241
Human leukocyte antigen 257, 258

Human serum albumin 254
Hyaluronic acid 35
Hybridoma 253
Hydrocarbon chain 133
Hydrochloric acid 114
Hydrocortisone 236
Hydrogen
   bonds 97, 99
   peroxide 262
Hydrogenation 222
Hydrolases 17
Hydrolyze 104
Hydrophobic interactions 99
Hydrophobic region 149
Hydroxyindoleacetic acid 389
Hydroxyl radical 262
Hydroxylase enzyme 120
Hyperaldosteronism 74, 325
Hyperbilirubinemia 203
   acquired 205
   inherited
      conjugated 206
      unconjugated 206
Hypercalcemia 235, 296
   signs 297
   symptoms 297
   treatment 297
Hyperchloremia 306, 327
   causes 327
Hypercholesterolemia 171
Hypergammaglobulinemia 256
   acquired 256
Hyperglycemia 76, 378
Hyperglycemic hormones 71
Hyperglycemic hyperosmolar nonketotic coma 75
Hyperinsulinism 77
Hyperkalemia 305, 326
   causes 305, 326
   signs 305, 326
   symptoms 305
   treatment 305
Hyperlipidemia 63, 75, 169
Hyperlipoproteinemia 169
Hypernatremia 302, 323, 324
   causes of 302
   deficiency 302
   signs 302
   symptoms 302
   treatment 302
Hyperparathyroidism
   primary 235, 296
   secondary 235
Hyperphosphatemia 298
Hypertension 361
Hyperthyroid diseases 234
   biochemical findings 234
   normal levels 234
   symptoms 234
Hyperthyroidism 372, 373, 379
   subclinical 374
   thyroxine-induced 374
Hyperuricemia 63
Hypervolemia 321
   symptoms of 320
Hypoadrenalism 77
Hypocalcemia 295

   symptoms 296
   treatment 296
Hypochloremia 306, 327
   causes 327
Hypocholesterolemia 171
Hypochromic microcytic anemia 308
Hypogammaglobulinemia 256
Hypoglycemia 78, 237
   fasting 63, 77, 78
   neonatal 78
   reactive 78
   severe 153
Hypoglycemic hormone 70
Hypokalemia 237, 304, 325
   mild 305, 326
   symptoms of 305, 326
   type of 305
Hyponatremia 237, 300, 301, 323, 324
   diagnosis of 301
   inadequate volume 301, 324
   normal volume 301, 324
   symptoms 301
   treatment option for 303f
   types of 323
Hypophosphatemia 297
Hypopituitarism 77
Hypothalamus 236
Hypothyroid diseases 233
   types of 233
Hypothyroidism 77, 372, 373, 379, 386
   neonatal 312
   subclinical 374
Hypovolemia 320
   symptoms of 320
Hypoxia 199

**I**

Ibuprofen 142
Iduronic acid 35
Immune system
   disorders 255
   protects 249
Immunity 250
   cellular 102, 249, 250
   humoral 102, 249, 250
   types of 102, 250
Immunochemistry 249
Immunoelectrophoresis 255
Immunoglobulin 99, 102, 250, 251, 253
   A 388
   amount of 253
   blood test 255
   functions of 251
   G 388
   largest 252
   levels, causes of 256
   M 388
   structure of 250, 250f
   test 253
   types of 250t, 251
Immunology 249
Immunotherapy 249
Infant and young child feeding 358
   guidelines 358
Infection 78
Inhibition, competitive 20f

# Index

Inhibits gluconeogenesis 70
Inhibits glycolysis 70
Insulin 70, 240
  action of 163
  causes, action of 181
  functions of 240
  inhibits gluconeogenesis 185
  lowers blood glucose 70
  mechanism of action of 71
  metabolic effects of 70
  receptor 71
  secretion
    factors inhibiting 70
    factors stimulating 70
Insulin-mediated
  enzyme synthesis 71
  glucose transport 71
Integrated Child Development Services Scheme 356
Intermittent porphyria, acute 204
Intestinal cells 149
Intestinal enzymes 149
Intestinal lymphangiectasia 256
Intestinal obstruction 24
Intestine
  digestion in 114
  small 148
Intracellular enzymes 13
Intracellular fluid 317, 322
Intrauterine hypothyroidism 312
Intravenous glucose tolerance test 78
Intrinsic proteins 5
Inulin 34
Iodine 312
  cretinism 312
  deficiency
    disorder, control of 357
    manifestation 312
  functions 312
  number 140
  signs of 340$f$
  sources 312
Ionic calcium 295
Ionic interactions 99
Iron 306, 355
  absorption 307
  and transport, mechanism of 307
    reducing 307$t$
  deficiency 355
    anemia 339
  functions 306
  overload 309
  sources 306
  sulfur protein 224
Irritable bowel 332
  syndrome 332
Islets of Langerhans 240
Isocitrate dehydrogenase enzyme 55
Isocitrate lyase 56
Isoenzymes 23, 25
Isohydric shift 212
Isoleucine 91
Isomaltose 34
Isonicotinic acid hydrazide 22, 284
Itching 383, 384

## J

Jamaican vomiting sickness 153
Jaundice 205, 206, 366, 386
  hemolytic 171, 205, 366
  hepatic 205, 366
  neonatal 205
  obstructive 24, 26, 171, 205, 366, 387
  physiologic 205
  posthepatic 205, 366
  prehepatic 205
  types of 205, 206, 206$t$, 367$t$

## K

Kayser-Fleischer ring 309
K-dependent carboxylase enzyme 277
Keratan sulfate 35
Keratin 270, 272
Keratomalacia 274, 274$f$
Ketoacidosis 214
Ketogenesis 71, 161
Ketogenic substances 162
Ketohexose 33
Ketolysis 161, 162$f$
Ketone body 161, 173, 214
  activation of 162
  breakdown of 161
  formation of 161
  synthesis 70, 162$f$
  utilization of 161
Ketonuria 161
Ketopentose 33, 64
Ketotriose 33
Kidney 234, 309
  cancer 296
  disease 126
  failure 324
  function of 213, 368
  pathological conditions of 370
  response 215
  role of 213$f$
Kreb's cycle 53, 55
Kreb's-Henseleit cycle 117
Kwashiorkor 329, 337-339, 339$t$
  symptoms of 338, 338$f$
Kynureninase 283

## L

Laboratory
  test 381-384
  values 386
Lacrimal glands, keratinization of 274
Lactase 43, 45
  deficiency 45
Lactate dehydrogenase 9, 23-25, 99, 190, 387
  enzyme 50
Lactic academia 63
Lactic acid 163, 210
  accumulation of 210
Lactic acidosis 78, 210, 214
Lactose 34
  intolerance 68, 69$f$
    cause for 68
Lactosuria 69
Laid-back breastfeeding 360

Laurell rocket technique 255
Lean body mass, amount of 335
Lecithin 135, 140
  cholesterol acyltransferase 160, 168
    role of 160
Lens 47
  protein 271, 272
Leptin 188, 189
  functions 189
Lethargy 118
Leucine 91
Leukemia 296, 370, 386
Leukocytes 258
Leukotrienes 141, 143
Liddle syndrome 325
Ligases 17
Lignoceric acid 137
Lineweaver-Burk
  equation 21, 23
  plot 19$f$
Linolenic acid 137, 138
Lipase 24, 26
Lipid 133, 148, 230, 364
  absorption of 150$f$
  amphipathic nature of 140
  chemistry of 133
  classification of 133, 134$t$
  compound 134
  derived 134, 137
  digestion of 148, 149$f$
  functions of 133, 134
  lipid 263
  metabolism 148, 182, 183, 184
    effects on 70
    regulation of 163
  peroxidation 263
  physical properties 139
  profile 170
  properties of 139
  protein 263
  synthesis of 163
Lipolysis 71, 154
Lipoprotein 134, 136, 164, 165$t$, 168
  abnormal form of 168
  function 136, 164
  intermediate-density 136, 165, 167
  metabolism 71
  separation of 136$f$, 165$f$
  structure of 136, 136$f$, 164
  viscous barriers 10
Lipotropic factors 143, 143
Live-attenuated vaccines 250
Liver 63, 64, 67, 182, 320
  alcohol dehydrogenase 310
  cancer of 25
  carcinoma 387
  cell 207
    damage 365
  cirrhosis 24
  disease 24, 25, 324, 365, 386, 387
    acute 24
    alcoholic 24
    diet for 360
    serum enzymes in 366
  disorder 387
  enzymes 206

function test 364
    indications of 364
    in lipid metabolism, role of 163
    in starvation 184
    mitochondria 161
    synthesized in 168
Lock and key model 16, 17f
Low-density lipoprotein 134, 136, 137, 165-167, 169, 266
    cholesterol 170, 386
    composition of 167f
    very 134, 136, 165, 166, 166f, 167, 168
Lung, cancer of 25
Lupus 255
Luteinizing hormone 230-232, 388
Lymphocyte count 390
Lymphocytic leukemia, chronic 256
Lymphocytosis 237
Lymphoma 256, 296
Lysine 92
Lysophospholipase enzyme 149
Lysosomes 1, 3, 9

## M

Magnesium 298, 389
    deficiency 298
    functions 298
    sources 298
Malabsorption 386
    syndrome 171
Malate dehydrogenase enzyme 55
Malate synthase 56
Male infertility 266
Malonyltransferase 157
Maltase 43
Maltose 34
Mammary gland 64
Manganese 310
    containing enzymes 310
    deficiency 310
    functions 310
    sources 310
Mannose 46
Mannosidase 9
Maple syrup urine disease 124
Marasmus 337-339, 339t
    features of 338f
Mass spectrometry 106
Massive liver enlargement 63
McArdle's disease 64
Meal planning 350, 350f
Mean corpuscular
    hemoglobin 390
        concentration 390
    volume 390
Megaloblastic anemia 287
Megaloblasts 339
Melanin 122, 127
Melatonin 265
Membrane
    functioning, proteins of 7f
    lipid bilayer of 140f
    phospholipids 263
Memory capabilities 266
Meningitis 389
Menkes' syndrome 310

Mental
    retardation 312
    stress, type of 236
Messenger ribonucleic acid 230
Metabolic acidosis 213-216
Metabolic alkalosis 213, 215, 216
Metabolic disorders 386
Metabolic fates 118f
Metabolic stress 183
Metabolic syndrome 361
    diabetes 329
Metabolism 142, 181f, 229
    after meal, integration of 188f
    during starvation 183
    hormonal regulation of 185, 187f
    integration of 181, 182f, 183f
    pathways of 182
Metalloenzymes 13
Metformin 214
Methanol 214
Methemoglobin 201
Methemoglobinemia, causes of 201
Methionine 92, 124, 125
    catabolism 125
    from homocysteine, formation of 126
Methyl donor 126
Methyl tetrahydrofolate, deficiency of 125
Methylcobalamin 14
Micelles, mixed 149
Michaelis-Menten equation 18f, 19, 20, 23
Milk and milk products 352
Millets 352
Mineralocorticoids 239, 378
Minerals 294, 349
Mitochondria 1, 3, 4, 9, 152, 154, 202, 227
Mitochondrial membrane 173, 223, 226
Mitochondrion 226f
    consists 223
    longitudinal section of 3f
Molecules, movement of 6
Molybdenum 311
    deficiency 311
    metabolic functions 311
    sources 311
Monoacylglycerol 134
Monoclonal antibodies 252, 253
Monoclonal components 256
Monocyte count 390
Mono-oxygenase system 155
Monosaccharide 33
    absorption of 45
    classification of 33t
    unit 34
Monounsaturated fatty acids 137, 155
Mouse's spleen 252
Mucin 43
Mucopolysaccharides 34, 35
Mucus cells 43
Multicellular organism 10
Multiple myeloma 256, 296, 387
Muscle
    cramps 384
    degeneration 386

glycogenolysis 62
hexokinase 50
Muscular dystrophy 24, 370
Mutarotation 37
Myasthenia gravis 370
Myocardial complications, risk of 143
Myocardial infarction 24, 25, 25f, 190, 190f, 386, 387
    diagnosis of 189
    laboratory tests in 189
Myoglobin 195, 196, 196f, 197, 225
Myosin 270, 272
    filament 271
    structure of 271f
Myxedema 171, 233

## N

N-acetyl galactosamine 35
N-acetyl glucosamine 34, 35
Nail, spooning of 309f
National Nutritional Programs 356
Nausea 118, 381
Nephritis, chronic 369
Nephron, structure of 368f
Nephropathy 74
    diabetic 370
Nephrosclerosis 369
Nephrosis 171
Nephrotic syndrome 24, 171, 256, 369-371
Neural tube defect 387
Neurological disorders 309
Neuropathy 74
Neutrophil count 390
Niacin 14, 282, 288
    coenzyme forms 282
    deficiency 282
    sources 282
Nicotin 76
Nicotinamide 288
    adenine dinucleotide 14, 48, 49, 181
        hydrogen 48, 49
        phosphate 14
Nicotinic acid 282, 288
Niemann-Pick disease 136
Night blindness 274
Ninhydrin reaction 94
Nitrogen
    balance 337
    state
        negative 337
        positive 337
Non-alcoholic fatty liver 360
Nonapeptide 95
Noncompetitive inhibition 22, 22f
Nonenzymatic antioxidants 265
Nonoxidative irreversible phase 64
Non-protein nitrogen 379
    excretion of 368
Noradrenaline 239, 379
Norepinephrine 121, 127, 186, 239, 379
Nucleated cells 154
Nucleic acids 297
Nucleotidase 43
Nucleus 4, 9
Nutrient preservation 346

Nutrients, preservation of 345
Nutrition 329
   calorie 329
   related diseases 337
Nutritional anemia 357
Nutritional assessments, methods of 339, 340
Nutritional deficiency, signs of 339, 340*t*
Nutritional indices 342
Nutritional status, assessing 339

## O

Obesity 188, 361
   and overweight 172
   diet for 360
Oleic acid 137
Oligomycin 227
Oligosaccharides 33
Oliguria 370
Optical activity 37
   carbohydrates 36
Oral contraceptives 76
Oral glucose tolerance test 75
Organ function tests 364
Organelle separation 9*f*
Organic acids 214
Organic compounds, group of 90
Organic solvents, precipitation by 102
Organophosphorus poisoning 24
Ornithine transcarbamoylase 117
Osmolality 386, 389
   determination 370
Osmotic pressure 298
Osteoporosis 234
Ovarian cancer 387
Ovarian hormones 230
Ovary 67, 241
   estrogen 241
   progesterone 242
Oxalate 389
Oxaloacetate 56
   lack of 161
Oxidation reactions 14, 22, 263
Oxidative deamination 116
Oxidative decarboxylation 14, 55
Oxidative irreversible phase 64
Oxidative phosphorylation 225, 226*f*
Oxidative stress 266
Oxidoreductases 17
Oxygen
   binding 196
      factors affecting 197
   dissociation 196
   species, reactive 262, 262*f*
   transports 194
Oxyhemoglobin 200
Oxytocin 233

## P

Paget's disease 24
Pain 382
   abdominal 381, 384
Palmitic acid 137, 152, 153*f*
   oxidation, energetics of 152
Palmitoleic acid 137

Pancreas 240
   alpha cells of 240
   tumor of 74
Pancreatic disease 73
Pancreatic hormones 230
Pancreatic juice 43
Pancreatitis 386, 24, 387
Pantothenic acid 14, 285, 289
   deficiency 285
   sources 285
Para-aminobenzoic acid 21
Paraldehyde 214
Paraprotein 256
Paraproteinemia, benign 257
Parathyroid gland 235
Parathyroid hormone 230, 234, 235, 235*f*, 295
   action of 295
   functions 234
   role of 296*f*
Parietal cells 43
Parkinson's disease 122
Passive transport 6
Pellagra 282
   signs of 283*f*
Penicillamine 310
Pentapeptide 95
Pentoses 33
Pepsinogen 14, 43
Peptide and peptide bond 94
Peptide fragments, digestion into 106
Peptide hormones 229
Peripheral neuritis 280
Peroxidas 307
Peroxidation 140
Peroxide 262
Peroxiredoxins 264
Peroxisomal fatty acid 154
   oxidation 154
Peroxisomes 3, 9
pH, effect of 15
Phagocytic cells 251
Phagocytosis 8
   process of 8*f*
Phenotyping 258
Phenyl acetate 121*f*
Phenylalanine 92, 120
   hydroxylase 120
Phenylketonuria 120
Phenyllactate, formation of 121*f*
Phenylpyruvate 121*f*
Pheochromocytoma 239, 296
Phosphatases 25
Phosphate 386
   buffer 217
      system 211
   group 140
Phosphatidyl ethanolamine 135
Phosphatidyl inositol 135
Phosphatidyl serine 135
Phosphatidylcholine 135, 149
Phosphoenolpyruvate carboxykinase 58, 185
Phosphoglucomutase enzyme 60, 61
Phosphohexose isomerase enzyme 47
Phospholipase 149

Phospholipids 134, 135, 140, 150
   types of 135
Phosphorus 297, 370, 389
   sources 297
Phosphotriose isomerase enzyme 47
Physical stress, type of 236
Pinocytosis 8
Pituitary gland comprises 231
Pituitary hormones 230, 231
   posterior 233
Plaque formation 169*f*
Plasma 263
   calcium
      level, high 275
      low 275
   cell 256
   cholesterol 160
   lipoproteins classes and functions 165
   membrane 1, 5*f*, 8, 9
   osmolality 299, 322
   proteins 100, 101*t*
      separation of 102
Plasmalogens 135
Plasmodium falciparum 199
Platelet
   aggregation and thrombosis 142
   count 390
Pneumonia 370
Polycythemia 311
   vera 370
Polydypsia 72, 301
Polypeptide 13, 95
   chains 194
Polyphagia 72
Polysaccharides 34, 44
Polyunsaturated fatty acid 137, 160
Polyuria 72, 233
Pompe's disease 63
Porphobilinogen 204
   deaminase 203
Porphyrias 203, 204
   causes of 204*t*
Postprandial glucose 386
Potassium 302, 325, 381, 386, 389
   and sodium, movement of 304*f*
   extracellular 303
   functions 304
   sources 304
Preproinsulin 240
Pre-renal disorder 386
Proenzymes 14
Progesterone 388
   levels of 241
Prokaryotic cell 4, 4*f*, 5
Prolactin 231, 232
   inhibiting factor 232
Proline 92, 94
Propionic acid 58, 59
Prostacyclins 141, 142
   synthesis, inhibition of 141
Prostaglandin 141
   biochemical actions of 142
   E1 187
   synthesis 141, 141*f*
Prostanoids 141

Prostate
  carcinoma of 24, 387
  specific antigen 387
Protection against radicals, mechanisms for 263
Protein 95, 330, 331, 337, 349, 354, 383, 389
  and weight
    gain 331
    loss 331
  buffer 217
    system 211
  building blocks of 124
  by salts, precipitation of 102
  chemistry of 90
  classification of 96
  complementary 331
  complete 331
  conformation 209
  conjugated 13, 96$t$
  denaturation of 99
  digestion of 114, 115$f$
  energy malnutrition 337, 340
  functions of 96
  general functions of 96
  incomplete 331
  losing enteropathy 256
  metabolism 71, 74, 182, 183, 184
  modification of 100
  primary structure of 97, 97$f$
  quantity of 104
  quaternary structure 99
  role of 331
  secondary structure 97
  sequencing 103
  specialized 268
  structure of 97, 268
  synthesis 364
  tertiary structure of 98, 98$f$
  tests for 107
Proteinuria 370
Proteoglycans 38, 268
Prothrombin time 365, 383
Proton gradient 225
Proteolytic enzymes 13, 14
Provitamin A carotenoids 273
Pruritus 383, 384
Pseudohyperkalemia 305, 326
Pseudohypoaldosteronism 326
Pseudohypokalemia 304, 325
  symptoms 325
  tests 326
  treatment 326
Pseudohypoparathyroidism 296
Pyelonephritis 370
Pyridoxal 288
  phosphate 14, 283
Pyridoxamine 288
Pyridoxine 14, 283, 288
  active form of 283
  antagonists 284
  deficiency
    manifestations 283
    signs of 284$f$
  sources 283
Pyruvate 53, 56, 223
  carboxylase 58
  dehydrogenase 53
  kinase 70
Pyruvic acid 163

## R

Raised free thyroxine 374$t$, 375$t$
Rancidity 140
Rapoport-Luebering cycle 52$f$
Random glucose 386
Reactive oxygen
  biological effects of 262
  species, formation of 262
Red blood cells 4, 371
  abnormal 339
  count 390
Reduction tests 37
Reduction-oxidation reactions, principles of 222
Refsum's disease 155
Renal disease, diet for 361
Renal disorder 386
Renal failure 370
  acute 369
  chronic 214, 369
Renal function
  influence on 142
  tests 368
Renal glycosuria 77
Renal kidney failure 322
Reproductive dysfunction 310
Respiratory acidosis 213, 215
Respiratory alkalosis 213, 215
Respiratory chain, structural organization of 223
Respiratory function, effects on 142
Resting metabolic rate 334
Retinoic acid 274
Retinoids 273
Retinopathy 74
Rheumatoid arthritis 255, 256, 387
Rheumatological disease 256
Rhodopsin 274
Riboflavin 14, 281, 288
  active form of 281
  deficiency of 281
Ribonuclease 43
Ribonucleic acids 4
Ribose 33
  5-phosphate keto-isomerase 64
Ribozymes 14
Ribulose 5-phosphate epimerase 64
Rickets 24
Rod cells 274
Rotor syndrome 207

## S

Saccharin 189
S-adenosyl methionine 125
  formation of 124
Safe food handling 346
  storage of food 346
Salicylates 214
Salivary amylase hydrolyses 44
Salt fractionation 102
Sanger's reagent 105
Sarcoidosis 297
Satiety hormone 189
Saturated fats 332
Saturated fatty acid 137
Scleroproteins 96
Scurvy 329
  symptoms of 279$f$
Seborrheic dermatitis 282
Secretin 114, 149
Selenium 265, 311
  absorption 311
  deficiency 311
  sources 311
Seminal vesicles 67
Sepsis 256, 370
Serine 92
Serotonin, synthesis of 123
Serotyping 258
Serum 322
  bilirubin 382, 383
  calcium level, regulation of 295
  chloride
    high 306
    low 306
  cholesterol 170
  content 308
  electrophoresis 103$f$
  enzyme 24, 24$t$, 206
    levels 190$f$
  glutamate pyruvate transaminase 116
  glutamic
    oxaloacetic transaminase 387
    pyruvic transaminase 387
  immunoglobulin 253
    quantitative determination of 254, 255
  inorganic phosphate level 297
  osmolality 299
  potassium 325
  protein 365
    electrophoresis 365
Shock 320, 369, 387
Shuttle pathways 51
Sialic acid 38
Sick euthyroid syndrome 375
Sickle cell 205
  anemia 199
  disease 198
  hemoglobin 199
    symptoms of 199
  red blood cell 199$f$
  trait 199
Sickling test 200
Simple lipids 133, 134
Singlet oxygen 262
Skeletal muscle 183
  diseases 25
Skinfolds 341
Slurred speech 118
Sodium 298, 322, 381, 386, 389
  balance 322
  functions 298
  sources 298
  thiopental 267
Solid food feeding 359
Solitary thyroid nodules 372
Solubility test 200

# Index

Somatomammotropin 232
Somatotropin 231
Sorbitol dehydrogenase 67, 68
Sorbitol pathway 67
Special Nutrition Program 356
Sphingomyelin 135
Sphingomyelinase enzyme, deficiency of 136
Sphingophospholipids 135
Spleen 67
Spoon feeding 359
Squalene 134
Starch 34, 330
Starvation hormone 189
Stearic acid 137
Stereoisomerism 36
Steroid 139, 229
   hormone 143, 242
   synthesis 64
Stevia 189
Sticky patch 199
Stomach, digestion in 114
Stroke 172, 349
Stuart-Prower factor 22
Subcellular fractions, marker enzymes of 9t
Subcellular organelles 154
Substrate concentration, effect of 16, 16f
Succinate dehydrogenase 9, 55, 224
Succinate thiokinase 55
Sucralose 189
Sucrase 43, 45
Sucrose 34
   and lactose 44
Sulfates 214
Sulfhemoglobin 201
Sulfite oxidase 311
Sulphanilic acid 204
Superoxide
   anion 262
   dismutase 264
Suprarenal cortical hormones 230
Suprarenal medullary hormones 230
Swelling, abdominal 383, 384
Swollen face, sign of 381
Synthesis 141, 158
Systemic lupus erythematosus 256

## T

Tachycardia 281
Target cell 229, 231
Taurochenodeoxycholic acid 160
Taurocholic acid 160
Testes 64, 242
Testicular hormones 229
Testosterone 229
Tetrahydrofolate 14
   formation of 286f
Tetrahydrofolic acid 21
Tetroses 33
Thalassemia 198
   causes of 198
Therapeutic diets 354
Thiaminase 281
Thiamine 14, 280, 288
   pyrophosphate 14

Thiazides 76
Thiokinase enzyme 150
Threonine 92
Thromboxanes 141
   synthesis of 143
Thymus 249
Thyroid
   binding globulin 374
   cancer 372
   cells 371
   disorder 387
   function tests 371, 371
   hormone 230, 233, 379
      biochemical findings 234
      deficiency 122
      functions of 233
      pathophysiology 233
      symptoms 234
   iodine uptake scan 376
   releasing hormone test 371, 375
   scan 376
   stimulating hormone 187, 230-232, 374t, 375t, 387
Thyroiditis 372, 374, 375, 379
Thyrotropin-releasing hormone 95, 229, 232
Thyroxine 72, 186
Tissue anoxia 214
Tocopherol 276
Total protein 365, 382, 386
Toxic liver cell necrosis 24
Toxic multinodular goiter 374, 379
Toxic waste product 203
Toxicity 310, 346
Toxoid vaccines 250
Trace elements 294
Trans fat 332
   risks 332
Transaminases 283
   serum 367
Transferases 17
Transferrin 265, 307
Transketolase
   reaction 14
   transfers 65
Transport across membrane 5
Triacylglycerol 133, 140, 150
   biosynthesis of 162
   fate of 151, 162, 163
   synthesis 162f
Tricarboxylic acid 181-222
   cycle 13, 53
   reactions of 54
Triglyceride 133, 134, 140, 386
   hydrolysis of 140
Triiodothyronine 374t, 375t
Trioses 33
Tripeptide 95
Tropoelastin 269
Tropomyosin 270
Troponin 270
Trypsin hydrolyzes peptide bonds 114
Trypsinogen 43
Tryptophan 92
   metabolic fate of 122
   metabolism of 122

Tuberculosis, treatment for 22
Tubular damage 309
Tubular disease 371
Tubular necrosis 369, 370
Twenty four-hour urinary free cortisol level 378
Tyrosinase deficiency 122
Tyrosine 92, 120
   catabolism of 120, 120f, 121f
   from phenylalanine, synthesis of 120f
   metabolic fate of 122
   metabolism of 120
   synthesis of 120
Tyrosinemia 121

## U

Ubiquinone 224
Ubiquitone 266
Urea 369, 381, 382, 386, 389
   cycle 117, 117f
      inborn errors of 117t
Uric acid 266, 370, 386, 389
Uridine diphosphate 204
Urinary tract
   infection 371
   obstruction 370
Urine 367, 389
   analysis of 124
   bile
      pigments 383
      salt 367, 383
   diluted 233
   glucose 76, 77
   ketone bodies 382
   osmolality 299, 322
   pH of 212
   sample collections 238
   sodium in 302
Urobilinogen 366, 367, 383
Urobilins 367
Uronic acid pathway 47

## V

Vaccine
   development 250
   types of 250
Valine 92
Van Den Bergh's reaction 366
Van Den Bergh's test 204, 205, 366
Van Der Waals forces 99
Vanillylmandelic acid 389
Vasopressin 233
Vertebrate hormones 229
Viral hepatitis 24
   acute 24
   types of 368
Viral infections 255
Vitamin 14, 273, 349, 364
   A 133, 273, 274, 278
      role of 274
   $B_1$ 280, 288
   $B_{12}$ 14, 287, 289
      active form of 287
      deficiency 286, 287, 339

roles of 286
sources 287
$B_2$ 14, 281, 288
$B_3$ 288
$B_5$ 289
$B_6$ 14, 288
$B_7$ 289
B-complex 280
C 140, 264, 265, 279, 288
   deficiency 279
   functions 279
   role of 279f
   signs 279
   sources 279
   symptoms 279
D 133, 273, 275, 278
   action of 295
   deficiency 276, 295, 340f, 361
   functions 275
   sources 275
$D_3$ 275
   deficiency, features of 276f
   formation of active 275f
dependent gamma carboxylation 277
doses of 279
E 133, 140, 264, 265, 276, 278, 311
   deficiency 276
   functions 276
groups of 273
K 22, 133, 273, 276, 278
   antagonists 278
   cycle 278f
   deficiency 278
   exception of 273
   functions 277
   sources 276
   water-soluble 273, 279, 287, 288t
Vomiting 118, 281, 381, 383
von Gierke's disease 63

## W

Waist circumference 343
Wald's visual cycle 274f
Waldenström's macroglobulinemia 257
Water balance 317
Water excess 321
   causes 321
   treatment 321
Wernicke-Korsakoff syndrome 280, 281
White blood cells 262
   count 390
William's syndrome 270
Wilson's disease 24

## X

Xanthine 389
   oxidase 21, 281, 311
Xanthochromatosis 171
Xylose 33
Xylulose 33

## Z

Zellweger's syndrome 154
Zinc 310
   deficiency 310
   functions 310
   sources 310
   turbidity 387
Zona fasciculata 235, 376
Zona glomerulosa 235, 376
Zona reticularis 235, 376
Zymogen 14
   activation 114

EU GSPR Authorised Reprsentative
Logos Europe, 9 rue Nicolas Poussin
1700, La Rochelle, France
Phone: +33 (0) 6 67 93 73 78
E-mail: contact@logoseurope.eu

www.ingramcontent.com/pod-product-compliance
Ingram Content Group UK Ltd.
Pitfield, Milton Keynes, MK11 3LW, UK
UKHW050429150426
5217IPUK00019B/1314